Human Auditory Evoked Potentials

Audiology Editor-in-Chief
Brad A. Stach, PhD

Human Auditory Evoked Potentials

Terence W. Picton

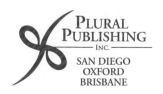

PLURAL
PUBLISHING
INC.

SAN DIEGO
OXFORD
BRISBANE

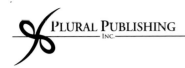

PLURAL PUBLISHING
INC.

5521 Ruffin Road
San Diego, CA 92123

e-mail: info@pluralpublishing.com
Web site: http://www.pluralpublishing.com

49 Bath Street
Abingdon, Oxfordshire OX14 1EA
United Kingdom

Typeset in 10.5/13 Palatino by Flanagan's Publishing Services, Inc.
Printed in the United States of America by Bang Printing

Library of Congress Cataloging-in-Publication Data

Picton, T. W. (Terence W.)
  Human auditory evoked potentials / Terence W. Picton.
      p. ; cm.
  Includes bibliographical references and index.
  ISBN-13: 978-1-59756-362-8 (alk. paper)
  ISBN-10: 1-59756-362-5 (alk. paper)
 1. Auditory evoked response. I. Title.
  [DNLM: 1. Evoked Potentials, Auditory. 2. Cochlear Implants. WV 270]
  RF294.5.E87P53 2010
  617.8'82—dc22
                                                              2010028377

Contents

Preface   *vii*

1 Introduction: Past, Present, and Potential   1

2 Recording Evoked Potentials: Means to an End   25

3 Frequency Domain: Music of the Hemispheres   59

4 Finding Sources: Forward and Backward   87

5 Acoustic Stimuli: Sounds to Charm the Brain   123

6 Interpreting the Waveforms: Time and Uncertainty   155

7 Electrocochleography: From Song to Synapse   189

8 Auditory Brainstem Responses: Peaks Along the Way   213

9 Middle-Latency Responses: The Brain and the Brawn   247

10 Auditory Steady-State and Following Responses: Dancing to   285
    the Rhythms

11 Late Auditory Evoked Potentials: Changing the Things Which Are   335

12 Endogenous Auditory Evoked Potentials: Attention Must Be Paid   399

13 Infant Hearing Assessment: Opening Ears   449

14 Neurotology and Neurology: From Cochlea to Cortex   493

15 Auditory Neuropathy: When Time Is Broke   535

16 Cochlear Implants: Body Electric   569

17 Concluding Comments: Beginning to Live   601

Index   *609*

Preface

This book is about the human auditory evoked potentials (EPs), the small electrical changes that can be recorded from the scalp following a sound. EPs are generated at all stations of the auditory system from the hair cells of the cochlea to the neurons of cerebral cortex. Recording auditory EPs can help us understand normal auditory perception and evaluate patients with disorders of hearing.

The point of view of the book is mine. What is offered therefore is consistent in its approach but flavored by my personal biases. Because I would like you, the reader, to share these, I often use the cajoling (rather than editorial) "we" when describing what you and I can record and how we might interpret these recordings.

However, as readers, you should make up your own minds and learn to see beyond me. In this regard, you should be aware that I have some commercial interest in the MASTER system for recording auditory steady-state responses that was licensed to Biologic Systems Corporation. My share of the patent-licensing fees is very small and I doubt that it affects my thinking. There are no other conflicts of interest.

The book is neither exhaustive in its review nor encyclopedic in its scope. Rather, it is a handbook in the original sense of the term, a book of essential information that comes to hand rather than stays on the shelf. The intended readers are those who record the auditory EPs in

order to find out how the human brain responds to sounds—audiologists, neurologists, psychologists, and physiologists.

As well as reviewing the published literature, the book contains occasional ideas and data that have not been published previously. Among the new ideas are the concepts of the "physiological threshold level" described in Chapter 5, and the suggestions about how to handle the statistical problem of evaluating responses to multiple simultaneous stimuli in Chapter 6. Among the new data are the studies of the effect of age on the auditory steady-state responses in Chapter 10 and the evaluation of temporal integration in the brainstem in the same chapter. The time-warped middle latency responses presented in Chapter 16 have been in my unpublished files for a decade.

This book is limited to the electrical potentials recorded in response to sounds from electrodes placed on the human scalp or in the external or middle ear. Changes in the magnetic fields evoked by sounds, and intracranial recordings of auditory EPs in animals and man are reviewed only as they relate to the scalp-recorded electrical potentials. Otoacoustic emissions and vestibular responses are covered briefly as they supplement the auditory EPs in clinical testing.

In writing this book, I have become acutely aware of the immensity of the scientific literature. Even in the limited field of the auditory EPs, thousands of papers jockey for attention every year. This contrasts strikingly with the early days of the field when I could be reasonably sure that I had read just about everything of importance. Today, it is impossible to digest fully more than a fraction of what is published—so many papers, so little time. This vast accumulation of knowledge requires condensation, theories that subsume what is known into essential representations. One of the main goals of the book is to summarize what is known and to organize it as simply as possible.

Each chapter in the book is self-contained, listing its own references and explaining its own abbreviations, which I have tried to keep to a minimum. Mathematical formulae are not used in the text. However, these equations sometimes insist on being properly presented. The compromise has been to include them occasionally in the figures. More mathematical rigor can be found by consulting the papers listed in the references.

Although the book is organized to be read from beginning to end, some of you may wish to go initially to the chapters in which you are most interested. It often is better to find out what responses can be recorded before learning how to record them. Cross-references to other chapters may then lead you to the other parts of the book. The epigraphs for each chapter are chosen to allude to general principles, and to bring in other views and other languages. We should not forget that there is much in the world beyond our particular field of science.

The book contains many figures. We cannot understand the EPs if we cannot see them. To be consistent, all of the figures are plotted so that positive is upward. The literature uses both positive-up and negative-up conventions. Sometimes, this is related to the background of the scientists who record the EPs; electroencephalographers have used negative-up whereas engineers have preferred positive-up. The plotting conventions also often relate to what is being recorded, as components are more easily recognizable when they point upward. Thus, the auditory brainstem response typically is plotted positive-up and the mismatch negativity negative-up. Because I have great empathy for people who have difficulty knowing which way is up, I decided one convention would be preferable to two. My intent was not to rewrite history but to make it easier to understand.

The picture on the cover is a pastiche of several visual aspects of recording auditory EPs. In it, you may hear an exponential stimulus, dive through the tuning curve, enter a two-sphere head-model, ride the waves of the auditory EP, and ultimately find the audiogram you seek.

A book cannot be written without help. I would particularly like to thank those colleagues who reviewed draft-chapters: Claude Alain, Manny Don, Andrée Durieux-Smith, Karen Gordon, Steven Hillyard, Risto Näätänen, David Stapells, Arnold Starr, and Jan Wouters. As well, I am indebted to the many people I have consulted about various issues and ideas: Chuck Berlin, Ken Campbell, Barbara Cone, Rafael Delgado, Jos Eggermont, Bill Gibson, Bob Harrison, Martyn Hyde, Sasha John, Nina Kraus, Eleftherios Papathanasiou, Rob Patuzzi, Marilyn Pérez Abalo, Curtis Ponton, Catherine Poulsen, Bernhard Ross, Yvonne Sininger, Margot Taylor, and Istvan Winkler. My reviewers and consultants are absolved from any residual defects; whatever remains incorrect or unclear is my fault.

Preface

This book is about the human auditory evoked potentials (EPs), the small electrical changes that can be recorded from the scalp following a sound. EPs are generated at all stations of the auditory system from the hair cells of the cochlea to the neurons of cerebral cortex. Recording auditory EPs can help us understand normal auditory perception and evaluate patients with disorders of hearing.

The point of view of the book is mine. What is offered therefore is consistent in its approach but flavored by my personal biases. Because I would like you, the reader, to share these, I often use the cajoling (rather than editorial) "we" when describing what you and I can record and how we might interpret these recordings.

However, as readers, you should make up your own minds and learn to see beyond me. In this regard, you should be aware that I have some commercial interest in the MASTER system for recording auditory steady-state responses that was licensed to Biologic Systems Corporation. My share of the patent-licensing fees is very small and I doubt that it affects my thinking. There are no other conflicts of interest.

The book is neither exhaustive in its review nor encyclopedic in its scope. Rather, it is a handbook in the original sense of the term, a book of essential information that comes to hand rather than stays on the shelf. The intended readers are those who record the auditory EPs in order to find out how the human brain responds to sounds—audiologists, neurologists, psychologists, and physiologists.

As well as reviewing the published literature, the book contains occasional ideas and data that have not been published previously. Among the new ideas are the concepts of the "physiological threshold level" described in Chapter 5, and the suggestions about how to handle the statistical problem of evaluating responses to multiple simultaneous stimuli in Chapter 6. Among the new data are the studies of the effect of age on the auditory steady-state responses in Chapter 10 and the evaluation of temporal integration in the brainstem in the same chapter. The time-warped middle latency responses presented in Chapter 16 have been in my unpublished files for a decade.

This book is limited to the electrical potentials recorded in response to sounds from electrodes placed on the human scalp or in the external or middle ear. Changes in the magnetic fields evoked by sounds, and intracranial recordings of auditory EPs in animals and man are reviewed only as they relate to the scalp-recorded electrical potentials. Otoacoustic emissions and vestibular responses are covered briefly as they supplement the auditory EPs in clinical testing.

In writing this book, I have become acutely aware of the immensity of the scientific literature. Even in the limited field of the auditory EPs, thousands of papers jockey for attention every year. This contrasts strikingly with the early days of the field when I could be reasonably sure that I had read just about everything of importance. Today, it is impossible to digest fully more than a fraction of what is published—so many papers, so little time. This vast accumulation of knowledge requires condensation, theories that subsume what is known into essential representations. One of the main goals of the book is to summarize what is known and to organize it as simply as possible.

Each chapter in the book is self-contained, listing its own references and explaining its own abbreviations, which I have tried to keep to a minimum. Mathematical formulae are not used in the text. However, these equations sometimes insist on being properly presented. The compromise has been to include them occasionally in the figures. More mathematical rigor can be found by consulting the papers listed in the references.

Although the book is organized to be read from beginning to end, some of you may wish to go initially to the chapters in which you are most interested. It often is better to find out what responses can be recorded before learning how to record them. Cross-references to other chapters may then lead you to the other parts of the book. The epigraphs for each chapter are chosen to allude to general principles, and to bring in other views and other languages. We should not forget that there is much in the world beyond our particular field of science.

The book contains many figures. We cannot understand the EPs if we cannot see them. To be consistent, all of the figures are plotted so that positive is upward. The literature uses both positive-up and negative-up conventions. Sometimes, this is related to the background of the scientists who record the EPs; electroencephalographers have used negative-up whereas engineers have preferred positive-up. The plotting conventions also often relate to what is being recorded, as components are more easily recognizable when they point upward. Thus, the auditory brainstem response typically is plotted positive-up and the mismatch negativity negative-up. Because I have great empathy for people who have difficulty knowing which way is up, I decided one convention would be preferable to two. My intent was not to rewrite history but to make it easier to understand.

The picture on the cover is a pastiche of several visual aspects of recording auditory EPs. In it, you may hear an exponential stimulus, dive through the tuning curve, enter a two-sphere head-model, ride the waves of the auditory EP, and ultimately find the audiogram you seek.

A book cannot be written without help. I would particularly like to thank those colleagues who reviewed draft-chapters: Claude Alain, Manny Don, Andrée Durieux-Smith, Karen Gordon, Steven Hillyard, Risto Näätänen, David Stapells, Arnold Starr, and Jan Wouters. As well, I am indebted to the many people I have consulted about various issues and ideas: Chuck Berlin, Ken Campbell, Barbara Cone, Rafael Delgado, Jos Eggermont, Bill Gibson, Bob Harrison, Martyn Hyde, Sasha John, Nina Kraus, Eleftherios Papathanasiou, Rob Patuzzi, Marilyn Pérez Abalo, Curtis Ponton, Catherine Poulsen, Bernhard Ross, Yvonne Sininger, Margot Taylor, and Istvan Winkler. My reviewers and consultants are absolved from any residual defects; whatever remains incorrect or unclear is my fault.

I am extremely grateful to my wife Nina Picton, my research-assistant Patricia van Roon, and my editor Casey Stach for their extensive help in getting the book into publishable form. I have enjoyed my interactions with Plural Publishing and especially thank Sandy Doyle and her production staff for their gentle attention to all the details. Finally, I would like to thank my most important teacher, Bob Galambos, and my main inspiration, Hallowell Davis.

This publication marks the passing earlier this year of two important figures. I shall miss the counsel of my mentor, Bob Galambos, and the encouragement of my publisher, Sadanand Singh. I hope the book is in tune with their spirit.

This book culminates my career in science. I have very fond memories of interacting with my students, fellows, and colleagues in the day-to-day work of science. One of my advisors, Baird Hastings, said that the important thing in science is to have fun in the laboratory. This book should not be read without recourse to a laboratory where you can record EPs, and I wish you as much enjoyment there as I have had. Much more needs to be figured out—and much fun can be had in the figuring.

Terry Picton
Toronto, September, 2010

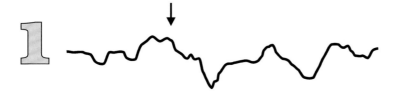

Introduction:
Past, Present, and Potential

> Glendower: I can call spirits from the vasty deep.
>
> Hotspur: Why, so can I, or so can any man;
>   But will they come when you do call for them?
>
> Shakespeare, *Henry IV*, Part 1, Act 3, Scene 1

This chapter introduces the human auditory evoked potentials (EPs)—the electrical changes that are generated in the human ear or brain in response to sounds. Because they typically are recorded from the scalp at some distance from their origin, these EPs can easily be considered as coming from the "vasty deep." First, we consider the meaning of the various terms we will be using. If we do not know what we are discussing, we soon will become lost. Different ways of classifying and naming the auditory EPs are then presented. These are the shelves on which to store what we learn. Some principles whereby we might distinguish different components of the EP waveforms are briefly mentioned. Finally, we review the historical background of our field. This allows us to refer to some of our great predecessors—another interpretation of

the spirits we can call upon. Even when we know what we are looking for, it is difficult to record the human auditory EPs. It was much more difficult to record these phenomena when they were unknown.

DEFINITIONS

The meanings of the words "auditory evoked potentials" need to be considered before we begin, if only so that we can tell our mothers what we do for a living. "Auditory" concerns that which is heard. "Potential" is the energy at a location within a field. For our purposes, both field and potential are electrical. Electrical potentials are measured in volts. The term "evoked" is complex. In olden days, magicians used to evoke spirits from the void. Both causality and capability are involved.

A response (effect) is called forth in something capable of responding (the depths of the brain) by a stimulus (cause). Some consistency of timing is usually part of evoking—the response should occur at approximately the same latency whenever the stimulus is presented. When the timing of the response changes from trial to trial or when the potentials change before rather than after the stimulus, a more general term "event-related potential" (ERP) is used. When the variability of timing is greater than the wavelength of a rhythmic response, we can consider the response "induced" rather than evoked, and we then need special measurement procedures. Auditory stimuli can induce event-related desynchronization (ERD) or synchronization (ERS) of the rhythms of the ongoing electroencephalogram (EEG). The term "evoked response," although once decried as a tautology (as all responses are evoked), has now returned as a way of discussing different kinds of responses—electrical, magnetic, hemodynamic, and otoacoustic.

CLASSIFICATION

Many different EPs can be recorded from the human scalp when sounds are presented. Some way of categorizing them is essential to any understanding. The first main classification of these potentials by Hallowell Davis (1976) was based primarily on latency, the time between the onset of the stimulus and the onset of the response. EPs were thus first, fast, middle, slow, or late. The first and fast responses are often considered "early" and the slow and late are often combined together as "late." One subsidiary categorization parameter was the recording technique (electrocochleography or vertex recordings). Most of the auditory EPs are best recorded from the vertex using a reference electrode on the mastoid or neck. Another subcategory was the probable source of the responses. In this way, we could describe the compound action potential (CAP) of the auditory nerve as part of the electrocochleogram (ECochG), and consider the fast response as the auditory brainstem response (ABR). In this book, we use ECochG for Davis's first response and ABR for his fast response. We continue with the term "middle-latency response" (MLR) and generally use "late auditory evoked potential" (LAEP) to describe Davis' slow and late responses.

Responses at all the different latencies can be evoked by the same stimulus —typically a click or brief tone. The different responses can then be plotted using several time bases, around 10 ms for the early responses, 50 ms for the middle-latency responses, and 500 ms for the slow and late responses. Another way to delineate the response is by using logarithmic axes to accentuate the earlier and smaller waves (Picton, Hillyard, Kraus, & Galambos, 1974). These approaches are illustrated in Figures 1–1 and 1–2.

As well as latency, time provides one other way to classify the EPs. "Transient" EPs that occur following a change in the stimulus—such as its onset or offset— can be distinguished from "sustained" responses that are evoked continuously throughout the stimulus. The term sustained potential (SP) has come to describe two different sustained responses: the summating potential of the cochlea and the sustained potential of the cortex. If the stimulus is changing regularly, a "steady-state" response can be evoked. In the auditory system, this type of response is termed the "auditory steady-state response" (ASSR). These different kinds of response are illustrated in Figure 1–3.

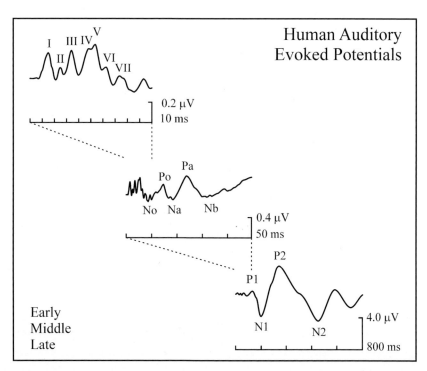

Figure 1–1. *Auditory EPs. This representation uses three different time-bases to show the early response (ABR), the middle-latency response (MLR), and the late response (LAEP).*

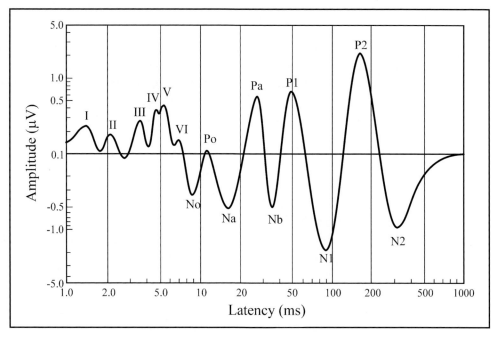

Figure 1–2. *Auditory EPs plotted using logarithmic axes. This allows the small early waves to be plotted in the same waveform as the large late waves. This approach to representing the auditory EP was first used by Picton and Galambos in 1972. The diagram, derived from Picton et al. (1974), shows the response to a 60 dB nHL click presented at a rate of 1 per s.*

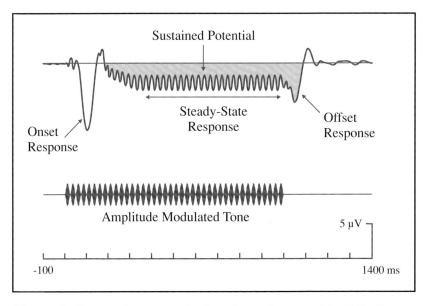

Figure 1–3. *Transient, sustained, and steady state EPs. This diagram shows the response to an amplitude-modulated tone lasting for 1 s. Transient responses occur at the onset and offset of the tone. A sustained potential (*shaded area*) occurs during the tone. The response to the modulations of the tone reaches steady-state after 200 to 300 ms.*

Table 1–1 presents a simple classification of the most common auditory EPs that uses both onset-latency and time-course.

NOMENCLATURE

The EPs have many names. Some names are related to where the responses are generated, for example, the ABR, which comes from the brainstem, and other names to where they are recorded, for example, the vertex potential. The negative or positive polarity of a wave and its location in a sequence lead to names such as P1, N1, P2, and N2 for the waves of the LAEP. Subcomponents of the main waves may require a secondary alphabetic sequencing, for example, N1a, N1b, and N1c. The MLR uses the alphabet as its sequence (Na, Pa, Nb). If all the waves are of the same polarity, a simple numbering can suffice (e.g., waves I–VII of the ABR). More specific than the location in a sequence is the latency in milliseconds of the wave at its peak (or trough). This leads to names such as P50, N100, P180, and N250. Because latency changes with different stimuli and different subjects, we often base the name on the typical latency in a young adult for a moderately intense stimulus. No one system of naming is either accepted by all users of the auditory EPs or obviously appropriate for all waves that can be recorded. We generally learn to use the names the waves were given when they were initially described. Some of these are more mysterious than others. The large response to sounds that was recognized in the EEG of a sleeping subject was called the "K-complex." This appears to have occurred because the technician knocked

Table 1–1. Classification of Auditory Evoked Potentials

Latency	Transient	Steady-State	Sustained
First (0–5 ms)	Cochlear Nerve Compound Action Potential (CAP: N1, N2)	Cochlear Microphonic (CM)	Summating Potential (SP)
Fast (1–15 ms)	Auditory Brainstem Response (ABR: I–VII)	Frequency Following Response (FFR); Fast (>70 Hz) Auditory Steady-State Response (ASSR)	Pedestal of frequency-following response
Middle (10–50 ms)	Middle-latency Response (MLR: Na, Pa, Nb)	40-Hz Potential	
Slow (30–500 ms)	Vertex Potential (P1, N1, P2, N2)	Slow (<30 Hz) Auditory Steady-State Response (ASSR)	Cortical Sustained Potential (SP)
Late (200–1000 ms)	Mismatch Negativity (MMN); Processing Negativity; Late Positive Waves (P3 or P300)		Contingent Negative Variation (CNV)

on the wall and wrote down "K" on the EEG record.

Crucial to any nomenclature is the polarity of the wave. However, polarity depends on the recording electrodes. All EEG recordings are between two electrodes, and what is negative at one electrode is positive at the other. In addition, there are two conventions about how negative and positive are plotted—the physicist's convention of positive-up and the EEG convention of negative-up. This latter counterintuitive convention derived from the fact that the most important phenomena in clinical EEG recordings, epileptic spikes, generally are negative. Both polarity conventions are used for plotting EPs, and we must learn to interpret both when reading the historical literature. In this book, we plot the waves positive-up. This has involved replotting many of the original records. Apologies may be due for allowing consistency to override history.

Auditory responses can be recorded from the human brain using magnetic instead of electric measurements, with magnetoencephalography (MEG) rather than EEG. Peaks and troughs in the magnetic waveform that are homologous to those recorded electrically generally are named by appending an "m" to the electrical name. For example the N1m is the MEG response that has many of the same features as the N1 of the LAEP. This obviates the "polarity" problem of MEG: if fields are given polarity on the basis of whether they are ingoing or outgoing, waveforms originating in the right and left auditory cortex have opposite polarity when recorded over homologous right and left scalp regions.

Sometimes the auditory EPs include the stimulus in the name. Thus, the "tone-ABR" is distinguished from the "click-ABR." This distinction is worthwhile because the responses have both a different waveform—the tone-ABR varies with the frequency and the rise-time of the tone—and a different audiometric interpretation —the tone-ABR can provide frequency-specific threshold. The ASSRs can be categorized as frequency-following responses (FFRs) and envelope-following responses on the basis of whether they are determined by the carrier frequency or the modulation frequency of a sound. When electrical stimuli are used instead of acoustic stimuli, it is customary to prepend an "E" to the name of the response (e.g., ECAP and EABR), and an "e" to the name of a wave (e.g., eIII and eV).

To save time, abbreviations are used to name the most common auditory EPs. In order not to overload memory, we will restrict ourselves to a small number of abbreviations. The abbreviations used in this chapter (and listed at the end) are essential and certainly worth remembering.

COMPONENTS

So far, we have considered the different components of the auditory EP in terms of the peaks and troughs in the waveform. However, different generators may contribute to what is recorded from the scalp at any one point in time. This becomes a particular problem for the later parts of the auditory response when multiple regions of the cortex may be simultaneously active. The peaks we pick in the scalp-recorded waveform then are not necessarily related to the peaks of activity in different cortical regions.

We often distinguish different components of the response by comparing recordings made under different experimental conditions. For example, when the ECochG is recorded at different stimulus rates, the SP component of the response remains stable whereas the CAP decreases at the more rapid rates. Following this idea, an EP component can be considered as "a source of controlled, observable variability" (Donchin, Ritter, & McCallum, 1978). One of the experimental variables that can distinguish components is the scalp topography. This can be interpreted in terms of sources within the brain. Thus, Scherg and von Cramon (1986) proposed that the components of scalp-recorded waveforms could be considered in terms of source potentials, each representing the "compound local activity of a circumscribed brain region." Näätänen and Picton (1987) melded these two approaches proposing that components were the sources of experimental variability that could be explained by localized physiologic activities. In recent years, we have begun to consider brain activity in terms of networks. The true components of a brain response may not necessarily be generated by a localized region of the brain. Instead, they might represent specific interactions between separate regions.

The type of component analysis used to evaluate the auditory EPs should be chosen so that the recorded data are most simply and meaningfully portrayed. For the early EPs, measuring the peaks and troughs of the waveform has been the usual approach. For the later EPs, we often assume overlapping components. A common technique to separate the components has been the subtraction of the waveforms recorded in one experimental condition from those recorded in a second condition to give the component that represents the processing that only occurs in the second condition. More formal mathematical component analyses can also be used; these are discussed in Chapter 2.

PRECEDENTS

History is important. Insight into present problems can come from learning how our mothers and fathers approached previous problems. In addition, a rapid tour through the past provides an overview of our current state of knowledge. The figures in this chapter, tracings of the auditory EPs as they were first recorded, can give flesh and bone to the abstract components listed in Table 1–1.

Early Electrical Recordings From the Human Brain and Ear

The electrical activity of the human brain —the EEG—was first recorded in the 1920s by Hans Berger in Jena, Germany. The most striking finding was an alpha rhythm, an oscillatory activity of 8 to 13 Hz. In his second published report on the EEG, Hans Berger (1930) noted that the alpha rhythm could be attenuated by loud sounds. EEG rhythms of frequencies near 10 Hz are generated when the cortex is in a state of idling and reflect many neurons firing rhythmically and synchronously. When the cortex has to process information, the neurons fire more rapidly and tend not to be synchronized. The decrease in the alpha rhythm following a sound might be caused by general arousal of the brain, which attenuates all rhythms of the brain, or by the more specific "desynchronization" of a tau rhythm that is generated in the auditory cortex (tau being the Greek letter "t" and indicating the temporal lobe). This rhythm is not easy to distinguish from other rhythms of similar frequency in EEG recordings, but can be seen using MEG (Lehtelä, Salmelin, & Hari, 1997). Our present understanding of the nature of the EEG rhythms thus derives from later times and different techniques than those of Berger, although he was the first to show that the brain was inherently both rhythmic and responsive.

At about the same time, scientists were trying to record the electrical activity of the human ear. In 1935, Fromm, Nylen, and Zotterman measured the cochlear microphonic (CM) from an electrode placed on the round window of a patient with a tympanic perforation. Both Fromm and Berger were trying to record in human subjects what had already been studied in animals. This has been a part of our history. What can be recorded in the animal ear or brain by direct recordings usually can be recorded in human subjects at the scalp or in the middle or external ear. However, the human recordings generally are more difficult and need more sensitive recording devices.

Berger's studies of the EEG soon became better known and developments in electronic amplification made the recordings more reliable—the signals were amplified prior to causing movement in a galvanometer. At Harvard, a skeptical Hallowell Davis suggested to his students Howard Simpson and Bill Derbyshire that they should try to see whether they could replicate this activity.

About three weeks later, Bill and Howard came to my office again, looking a bit sheepish, "You are right, chief" said Bill. "We have stuck needles in each other's scalps. The base line is unsteady, but we can't see anything rhythmic on the scope . . . " I went with them to the lab and Bill stuck needles into Howard's scalp. Howard sat in the shielded room and closed his eyes. The spot wobbled unsteadily across the scope. "That's what I thought," said I, "but three heads are better than two. Put the electrodes on my head." They did, and I sat in the room and closed my eyes. Immediately there were shouts outside: "There it is! There it is." It seems I have very strong alpha waves. (Davis, 1975, pp. 316–317)

Scientists began to investigate more fully how the EEG rhythms changed with stimulation. The typical change was the attenuation of the alpha rhythm that Berger had noted. However, occasionally brief transient responses could also be recorded. In 1939, Pauline Davis, the wife of Hallowell Davis, recorded consistent changes in the EEG in response to sounds. However, these responses varied from trial to trial and were often obscured by other waves in the electroencephalogram. Some of her recordings are shown in Figure 1–4. A companion paper with her husband and others (Davis, Davis, Loomis, Harvey, & Hobart, 1939) showed that the responses were much larger during sleep, although still very variable in the changing background activity of the EEG. The large responses that occurred during sleep were

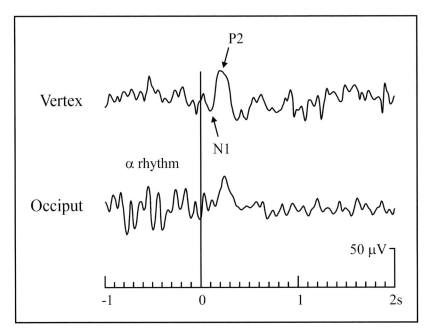

Figure 1–4. *First recordings of human auditory EPs. These data were traced from Figure 1E of Pauline Davis' paper (1939). The stimulus was a loud tone. Recordings were obtained using a linked-ear reference. The N1 and P2 labels (reflecting a later nomenclature) were not used in the original paper. The sound attenuated the occipital alpha rhythm as well as evoking the vertex transient response.*

often associated with spindles and were called K-complexes.

Averaging

The first clear approach to distinguishing the responses from the background EEG was by George Dawson (1950), who photographically superimposed multiple traces of somatosensory evoked potentials (following electrical stimulation of the median nerve at the wrist). The most intense part of the tracings showed the modal waveform, the "mode" being a measurement of the central tendency of a set of numbers that shows the most common values (those that are in fashion). My own introduction to the EPs was through John Scott, who had worked with Dawson on these recordings. Such are my tenuous links to history. Dawson went on to design a computer that could convert incoming signals into discrete values and average these together over many different responses (giving the mean rather than the modal response). Basically, the amplified EEG signal was mechanically directed by a rotating switch to a bank of capacitors that could store the sum of the charge at each point in time.

The averaging process increased the signal-to-noise ratio (SNR) of the EP recording. Averaging preserved the EP, which was the same from one stimulus to the next, while decreasing the background EEG activity, which varied from recording to recording. The EP was the signal and the EEG the noise.

New averaging computers were soon constructed that used electronic rather than mechanical switching. These allowed Geisler, Frishkopf, and Rosenblith in 1958 to record auditory EPs from the scalp that appeared to be generated in the auditory cortex. Much controversy soon erupted about whether these potentials were really generated in the brain or were just artifacts generated by reflexes in the scalp muscles. Geisler gave up his human recordings and returned to a very productive career studying the auditory system in animals. The current consensus is that most of what is recorded from the scalp in a relaxed subject is generated in the brain. If we look back at the original Geisler recordings, we can see clear MLR waveforms with a positive wave peaking at 30 ms. Some of these responses are shown in Figure 1–5.

Just to show that artifacts can contaminate a recording does not mean that artifact is all that can be recorded; we must always try to distinguish both the real and the artifactual. Both brain and muscle responses are interesting and both can tell us much about how the auditory system works. The waves of Geisler and his colleagues were pursued by others such as Goldstein and Rodman (1967), who used an alphabetical sequence for naming the waves (the numerical sequence having already been used for the late auditory EPs). Raising the upper frequency cutoff of the amplifiers from 50 to 150 Hz (Mendel & Goldstein, 1969) showed an earlier negative-positive wave complex, giving necessary birth to the complex nomenclature of No-Po-Na-Pa-Nb.

Attention then switched to the LAEPs (and to the effects of attention). These late waves were not distorted by muscle activity but were affected by attention and changed dramatically with sleep. Williams, Tepas, and Morlock (1962) had shown the changes with sleep and provided the P1-N1-P2-N2 nomenclature that we still use. (They who first named the waves deserve to be remembered.) Some of their

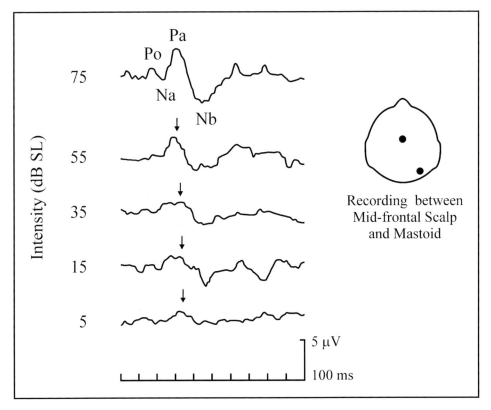

Figure 1–5. First recordings of the human auditory EPs using averaging. The stimuli were clicks presented at a rate of 1 per 1.5 s. The intensity is listed relative to sensation level (the subject's own threshold). Data traced from Geisler et al. (1958), with labels added from later nomenclature. The Pa wave is recognizable down to 5 dB above threshold (arrows).

waveforms are shown in Figure 1–6. Several investigators began to publish the results of recording the LAEPs from the scalp of waking human subjects, most clearly by McCandless and Best (1964) and Rapin (1964). Davis and Zerlin published their classic paper on the auditory vertex potential in 1966.

Brain and Mind

Since the days of Berger, the possibility that the electrical waves generated by the brain might tell us about the human mind had always fascinated scientists. In the mid-sixties, several new findings made this possibility even more exciting. In 1964, Walter, Cooper, Aldridge, McCallum, and Winter described a slow negative wave associated with expectancy—the contingent negative variation (CNV). In 1965, Sutton, Braren, Zubin, and John showed how a late positive wave in the auditory evoked potential could indicate the resolution of uncertainty. Following after the usual P1-N1-P2 complex, the late positive wave occurred with a peak latency of about 300 ms. Sutton et al. (1965) considered this wave to be an "endogenous"

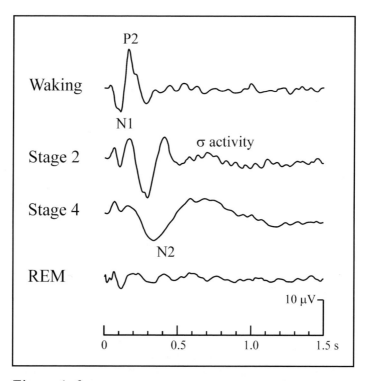

Figure 1–6. *Late auditory EPs recorded during sleep. There are marked changes in the auditory EPs when a subject falls asleep. In stage 2 and 4 sleep, the N1 wave of the response becomes smaller and the N2 wave becomes prominent. In Stage 2 sleep spindles (σ activity) often follow the response (the combination of the large response and the sleep spindle being known as the K-complex). These spindles can show up even in the averaged response. In rapid-eye-movement (REM) sleep, the response returned to the same morphology as during wakefulness but was much smaller in amplitude. These waveforms were traced from Williams et al. (1962).*

EP component, related to the attitude of the subject to the stimulus, as opposed to the earlier "exogenous" EP components, related to the physical nature of the stimulus. In this manner, the late EPs could show the interaction between the physical stimulus and its psychological perception. A follow-up paper (Sutton, Tueting, Zubin, & John, 1967) showed that the late positive wave occurred about 300 ms after the delivery of information, whether this was signaled by a stimulus or by its omission.

The wave has been variously called the P3 (from its position in the sequence) or the P300 (from its typical latency). Figure 1–7 shows the waveforms of two of the subjects in the first paper.

Recordings From the Ear and Brainstem

At about this time, the first nonsurgical recordings of the human cochlear nerve

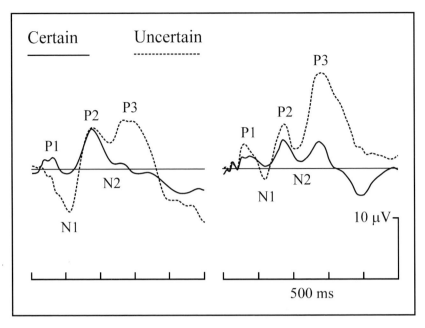

Figure 1–7. *The late positive wave of the auditory EP. In this experiment the subjects were asked to predict whether the next stimulus would be a click or a flash of light. In the "certain" condition, they knew what the stimulus would be and in the "uncertain" condition they did not. Recordings were obtained in response to the sound from an electrode in the left central region relative to the linked ears. Responses from two different subjects are shown. A large late positive wave occurred when the click resolved uncertainty. These waveforms were traced from Sutton et al. (1965), and labeling was added.*

action potential were made. Three papers were published: from Japan by Yoshie, Ohashi, and Suzuki (1967) using an electrode in the external auditory meatus; from France by Portmann, Le Bert, and Aran (1967) using a needle electrode that was inserted through the tympanic membrane onto the cochlear promontory; and from Israel by Sohmer and Feinmesser (1967) who used an electrode on the earlobe. All showed the N1 and N2 waves of the cochlear nerve action potential and demonstrated the characteristic increase in latency and decrease in amplitude with decreasing intensity. Figure 1–8 shows the results from Japan.

Sohmer and Feinmesser also described some late waves in their recordings of the electrocochleogram, and considered the possibility that these might have been generated in the brainstem rather than the cochlea. However, it was Jewett and his colleagues (Jewett, Romano, & Williston, 1970; Jewett & Williston, 1971) who finally clearly described what was to become the "auditory brainstem response" (ABR) and proposed our current nomenclature using Roman numerals. Interestingly, Jewett had first seen the waves in recordings from the cat cortex in Galambos' laboratory during some studies examining the possibility of glial-neuronal communication. However,

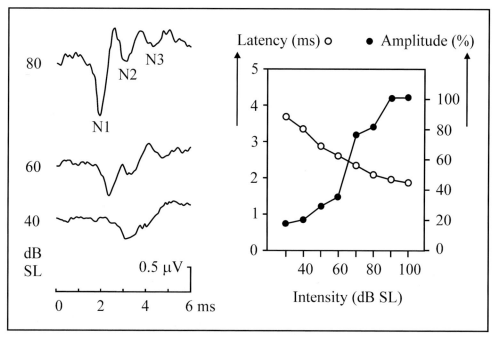

Figure 1–8. *Cochlear nerve compound action potentials (CAP) recorded from the external auditory meatus. The left of the figure shows sample waveforms in response to a click. The graph on the right shows the effects of stimulus intensity on the peak latency of the N1 and its amplitude. The amplitude is on an arbitrary scale. In meatal recordings, the responses are one to several microvolts in amplitude. In transtympanic recordings they are about five times larger and in earlobe recordings about five times smaller. Data from Yoshie et al. (1967).*

the waves were earlier than expected for the cortical recordings, just like the waves were later than expected by Sohmer and Feinmesser for their cochlear recordings. In his own words:

By pushing the averager to its limits, I was able to get small early potentials throughout the brain, whether I probed the cortex or deeper into the thalamus and then into the midbrain. What were they? After some initial puzzlement, I had gotten a recording from the cortex in which the waves were exactly time synchronous with the N1 response at the round window, so it was pretty

clear that the generator of this response was the eighth nerve and that the potentials were nothing but the result of distant current flow in a volume conductor. And then I made a major error—those of you who are sensitive to nuances will have caught it in the preceding sentence: the words "nothing but" bespeak an attitude that determined my behavior. (Jewett, 1983, pp. xxv–xxvi)

Several years were to pass before Jewett realized that these potentials could be reliably recorded from the human scalp. Figure 1–9 shows some of the early

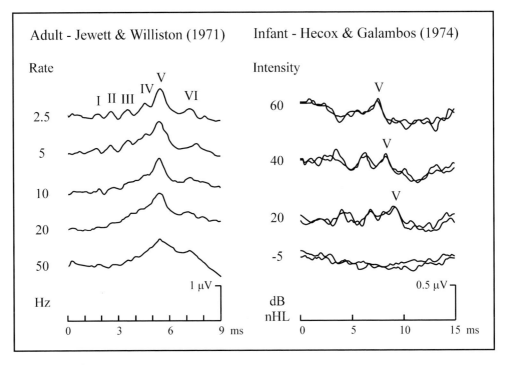

Figure 1–9. *Early recordings of the auditory brainstem response (ABR). On the left are shown ABR waveforms traced from Jewett and Williston (1971). Binaural clicks were presented at rates between 2.5 and 50 Hz. Responses were recorded from the vertex using the right earlobe as a reference. With increasing rate, wave V remains prominent whereas the other components of the response become less defined. On the right are shown recordings from a 5-week-old infant from Hecox and Galambos (1974). Clicks were presented monaurally at 30 Hz and responses recorded between vertex and ipsilateral mastoid. With decreasing intensity, the latency of the response increased. No response was recognizable below threshold.*

recordings. These tiny early waves in the auditory evoked potential, fondly called the Jewett "bumps," quickly found applications in audiology (Hecox & Galambos, 1974), neurology (Starr & Achor, 1975), and psychology (Picton & Hillyard, 1974). Stimulated by Jewett's work, Moushegian, Rupert, and Stillman (1973) reported brainstem responses to low-frequency tone-pips and showed how the response tracked the acoustic waveform, a human "frequency following response" (FFR). (Figure 1–10)

Attention

Selective auditory attention, the cocktail-party ability to ignore the boring person in front of you while closely following some far more interesting conversation at another location in the room, led to many experiments in the 1970s. Hillyard, Hink, Schwent, and Picton (1973) used a dichotic listening task to show that the N1 potential was enhanced by attending to a particular channel of sounds ("stimulus set"), whereas the P3 wave only occurred when

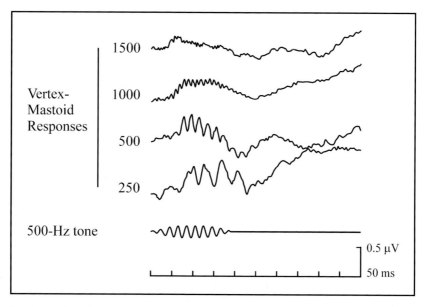

Figure 1–10. *First recordings of the human frequency-following response* **(FFR).** *The lowest tracing shows the stimulus waveform for the 500-Hz tone. Tones of other frequency had a similar stimulus envelope. The FFR has a waveform similar to that of the stimulus but is delayed by about 8 ms and rides on a slight baseline shift or pedestal (most clearly seen at 1000 Hz). The response decreases with increasing frequency. Data traced from Moushegian et al. (1973).*

the subject detected a target in the attended channel that required some response ("response set"). Figure 1–11 illustrates the N1 effects in one subject.

In 1978 Näätänen, Gaillard, and Mäntysalo used a new approach to determining the component structure of the evoked potential during attention: subtracting responses recorded in one condition from those recorded in a different condition to give a "difference curve." This procedure showed a "mismatch negativity" (MMN), which was a small negative wave superimposed on the N1-P2 response to a deviant stimulus occurring in a train of standard stimuli. This occurred whether or not the subject was attending to the stimuli, and therefore seemed to represent an auto-

matic discrimination-process closely related to the orienting response. These results are illustrated in Figure 1–12. Attending to the stimuli also resulted in a second superimposed slow negative wave that lasted much longer. In the figure, this can be seen by comparing the standard response when the stimulus was attended and when it was ignored (middle tracings). The authors named this the "processing negativity," because it appeared to represent the additional processing of stimuli that subject was asked to attend to in order to discriminate occasional targets. Later studies by the Hillyard group showed that this difference negativity (which they called the Nd) could be composed of both an enhanced N1 and a slower negative wave.

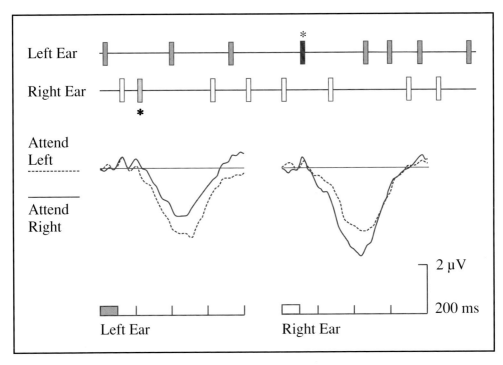

Figure 1–11. Effect of selective attention on the auditory EPs. *The upper part of the figure shows the stimuli. Brief tones of 1500 Hz were presented to the left ear and tones of 500 Hz to the right ear according to a random schedule with a stimulus onset asynchrony between 100 and 800 ms. The subject was asked to attend to one ear and to detect occasional increases in the frequency of the tone (*). The lower part of the figure shows the EPs recorded between vertex and mastoid. The N1 wave peaking between 100 and 150 ms was larger when the stimulus was attended. Data from Hillyard et al. (1973).*

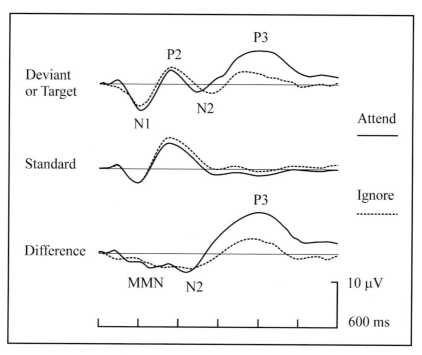

Figure 1–12. Mismatch negativity (MMN). *This figure combines data from Figures 1 and 4 from Näätänen et al. (1978). The subject was asked to attend to one ear while stimuli were presented concurrently to the two ears in a paradigm similar to that described in Figure 1–11 except that the stimulus onset asynchrony was constant at 800 ms. There was a small sustained difference between the responses to attended and ignored standard stimuli (middle tracings), beginning after the N1 and lasting for the duration of the recording. This later became known as the "processing negativity." The deviant or target stimuli (called "signals" in the original paper) showed an early negative shift that occurred whether or not the stimulus was attended. This later became known as the MMN.*

David, Finkenzeller, Kallert, and Keidel (1969) followed up some suggestive earlier work by the psychologist Köhler to make the first clear direct-coupled recordings from the human scalp of the human auditory sustained potentials (SPs). As shown in Figure 1–13, these small verterx-negative potentials lasted through the duration of a tone. They often finished with an offset response that was similar to the onset response in its morphology but smaller in amplitude.

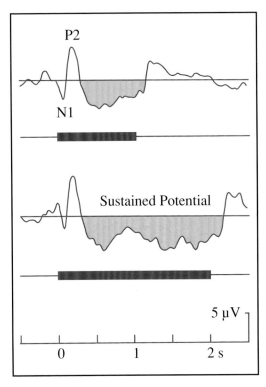

Figure 1–13. Auditory sustained potentials (SPs). When long-duration tones are presented, direct-coupled recordings show a small sustained negative deflection that follows the N1-P2 onset response and lasts the duration of the stimulus. Figure shows the responses to tones of two durations—1 and 2 s. Data traced from David et al. (1969).

Rhythmic Responses

While trying out a new system for recording the ABR, Galambos and his colleagues discovered that the brain responds particularly well at rates near 40 Hz:

> I was asked by my penultimate graduate student, Peter Talmachoff, what click stimulus rate to use . . . I told Peter to use 40/s, which he did, and he returned a few days later to show me records from several of his student subjects with the expected ABRs riding on top of a very large 40-Hz sine-wave-like deflection. We thought at first that the sine waves must be artifacts, but quickly convinced ourselves they were real physiological events. The explanation: Peter's new amplifiers passed more low-frequency EEG energy than the ones we and others had been using. (Galambos, 1992, p. 266)

Galambos, Makeig, and Talmachoff (1981) proposed that the prominent 40-Hz response represented the superimposition of the responses which lasted longer than the interval between the stimuli. This idea is illustrated in Figure 1–14. Galambos et al. (1981) suggested that this new 40-Hz potential might be useful in objective audiometry. However, they soon found that the response was not prominent in infants and decreased significantly with sleep. Although the response could be used to assess hearing in adults and older children, it was not reliable in infants.

Rickards and Clark (1984) in Australia followed up on some of the ideas about steady-state responses that Regan (1966, 1977) had developed in the visual system. They looked at the auditory EPs in the frequency domain rather than the time domain, a different point of view that

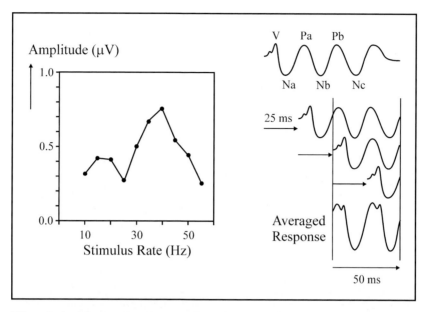

Figure 1–14. ***Auditory 40-Hz potential.*** *The left side of the figure shows how the amplitude of the response changes with different stimulus rates. The right side of the figure shows a proposed mechanism for the generation of the 40-Hz response. The top line shows the response to a stimulus presented at a rate of 10 Hz. The different waves of the response are separated by interpeak latencies of about 25 ms. If stimuli are presented at a rate of 40 Hz (once every 25 ms), the waves of the response superimposed. For example, the Na wave of one response will occur at the same time as the Nb wave of the preceding response. The responses will thus sum to give an average response that is several times larger than the response to a single stimulus. Data traced from Figures 1 and 2 of Galambos et al. (1981).*

appropriately came from the other side of the world. Cohen, Rickards, and Clark (1991) found that, although the ASSRs at rates near 40 Hz decreased dramatically in amplitude with sleep, ASSRs at rates near 80 Hz were little affected by the subject's state of arousal. Their amplitude did decrease a little during sleep but this was likely due to the decreased background EEG noise in the sleep recordings—all recordings (as we shall see in the next two chapters) representing a combination of both residual response and noise. Figure 1–15 illustrates some of their results.

Lessons of History

What can we learn from this rapid run through the history of recording human auditory EPs? What do the spirits we have evoked from the past have to say?

First is our dependence on technology. Clearly demonstrating the EEG required improving our instruments to detect tiny electrical changes. Recording EPs could not be reliably performed until the advent of computers that convert electrical input to numbers and average these numbers in relation to the presentation of stimuli.

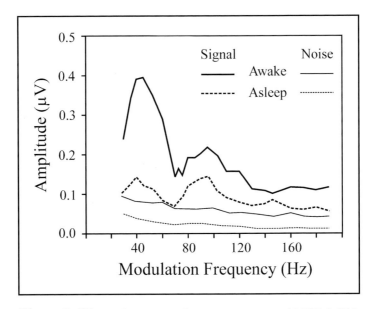

Figure 1–15. *Auditory steady-state responses (ASSRs). This figure shows the amplitudes of the ASSR to binaural tones of 2 kHz amplitude-modulated at rates between 30 and 185 Hz. The responses near 40 Hz are much more decreased by sleep than the responses at more rapid modulation rates. The noise levels (residual EEG and muscle activity) in the recording also are decreased by sleep. Data are replotted from Figure 7 of Cohen et al. (1991).*

Looking back on the difficulties of the early recordings, we cannot but admire both the insight and the persistence of the early researchers. They were able to discover things not previously known using techniques not previously tried.

As well, we learn new things by pushing the limits of our methods. The ABR was seen when scientists looked for auditory EPs at shorter and shorter latencies. The ASSRs were recorded when they presented stimuli at faster rates than they were accustomed to.

The argument that something is an artifact should be treated with caution. Our recordings seldom pick up only artifact or only brain-response. As Jewett remarked, we should always be careful of the "nothing but" argument. Explaining the meaning of something is better than explaining it away.

The study of human EPs will always be indebted to studies made in animals. Many of the early experiments sought to record from human subjects what had already been recorded in animals. Sometimes the direction needs to be reversed. Some responses that can be more easily recorded in human subjects—the P300, for example—need further study in animals.

The interstices between fields of study are fruitful areas for science. Psychoacoustics provides stimuli to perceive and models for their perception. Physiology describes the neuronal processes that evaluate auditory information. EP studies can gain from both. Hallowell Davis worked productively among many different fields.

He is the only person to have served as President for the American Electroencephalographic Society (1949–1950), the Acoustical Society of America (1953–1954), and the American Physiological Society (1958).

Always notice things beyond your focus. Science proceeds by testing hypotheses but must not become hypothesis-bound. We do not know enough to propose hypotheses that cover all eventualities. If there is something in your results that is not covered by your hypotheses, figure out what it is. Serendipity plays a role in many scientific discoveries. Näätänen and his colleagues (1978) discovered the MMN (which is relatively resistant to attention) while trying to understand the effects of selective attention. However, the benefits of a chance finding occur only if the experimenter notices the unexpected and interprets its meaning.

ABBREVIATIONS

ABR	Auditory brainstem response
ASSR	Auditory steady-state response
CAP	Compound action potential
CM	Cochlear microphonic
EEG	Electroencephalography
EABR	Electrical auditory brainstem response
ECAP	Electrical compound action potential
ECochG	Electrocochleography
EP	Evoked potential
ERD	Event-related desynchronization
ERP	Event-related potential
ERS	Event-related synchronization
FFR	Frequency-following response
LAEP	Late auditory evoked potential
MEG	Magnetoencephalography
MLR	Middle-latency response
MMN	Mismatch negativity
SNR	Signal-to-noise ratio
SP	Summating potential (cochlea)
	Sustained potential (cortex)

REFERENCES

Berger, H. (1930/translated by Gloor, P., 1969). On the electroencephalogram of man. Second report. In P. Gloor, *Hans Berger on the electroencephalogram of man. Electroencephalography and Clinical Neurophysiology,* Supplement 28 (pp. 75–93). New York, NY: Elsevier.

Cohen, L. T., Rickards, F. W., & Clark, G. M. (1991). A comparison of steady-state evoked potentials to modulated tones in awake and sleeping humans. *Journal of the Acoustical Society of America, 90,* 2467–2479.

David, E., Finkenzeller, P., Kallert, S., & Keidel, W. D. (1969). Akustischen Reizen zugeordnete Gleichspannungsänderungun am intakten Schädel des Menschen. [Sound correlated d-c changes from the intact head of human subjects]. *Pflügers Archiv, 309,* 362–367.

Davis, H. (1975). Crossroads on the pathways to discovery. In F. G. Worden, J. P. Swazey, & G. Adleman (Eds.) *The neurosciences: Paths of discovery* (pp. 309–321). Cambridge, MA: MIT Press.

Davis, H. (1976). Principles of electric response audiometry. *Annals of Otology, Rhinology and Laryngology, 85*(Suppl. 28*),* 1–96.

Davis, H., Davis, P. A., Loomis, A. L., Harvey, E. N., & Hobart, G. (1939). Electrical reactions of the human brain to auditory stimulation during sleep. *Journal of Neurophysiology, 2,* 500–514.

Davis, H., & Zerlin, S. (1966). Acoustic relations of the human vertex potential. *Journal of the Acoustical Society of America, 39,* 109–116.

Davis, P. A. (1939). Effects of acoustic stimuli on the waking human brain. *Journal of Neurophysiology, 2,* 494–499.

Dawson, G. D. (1950). Cerebral responses to nerve stimulation in man. *British Medical Bulletin, 6,* 326–329.

Donchin, E., Ritter, W., & McCallum, W. C. (1978). Cognitive psychophysiology: The endogenous components of the ERP. In E. Callaway, P. Tueting, & S. H. Koslow. (Eds.), *Event-related brain potentials in man* (pp. 349–411). New York, NY: Academic Press.

Fromm, B., Nylen, C. O., & Zotterman, Y. (1935). Studies in the mechanism of the Wever and Bray effect. *Acta Otolaryngologica, 22,* 477–486.

Galambos, R. (1992). A career retrospective. In F. Samson & G. Adelman (Eds.), *The neurosciences: Paths of discovery II* (pp. 260–280). Cambridge, MA: Birkhäuser Boston.

Galambos, R., Makeig, S., & Talmachoff, P. J. (1981). A 40-Hz auditory potential recorded from the human scalp. *Proceedings of the National Academy of Sciences (USA), 78,* 2643–2647.

Geisler, C. D., Frishkopf, L. S., & Rosenblith, W. A. (1958). Extracranial responses to acoustic clicks in man. *Science, 128,* 1210–1211.

Goldstein, R., & Rodman, L. B. (1967). Early components of averaged evoked responses to rapidly repeated auditory stimuli. *Journal of Speech and Hearing Research, 10,* 697–705.

Hecox, K., & Galambos, R. (1974). Brain stem auditory evoked responses in human infants and adults. *Archives of Otolaryngology, 99,* 30–33.

Hillyard, S. A., Hink, R. F., Schwent, V. L., & Picton, T. W. (1973). Electrical signs of selective attention in the human brain. *Science, 182,* 177–180.

Jewett, D. L. (1983). Introduction. In E. J. Moore (Ed.), *Bases of auditory brain-stem evoked responses* (pp. xxi–xxx). New York, NY: Grune and Stratton.

Jewett, D. L., Romano, M. N., & Williston, J S. (1970). Human auditory evoked potentials: Possible brain stem components detected on the scalp. *Science, 167,* 1517–1518.

Jewett, D. L., & Williston, J. S. (1971). Auditory-evoked far fields averaged from the scalp of humans. *Brain, 94,* 681–696.

Lehtelä, L., Salmelin, R., & Hari, R. (1997). Evidence for reactive magnetic 10-Hz rhythm in the human auditory cortex. *Neuroscience Letters, 222,* 111–114.

McCandless, G. A., & Best, L. (1964). Evoked responses to auditory stimuli in man using a summing computer. *Journal of Speech and Hearing Research, 83,* 193–202.

Mendel, M. I., & Goldstein, R. (1969). The effect of test conditions on the early components of the averaged electroencephalic response. *Journal of Speech and Hearing Research, 12,* 344–350.

Moushegian, G., Rupert, A. L., & Stillman, R. D. (1973). Scalp-recorded early responses in man to frequencies in the speech range. *Electroencephalography and Clinical Neurophysiology, 35,* 665–667.

Näätänen, R., Gaillard, A. W, & Mäntysalo, S. (1978). Early selective-attention effect on evoked potential reinterpreted. *Acta Psychologica, 42,* 313–329.

Näätänen, R., & Picton, T. (1987). The N1 wave of the human electric and magnetic response to sound: A review and an analysis of the component structure. *Psychophysiology, 24,* 375–425.

Picton, T. W., & Hillyard, S. A. (1974). Human auditory evoked potentials. II. Effects of attention. *Electroencephalography and Clinical Neurophysiology, 36,* 191–199.

Picton, T. W., Hillyard, S. A., Krausz, H. I., & Galambos, R. (1974). Human auditory evoked potentials. I. Evaluation of components. *Electroencephalography and Clinical Neurophysiology, 36,* 179–190.

Portmann, M., Le Bert, G., & Aran, J. M. (1967). Potentiels cochléaires obtenus chez l'homme en dehors de toute intervention chirurgicale. [Cochlear potentials obtained in man without surgical intervention.] *Revue de Laryngologie Otololgie et Rhinologie (Bordeaux), 88*, 157–164.

Rapin, I. (1964). Evoked responses to clicks in a group of children with communication disorders. *Annals of the New York Academy of Sciences, 112*, 182–203.

Regan, D. (1966). Some characteristics of average steady-state and transient responses evoked by modulated light. *Electroencephalography and Clinical Neurophysiology, 20*, 238–248.

Regan, D. (1977). Steady state evoked potentials. *Journal of the Optical Society of America, 67*, 1475–1489

Rickards, F. W., & Clark, G. M. (1984). Steady-state evoked potentials to amplitude-modulated tones. In R. H. Nodar & C. Barber (Eds.), *Evoked potentials II* (pp. 163–168). Boston, MA: Butterworth.

Scherg, M., & von Cramon, D. (1986). Evoked dipole source potentials of the human auditory cortex. *Electroencephalography and Clinical Neurophysiology, 65*, 344–360.

Sohmer, H., & Feinmesser, M. (1967). Cochlear action potentials recorded from the external ear in man. *Annals of Otology, Rhinology and Laryngology, 76*, 427–435.

Starr, A., & Achor, J. (1975). Auditory brain stem responses in neurological disease. *Archives of Neurology, 32*, 761–768.

Sutton, S., Braren, M., Zubin, J., & John, E. R. (1965). Evoked-potential correlates of stimulus uncertainty. *Science, 150*, 1187–1188.

Sutton, S., Tueting, P., Zubin, J., & John, E. R. (1967). Information delivery and the sensory evoked potential. *Science, 155*, 1436–1439.

Walter, W. G., Cooper, R., Aldridge, V. J., McCallum, W. C., & Winter, A. L. (1964). Contingent negative variation: An electric sign of sensorimotor association and expectancy in the human brain. *Nature, 203*, 380–384.

Williams, H. L., Tepas, D. I., & Morlock, H. C., Jr. (1962). Evoked responses to clicks and electroencephalographic stages of sleep in man. *Science, 138*, 685–686.

Yoshie, N., Ohashi, T., & Suzuki., T. (1967). Non-surgical recording of auditory nerve action potentials in man. *Laryngoscope, 77*, 76–85.

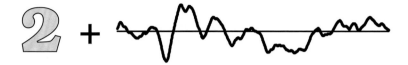

Recording Evoked Potentials: Means to an End

Qu'est-ce que l'homme dans la nature? Un néant à l'égard de l'infini, un tout à l'égard du néant, un milieu entre rien et tout.

(What is man in nature? Nothing in relation to the infinite, everything in relation to nothing, a middle between nothing and everything.)

Blaise Pascal, *Pensées, 72*

Recording evoked potentials (EPs) requires the application of several important techniques. Any practitioner of the art of evoked potentials must become acquainted with the principles underlying these techniques. This chapter introduces these principles as simply as possible and provides some examples of their application. We begin with the concepts of time and frequency, and then look closely at how we evaluate the auditory EPs from the perspective of the time domain. Techniques available in the frequency domain follow in Chapter 3. In the time domain, averaging—taking the mean of a set of time-waveforms—is the technique around which everything revolves.

TIME AND FREQUENCY

Underlying much of how we record the EPs are the concepts of time and frequency. All signals that occur in the time domain can be transferred without loss of information into the frequency domain. Thus, a potential that changes over time also can be considered as a spectrum of potentials at different frequencies. In 1822, Jean-Baptiste Joseph Fourier first showed that any signal can be expressed as the sum of a series of sine waves with frequencies harmonically related to the original signal. The Fourier transform can convert time signals to frequencies (Fourier analysis). It can also operate inversely (Fourier synthesis) to convert frequencies to time signals. For our purposes, we use the "discrete" Fourier transform wherein the signals are represented as sets of numbers rather than continuous variables. A common algorithm for the discrete transform is the Fast Fourier Transform (FFT) of Cooley and Tukey (1965), which can be applied to data sets wherein the number of values is equal to a power of 2 (e.g., 64 or 1024).

Figure 2–1 illustrates how the Fourier transform operates on a scalp-recording of the electrical activity of the brain, the electroencephalogram (EEG). As shown in the upper part of the figure, the recorded potential changes over time. At the begin-

ning of the tracing, it oscillates between positive and negative at a rate near 10 Hz. This is the most prominent of the EEG rhythms, the alpha rhythm. At other times in the recording, the potential changes more slowly or more rapidly. Converting the EEG time signal into the frequency domain gives a spectrum of potential amplitudes at different frequencies. These are plotted in the histogram at the bottom of the figure. In this particular example, the EEG shows alpha activity (8–13 Hz), beta activity (14–30 Hz), delta activity (0–3 Hz), and theta activity (4–7 Hz).

The figure does not show all of the data available in the frequency domain. At each frequency, the transform provides

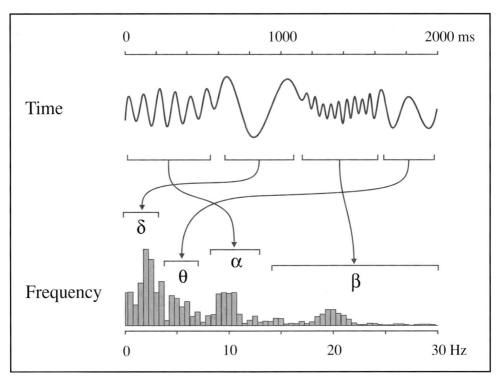

Figure 2–1. Time and frequency domains. At the top is a sample EEG signal recorded over 2 seconds. At the bottom is the amplitude spectrum of this EEG activity obtained by applying the Fourier transform to the time-domain signal. In the frequency domain, EEG activity typically is considered in terms of different frequency bands: alpha, beta, theta, and delta.

both real and imaginary values. These paired values can be converted to amplitude and phase. The phase at each frequency represents the point in the cycle of a cosine wave at the beginning of the analysis time. The phases of the different frequencies in the spectrum can represent their timing in the waveform. Thus, multiple different time-waveforms could have the same amplitude spectrum, but their phase spectra would be different. In addition to the absence of any phase information, the amplitude spectrum in the figure only shows the lower range of the available frequencies. For this particular signal, the values at higher frequencies were essentially zero. The number of values in each of the amplitude and the phase spectra is one half the number of time points in the original signal. The resolution of the frequency spectrum, the frequency difference between adjacent bins in the spectrum, is the reciprocal of the duration of the signal analyzed. For this particular analysis of a 2-s sample, the resolution is 0.5 Hz. The full spectrum therefore extends from zero to the Nyquist frequency, which is one half of the rate at which the time-domain values were collected. In this particular example, that rate was 250 Hz (once every 4 ms); therefore, the Nyquist frequency is 125 Hz. The amplitude spectrum in the figure plots only the initial 61 values (from 0 to 30 Hz) rather than the full 250 values (from 0 to 124 Hz).

EPs typically are represented as time-waveforms, potentials with peaks and troughs at different latencies after the stimulus. However, like the EEG, these waveforms also can be considered in the frequency domain. The left side of Figure 2–2 shows the fast, middle, and slow auditory EPs in response to a brief transient stimulus such as a click. The figure is diagrammatic, based on the amplitudes and latencies

reported in Picton, Hillyard, Krausz, and Galambos (1974). The right side of the figure shows the associated spectra. Some consideration of how rapidly the time waveform changes will explain the spectral patterns (e.g., Boston, 1981). The fast EP (or ABR) contains peaks that occur at about once a millisecond. This causes the activity in the spectrum at frequencies near 1000 Hz. The double peak IV–V complex is broader than the other peaks and this is transformed into the spectral activity near 500 Hz. In addition, there is a broad wave underlying the peaks that goes to positive near 5 ms and back to negative near 10 ms, thus going through a full cycle in about 10 ms. This would explain the spectral activity near 100 Hz. In the middle-latency response (MLR), the intervals between adjacent latency peaks of the same polarity are near 25 ms and the main activity in the spectrum occurs between 30 and 50 Hz. Most of the activity in the late auditory EP (LAEP) is near 5 Hz.

RECORDING EEG SIGNALS

Electrodes

The EEG is recorded from the scalp using special connections called electrodes. Two main kinds of electrodes are used. Reversible electrodes, such as a pellet made by sintering together silver and silver-chloride, are able to measure long lasting potentials without any loss of stability. Simple metal electrodes set up an electrode double layer when current passes through them and this double layer acts as a high-pass filter, slowly returning any sustained potential to zero. The amount of filtering depends on the metal and the amount of current drawn by the amplifier. This filtering can be reduced by using gold-plated electrodes

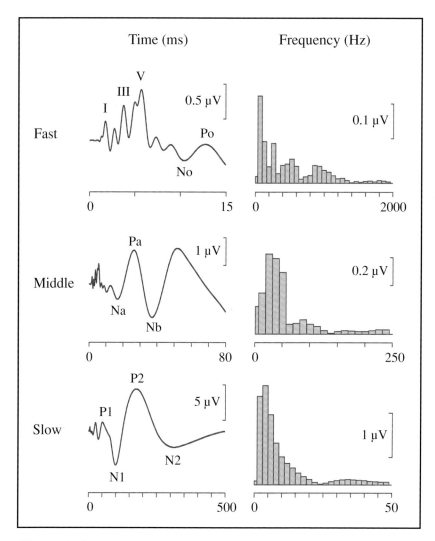

Figure 2–2. Auditory EPs in both the time and frequency domains.
The waveforms on the left represent the typical transient auditory EPs, evoked by a click presented once a second. The fast EPs are seen at the beginning of the waveforms for the middle EPs and the middle EPs are seen at the beginning of the slow EPs. The spectra on the right represent the frequencies present in the time waveforms. The amplitude calibration of the spectra is based on the baseline-to-peak amplitude of the sinusoidal component.

rather than simple copper electrodes, and by connecting the electrodes to amplifiers with high input impedance.

Fixing an electrode in place on the scalp may be achieved in many ways. We can use a sticky paste under the electrode, provided the paste is also conductive. A gauze pad is then placed over the electrode to prevent it sticking to the earphones or the pillow. Another approach to fixation is to use a collodion-soaked gauze pad. This technique is more secure and therefore better for long-duration recordings or intraoperative studies. Collodion can be removed after the recording using a diluted acetone solution. Electrodes also can be held in position within a tight-fitting elastic cap, or be part of a geodesic structure. This approach is essential when using many electrodes. Electrodes for electrocochleography (ECochG) can be held in place in the external auditory meatus by the foam around the ear insert that conducts sound to the ear, or can be inserted as sterile needles either into the skin of the meatus or transtympanically onto the cochlear promontory in the middle ear.

A conducting connection is essential to making any electrical recording. Typically, this is achieved using a saline jelly. Even a dry electrode will work if there is sweating, but this may not give a continuous connection, particularly on a hairy scalp. The skin of the scalp is also a barrier to conduction between the subcutaneous fluid and the electrode. The skin can be abraded with a blunt needle or with a mildly abrasive pad containing alcohol, which dissolves fat and acts as an antiseptic. The connectivity between the electrode and the subcutaneous tissue is assessed by measuring the electrode impedance. Impedance is a measurement of resistance appropriate for alternating current signals (where phase as well as amplitude can be affected). In order to measure the electrode impedance, a tiny current is applied across the electrodes at a frequency appropriate to the recording (e.g., 10 Hz for recording the EEG). Electrode impedances of less than 10 kOhms are recommended. Some new amplifiers do not need impedances this low to make reasonable recordings. However, the amplitude of any artifactually induced voltage differences between electrodes increases as the interelectrode impedance increases.

In recent years, small preamplifiers have been placed right on the electrodes (e.g., Taheri, Knight, & Smith, 1994). These increase the power of the signal transmitted from the scalp to the EEG amplifier. This approach does not change the artifacts that can be recorded at the electrode-scalp interface (such as electrode "pops" or skin potentials). However, preamplifiers significantly decrease the amount of electromagnetic noise picked up in the electrode wires (connecting the electrodes to the amplifier) relative to the EEG signal. The noise is about the same, but now it is relative to an amplified EEG signal. Another recent development is wireless transmission between the electrodes and the recording system (Sokolov, 2007).

Electrode Locations

Electrodes should be positioned on the scalp according to conventions that can be applied to different head shapes and sizes. The most widely used convention is the 10-10 system promulgated by the American Clinical Neurophysiology Society (2006). This system of electrode placement is designed to place electrodes at approximately equal distances from each other over the scalp. It uses a combined alphanumeric nomenclature with letters denoting locations on sagittal (front-to-back) lines and numbers indicating locations on coronal (side-to-side) lines. The first defining measurement is the distance from nasion (Nz) to inion (Iz) across the top to the head. The nasion is the notch between the nose and forehead and the inion is the small bump where the posterior neck muscles attach to the skull. The midline electrode positions are then located every tenth of this distance from nasion to inion. These locations are named with "z" to denote the midline. The frontal electrode Fz is located at three tenths of the distance and central electrode Cz is located halfway (at the vertex). A horizontal circumferential measurement at the level of the frontal pole (Fpz, one tenth the distance from nasion to inion) and the occiput (Oz, nine tenths the distance) is divided into tenths on each side. Electrodes between the midline and the circumference are named using the midline alphabetic abbreviation and numbers to denote how far away from the midline. Odd num-

bers are used on the left and even numbers on the right. The only exceptions to this nomenclature are the electrodes over the temporal lobes which are denoted FT for frontotemporal, T for midtemporal and PT for parietotemporal. The midtemporal electrodes (T7 on the left and T8 on the right) are located on the circumference halfway between Fpz and Oz. Further details are provided in Figure 2–3.

Other approaches to locating scalp electrodes can be used, and many caps (particularly those with many electrodes)

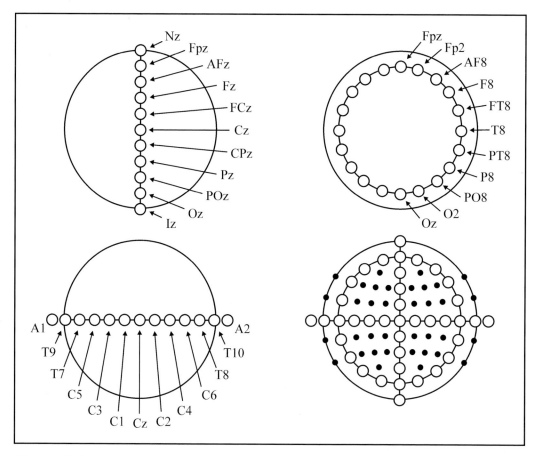

Figure 2–3. Electrode locations in the 10-10 system. The electrodes are named using an alphabetic notation to denote front to back location (upper left) and a numerical notation to denote left to right location (lower left). Electrodes over the temporal lobe are named differently from those close to the midline (upper right). A1 and A2 are the left and right earlobes. The full system is illustrated in the lower right.

use their own coordinate system. Wherever possible, however, to maintain consistency across publications some reference should be made to the 10-10 system (e.g., by identifying those electrode locations homologous to locations in the 10-10 system).

Amplification

EEG potentials recorded at the scalp are tiny. They are measured using units such as millivolts (thousandths of a volt, mV), microvolts (millionths of a volt, μV), or even nanovolts (billionth of a volt, nV). In order to be evaluated in computers or viewed on displays, the EEG signals must be amplified to the level of volts. This typically requires an amplification of 10,000 to 1,000,000 times. The actual amount of amplification should make the recorded signal span as much as possible of the range that the analog-to-digital (AD) converter of the computer can handle without blocking. Thus, if the recorded signal varies between a maximum of +20 μV and a minimum of −20 μV and the AD converter has an input range of ±10 V, the amplification should be 500,000 times. Note that we are considering the amplitude of the recorded EEG and not that of the EP, which may be much smaller. For example, an ABR with an amplitude of 1 μV may be occurring in the EEG that varies between +20 and −20 μV. Computer procedures such as averaging will be needed to distinguish these tiny EPs from the background EEG

Many other potentials occur at the level of the recording electrodes in addition to those generated in the brain. The largest of these are related to our electric power systems, which create electric currents at 60 Hz (in North America) or 50 Hz (in Europe and most of Asia and Africa).

These currents can cause magnetic fields, and these in turn can induce currents in the recording circuits, which are seen as periodic potentials at the frequency of the power system and its harmonics. These potentials often go by the names of "line noise" or "mains hum," the latter term coming from descriptions of what the noise sounds like when the amplified signals are monitored on a speaker. Most of the potentials generated from such sources are similar in locations that are close to each other. The main approach to distinguishing EEG potentials from power-line potentials therefore is the differential amplifier. Rather than measuring the potential at one electrode (relative to some general reference level considered as "ground"), a differential amplifier measures the difference in potential between one electrode (input 1) and a second electrode (input 2). Input 1 is also called "noninverting" or "+," and input 2 "inverting" or "−." In most EP studies, recordings are made from an "active" electrode connected to input 1 and a "reference" electrode connected to input 2. Potentials such as line noise that are the same at each electrode cancel themselves out by a process called common-mode rejection. How well this is done is assessed by measuring the "common mode rejection ratio," usually expressed logarithmically and typically over 80 dB in EEG amplifiers.

Filtering

Filtering is used to attenuate frequencies in the recorded signal that contribute little to the signal that we are interested in but which, nevertheless, obscure its recognition or measurement. The obscuring activity can be considered electrical noise, as it can prevent any understanding of electrical signals in the same way that acoustical noise prevents our understanding of speech signals. In the context of rapidly recognizing a signal, an optimum filter reduces frequencies in the recording in inverse proportion to the signal-to-noise ratio (SNR) at that frequency (Doyle, 1977). This optimum filter is called the Wiener filter after Norbert Wiener, who first described it and also founded the field of cybernetics.

The concept of optimal filtering can be illustrated by recording an EP in the presence of so much line noise (mains frequency) that common mode rejection is ineffective and the signal is overwhelmed by the noise. If we are recording the MLR, the frequency content of which is between 10 and 100 Hz, the recording can be clarified by using a notch filter that attenuates the line-noise frequency. This is illustrated using simulated data in Figure 2–4. In the example in the figure, the mains frequency is 50 Hz. The signal-to-noise ratio (SNR) is lowest at 50 Hz and therefore an optimum filter would cause more attenuation of the activity at this frequency than at other frequencies. Although the response is made recognizable by filtering, we also should note that the morphology of the response has changed a little—the amplitude of the Pa wave is smaller after filtering. The original response contained energy at the same frequency as the line noise and this was removed by the filter. A notch filter is a very simple optimum

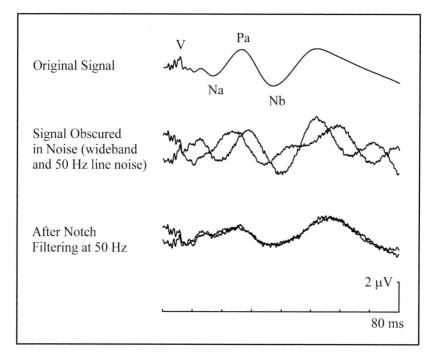

Figure 2–4. Notch filtering. *The original signal shown in the upper part of the figure was mixed with noise consisting of low-level wideband noise and high-amplitude line noise at 50 Hz. The response is not reliably recognized in the replicated waveforms* (middle). *Notch filtering removes the line noise and makes the response clear* (lower tracings).

filter. More complicated optimum filters would have different attenuation amounts at different frequencies based on the differences between the spectrum of the electrical noise and the spectrum of the EP. Unfortunately, we may not know these spectra for an individual subject until we start to record the responses. Part of the recording therefore must be used to estimate these spectra before the optimum filter can be applied.

Filtering can be performed using analog circuits or digital programs. Any analog filter can be instantiated in digital form. However, digital filters can be created that cannot be set up easily in analog circuits. Digital filters are applied once data are collected, but with the speed of modern computers, such filtering usually can be performed on one recording before the next recording is obtained. Digital filters have a major advantage over analog filters in that they can be designed to preserve the phase relations between the different components of the signal. The simplest approach is to apply the filter to the signal twice, once in the normal time direction and once with time reversed. Preserving phase information leads to much less distortion of the response waveform. This is illustrated in Figure 2–5. Using the digital filter maintains the general morphology of the response—Wave V continues to appear as a positive wave. With an analog

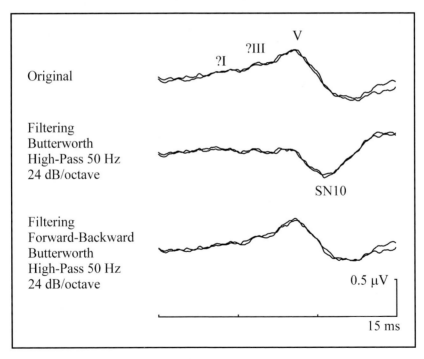

Figure 2–5. *Waveform distortion with analog filtering. The original waveforms were filtered in two ways. Analog high-pass filtering with a steep slope distorts the waveform and makes the slow negative wave at 10 ms (SN10) the most prominent component. A similar amount of filtering but applied in a forward and backward manner (only possible with digital filtering) does not distort the waveform.*

high-pass filter with a cutoff of 40 Hz and a relatively steep slope, the phase of the activity underlying this wave is altered and the negative wave following Wave V becomes more prominent (Stapells & Picton, 1981). This wave, called the SN10 or the slow negative wave at 10 ms, can be used to assess ABR thresholds in evoked potential audiometry (Davis, Hirsh, Turpin, & Peacock, 1985), but it is easier (and less confusing) to evaluate the digitally filtered waveform.

Analog filtering is applied to the signal before it is converted to digital format. The main purpose of analog high-pass filtering is to maintain the signal within the range of the computer's AD converter. Low-pass filtering prevents high-frequency signals from "aliasing" back into the signal during AD conversion (a phenomenon that we consider in the next section). The bandpass of such an analog filter can be approximated using two very simple rules of thumb (Picton & Hink, 1974). The low-frequency cutoff (in Hz) is set to one divided by four times the recording duration (in seconds), and the high-frequency cutoff to one divided by four times the digitization interval (in seconds). Thus, if we are recording the ABR with a sweep of 15 ms and a digitization interval of 0.05 ms (equivalent to an AD conversion rate of 20 kHz), we can set the filters to pass frequencies between 16 Hz and 5000 Hz. If we know the content of the EP signal beforehand, we can restrict the bandpass even further, and we normally use a bandpass between 30 and 3000 Hz for recording the ABR. Typical frequency bandwidths for recording the different auditory EPs are given in Table 2–1 together with the recommended AD conversion rates and recording durations.

Further filtering of the EP can then be performed using digital filters. In general,

the frequency content of the EP waveform is similar to that of the background EEG in which it is recorded. Optimum filters, based on comparing the spectrum of the EP to the spectrum of the EEG, usually are not that helpful in enhancing the SNR, and may cause distortion of the response waveform. This is not a problem when the intent is only to recognize whether a response is present or not, but it is a problem when comparing latencies and amplitudes to normal values. Generally, we therefore use simple bandpass filters.

Occasionally, time-varying filters may be helpful (de Weerd, 1981). For example, we may wish to record both the ABR and the MLR simultaneously. If so, it may be advantageous to filter the response with a bandpass that moves from high to lower frequencies as the latency increases (Picton, Lins, & Scherg, 1995).

Analog to Digital (AD) Conversion

Before being analyzed in the computer, the recorded data must be converted from a continuous waveform to a set of discrete values, the process of AD conversion. This process has two main parameters: the rate at which the conversion occurs and its amplitude resolution. The rate must be sufficient to reproduce the frequencies present in the recorded response. Because the Fourier transform allows us to measure only frequencies that are lower than one half the conversion rate, the rate of AD conversion must be at least twice the maximum frequency that we anticipate recording in the EP signal (and preferably at least four times).

The problem of aliasing must be considered when setting the AD conversion rate and the analog filters that precede the

Table 2–1. Recording Parameters for Human Auditory Evoked Potentials

Potential	Component	Electrodes[1]	Filter (Hz)	A–D (kHz)	Stimulus Rate (Hz)[2]	Epoch (ms)[3]	Averages
ECochG	CAP, CM	EAM-Mc TT-Mc	100–3000	20–50	5–20	5–10	500–2000 100–500
ABR	I V	Cz-Mi	30–3000	20–50	5–20 10–80	15–20	1000–5000
	80-Hz ASSR	Cz-Nz	30–300	1	80–100	1000	100–5000
MLR	Pa	Cz-Mi	5–500	1–2	5–20	50–100	200–1000
	40-Hz ASSR	Cz-Nz	10–100	0.2–0.5	30–50	1000	20–1000
Slow EP	N1 SP	Cz-Mc Fz-Mc	1–30 0.1–15	0.25–0.5	0.25–1	500–1000	50–200 100–200
Late EP	MMN P3	Fz-Mc Pz-Mc	0.1–15	0.25–0.5	0.1–0.5 0.05–0.25	500–1000	200–1000 20–100

[1]EAM is an electrode in the external auditory meatus; TT is a needle electrode inserted transtympanically onto the cochlear promontory in the middle ear; Mc and Mi are the contralateral and ipsilateral mastoids; Nz is a midposterior neck electrode; Cz is the vertex; Fz and Pz are midfrontal and midparietal electrodes.

[2]For the late EPs we have given the rates at which the deviants or targets occur. Between these stimuli are the standard stimuli that occur at rates that are 5 to 10 times faster.

[3]For the auditory steady-state response (ASSRs), we have listed a typical recording epoch that then can be analyzed in the frequency domain, often after being concatenated to increase the resolution of the analysis. The 40-Hz ASSR also can be evaluated in the time domain, typically using sweeps of 50 to 100 ms and averages of 100 to 500.

conversion. As shown in Figure 2–6, frequencies that are greater than the Nyquist frequency can appear as lower frequencies after conversion. This process is known as aliasing—higher frequencies masquerading as lower frequencies. A visual example of aliasing is the apparent slow reverse motion of the spokes when wheels are rotating more quickly than a movie's frame rate. Aliasing is prevented by setting the low-pass filters below the Nyquist frequency and ensuring that their slope is sufficiently steep to attenuate higher frequencies down to a level that an aliased version of these frequencies would be too small to be recognized in the digitized data.

The amplitude resolution of the AD converter is expressed in bits, the information given by a choice between two equally probable events. A one-bit converter tells only whether the recorded value is positive or negative, provided that the signal is set up so that the level at which the AD converter changes from 0 to 1 is the same as zero in the recorded signal. Most AD converters are 12 bits or more; they provide at least 2^{12} or 4096 possible levels. Thus, if a 12-bit AD converter receives an EEG signal that has been amplified so that the maximum range of the converter spans an EEG signal with an amplitude (before amplification) of between −100

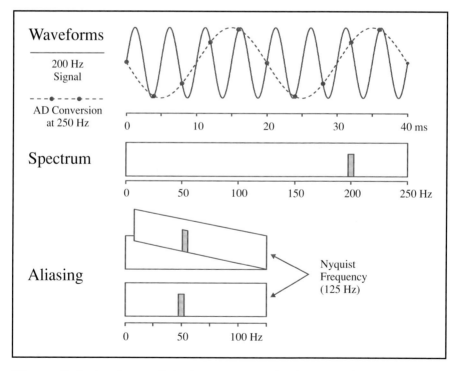

Figure 2–6. *Analog to digital conversion. This figure illustrates the aliasing of frequencies higher than the Nyquist frequency. The continuous line in the upper tracing represents the original 200-Hz signal. The dashed line represents the 50-Hz signal that is seen after this has been analog-to-digital converted at 250 Hz. The lower part of the figure shows how this process can be considered as a folding of the original spectrum into the frequency range that is covered by the digitized data.*

and +100 µV, the resolution of the AD converter can also be described as 200/4096 or .05 µV/bit. This parameter combines both the amount of amplification and the resolution of the AD converter.

AVERAGING

Averaging is a procedure that can distinguish a signal hidden in noise. Multiple measurements are required. If the signal is always the same and if the electrical noise varies randomly from measurement to measurement, averaging will increase the SNR. As discussed by Dawson (1954) in his classic paper on averaging EPs, averaging was first used to demonstrate a lunar tide in the atmospheric pressure. The effect of the moon on the atmospheric pressure is tiny compared to the ongoing fluctuations in this pressure caused by the weather. By making measurements over many months and averaging these together in relation to the earth's rotation relative to the moon (the tidal day), the small effects of the moon on the atmospheric pressure could be recognized.

Like the atmospheric tide, most auditory EPs are significantly smaller than the background activity in which they are recorded. The background activity consists of the EEG activity from the brain and electromyographic (EMG) activity generated in the muscles of the head and neck. The EPs usually remain smaller than the background activity even when filtering optimally attenuates EEG/EMG activity at frequencies not present in the EP.

Therefore, averaging is necessary to decrease the amplitude of the background activity while preserving the EP signal. This is illustrated in Figure 2–7. The stimulus is repeated for many "trials" to provide multiple recordings of the EP and background EEG. If a single noise potential occurs on one of the trials, it will decrease by a factor equal to the number of trials. If a randomly distributed EEG noise occurs on all trials, its root-mean-square amplitude decreases during averaging by a factor equal to the square root of the number of trials. This is akin to what occurs in statistics when the standard deviation of a sample is converted to the standard error of the mean by dividing by the square root of the number of samples. The background EEG never becomes zero. If we wish to halve the noise, we need to average four times as many trials. Given this, we realize how important it is to reduce the noise level of the recording (either by filtering or by getting the subject to relax) before averaging begins.

The use of averaging to distinguish EPs (signal) from the background EEG (noise) is based on three assumptions (Glaser & Ruchkin, 1976). First, the signal should remain constant from one trial to the next; second, the noise should vary randomly across trials; and third, the signal and noise should sum linearly to produce the activity recorded on each trial. EPs do not always fulfill these assumptions. The EP signal may vary from trial to trial. This is especially true of the later components of the response. Variations in amplitude do not disrupt the averaging process much; the final average EP is the average of the amplitudes.

Latency Jitter

Variations in the latency or phase of an EP from trial to trial are much more problematic. If a negative wave on one trial occurs at the same latency as a positive wave on another trial, averaging can lead to cancellation. Techniques exist to compensate for

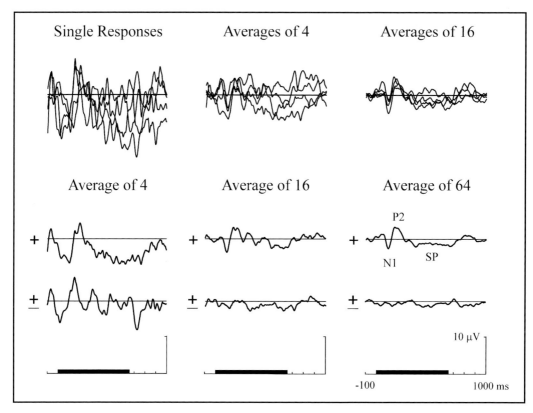

Figure 2–7. Averaging. *This figure shows how multiple single responses can be averaged together to provide a clear EP. Each response was evoked by a 650 ms tone at 65 dB SPL presented with an interstimulus interval between 1 and 3 seconds. The responses were recorded from the vertex relative to an average reference. The upper left shows four superimposed single responses. When these are averaged together, the morphology of the response becomes apparent but the response is only at the same level as the background EEG, shown by the ± average (which is discussed further in Chapter 5). Averages of 4 and 16 are clearer and the average of 64 shows a LAEP (with N1-P2 onset response and SP) that is much larger than the residual background EEG.*

such latency "jitter," but these techniques (reviewed by Ruchkin, 1988) require that the EP be to some degree recognizable in each single trial. Latency compensation techniques can work when averaging occurs over a few trials (perhaps less than 100) but not when the EP is so much smaller than the background EEG that averaging over thousands of trials is required.

A simple technique to compensate for the effects of latency jitter is the Woody filter (Woody, 1967). Basically, each single-

trial recording is cross-correlated to the average waveform, and the latency at which the maximum correlation occurs is used to shift the timing of the EP for that trial when computing a subsequent average (which may then serve as the template for a further set of cross-correlations). The process can iterate until there is little or no further change in the averaged waveform. Figure 2–8 shows the operation of a Woody filter (with no iteration). The simulated LAEP is what might be expected when one detects an auditory target that differs

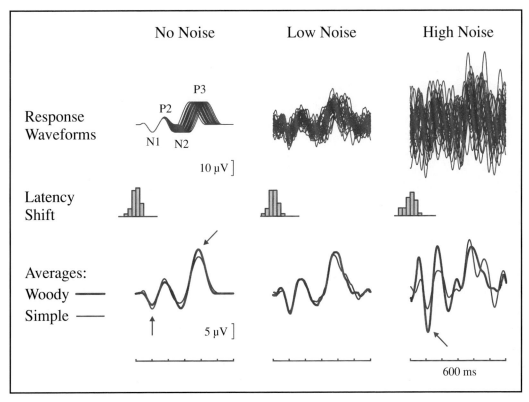

Figure 2–8. Latency jitter and the Woody filter. *For this simulation, 30 EPs were constructed with the N1-P2 waves having constant latency and the N2-P3 complex varying in latency from trial to trial. The latency shift estimated by the Woody filter is shown in the histogram. With no noise, the average waveforms obtained after Woody filtering correctly show the amplitude of the N2-P3 complex (diagonal downward arrow) but attenuate the N1-P2 waves (upward arrow). With high levels of noise the Woody filter can create spuriously large EPs (diagonal upward arrow). The averages are plotted using a more sensitive scaling than the single-trial response waveforms.*

in frequency from a standard stimulus. An N1-P2 onset response occurs with a stable latency and is followed by an N2-P3 complex that varies in latency with how difficult the subject finds the discrimination. When there is no EEG noise, the Woody filter works well to record the larger N2-P3 complex, but attenuates the smaller N1-P2 complex. With low levels of noise, the Woody filter provides a good representation of the large N2-P3 complex. However, when the recordings contain large amounts of background EEG noise, the Woody filter may lock onto potentials

in the noise and give a spuriously large response, such as the unusual N1-P2 response (indicated by the diagonal arrow in the lower right of Figure 2–8).

High-Noise Trials

In many recording situations, the background EEG/EMG noise fluctuates from trial to trial. Subjects have an intrinsically human need occasionally to move, swallow, blink their eyes, and otherwise interfere with the smooth progress of averaging.

There are three main ways to deal with the problem of noisy trials. The first is to select some criterion level of noise and to reject all trials which exceed that level from being averaged. Because the EP recorded in a single trial generally is much smaller than the background EEG/EMG noise, the amplitudes recorded in that trial are taken to represent the noise (even though they actually represent signal+ noise). The criterion for rejection typically is a simple amplitude setting—if the amplitude of the recorded signal exceeds the criterion at any time, the trial is rejected. If we do not want to exclude trials in which there is only a brief spell of high noise levels, we can use a criterion based on the root-mean-square amplitude of the recording. If there are brief stimulus artifacts, the criterion may be limited to regions of the recording that are unaffected by stimulus artifact. For example, when recording the click ABR, we can restrict the noise evaluation to the latency range 1 to 15 ms rather than to 0 to 15 ms, as the first millisecond may contain a large stimulus artifact (especially if we are using a bone-conduction transducer). If we applied our rejection-criterion to the first millisecond, all trials might be rejected.

If we record and store all the single trials prior to averaging, the criterion for rejecting noise-contaminated trials may be determined post hoc. In the process of "selective" or "sorted" averaging (Mühler & von Specht, 1999), we can sort the individual trials on the basis of the recorded amplitude (taken as an estimate of the background EEG/EMG noise). We then can reject the 5 or 10% with the highest levels, or we can reject those with noise levels that are determined as outliers (e.g., by exceeding the mean noise value by more than two standard deviations). An adaptive approach computes multiple different averages each missing one trial, thereby determining which trials contribute the least noise to the overall average and then averaging these (Talsma, 2008). Another technique averages only the trials that correlate best with the initial overall average (Abrams, Nicol, Zecker, & Kraus, 2008). This should be applied only after high-noise trials have been removed; otherwise, trials with artifact that spuriously correlate with the response might cause distortion.

The second approach to the problem of noisy trials does not reject trials from averaging but weights each trial on the basis of the estimated noise level prior to averaging. In this process of "weighted averaging" (Elberling & Wahlgreen, 1985; Hoke, Ross, Wickesberg, & Lütkenhöner, 1984), trials containing more noise contribute less to the final average waveform than those containing less noise. One advantage of weighted averaging is that it can easily be performed online. The computational load of selective averaging makes it difficult to perform online at rapid stimulus rates.

Figure 2–9 shows the averaging of a set of 100 responses to a 650-ms tone. The stimuli and subject are the same as in Figure 2–7. The averages shown in the upper left are based on simple averaging. Two averages (each of 50 responses) are superimposed to give some sense of the reliability of the response. As shown in the middle top graph, the background noise on some trials was higher than on others. Rejecting the 10 trials with the most background noise (arrows) as artifact-contaminated gave the responses shown in the middle lower graph. The correlation between each of the 100 responses and the average waveform is shown in the upper right. After artifact-contaminated trials have been rejected, the 10 further trials with

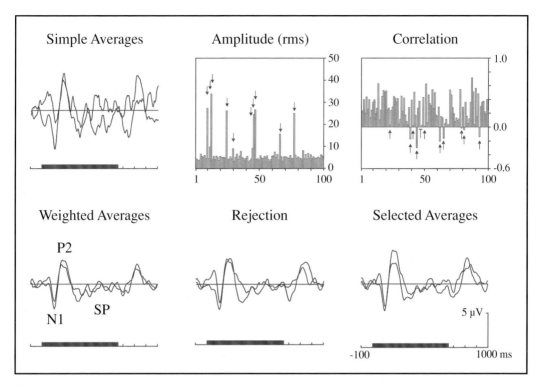

Figure 2–9. Weighted averaging, artifact rejection, and selective averaging. The upper left shows replicate averages (50 each) of responses to the same stimuli as used in Figure 2–7. The responses show the N1-P2 onset response and a small sustained potential (SP). The upper middle graph shows the root-mean-square amplitude of all 100 single responses. The weighted averages (lower left) were obtained after weighting each response by the reciprocal of the variance (the square of the root mean square value) on each trial. The rejection average (lower middle) was obtained after eliminating from the average the ten trials with the greatest amplitude (downgoing arrows). The graph in the upper right shows the correlation between each single response and the average response. The "selected averages" (lower right) show the responses obtained after eliminating ten trials (remaining after the artifact rejection) with the lowest correlation value (upgoing arrows). The blunt arrow indicates a trial with low correlation that was already rejected.

the lowest level of correlation were also rejected, to obtain the selective averages in the lower right.

SCALP TOPOGRAPHY

Auditory EPs can be recorded from many different locations on the scalp. Many early potentials are generated in a single region of the brain and are maximally recorded using a single channel, measuring the difference between two locations on the scalp. However, as the latency increases, many different regions of the brain become simultaneously active and this can lead to a complicated distribution of potentials over the scalp. Multichannel recordings then can help to distinguish different responses coming from different regions of the brain.

Figure 2–10 shows the scalp topography of the LAEP in response to a tone.

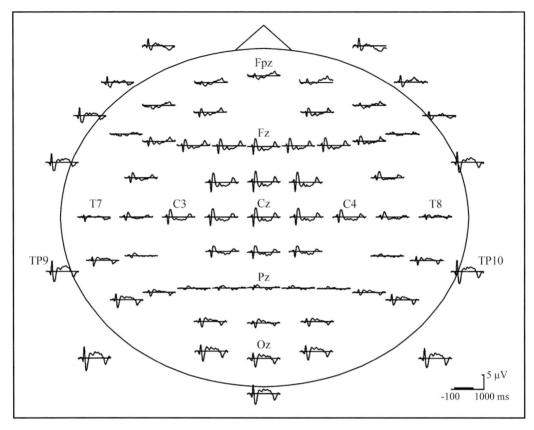

Figure 2–10. *Scalp topography of the LAEP. The EPs were obtained by averaging 100 artifact-free responses to the stimulus described in Figure 2–7. All recordings are relative to an average reference. The scalp is viewed from the top with the nose anterior. The waveforms are located on the graph using an azimuthal equidistant projection (the distances along the meridians are to scale, although the vertical scale is less than the horizontal scale).*

Responses were recorded from 65 different scalp areas. Waveforms at selected scalp locations are shown in larger size in Figure 2–11.

The setup of the electrodes in a multi-channel recording is called the montage. When only a few channels of data are recorded, we can choose whichever electrode-pairs we find most helpful. For example, the ABR typically is recorded using two channels: vertex to ipsilateral mastoid and vertex to contralateral mastoid. When recording from many different scalp loca-tions, we customarily refer the recordings to a single reference. Otherwise, it is too difficult to keep the nature of the different channels in mind.

Many different references have been used to record the scalp topography of the auditory EPs. Early multichannel record-ings used the mastoids, the nose or a "noncephalic" reference. The last consisted of two electrodes on the front and back of the chest, with their contributions to the reference balanced through a potenti-ometer to decrease the amount of electro-

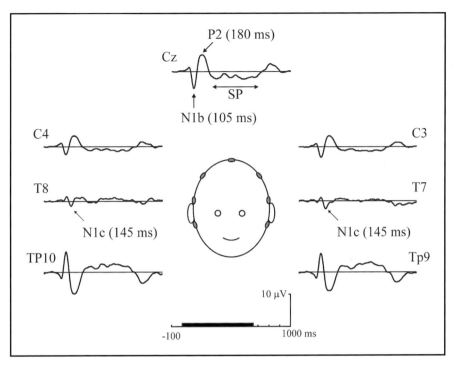

Figure 2–11. *EP waveforms at different scalp locations. Waveforms from Figure 2–10 are plotted for electrodes located along the meridian passing through the midcoronal plane of the head. The main responses are inverted in polarity between the vertex (Cz) and the left and right mastoids (TP9 and TP10). In the midtemporal electrodes (T7 and T8), there is a small N1c component with a latency between the latencies of N1 and P2.*

cardiographic (ECG) artifact (Wolpaw & Wood, 1982). When a large number of electrodes is used, and when they cover the scalp in a relatively even-spaced way, an average reference is the least biased of all electrodes (Bertrand, Perrin, & Pernier, 1985; Dien, 1998). In an N-channel referential recording, the average reference is calculated by averaging together all the simultaneous recordings and dividing by N+1. This is then subtracted away from each of the recorded channels and from the reference (deemed to be zero) to give an N+1 channel recording. If the original reference is complicated, for example, a linked-mastoid electrode wherein one does

not know how much is recorded from each mastoid, one can divide by N (rather than N+1) and not compute the activity at the reference. The main consequence of an average-reference recording is that the sum of all the voltages across all of the electrodes is zero at any point in time. Indeed, the logical justification for the reference is that the charge distributed over the surface of a spherical volume-conductor must sum to zero (Bertrand et al., 1985). This justification thus requires electrodes over all regions of the spherical surface. When we make multichannel scalp recordings, some electrodes must be located over the lower portion of the scalp—below the equator running through Fpz, T8, Oz, and T9—or our interpretation of the fields may become distorted.

As well as displaying the EPs from different channels on an outline of the scalp (as in Figures 2–10 and 2–11), all of the data may be superimposed. If the channels are average-referenced, this type of plot will show simultaneous positive and negative deflections at peaks in the waveform. This gives a "butterfly" plot, with antennae at the onsets and wings during the sustained potentials (SPs). Such a plot is given in the upper part of Figure 2–12. Calculating the variance across all the scalp electrodes at each point in time gives a plot of how the "global field power" changes over time (Lehmann, 1987). A similar measure is the root-mean-

square amplitude of all recordings at each point in time. This is shown in the lower part of Figure 2–12. Peaks in this waveform may be a better way to identify peak activity in a response than relying only on the waveform at one scalp location.

Multichannel recordings provide a measurement that has both temporal and spatial dimensions. The spatial dimension of the measurement can be shown with topographic maps. At any one point in time, the potential at multiple points in space can be plotted as a contour plot. Measurements at locations intervening between the recording locations can be estimated using different interpolation algorithms. Contours are then drawn to link points of the same voltage. The most appropriate mapping algorithm for scalp-

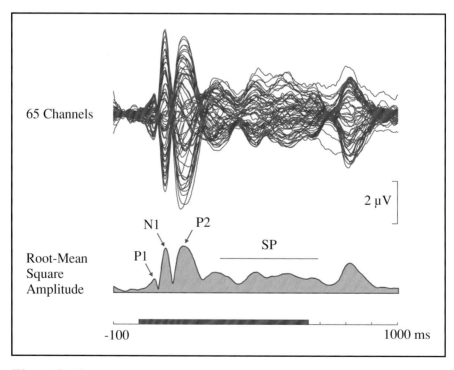

Figure 2–12. **Butterfly and root-mean-square plots.** *Same data as in Figure 2–10 except all 65 channels of data are superimposed in the upper plot. The root-mean-square amplitude at each time point is plotted below.*

recorded EPs uses spherical splines (Perrin, Pernier, Bertrand, & Echallier, 1989). These algorithms also allow the calculation of the second derivative of the topography, which estimates the current source density at each point of the scalp. Current source density maps tend to show the polarity inversion that occurs with dipole generators more precisely. The principles allowing us to analyze topographic maps in terms of the intracerebral generators are considered in Chapter 4. Figure 2–13 illustrates contour plots for both the potential and the current source density for two separate time points (the N1 and P2 peaks) for the EPs plotted in Figures 2–10 and 2–11. Typically, topographies are displayed using color scales (e.g., going from red as positive through green at zero to blue as negative). Gray scale topographies are not as easy to visualize. This chapter uses light gray to represent near-zero values and darker gray to show maxima and minima, with signs to identify which is which.

COMPONENT ANALYSIS

Peak Measurements

In order to measure the EPs that we have recorded, we must decide how to recognize the different components. The simplest way is to identify different peaks and troughs in the waveform. Generally, one takes the maximum (or minimum) measurement within a predefined latency range. Sometimes the latency can be defined on the basis of a preceding component. Thus, N1 may be defined as the maximum negative peak within the latency range 50 to 150 ms and P2 the maximum positive peak between N1 and 250 ms.

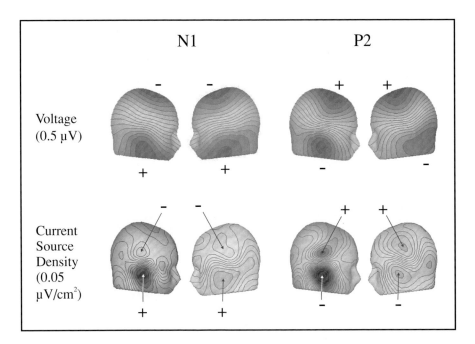

Figure 2–13. *Voltage and current source density maps. This are for the N1 and P2 peaks of the data shown in Figure 2–10.*

Peak-picking sometimes causes headaches. When there are several peaks in a latency range, even when they are not equal we may be loath to pick one over the others. One approach to this problem is to low-pass filter until there is only one peak, and then to measure this filtered peak. Sometimes, the waveform of a peak is temporally asymmetric with a fast rise and slow fall. In this case, we might decide to choose the latency at the half-area measurement (Luck, 2005). Sometimes, the peak rides on a slower wave and cannot be picked as the maximum or minimum within the defined latency region. At other times, it may show up as a deflection rather than as a definite peak. In both cases, we can pick the deflection visually, or we can high-pass filter the waveform (or take its second derivative) to remove the slower wave. Figure 2–14 illustrates some of the approaches to measuring peaks.

Peaks in an EP waveform may or may not be associated with specific intracerebral processes. Multiple locations in the brain may generate potential fields that are recorded at the scalp. Because these different fields add to each other at each point on the scalp and at each point in time, a peak at a particular electrode may not necessarily represent a peak in a particular generator process.

Difference Waveforms

One way to check how a waveform might represent two different underlying pro-

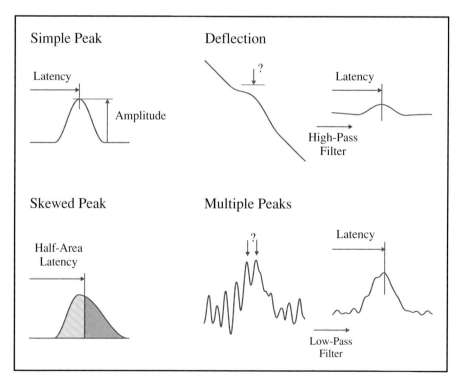

Figure 2–14. Measurement of peaks. This figure shows some simple techniques to measure the latency of peaks (or troughs) in an EP waveform. For the skewed peak, the latency is chosen to equalize the areas under the curve before and after the chosen latency.

cesses is to calculate difference waveforms. EPs are recorded in two different conditions. In the first, the response is hypothesized to contain two waveforms and in the second only one. Subtracting the second from the first will give a difference waveform that represents the activity that is present in the first but not in the second. A simple example is to subtract the response to a standard stimulus from the response to a deviant to get the mismatch negativity (MMN). This is illustrated in Figure 1–12 in Chapter 1. Two aspects of difference waveforms need to be kept in mind. First, they only represent a true additive factor in the recording if the activity or activities shared in common between the two original waveforms can be assumed to be the same in the two recording conditions. Second, the difference waveform will be noisier than the original waveforms as the subtraction process effectively adds the noise in the two recordings. We cover these issues in Chapter 5 where signals and noise are discussed at greater length.

Mathematical Component Analyses

Difference waveforms are useful only when the number of components in a waveform is small. When multiple components contribute to our recordings, more complicated procedures are necessary to decompose the recorded waveforms into components. Some idea of the basic waveforms that are adding together to make the scalp waveforms can be obtained by a principal components analysis (PCA), a method for linearly decomposing a multivariate data matrix into a set of components, each of which explains a portion of the variance in the data. When applied to a set of EP waveforms, the analysis most commonly is set up as a temporal PCA to give components that have the same structure as the EP in terms of being a waveform that changes over a particular period of time (Dien, Beal, & Berg, 2005; Donchin & Heffley, 1978; Möcks & Verleger, 1991). Each component is then associated with an array of "coefficients," each of which specifies the estimated contribution of that particular component to each of the waveforms in the original matrix. The EPs that are entered into the PCA may be from different locations on the scalp and/or from different experimental conditions. The simplest analysis would be using just one set of recordings from multiple electrode locations. This is illustrated in Figure 2–15.

The nature of the PCA components can be interpreted by seeing how they are reflected at the different electrode locations. By point-by-point multiplying the component waveform by the actual waveform recorded at each scalp location, we can calculate electrode "scores"—how well the component is seen at that electrode. From these scores, we can determine a topography for the component (right side of Figure 2–15). In the example used for the figure, the first component reverses polarity over the Sylvian fissure, being positive at the vertex and negative at the mastoids. The polarity of a component is arbitrary. Everything would be the same if the component waveform were inverted and the topography negative at the vertex and positive at the mastoid. As explained in Chapter 4, this type of topography means that activity in the auditory cortex on the superior surface of the temporal lobe probably is the main generator. The second component shows a topography that is negative above the eyes and positive below. This likely represents artifact

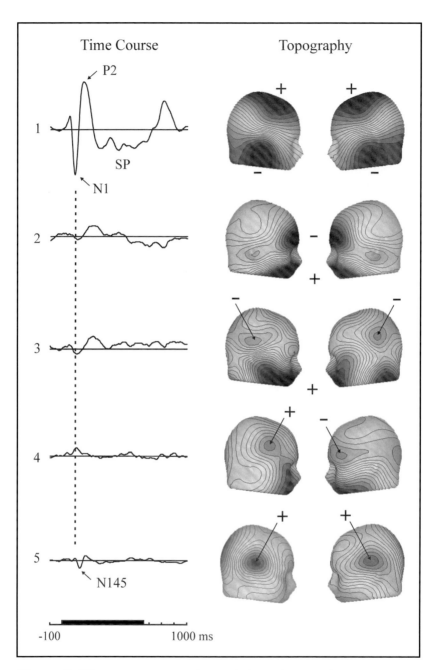

Figure 2–15. *Component analysis of the scalp waveforms of the late auditory EP. The data from Figure 2–10 were submitted to a principal component analysis. The first five components shown on the left accounted for 85.7, 7.5, 3.3, 1.3, and 1.0% of the total variance. The vertical dotted line is at the latency of the N1 wave. The first component contains most of the waves seen at the vertex. The fifth component contains the N145 wave seen in the mid-temporal electrodes. The maps derived from the electrode scores for each component are shown on the right.*

from eyeblinks or vertical eye movements. These artifacts are considered a little more closely later in this chapter. The third component is positive anteriorly and negative posteriorly. This is likely the result of activity in the walls of the sulci on the top of the temporal lobe. The fourth component has a topography that is negative over the left anterior regions and positive on the right. This is likely a result of lateral eye-movements (see next section). The fifth component is maximally picked up over the midtemporal area. It reflects the N145 component of the waveforms recorded at T8 and T9. Although it explains only a small amount (1%) of the overall variance in the data, this remains a clearly defined component. The small percentage is mainly because the component is only active over a brief period of time.

If we enter EPs into the PCA using both electrode locations and experimental conditions as sources of variance, the resultant components may reflect variance caused by either or both these parameters. Sometimes the components may not make sense. This is particularly true when a component changes both in its scalp topography and in its relationship to the experimental variables. The technique of "Partial Least Squares" limits the components to explaining only part of the variance in the data (Lobaugh, West, & McIntosh, 2001). This analysis can be set up to determine components that are specifically affected by the different experimental conditions. Each component then has a design "salience," which indicates how much a component is present in a particular experimental condition, and an electrode salience, which indicates how prominently the component is seen at each electrode.

The data matrix of recorded EPs is composed of multiple time points at multiple locations. A spatial PCA can be set up so that the basic structure of the derived components is the topography—values at the different electrodes—rather than the time waveform that is the basis of the temporal PCA. Both spatial and temporal PCAs can be performed on the same dataset. One approach might be to perform a spatial PCA to derive a set of topographies that can act like virtual electrodes in order to analyze the different temporal components in the original data set (Spencer, Dien, & Donchin, 2001).

Independent component analysis performs a linear decomposition of a data set but distinguishes components in terms of their statistical independence rather than their contribution to the variance (Makeig, Jung, Bell, Ghahremani, & Sejnowski, 1997; Van Dun, Wouters, & Moonen, 2007). Components are independent if knowledge about one does not provide any information about the other. Independence involves the evaluation of higher order statistical properties in addition to the variance used in the calculation of principal components.

ARTIFACTS

Many different phenomena can be recorded from electrodes placed on the scalp when auditory stimuli are presented. Many of these potentials are not generated in the auditory nervous system. If our intent is to record the auditory EPs coming from the cochlea or brain, these potentials are considered artifacts (Barlow, 1986). Artifacts can be classified initially on the basis of whether they originate in the subject (physiologic) or in the environment (physical), and secondarily on the basis of whether they are stimulus-related or stimulus-independent. Table 2–2 provides the essential features of many of these artifacts.

Table 2–2. Artifacts During the Recording of Human Auditory Evoked Potentials

	Source	Mechanism and Frequency Content	Control
Physical	Power cables and transformers	Electromagnetic fields at the frequency of the power source, and its harmonics	Shielding, braided electrode wires, active electrodes, decreasing interelectrode impedance
	Stimulus Transducers	Electromagnetic field at frequency of the stimulus	Alternating polarity of stimulus, shielded transducers, distancing transducer from ear
	Electrodes	Electrode pop due to changing electrode-impedance; all the frequencies in amplifier band-pass	Decreasing interelectrode impedance
	MRI imaging	Multiple frequencies generated by the imaging protocol	Averaging on the artifact and subtracting
	Movement	Movement of electrodes through static magnetic fields: 0–100 Hz	Artifact rejection (remove any trials contaminated by large potentials from the analysis).
Physiologic	Eye Movements	Rotation the eyeball: 0–50 Hz	Voluntary fixation, ocular source components, topographic regression
	Eye Blinks	Eyelid moving over the cornea: 1–5 Hz	Ocular source components, artifact rejection ocular source components
	Muscle	Spontaneous muscle activity is mainly in range 10–500 Hz	Relaxation , sleep, filtering provided that the EP is slow or late
	Muscle Reflexes	Scalp microreflexes: mainly 20–50 Hz	Relaxation, sleep
	Tongue	Movement of tongue in oral cavity: 0.1–20 Hz	Ask subject not to move tongue, artifact rejection
	Skin	Activation of skin and sweat glands: 0.1–2 Hz	Cooling, abrasion or puncturing of skin.
	Electrocardio-gram (ECG)	Depolarization of cardiac muscle: 1–50 Hz	Averaging on the ECG and subtracting
	Blood Vessel	Potentials related to blood flow or in fMRI to small movements in a magnetic field: 0.1–20 Hz	Averaging on the ECG and subtracting

Artifacts can be handled in several ways. Like diseases, artifacts can be prevented, survived, treated, or quarantined. For example, muscle artifacts can be prevented by relaxing the subject, survived by averaging more trials, treated by compensating for their effects in the recording, or quarantined by rejecting trials with high levels of muscle activity from the averaging process.

Artifacts that are not specifically related to the stimulus can be removed by averaging. However, if they are large and/or frequent, the amount of extra averaging needed to attenuate them sufficiently could take too long. If this is true, one approach is to decrease the artifacts before they are recorded. Decreasing physical artifacts might be done by using a shielded room or specifically shielding power cables and equipment. Muscle artifacts can be decreased by relaxing the subject. If the EP of interest is unaffected by sleep, recordings should be obtained when the subject is asleep and muscle activity is minimized. Eyeblinks and eye movements can be reduced by having the subject stare at a fixation point and try not to blink during the recording. Skin potentials can be decreased by cooling the room, trying to decrease the subject's anxiety about the test, and finally by puncturing the skin with a sterile needle to short-circuit the generation of the potentials (Picton & Hillyard, 1972).

Sometimes the artifact can be accurately estimated and then subtracted out of the EEG recording. The ECG artifact recorded together with the EEG at a particular location on the scalp is similar on each cardiac cycle. Beat-to-beat differences related to small shifts in the heart position during respiration are small. We therefore can obtain an average ECG waveform at any scalp location by triggering on a concomitantly registered ECG (e.g., one recorded between the shoulders). Averaging the EEG signals using this trigger attenuates the EEG but leaves a good representation of the ECG at each scalp location. This averaged scalp ECG artifact then can be subtracted from the recorded EEG on each heartbeat.

When recording the EEG or EPs during magnetic resonance imaging (MRI), large "pulse artifacts" occur because of the tiny movements of the scalp electrodes within the large magnetic field of the MRI. These also can be estimated and removed by calculating an ECG-triggered average and subtracting this from the recording after each heartbeat (Allen, Polizzi, Krakow, Fish, & Lemieux, 1998); the averaged waveform will contain both the ECG artifact and the pulse artifact. During functional MRI studies, the EEG is also obscured by a huge imaging artifact. Provided the EEG amplifiers have a sufficiently large input range so that they can accurately record both the artifact and the EEG, even this artifact can be removed by averaging on the imaging signal and then subtracting the averaged imaging artifact from the recording (Allen, Josephs, & Turner, 2000). Independent component analysis also can be used to remove artifacts during functional MRI (Debener et al., 2007; Mantini et al., 2007).

A particular trick that might be useful with line noise (or any periodic noise of known frequency) is to ensure that the stimulus occurs alternately on exactly opposite points in the line- noise cycle. For example, if the line noise is 60 Hz, each cycle lasts 16.67 ms. If the interval between stimuli is set to be any odd-numbered multiple of a half-cycle (8.33 ms), then the line noise will reverse in polarity on alternate trials and thus continually cancel itself out in the ongoing average. This logic gives stimulus onset asynchronies of 8.33, 25, 41.67, 58.33 ms, and so on, equivalent to stimulus rates of 120, 40, 24, 17.1 Hz, and so on. We also could actually trigger on a particular phase of the line noise (or on that particular phase of the line noise following a desired stimulus onset asynchrony) and alternately add a delay of 8.33 ms or not (Sgro & Emerson, 1985).

Stimulus artifact associated with the sound is a particular problem when recording auditory EPs. If the artifact is over before the response occurs, it can just be ignored. Moving the electroacoustic transducer away from recording electrodes by using a tube to conduct the sound to an ear insert has two effects. First, the artifact is decreased in size. Second, the artifact is moved in time, occurring earlier than the time when the sound reaches the ear. When the stimulus artifact occurs during the response, we need an approach that removes the artifact without affecting the response. When recording the LAEPs evoked by tones, a low-pass filter with a cutoff below the frequency of the tone will remove the artifact it causes. Reversing the polarity of the stimulus on alternate trials will cancel out the stimulus artifact, and leave the EP unchanged if its morphology is the same for either polarity of stimulus. When cochlear implants are used, the stimulus artifact is very troublesome as electrical current time-locked to the stimulus is being injected directly into the cochlea. Specialized techniques used to separate electrical stimulus artifact from the responses recorded from the cochlea or brain are reviewed in Chapters 7 and 16.

Artifacts that are time-locked to the stimuli cannot be removed by averaging. Trials occasionally contaminated by time-locked artifacts can be rejected. This runs the risk that the remaining trials might be too few for a reliable average recording.

Another approach is to estimate the contribution of the artifact to the recording and to subtract this estimate from the recorded activity. For example, the electro-oculogram can be monitored by electrodes placed around the eye, and the amplitude of the artifact at scalp electrodes can be estimated by calculating a regression between the scalp-recording and the monitored activity. Unfortunately, because the monitoring electrodes also pick up brain activity, this approach will also subtract out some portion of the brain activity, particularly in the scalp electrodes near the eyes.

Ocular Artifacts

Artifacts deriving from the eyes are especially problematic when recording the LAEPs. Such artifacts tend to be evoked by the stimuli. The subject may blink in response to loud sounds or may look toward the source of a sound. Even when not specifically evoked by the sound, such ocular artifacts can be so large that they are difficult to average away. The potential associated with a blink recorded in the midfrontal electrodes has an amplitude of about 200 µV. Even if only one blink occurred during the recording of 100 trials, this would still persist in the average with an amplitude of 2 µV and distort the recorded EP. Typically, multiple blinks occur and it becomes impossible to determine what is blink and what is brain.

Ocular artifacts are of two main kinds (Lins, Picton, Berg, & Scherg, 1993a). The first is related to the rotation of the eye (around a horizontal or vertical axis) as it looks in different directions. The eye is electrically polarized with the cornea positive relative to the back of the retina. When the eye rotates, the scalp near where it moves becomes positive and the opposite region of the scalp becomes negative. Thus, an upward movement causes the forehead to become positive and the cheek to become negative. The second type of ocular artifact is caused by movement of the eyelid relative to the eye. When the eyelid moves over the positive cornea, the region of the scalp above the eyelid becomes positive. This is like connecting the forehead to the positive pole of a battery. An old idea that the blink artifact was caused by the upward rotation of the eyeball is not correct—the blink artifact occurs even when the eyeball does not rotate (Matsuo, Peters, & Reilly, 1975). As seen in Figure 2–16, the scalp topography of the eyeblink thus differs from that of the upward saccade and these two phe-

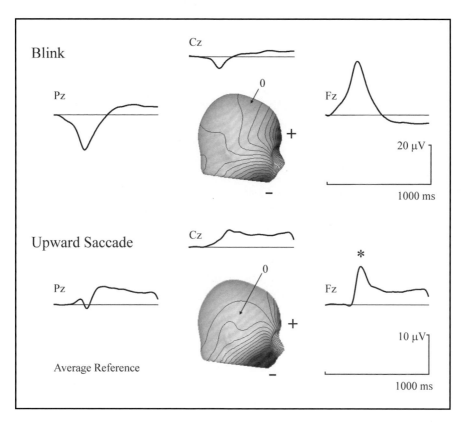

Figure 2–16. Ocular artifacts. This figure shows the scalp topographies for a blink and an upward saccade, together with waveforms from three midline electrode locations (referred to an average reference). Both topographies show a positive maximum above the eyes and a negative minimum below. However, the potential associated with the saccade extends further back on the scalp than that associated with a blink. The zero area (indicated by 0) is in the midtemporal region for the saccade but loops up just in front of the vertex for the blink. The vertex recording of a blink is thus negative when recorded using an average reference. The vertex recording of an upward saccade is positive. At the very beginning of an upward saccade, the eye moves briefly under the eyelid before the eyelid is also raised. This causes a small blink-like artifact called the rider-artifact (asterisk).

nomena must be distinguished in any protocol for artifact compensation. As the eye moves upward, there might be a slight lag in the upward movement of the lid. This can cause the eye to slide briefly under the lid and result in a "rider artifact" at the beginning of an upward saccade (Lins et al., 1993a)

The various techniques of component analysis that we discussed in the previous section of this chapter also can be used to subtract out ocular artifacts. Basically, the artifact is identified as a component with a different topography from the brain activity, and then eliminated. Two main approaches are available. A spatial PCA can give the particular topography or topographies that are associated with an artifact. The recorded EEG then can be decomposed into the artifact components and concomitant components that model the activity coming from intracerebral sources (Berg & Scherg, 1994; Ille, Berg, & Scherg, 2002; Lins, Picton, Berg, & Scherg, 1993a; Picton et al., 2000). Independent component analysis can be used to distinguish artifactual components related to blinks and saccades on the basis of both topography and morphology (Hoffman & Falkenstein, 2008; Jung et al., 2000).

Muscle Artifact

Muscle activity can be part of the ongoing background noise or it can be evoked by the auditory stimulus. Ongoing muscle activity can be removed by relaxing the subject or by filtering. Filtering is helpful only for the LAEPs. The spectra of the ABR and MLR are not that different from the spectra of muscle activity and it is difficult to set up filters that will remove the muscle without significantly distorting

the EPs. Muscle reflexes occur in the muscles of the head such as the postauricular muscle and temporalis muscle. These occur at the same time as the MLRs and need to be identified so as not to be mistaken for brain responses. As discussed in Chapter 1, early studies of the auditory EP caused controversy about the relative role of muscle and brain in these recordings. The many different muscle reflexes are considered in Chapter 9.

CONCLUDING COMMENTS

The auditory EP viewed in the time-domain is a series of peaks and troughs that follow the onset of an auditory stimulus and a sustained baseline shift during the continuation of a stimulus. The EP waveform typically is much smaller than the other activity that can be recorded from the scalp. As well as hearing the sound, the brain must take care of all its other tasks—staying awake, sitting still, thinking about what happened yesterday, and predicting what might occur tomorrow. Each of these tasks generates electrical activity. However, when the stimulus is repeated, only the hearing will be the same; the brain will have moved on to other thoughts and tasks and the electrical activity associated with them will be different than before. Whereas the EP is time-locked, the other activity is random relative to the stimulus. Therefore, the process of averaging can be used to cancel out the other activity, and leave the average EP waveform. The response is not perfect—there is always some residual background activity. It is not everything we might hope for, but it is much more than nothing, like Pascal's man in the middle.

ABBREVIATIONS

ABR	Auditory brainstem response
AD	Analog-to-digital
ASSR	Auditory steady-state response
EAM	External auditory meatus
ECG	Electrocardiogram
ECochG	Electrocochleography
EEG	Electroencephalogram
EMG	Electromyography
EP	Evoked potential
FFT	Fast Fourier Transform
LAEP	Late auditory evoked potential
MLR	Middle-latency response
MMN	Mismatch negativity
MRI	Magnetic resonance imaging
PCA	Principal component analysis
SNR	Signal-to-noise ratio
SN10	Slow negative wave at 10 ms
SP	Sustained potential
TT	Transtympanic

REFERENCES

Abrams, D. A, Nicol, T., Zecker, S., & Kraus, N. (2008). Right-hemisphere auditory cortex is dominant for coding syllable patterns in speech. *Journal of Neuroscience, 28*, 3958–3965.

Allen, P. J., Josephs, O., & Turner, R. (2000). A method for removing imaging artifact from continuous EEG recorded during functional MRI. *NeuroImage, 12*, 230–239.

Allen, P. J., Polizzi, G., Krakow, K., Fish, D. R., & Lemieux, L. (1998) Identification of EEG events in the MR scanner: The problem of pulse artifact and a method for its subtraction. *NeuroImage, 8*, 229–239.

American Clinical Neurophysiology Society. (2006). Guidelines for standard electrode position nomenclature. *Journal of Clinical Neurophysiology, 23*, 107–110.

Barlow, J. S. (1986). Artifact processing (rejection and minimization) in EEG data processing. In F. H. Lopes da Silva, W. Storm van Leeuwen, A. Rémond (Eds.), *Handbook of electroencephalography and clinical neurophysiology, Revised Series, Volume 2: Clinical applications of computer analysis of EEG and other neurophysiological signals* (pp. 1–62). New York, NY: Elsevier.

Berg, P., & Scherg, M. (1994). A multiple source approach to the correction of eye artifacts. *Electroencephalography and Clinical Neurophysiology, 90*, 229–241.

Bertrand, O., Perrin, F., & Pernier, J. (1985). A theoretical justification of the average reference in topographic evoked potential studies. *Electroencephalography and Clinical Neurophysiology, 62*, 462–464.

Boston, J. R. (1981). Spectra of auditory brainstem responses and spontaneous EEG. *IEEE Transactions in Biomedical Engineering, 28*, 334–341.

Cooley, J. W., & Tukey, J. W. (1965). An algorithm for the machine calculation of complex Fourier series. *Mathematics of Computation, 19*, 297–301.

Davis, H., Hirsh, S. K., Turpin, L. L., & Peacock, M. E. (1985). Threshold sensitivity and frequency specificity in auditory brainstem response audiometry. *Audiology, 24*, 54–70.

Dawson, G. D. (1954). A summation technique for the detection of small evoked potentials. *Electroencephalography and Clinical Neurophysiology, 6*, 65–84.

Debener, S., Strobel, A., Sorger, B., Peters, J., Kranczioch, C., Engel, A. K., & Goebel, R.

(2007). Improved quality of auditory event-related potentials recorded simultaneously with 3-T fMRI: removal of the ballistocardiogram artefact. *NeuroImage, 34,* 587–597.

de Weerd, J. P. (1981). A posteriori time-varying filtering of averaged evoked potentials. I. Introduction and conceptual basis. *Biological Cybernetics, 41,* 211–222.

Dien, J. (1998). Issues in the application of the average reference: Review, critiques, and recommendations. *Behavioral Research Methods, Instruments, and Computers, 30,* 34–43.

Dien, J., Beal, D. J., & Berg, P. (2005). Optimizing principal components analysis of event-related potentials: Matrix type, factor loading weighting, extraction, and rotations. *Clinical Neurophysiology, 116,* 1808–1825.

Donchin, E., & Heffley, E. F. (1978). Multivariate analysis of event-related potential data: a tutorial review. In D. A. Otto (Ed.), *Multidisciplinary perspectives in event-related brain potential research. U.S. Environmental Protection Agency EPS 600/9-77-043* (pp. 555–572). Washington, DC: Government Printing Office.

Doyle, D. J. (1977). A proposed methodology for evaluation of the Wiener filtering method of evoked potential estimation. *Electroencephalography and Clinical Neurophysiology, 43,* 749–751.

Elberling, C., & Wahlgreen, O. (1985). Estimation of auditory brainstem response, ABR, by means of Bayesian inference. *Scandinavian Journal of Audiology, 14,* 89–96.

Fourier, J.-B. J. (1822/translated by Freeman, A., 1878, reprinted 2009). *The analytical theory of heat.* Cambridge, UK: Cambridge University Press.

Glaser. E., & Ruchkin, D. (1976). *Principles of neurobiological signal analysis.* New York, NY: Academic Press.

Hoffmann, S., & Falkenstein, M. (2008) The correction of eye blink artefacts in the EEG: A comparison of two prominent methods. *PLoS One, 3*(8), e3004.

Hoke, M., Ross, B., Wickesberg, R., & Lütkenhöner, B. (1984). Weighted averaging—theory and application to electric response audiometry. *Electroencephalography and Clinical Neurophysiology, 57,* 484–489.

Ille, N., Berg, P., & Scherg, M. (2002). Artifact correction of the ongoing EEG using spatial filters based on artifact and brain signal topographies. *Journal of Clinical Neurophysiology, 19,* 113–124.

Jung, T. P., Makeig, S., Humphries, C., Lee, T. W., McKeown, M. J., Iragui, V., & Sejnowski, T. J. (2000). Removing electroencephalographic artifacts by blind source separation. *Psychophysiology, 37,* 163–178.

Lehmann, D. (1987). Principles of spatial analysis. In A. S. Gevins & A. Rémond (Eds.), *Handbook of electroencephalography and clinical neurophysiology (Revised series). Volume 1. Methods of analysis of brain electrical and magnetic signals* (pp. 309–354). Amsterdam, The Netherlands: Elsevier.

Lins, O. G., Picton, T. W., Berg, P., & Scherg, M. (1993a). Ocular artifacts in EEG and event-related potentials. I. Scalp topography. *Brain Topography, 6,* 51–63.

Lins, O. G., Picton, T. W., Berg, P., & Scherg, M. (1993b). Ocular artifacts in recording EEGs and event-related potentials. II. Source dipoles and source components. *Brain Topography, 6,* 65–78.

Lobaugh, N. J., West, R., & McIntosh, A. R. (2001). Spatiotemporal analysis of experimental differences in event-related potential data with partial least squares. *Psychophysiology, 38,* 517–530.

Luck, S. J. (2005). *An introduction to the event-related potential technique.* Cambridge, MA: MIT Press.

Makeig, S., Jung, T. P., Bell, A. J., Ghahremani, D., & Sejnowski, T. J. (1997). Blind separation of auditory event-related brain responses into independent components. *Proceedings of the National Academy of Sciences (USA), 94,* 10979–10984.

Mantini, D., Perrucci, M. G., Cugini, S., Ferretti, A., Romani, G. L., & Del Gratta, C. (2007). Complete artifact removal for EEG recorded during continuous fMRI using independent component analysis. *NeuroImage, 34,* 598–607.

Matsuo, F., Peters, J. F., & Reilly, E. L. (1975). Electrical phenomena associated with movements of the eyelid. *Electroencephalography and Clinical Neurophysiology, 38,* 507–511.

Möcks, J., & Verleger, R. (1991). Multivariate methods in biosignal analysis: Application of principal component analysis to event-related potentials. In R. Weitkunat (Ed.), *Digital biosignal processing* (pp. 399–458). Amsterdam, The Netherlands: Elsevier.

Mühler, R., & von Specht, H. (1999). Sorted averaging—principle and application to auditory brainstem responses. *Scandinavian Audiology, 28,* 145–149.

Perrin, F., Pernier, J., Bertrand, O., & Echallier, J. F. (1989). Spherical splines for scalp potential and current density mapping. *Electroencephalography and Clinical Neurophysiology, 72,* 184–187.

Picton, T. W., & Hillyard, S. A. (1972). Cephalic skin potentials in electroencephalography. *Electroencephalography and Clinical Neurophysiology, 33,* 419–424.

Picton, T. W., Hillyard, S. A., Krausz, H. I., & Galambos, R. (1974). Human auditory evoked potentials. I Evaluation of components. *Electroencephalography and Clinical Neurophysiology, 36,* 179–190.

Picton, T. W., & Hink, R. F. (1974). Evoked potentials: How? what? and why? *American Journal of EEG Technology, 14,* 9–44.

Picton, T. W., Lins, O., & Scherg, M. (1995). The recording and analysis of event-related potentials. In F. Boller & J. Grafman (Eds.). *Handbook of neuropsychology. Volume 10. Section 14. Event-related brain potentials and cognition* (pp. 3–73). Amsterdam, The Netherlands: Elsevier.

Picton, T. W., van Roon, P., Armilio, M. L., Berg, P., Ille, N., & Scherg, M. (2000). The correction of ocular artifacts: a topographic perspective. *Clinical Neurophysiology, 111,* 53–65.

Ruchkin, D. S. (1988). Measurement of event-related potentials: signal extraction. In T. W.

Picton (Ed.), *Handbook of electroencephalography and clinical neurophysiology (Revised series). Volume 3. Human event-related potentials* (pp. 7–43). Amsterdam, The Netherlands: Elsevier.

Sgro, J. A., & Emerson, R. G. (1985). Phase synchronized triggering: a method for coherent noise elimination in evoked potential recording. *Electroencephalography and Clinical Neurophysiology, 60,* 464–468.

Sokolov, Y. (2007). ABR testing in children made easy. *Hearing Review, 2007 International Edition.* Available from: http://www.hearingreview.com/issues/articles/2007-IN_05.asp

Spencer, K. M., Dien, J., & Donchin, E. (2001). Spatiotemporal analysis of the late ERP responses to deviant stimuli. *Psychophysiology, 38,* 343–358.

Stapells, D. R., & Picton, T. W. (1981). Technical aspects of brainstem evoked potential audiometry using tones. *Ear and Hearing, 2,* 20–29.

Taheri, B. A., Knight, R. T, & Smith, R. L. (1994). A dry electrode for EEG recording. *Electroencephalography and Clinical Neurophysiology, 90,* 376–383.

Talsma, D. (2008). Auto-adaptive averaging: Detecting artifacts in event-related potential data using a fully automated procedure. *Psychophysiology, 45,* 216–228.

Van Dun, B., Wouters, J., & Moonen, M. (2007). Improving auditory steady-state response detection using independent component analysis on multichannel EEG data. *IEEE Transaction in Biomedical Engineering, 54,* 1220–1230.

Wolpaw, J. R., & Wood, C. C. (1982). Scalp distribution of human auditory evoked potentials. I. Evaluation of reference electrode sites. *Electroencephalography and Clinical Neurophysiology, 54,* 15–24.

Woody, C. D. (1967). Characterization of an adaptive filter for the analysis of variable latency neuroelectric signals. *Medical and Biological Engineering, 5,* 539–553.

3 Frequency Domain: Music of the Hemispheres

> Swiftly the head-mass becomes an enchanted loom where millions of flashing shuttles weave a dissolving pattern, always a meaningful pattern though never an abiding one; a shifting harmony of sub-patterns.
>
> Charles Sherrington, *Man on His Nature*, 1940

The human brain generates many different rhythms. Some occur spontaneously and some are evoked by external stimuli. These various brain rhythms overlap and interact to form the human electroencephalogram (EEG). Sherrington likened the human brain to an enchanted loom where the rhythms of the nervous impulses create a "shifting harmony of sub-patterns." These EEG rhythms are most efficiently evaluated in the frequency domain. This chapter evaluates techniques that look at the auditory evoked potentials (EPs) from the point of view of their frequency rather than their timing.

TIME AND FREQUENCY DOMAINS

In the preceding chapter, we considered how any signal recorded in the time domain can also be considered in the frequency domain. In the time domain, the signal is represented as a waveform that changes in amplitude over time; in the frequency domain, the signal is represented as a spectrum of amplitudes and phases that change with frequency. A signal that changes more or less rapidly in time shows up as higher or lower frequencies in the spectrum (see Figure 2–1 in Chapter 2).

When we convert a time waveform to a frequency spectrum using the discrete Fourier transform, we obtain a series of complex numbers—half as many as there are time-points in the original waveform. Each complex number has both a real and an imaginary value. A complex number represents a vector with both magnitude and direction. Vectors can be represented as a point on a two-dimensional graph:

the real value is plotted relative to the x-axis and the imaginary value relative to the y-axis. The magnitude of the vector is the length of the line from the point to the origin, and the phase of the vector is the angle that that line makes with the x-axis (customarily measured in a counterclockwise direction). Such a graph is often called a polar plot because it is similar to a map that views the earth from the North or South Pole, where the lines of longitude intersect. Real and imaginary values can be converted into amplitude and phase using the formulae in the lower right of Figure 3–1. Phase is related to latency but the relationship is not simple.

The lower left of Figure 3–1 illustrates the spectra that can be derived from the Fourier Transform. The time-frequency transformation can be performed on continuous values or on discrete values that have been digitized using an analog-to-digital (AD) converter. As discussed in Chapter 2, a discrete transformation, such as the Fast Fourier Transform (FFT), represents discrete frequencies at a frequency resolution of $1/T$ (where T is the total time of the analyzed waveform). The discrete transform gives real and imaginary values for each of a set of frequencies that begin at 0 Hz and occur at multiples of $1/T$ up to the Nyquist frequency, which is one half of the rate at which the time waveform was sampled. The discrete frequencies are often called bins—from the idea that a spectrum contains multiple storage bins, each one for a specific frequency.

Figure 3–1 shows the FFT of a simple sine wave with a frequency of 5 Hz. In this example, the duration of the time waveform T is 1 second. The resolution of the spectrum is therefore 1 Hz. Because the AD conversion occurs 50 times in 1 second, the Nyquist frequency is 25 Hz.

Thus, the spectrum produced by the FFT of the signal has frequencies at 0, 1, 2, 3 . . . 24 Hz. Since the time waveform was a pure sine wave at 5 Hz, the spectra have zero values at all frequencies except 5 Hz. The real and imaginary values can be plotted on the polar plot shown on the lower right of the figure. The real value at 5 Hz is negative and thus the 5-Hz vector goes to the left of the y-axis. Similarly, the positive imaginary value directs the vector above the x-axis. From the real and imaginary values, we can calculate amplitudes and phases at each frequency. The most commonly represented spectra are the amplitude or power spectra. Power is simply the square of the amplitude. Although phases can be calculated for important parts of the spectra, it is not common to plot phase spectra.

Different waveforms in the time domain may have the same amplitude spectrum. This occurs when different frequency components have different phases, as illustrated in Figure 3–2. Often, we do not display the full range of the spectrum. In Figure 3–2, the Nyquist frequency was 250 Hz and we could have displayed frequencies up to 249 Hz. However, only the frequencies 0 to 20 Hz are shown in the plotted spectra. The values at higher frequencies were zero.

EVOKED POTENTIALS IN THE FREQUENCY DOMAIN

Auditory Steady-State Responses

The auditory steady-state responses (ASSRs) provide a simple example of how the auditory EPs can be considered in the

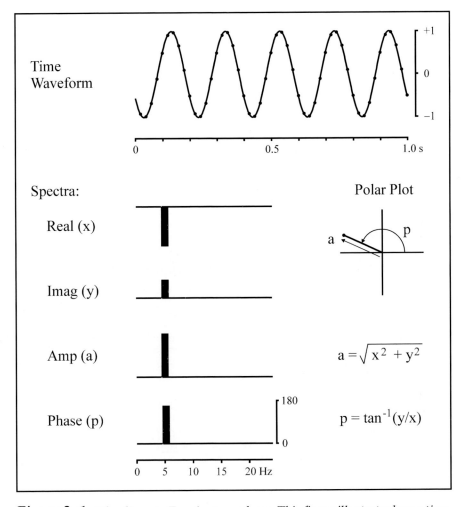

Figure 3–1. **The discrete Fourier transform.** *This figure illustrates how a time-waveform—a 5-Hz sine wave recorded for 1 s—can be evaluated in the frequency domain using a Fourier transform. The upper section of the figure shows the waveform in a continuous line and its conversion into a set of numbers (dots) at a rate of 50 Hz. On the lower left are shown the spectra that can be obtained. These go from 0 to 24 Hz, and have discrete values at multiples of 1 Hz. Because the time waveform contains only activity at 5 Hz, the only non-zero values in the spectra are in the 5-Hz bin. The transform initially gives a set of 25 real and 25 imaginary numbers. These can be plotted on the polar plot on the right; the dot is plotted at an x-position (left-right) equal to the real value and a y-position (up-down) equal to the imaginary value. The line from the origin to the dot represents the two-dimensional vector, which has an amplitude (a) and a phase (p, circling arrow). These can be calculated from the x and y values as shown in the lower right. The lower left shows the amplitude and phase spectra.*

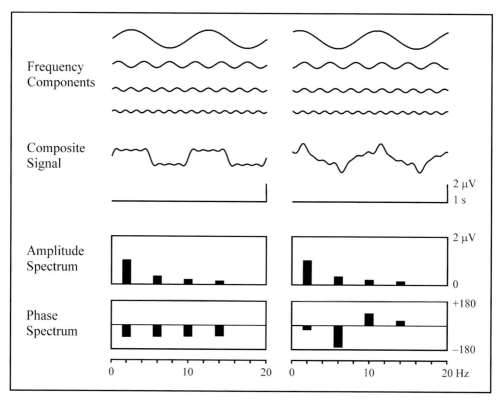

Figure 3–2. Amplitude and phase spectra. This figure illustrates how complex patterns of activity in the time domain can be built up from different frequency components. The set of waveforms in the left upper part of the figure show the odd numbered harmonics of a basic 2-Hz frequency: 2 Hz (first harmonic), 6 Hz (the third harmonic), 10 Hz (fifth harmonic), and 14 Hz (seventh harmonic) with amplitudes decreasing as the number of the harmonic. Thus, the seventh harmonic waveform is one seventh the amplitude of the first harmonic. All waveforms start at the same phase (–90° in terms of the cosine). The sum of these harmonic waveforms starts to look like a square wave. If we continued to add odd number harmonics the sum would approximate the square wave even more closely. However, if the components have different phases, as shown in the right section of the figure, the sum of the activities no longer looks like a square wave. The amplitude spectrum is the same but the phase spectrum is different.

frequency domain. A typical ASSR follows the modulation frequency of an amplitude-modulated tone. In the time domain, we record a sine wave at the frequency of the modulation, delayed by some latency from the stimulus modulation. In the frequency domain, we see a peak at the frequency of modulation. Figure 3–3 shows the ASSR to a tone that is amplitude-modulated at 40 Hz. The upper part of the figure shows the time waveform and its relation to the stimulus. The response is a sine wave that is follows after the stimulus by a delay. The lower left part of the figure shows the spectrum. Most of the energy in the response is at the modulation-frequency of the stimulus; in the spectrum, this shows as the peak at 40 Hz.

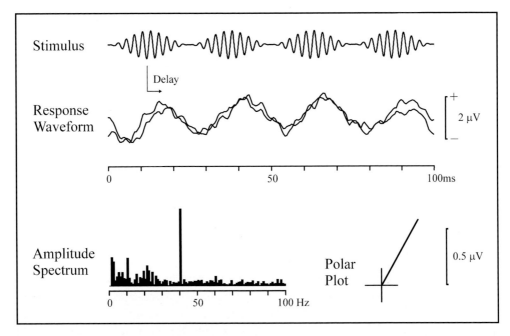

Figure 3–3. **Auditory steady-state responses (ASSRs).** *The time waveforms in the upper part of the figure were recorded in response to a 400-Hz tone amplitude-modulated at 40 Hz (upper line). The EEG data were recorded over 5 minutes and averaged every 100 ms to give the replicated waveforms in the second line. The response shows as a 40-Hz sinusoidal wave, delayed after the stimulus-envelope by about 4 ms. The lower left of the figure shows the spectrum of the activity. This was obtained after averaging the EEG every 1000 ms and then submitting the 1-s average waveform to an FFT. The amplitude spectrum shows as a peak at 40 Hz. The spectrum is calibrated to give the baseline-peak amplitude of the response. The bottom right of the figure shown the response at 40 Hz plotted in polar format.*

This ASSR example allows us to discuss several issues about time-to-frequency transformation. The first issue concerns the concepts of signal and noise. In the time domain, we can check the reliability of a recording by how well two responses superimpose. The noise is represented by the variability in the replications. In the frequency domain, the noise is represented by the amount of energy in the spectrum at frequencies other the response frequency. The ASSR illustrated in Figure 3–3 is highly reliable—the response waveform replicates well in the time-domain and its spectral peak is much larger than the

activity at adjacent frequencies in the frequency domain. We return to these ideas later in this chapter and explore them more fully in Chapter 6.

A second issue is the relationship between phase and latency. The response waveform in the time domain is shifted to the right relative to the envelope of the stimulus by about a sixth of a cycle. In the polar plot, the phase is actually 58 degrees. This could represent a latency of 4 ms (one cycle being 25 ms). However, phase is inherently ambiguous and the response may actually be shifted by an additional cycle (i.e., the peak of the stimulus envelope evokes not the first following positive wave but the subsequent one). If this were so, the actual latency would be 29 ms. This ambiguity may be resolved by recording responses to stimuli with different modulation frequencies and calculating the "apparent latency" (which we discuss later).

A third issue concerns the representation of the response after a discrete Fourier transform like the FFT. The spectrum from the FFT accurately measures only frequencies that are integer multiples of the resolution. Other frequencies will be spread out over several nearby spectral bins—"spectral leakage." This makes it very difficult to measure the amplitude at a frequency that is not an integer multiple of the resolution. When recording ASSRs, therefore, we must be careful to make the stimulus-frequency (and thus the frequency of the response) one of the frequencies that are accurately represented in the FFT. This is done by having an integer number of cycles within the recording period. Otherwise, the response will show up in several frequency bins rather than just one, and we cannot measure it accurately.

As well as reducing the signal (if it does not occur at one of the represented frequencies), spectral leakage also can increase the noise of the recording. If there are high-amplitude low-frequencies in the recording (from the EEG rhythms, for example), these might leak into the frequency region of the response and hamper its recognition. The amount of spectral leakage can be controlled by using a window to adjust the time signal prior to the FFT. Windows such as the Hanning window decrease the amplitude of the signal at the beginning and end of the recording. This does not affect the response if there is an integer number of cycles in the recording period, but it will decrease the amount of noise that leaks into the re-

sponse bin from other frequencies. Lyons (2004, Chapters 3 and 4) and John and Purcell (2008) provide reviews of this and other issues that must be considered when using the discrete Fourier transform.

Evoked and Induced Activity

Stimuli can change EEG rhythms in two ways: the changes can be specifically "evoked" or they can be "induced" (Galambos, 1992). When rhythmic activity is "evoked," the timing and the phase relationship between the stimulus and response are the same for each presentation of the stimulus—the response is thus considered to be "phase-locked" to the stimulus. Repeating the stimulus and averaging the responses in the time domain yields an average EP with the same waveform as any individual response. Phase-locking in the frequency domain is similar to time-locking in the time domain. If single responses are obscured by background EEG activity that is random in relation to the stimuli, averaging can be used to distinguish the evoked activity from the background activity. Evoked rhythmic activity may be either transient when a brief burst of activity follows a single stimulus (e.g., the gamma-band response), or steady-state when the rhythmic activity becomes phase-locked to a repeating stimulus (e.g., the 40-Hz response) (Pantev et al., 1993).

Induced activity is a change in EEG rhythms that is not phase-locked to the stimulus. Two types of phase-unlocking may occur: the burst may occur at the same time for every stimulus but the rhythmic activity within the burst may have a different phase each time, or each burst may contain activity that is exactly the same on each trial but the onset-latency of the burst may vary from one stimulus to another. These two kinds of induced activity are illustrated in Figure 3–4. If we average the responses in the time domain, these induced bursts of rhythmic activity will cancel themselves out, and little or no activity will be seen in the average.

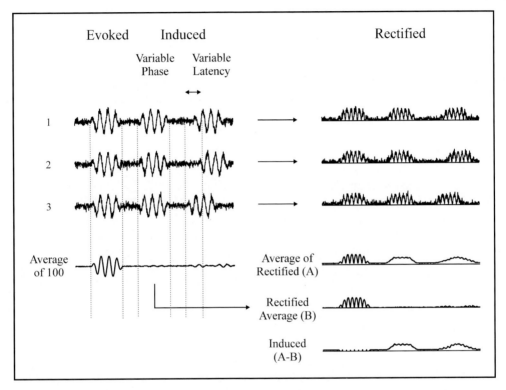

Figure 3–4. Evoked and induced activity. The left half of the figure shows some rhythmic responses to a stimulus, intermixed with a small amount of background noise. The data are modeled to represent EPs in background EEG, with the stimulus occurring at the beginning of the traces and recording-time represented on the x-axis. The earliest response ("evoked") is exactly the same each time the stimulus is presented (3 of the 100 different presentations are illustrated one below the other). The two next responses represent two kinds of induced activity. The first occurs at the same time relative to the stimulus but has a random phase—the response to the second stimulus is almost inverted relative to the first. The second has exactly the same waveform but occurs with a latency that varies over the region spanned by the arrow. If we average 100 responses, the background EEG decreases (by a factor of 10), the evoked response remains, and the two types of induced activity are no longer apparent. The right side of the figure shows one approach to recording the induced activity. Each recording is full-wave rectified and then the rectified activity is averaged. Now the recording (A) shows both the evoked and the induced activity. If we then rectify the average response (B) and subtract it away from the average of the rectified waveforms we get a representation of the induced activity as shown at the bottom right. Note that the noise interferes with the procedures a little —it can alter the rectified signals—and there are small signals left over after the subtraction. These problems would be attenuated by bandpass-filtering the signals prior to rectification, as recommended in the text.

However, if we evaluate the envelope of the activity on each trial and then average the envelope from stimulus to stimulus we can obtain evidence for an "induced" response. A simple way would be to filter each response using a bandpass that eliminates activity at frequencies other than those within the burst, to rectify the filtered waveforms and to average the rectified waveforms. The final average then shows the rectified representation of both the evoked and the induced activities. If we rectify the normal averaged waveform and subtract this from the average of the rectified responses, we can get a waveform that shows just the induced activity. These procedures are illustrated in Figure 3–4.

Probably the most common approach to the filtering and rectification is to calculate a "spectrogram" on each trial. A spectrogram plots how the activities at different frequencies change over time. Multiple transformations of the time domain activity into spectra are performed at each time during the recording. The power of the activity in each frequency band then can be plotted at each point in time. Calculating the amplitude as the square root of the power will give a rectified response. Performing this calculation for each of the frequencies resolved in the spectrum will serve as a bank of bandpass filters. In this way, we can estimate the time course of activity at each of the resolved frequencies.

Using the spectrograms, we can calculate an average response that contains both the evoked and the induced activity. If we average in the time domain, we obtain just the evoked activity. This can be treated in the same way as the single trials to get a spectrographic representation of the evoked activity. We can then subtract the evoked activity away from the combined evoked and induced activity to get the induced activity by itself. A cryptic mantra for evaluating induced activity is then "take the spectrogram of the average away from the average of the spectrograms."

This approach is not without controversy, however. The evoked potentials themselves may represent synchronization of the background rhythms. Therefore, we could also be justified in looking at the average of the single-trial spectrograms without any subtraction. Mazaheri and Picton (2005) and David, Kliner, and Friston (2006) provide fuller discussion of these issues, to which we return later in this chapter.

SPECTROGRAMS

In a spectrogram, the frequency is plotted along the y-axis instead of the x-axis typically used when a single spectrum is examined. Multiple spectra are calculated at different points in time and the results are plotted with time along the x-axis. The power or amplitude of the activity at each frequency is indicated by a color scale, which could involve distinct colors or different shades of gray. This scale could use just two levels, for example, black and white, or involve many levels. Color is basically the third dimension of the graph or the z-dimension.

Frequency transformations are performed at multiple points in time during the recording. Each spectrum is assessed over a brief period of time and the frequency resolution of the spectrum will be the reciprocal of this time. Thus, if each spectrum is based on 500 ms of the recording, the frequency resolution of the spectrum is 2 Hz. This will be the resolution of the spectrum in the y-axis. We can assess the spectra at a rate faster than that determined by the duration of the spectrum. For example, in Figure 3–5, the spectra are

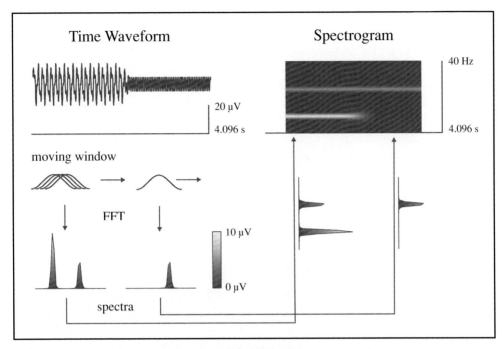

Figure 3–5. *Constructing a spectrogram. This time waveform in the upper left represents a combination of two activities: a 10-Hz rhythm that stops halfway across the recording period and a continuous 25 Hz rhythm. The waveform is sampled every 4 ms using periods of 1.024 second and a Hanning window. At each point in time, a spectrum is calculated using the Fast Fourier Transform (FFT); two such spectra are illustrated. The amplitude is converted from a measurement on the y-axis to a level on the gray color scale with light colors representing higher values. Each of the spectra (only two are illustrated) is then inserted into the spectrogram shown in the upper right. The raw spectrogram has been smoothed a little prior to representation. Because each spectrum is based on periods from 512 ms before to 512 ms after a particular point in time, the spectrogram can only start 512 ms after the beginning of the waveform and must stop 512 ms before the end. In the final spectrogram, frequency is on the y-axis of the spectrogram, time on the x-axis, and amplitude on the z-axis (shown using a gray scale with lighter gray indicating higher amplitude).*

based on 500-ms periods and are calculated every 4 ms (instead of every 500 ms). However, the temporal resolution along the *x*-axis is still determined by the time-period over which the frequency transform is calculated. If we are evaluating each spectrum over 500 ms, the real temporal resolution of the recording is approximately 2 Hz even though we may be performing these assessments at a much faster rate.

Spectograms From Short-Term Fourier Transforms

One way to calculate a spectrogram is to perform multiple short-term Fourier transforms, each assessing a brief time and each plotted at the center point of that brief time period. The parameters of such a spectrogram are therefore the duration of the Fourier transform (which determines both the resolution along the frequency axis and the resolution along the temporal axis) and the rate at which each transform is calculated (which determines how many points are actually plotted along the time axis). This process of constructing a spectrogram is illustrated in Figure 3–5.

When we are constructing a spectrogram, we are confronted with the time-frequency uncertainty principle (Schniter, 2005). The more accurately we wish to consider the timing of a signal, the less accurately we can assess its frequency content. This principle is illustrated in Figure 3–6. When we increase the duration over which the time-frequency transformation is calculated, we increase the frequency resolution of the spectrogram but decrease its temporal resolution. We must choose the best settings for the informa-

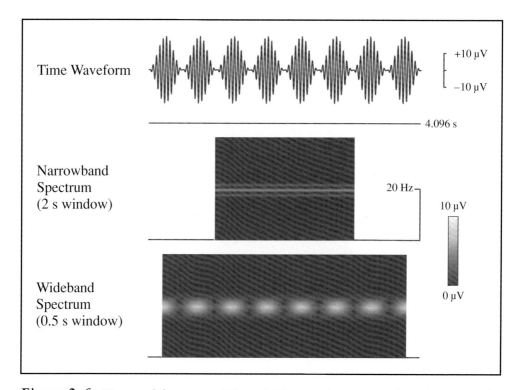

Figure 3–6. Time and frequency. When plotting spectrograms we have to compromise between time and frequency, both of which are determined by the duration over which the individual spectra are calculated. A longer time results in more precise frequency discrimination (giving a narrowband spectrogram) but less temporal resolution. A shorter time allows us to see how the signal is changing over time but loses frequency resolution. In this figure, a narrowband spectrogram shows the frequency spectrum of an amplitude modulated sine wave, with the center band at the carrier frequency (19.5 Hz) and side bands separated from this frequency by the modulation frequency (1.95 Hz). The wideband spectrogram at the bottom of the figure shows how the recorded waveform changes in amplitude over time but the frequency content of the signal is blurred over a wide range. Both views of the signal are valid. The choice between them depends on whether we want to consider the frequency patterns or the temporal changes of the recorded signal.

tion in which we are interested. Human knowledge is full of uncertainty and scientific experiment always requires some degree of compromise.

The spectrogram thus is an array of amplitudes or powers, with the x-dimension equal to the number of time points at which the spectra were calculated and the y-dimension equal to the number of frequencies in each spectrum. The color scale that provides the amplitude or power values should be chosen so that the spectrogram best represents the data. EEG signals have values that tend to decrease with increasing frequency and, unless the amplitudes are scaled to counteract this, anything occurring at higher frequency will vanish into the dark of a gray scale or the deep blue of a rainbow scale. One approach might be to relate the values to some baseline value. For example, when we are determining the changes related to a stimulus, we can use as a baseline the mean amplitude of the activity within each frequency line occurring before the stimulus. The scale can then be expressed as a ratio (often logarithmic) of this baseline. When evaluating evoked activity, this will give the signal-to-noise ratio (SNR) of the response. When evaluating induced activity, this will allow us to look at both increases and decreases in activity: synchronization and desynchronization. Another approach to scaling would be to multiply each value by the frequency at which it is calculated—this accentuates the activity at higher frequencies.

Spectrograms Calculated Using Wavelets

The short-term FFT approach to constructing the spectrogram is limited in terms of its frequency or temporal resolution. In order to consider frequencies as slow as 1 Hz (and higher frequencies with a resolution of 1 Hz), we must perform each FFT over at least 1 second. This makes the temporal resolution of the spectrogram near 1 second. We can perform multiple FFTs within each second but the results will change much more slowly than the rate of the FFT calculations. At higher frequencies, if we calculate the spectrum over such a long time, we will not see rapid changes in the activity at these frequencies. Various techniques have been used to optimize the spectral and temporal resolution of the spectrogram. For example, at high frequencies, we can analyze activity with greater temporal resolution and less frequency resolution than at lower frequencies. One of the most popular approaches uses a Morlet wavelet to calculate the activity at different frequencies with a resolution equal to several cycles of that frequency (Tallon-Baudry & Bertrand, 1999; Tallon-Beaudry, Bertrand, Delpuech, & Permier, 1997). We use this approach in our next analysis.

Spectrographic Evaluation of Auditory EP

The spectrogram allows us to distinguish two kinds of stimulus-evoked activity in the frequency domain: steady-state and transient. Steady-state responses maintain the same amplitude and phase relationship to the stimulus over time, whereas transient responses have changing relationships. An auditory stimulus can elicit a transient burst of activity with frequencies near 40 Hz—the "gamma-band response" (GBR: Pantev et al., 1991, 1993). This response is particularly evident when the stimuli occur infrequently (at interstimulus intervals of more than several seconds) or irregularly. In addition, if the stimulus recurs at rates near 40 Hz or if a continuous stimulus is modulated at such rates, a steady-state response at the frequency of stimulation occurs.

Transient and steady-state responses to an amplitude modulated tone are shown in Figure 3–7. The tone lasted 1 second but the amplitude-modulation only began after 100 ms. The average EP shows the onset response followed by a sustained potential (SP) on which is superimposed the ASSR. Filtering the waveform to show only activity at 40 Hz shows a transient GBR evoked by the onset of the tone and then a prolonged ASSR evoked by the modulation.

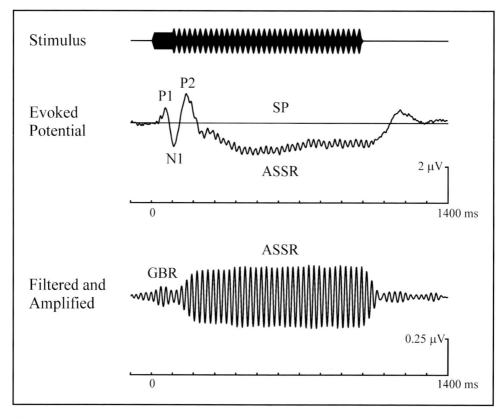

Figure 3–7. Transient and steady state responses. *The upper section of the figure shows an amplitude-modulated stimulus and its response. The evoked potential represents the grand-mean for eight subjects (each subject having 200 responses) to 1000-Hz tones lasting 1 s presented binaurally every 2 s at an intensity of 60 dB HL. Each stimulus was amplitude-modulated at 40 Hz, beginning 100 ms after the onset of the stimulus. The onset of the tone elicits a P1-N1-P2 complex and then a sustained potential (SP) lasting through the tone. Riding on the sustained potential is a small auditory steady-state response (ASSR). The lower section of the figure shows the evoked potential filtered using a narrow bandpass filter centered at 40 Hz and amplified to show the response more clearly. Near the beginning is a brief burst of activity—the gamma band response (GBR). This is followed by the ASSR which takes about 200 ms to build up to true steady state levels after the onset of the modulation. The ASSR falls back to baseline within about 50 ms after the stimulus ends.*

The frequency components of this EP can be viewed in a spectrogram, as shown in Figure 3–8. In the spectrogram, the transient response occurs for a brief time and the steady state response continues for the duration of the stimulus. Because the spectrogram was calculated using Morlet wavelets, it displays the low frequencies with low temporal resolution and the high frequencies with high temporal resolution. We can track the time course of activity by plotting selected lines of the spectrogram as shown in the upper right of the figure. At 40 Hz we see the GBR to the onset of the tone followed by an ASSR that grows in amplitude for about 200 ms after the onset of the modulation until finally "achieving steady-state" (cf. Ross, Picton, & Pantev, 2002). The P1-N1-P2 onset response to the tone is represented in the spectrogram by a burst of activity in the lower frequencies (around 8 Hz), and the SP shows up as activity in the very low frequencies (1-2 Hz). The scaled spectrogram at the lower left accentuates the responses at the higher frequencies—the brief GBR containing activity from 40 to 60 Hz and the straight line of activity at 40 Hz representing the ASSR to the modulated tone. On a spectrogram, transient responses

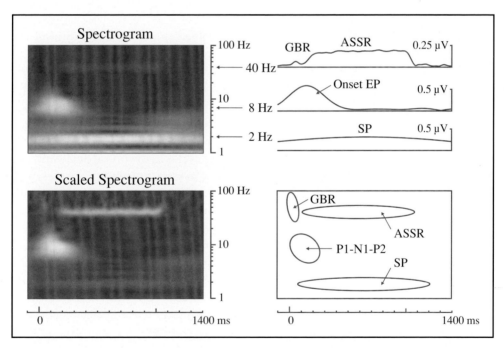

Figure 3–8. *Spectrogam of an auditory EP. The upper left of the figure shows the spectrogram of the amplitudes of the auditory EP shown in Figure 3–7. The spectrogram was calculated using the Morlet wavelet. This gives a finer temporal resolution for the higher frequencies. The gray color-scaling is set to span from minimum to maximum amplitude values. The frequency scale is logarithmic. On the right are shown the amplitude plots over time for 40 Hz, 8 Hz, and 2 Hz. The bottom left shows the spectrogram rescaled to accentuate the activity at the higher frequencies (by multiplying each pixel by the frequency at which it was calculated). This makes the gamma-band response (GBR) and the 40-Hz ASSR more clearly visible. The main components of this scaled spectrogram are diagrammed on the lower right.*

show up as blobs and steady-state responses as horizontal lines.

The distinction between transient and steady-state is not always as clear cut as we might wish as it depends on the time over which the response is evaluated. If a stimulus occurs regularly at a slow rate, the frequencies contributing to the transient evoked potential may be quite stable when viewed over time periods substantially longer than the interstimulus interval. Such a view will simply indicate that activity in a particular frequency band is being evoked by the stimulus but will not show its transient nature or give its timing.

PHASE AND LATENCY

Although phase is an essential part of the information contained in the signal, its evaluation is not as simple as the measurement of amplitude. Phase is circular rather than linear—phase goes round and round and often makes us dizzy. Phase is measured either in degrees or in radians, with 360° or 2π radians making a full cycle. Phase usually is measured in terms of the cosine waveform. The onset phase is the phase of the waveform at the onset of the response. A phase delay can be calculated by subtracting this measured phase from the phase of the stimulus at the onset of the recorded waveform. Often, the stimulus also is a cosine stimulus, in which case the phase delay is 360° minus the onset phase of the response. This is illustrated in Figure 3–9 where a stimulus beginning at 0° cosine phase evokes a response with a cosine onset phase of 240° or a phase delay of 120°. This delay can be converted to a latency using the simple formula presented in the figure. However, the interpretation of this latency is beset

with ambiguity. First, we are uncertain about which cycle of the stimulus is related to which cycle of the response. This is illustrated in Figure 3–9. Is a peak in the response related to the immediately preceding peak in the stimulus waveform (continuous arrow), the one in the preceding cycle (dashed arrow), or the one two cycles before? Second, we do not know which part of the stimulus waveform is specifically evoking a positive or negative peak in the response. The polarity of the response recorded from two electrodes is arbitrary; reversing which electrodes go into which input of the differential amplifier alters the phase of the response by 180°. Indeed, a peak in the response may be most closely related to a peak in the derivative (slope) of the stimulus envelope rather than its amplitude.

When the ASSR is dominated by a positive wave (such as wave V of the brainstem response recorded between vertex and neck electrodes), we sometimes can calculate the response latency by adding cycles to the phase delay and determining which number of cycles makes the most sense in terms of other information. John and Picton (2000) evaluated this approach for the 80- to 100-Hz ASSR. They found that at moderate intensities the latency of the responses varied from 15.8 ms for 6000-Hz carriers to 21.5 ms for 500 Hz. These estimates involved choosing how many extra cycles to add to the measured phase so that the resultant latencies made sense in terms of what might be expected from the traveling wave delay in the cochlea (e.g., Elberling, Don, Cebulla, & Stürzebecher, 2007; Neely, Norton, Gorga, & Jesteadt, 1988). As already noted, however, the technique of adding missing cycles depends on the fact that the main component contributing to the ASSR is measured as a positive

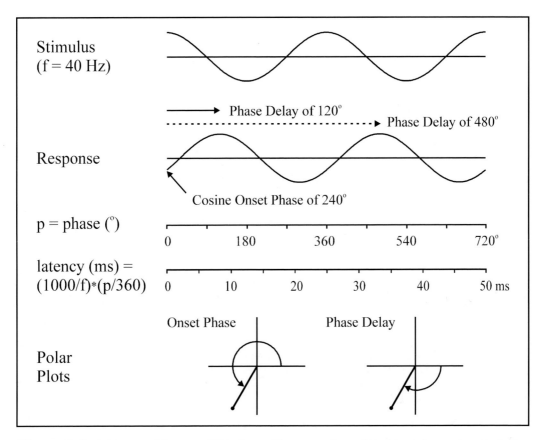

Figure 3–9. Phase and latency. This figure illustrates the ambiguities inherent in calculating a latency from phase. As shown in the center of the figure, phase can be converted to latency simply by making a cycle of phase equivalent to the period of the waveform at that frequency. In this example, a 40-Hz waveform goes through a full cycle of 360° in 25 ms. The upper diagrams illustrate how we cannot determine whether a peak in the stimulus is related to the immediately following peak in the response—giving a phase delay of 120° and latency of 8.3 ms—or the subsequent peak giving a phase delay of 480° and latency of 33.3 ms. The polar plots at the bottom of the figure show that the phase delay of the response can be calculated as 360° minus the onset phase of the response (provided the onset phase is measured relative to the cosine and the stimulus begins at cosine 0°). The formula for converting phase to latency is set up to give latency in ms and to use phase in degrees. It basically multiplies the period of the waveform (1000/f) by the proportion of the full cycle represented by the phase (p/360). If the units were seconds and radians, the formula would be latency = (1/f)*(p/(2π)).

wave (and thus similar to the stimulus at zero phase). For the 80- to 100-Hz ASSRs measured from the vertex using a neck reference, this is likely the case. If the response were inverted (e.g., by measuring from the neck relative to the vertex), the procedure would not work.

Apparent Latency

Another approach to estimating the latency of a steady-state response is to calculate the "apparent latency" by measuring the slope of the relationship between the response phase and the stimulus rate (Regan,

1989, pp. 42-43). In engineering, this value is called the "group delay" (e.g., Schoonhoven, Boden, Verbunt, & de Munck, 2003). The phase delay of the response is measured at different stimulus rates, and the slope of their relationship is then estimated by regressing phase against rate. If we only have two values, the slope is the difference in phase divided by the difference in rate. Apparent latency obviates the requirement that the main component of the response be related in polarity to the stimulus. Diamond (1977) proposed an interesting graphic way to estimate the latency of a steady-state response using time-domain peak measurements. This is essentially the same as the apparent latency estimations (John & Picton, 2000, Appendix). Figure 3–10 illustrates the calculation of apparent latency.

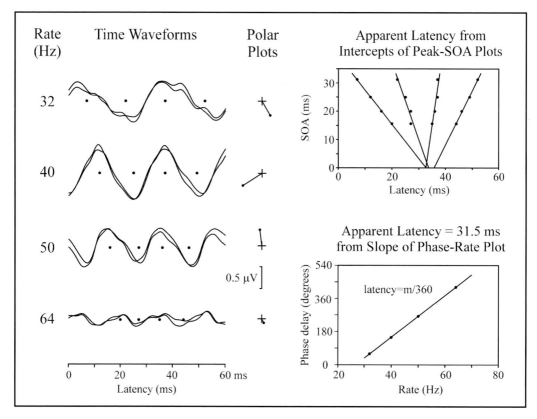

Figure 3–10. Apparent latency. The left side of the figure shows ASSRs evoked by amplitude modulated tones with different modulation rates and viewed in the time domain. As shown in the polar plots to the right of the time-waveforms, the phases of the responses vary with the rate of modulation. The dots represent the estimated latencies for peaks and troughs in the waveforms. The diagram at the upper right shows the technique of Diamond (1977) for graphically estimating the apparent latency from the timing of these peaks and troughs. The latencies are plotted against the stimulus onset asynchrony (SOA)—the time between the onsets of each period of modulation. The lines joining the dots reach the x-axis at latencies between 32 and 36 ms. The diagram at the lower right shows how the apparent latency (or group delay) can be calculated from the slope of the regression line for plotting the phase of the response (in degrees) against the frequency of the stimulus (and response). In this estimate the apparent latency was 31.5 ms.

The interpretation of the apparent latency, nevertheless, is still not simple (Hari, Hämäläinen, & Joutsiniemi, 1989). The concept depends on the idea that the response is evoked at a single latency. However, the ASSRs recorded from the scalp often reflect the activity of multiple different sources, each having its own latency. In addition, filtering within the brain and in the electronic amplifiers alters the phases of the recorded activity (Bijl & Veringa, 1985). If we evaluate the responses over only a brief range of stimulus rates, and if the responses at these rates are dominated by one source, the apparent latencies may make sense. In other situations, the results may not be interpretable.

SIGNALS AND NOISE IN THE FREQUENCY DOMAIN

Just like transient auditory EPs recorded in the time domain, ASSRs recorded in the frequency domain can be obscured by background EEG activity. In the frequency domain, the background EEG and EMG show up as activity in broad regions of the spectrum. When the amplitude of this noise increases, the ASSR is no longer visible as a distinct peak higher than its surroundings. Time must be invested to decrease the background noise. Multiple short recordings phase-locked to the stimulus can be averaged prior to the FFT, or the recordings can be concatenated together and the FFT applied over a longer period of time. In the latter approach, the background noise is divided up into a larger number of frequency bins. The number of frequency bins in the analysis is equal to one half the number of discrete time points in the recording and this number will increase as the duration increases. With the increased number of frequency bins, the amount of noise activity in any single bin decreases. If the response is exactly time-locked to the stimulus and if there is an integer number of stimuli (or stimulus modulations) in the recording sweep, the response energy remains in a single bin and is unaffected by the increased duration of the recording. In practice, we often combine both averaging and concatenation in evaluating the ASSR. A judicious compromise between the two approaches is necessary because the time for calculating the FFT becomes very slow when the sweep becomes very long. The processes are illustrated in Figure 3–11 using the auditory 40-Hz response. Both procedures follow the same rules of noise reduction. The amplitude of the residual noise decreases by the square root of the number of trials either averaged or concatenated (John, Lins, Boucher, & Picton, 1998).

Coherent Averaging and Spectral Averaging

When averaging together the different recordings in order to reduce the background noise, we must be sure to average both the real and imaginary components of the response (Picton, John, Purcell, & Plourde, 2003). This "coherent averaging" (Lyons, 2004, Chapter 11) ensures that the final response represents activity that has the same phase from one trial to the next (i.e., is phase-locked to the stimulus and a true evoked potential). This process can be performed by averaging each component of the real and imaginary spectra and then recomputing the amplitudes and phases. However, it is more easily performed by averaging the time-domain recordings and then performing the FFT on the averaged waveform. Averaging just the amplitude or the power of the response on each trial without regard to the phase

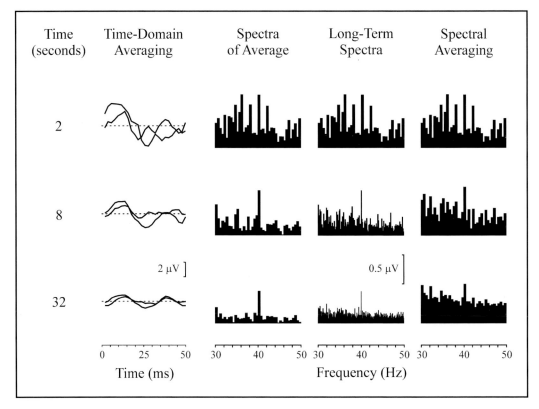

Figure 3–11. *Effects of recording time on ASSR detection. This figure shows responses to 75 dB pSPL 1000-Hz 5-ms tones presented at 40 Hz. Data over 2, 8, and 32 seconds were analyzed using four different techniques. Replicate time-domain averages of the responses over a 2-cycle period are shown in the leftmost data column. The response becomes reliably replicable after 32 seconds. Spectra calculated from the average time waveforms over a 2-s sweep are shown in the "spectra of average" columns. Taking spectra of the time domain averages is the same as "coherent averaging." Although the response at 40 Hz is visible after 2 s (one sweep), it is not higher than the activity at all other frequencies. However, when the spectrum is calculated after averaging 4 or 16 sweeps (8 or 32 s), the response at 40 Hz remains but the activity in adjacent frequency bins decreases. A similar effect is noted if the recordings are just concatenated (to give a sweep of 8 or 32 s) prior to the FFT—"long-term spectra." Here the resolution of the spectrum becomes finer; the width of the bins moves from 0.5 to 0.125 to 0.0325 Hz. Simply averaging the spectra without regard to phase ("spectral averaging," rightmost column) does not decrease activity in the adjacent bins but simply makes it less variable from bin to bin. The spectra are calibrated to represent the baseline-to-peak amplitude of the response.*

—"spectral averaging"—will not decrease the background EEG noise (although it will become less variable from one frequency bin to the other). The effects of spectral averaging are shown in the far right column of Figure 3–11. Spectral averaging can be used if we are interested in the pattern of the background EEG, but not if we wish to distinguish the EPs from that background EEG.

SYNCHRONIZATION AND DESYNCHRONIZATION

Although not appropriate for evoked responses, spectral averaging is the most common way to evaluate induced responses. Typically, we are interested in both the timing and the frequency of the induced activity and so we calculate a full spectrogram for each trial, a time period lasting from just before to some period after the stimulus. We then average the spectrograms over the multiple trials wherein the stimulus is presented, without considering the phases of this activity on each trial. The averaged spectrogram then plots the recorded activity in terms of both its frequency and its time course. Calculating the amplitude spectrograms for each trial and then averaging the spectrograms (without considering phase) gives the sum of both the evoked and induced activity. This shows changes in the background rhythms that occur in response to a sound, whether or not the rhythmic activity itself is precisely phase-locked to the stimulus. If we want to consider the induced activity by itself, we can eliminate the evoked activity by taking the spectrogram of the average waveform away from the average of the spectrograms obtained on each individual recording. However, this depends on how we conceptualize the responses: we might also conceive of the evoked activity as a specific phase-locked component of the more general category of induced activity.

Induced responses are of two kinds: the EEG activity in a particular frequency band can either increase (event-related synchronization, ERS) or decrease (event-related desynchronization, ERD) (Pfurtscheller & Lopes da Silva, 1999). Rhythmic activity is recorded in the EEG at the scalp or cortical surface when many neurons fire synchronously at a rate intrinsic to a particular region of the cortex or grouping of its neurons. When this occurs, the electric fields generated in the cortical pyramidal cells add together to produce a large surface-recorded rhythm. The most widely studied EEG rhythm is the alpha rhythm in the visual areas of the brain. When the eyes are closed, the neurons of the visual cortex tend to synchronize with each other by means of feedback interconnections and/or thalamic pacemakers. This synchronization creates a rhythm with a frequency near 10 Hz. The alpha rhythm is considered an "idling" rhythm—it occurs when the neurons of the visual cortex have nothing to do but dance together. When the eyes are open, visual information arrives at the cortex and the neurons become involved in processing that information; the demands of the input override any intrinsic rhythmicity and the neurons become "desynchronized." A similar change occurs in the mu-rhythm that occurs in the somatosensory and motor areas of the cortex. This rhythm desynchronizes when the cortex processes somatosensory input or initiates movement. Also, there likely is a tau rhythm in the temporal lobes that desynchronizes when auditory input is processed, but this is clearly recorded only by magnetoencephalography (Hari, Salmelin, Mäkelä, Salenius, & Helle, 1997).

Sometimes a stimulus will trigger a burst of rhythmic activity. Rhythmic synchronization between neurons may serve to link information being processed in different areas when processing sensory input or to facilitate associations when forming memories (Engel & Singer, 2001; Jensen, Kaiser, & Lachaux, 2007). In the auditory system, probably the most widely studied human ERS is the GBR—the burst of gamma activity that follows an auditory stimulus (Pantev et al., 1993).

A burst of frontal theta activity also may occur in relation to processing information from an auditory stimulus (Mazaheri & Picton, 2005).

Most of the research on human ERS and ERD has been carried out in the visual and somatosensory modalities. In these modalities, the background EEG rhythms—the posterior alpha rhythm and the central mu rhythm—are more prominent than in the auditory modality. Cacace and McFarland (2003; also McFarland & Cacace, 2004) have compared the spectra recorded when auditory stimuli are processed, and found ERS in the theta frequencies and ERD in the alpha and beta frequencies. Mazaheri and Picton (2005) examined the single-trial spectrograms when auditory targets are discriminated, thus giving some timing to the frequency changes—"spectral dynamics." Figure 3–12 shows the changes in the activity at different frequencies when a target tone is discriminated from a standard. The maps are derived from averaged single-trial spectrograms. Because the spectrogram of the average has not been subtracted, the activity represents both evoked and induced activity. The bursts of activity at theta and alpha frequencies likely represent both the evoked potentials and some theta ERS. During the processing of stimulus information there is also an alpha ERD. As shown in Figure 3–12, this may be more anterior than the alpha ERD that accompanies visual processing (maximal at the back of the head) and may perhaps represent changes in the tau rhythm.

Relations Between EPs and the Background EEG

Over many years there has been controversy about whether the sensory evoked potentials themselves represent the transient synchronization of background rhythms instead of additional activity superimposed on the background rhythms of the EEG. Sayers and his colleagues (Sayers & Beagley, 1974; Sayers, Beagley, & Henshall, 1974) found that a frequency transform of the late auditory evoked potential (LAEP) showed a similar amplitude spectrum to the background EEG but a specific phase spectrum. They therefore suggested that the LAEP might represent phase resetting of the different frequencies in the background EEG rather than an addition of extra activity. As we have already seen (Figure 3–2), the waveform of a signal in the time domain clearly depends on the phases of its component frequencies. The EP waveform could then represent a change in the phases of the frequencies that compose the EEG.

The advent of rapid computer programs to calculate the spectrograms of single-trial EPs have extended our ideas of the relations between EP and EEG (e.g., David et al., 2006; Makeig et al., 2002; Makeig et al., 2004; Shah et al., 2004). The view that we have been following so far is that these two activities are independent and additive. Stimulus-locked averaging then can then attenuate the background EEG and leaves the EP waveform. On single trials, the EP should be seen in the frequency transform as a transient increase in amplitude. Therefore, this view can be considered as an amplitude-modulation theory of EP generation. Clearly, the background EEG also might be independently affected by the stimulus. Thus, ERS or ERD could occur simultaneously with the EP. The alternative view, originally proposed by Sayers and Beagley (1974), is that nothing is added to the EEG, but that the EP is determined by a resetting of the phases of the ongoing EEG frequencies.

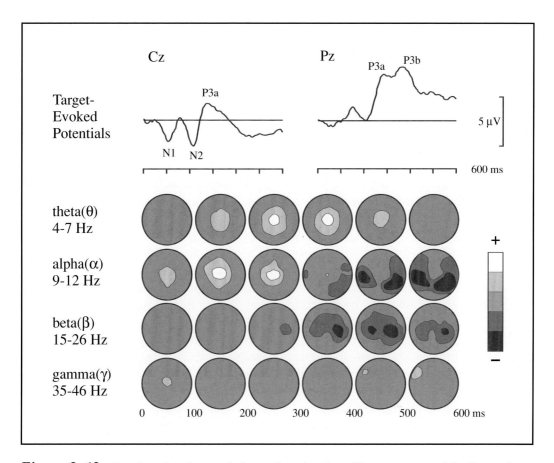

Figure 3–12. Synchronization and desynchronization. *The upper part of the figure shows the EP waveforms to occasional 1500-Hz targets occurring with a probability of 0.2 in a train of 1000-Hz standards. EPs at only 2 of the 65 electrode locations are shown: the vertex (Cz) and the midparietal (Pz). The lower part of the figure shows the full scalp topographies for each frequency band in the averaged single-trial spectrograms. The activity represents both evoked and induced potentials as the spectrogram of the average waveform was not subtracted. The full scalp topography of the waveforms was calculated sequentially using 100-ms intervals for the duration 0 to 600 ms after the stimulus, and plotted using an equi-azimuthal polar projection that descends to 20 degrees below the midtemporal equator. The gray scale has only 5 levels, increases in activity (ERS) being light and decreases (ERD) being dark. The maps show the percentage change in activity from the baseline period preceding the stimulus and are scaled differently for each frequency band: ±50% for theta, ±25% for alpha and beta, and ±50% for gamma. The theta activity shows ERS (white shading) maximal at 200–400 ms in the central areas. The alpha activity showing an ERS maximal at 100–300 ms. Both synchronizations likely represent a combination of the evoked potential and some induced activity. Both the alpha and the beta activity show ERD (black shading) toward the end of the tracing (when the target has been discriminated). These desynchronizations are more anterior than those that occur with visual processing and the alpha ERD may indicate a change in the temporal tau activity. The gamma activity shows a small brief burst of ERS within the first 100 ms—perhaps the gamma-band response. There also is some activity laterally at the end of the tracing, most likely some muscle or ocular artifact. Figure adapted from Mazaheri and Picton (2005).*

This proposal therefore can be considered the phase-modulation theory of EP generation. As well as demonstrating the specific phase pattern that causes the EP, we can also examine the trial-to-trial phase coherence of the EEG recordings. After the stimulus, this phase coherence is significantly different from the random phases that occur before the stimulus.

Unfortunately, it is not a simple matter to distinguish between these two views. Simply adding an EP waveform (with set phases for each of its component frequencies) to a randomly phased EEG causes the recorded phases to move toward the phases of the EP waveform. When the EP is smaller than the ongoing background activity, the overall amplitude (or energy) of the recording might not change significantly. On the trials when the added signal is inverted in polarity with the background EEG, the trial will actually show a decrease in energy. The addition of a signal to an unchanging background therefore can look much the same as a phase-locking of the background activity. Phase-synchronization during the EP is not proof that the ERP is generated by phase-resetting of the EEG.

Some features entailed by phase-resetting are not met in all examples of EPs. One key requirement of the phase modulation theory is that the existence of ongoing EEG rhythms whose phases can be modulated. Intracortical animal recordings have shown the visual-evoked ERP can occur when there is little background EEG activity (Shah et al., 2004). Measurements of the amplitude variance (Mäkinen, Tiitinen, & May, 2005) and comparisons between the phases of the EEG frequencies before and after the stimulus (Mazaheri & Jensen, 2006) do not support the phase-resetting explanation of the EP. Nevertheless, human cortical recordings sometimes show clear phase-resetting of EEG rhythms

without any consistent increase in amplitude (Rizzuto et al., 2003).

Neither the phase-modulation nor the amplitude-modulation theory fully accounts for the brain's response to stimuli. The EPs that originate in the cerebral cortex probably combine additive waveform and EEG resetting. The fact that the EPs and the EEG rhythms share neuronal generators probably accounts for this complex mixture (Mazaheri & Picton, 2005). Some neurons may generate only EEG rhythms and some may generate only EPs. However, given the set of stimuli that can activate a particular region of cortex, most neurons are involved in the generation of both EEG rhythms and EPs. Thus, a stimulus may cause several changes. First, the stimulus may activate cells that are quiescent. Activation may be precisely time-locked to the stimulus and show as a distinct EP, or not precisely time-locked to the stimulus showing as an induced ERS. Second, the stimulus may cause neurons that are already part of some ongoing EEG rhythm to lock themselves to the stimulus (phase-resetting). Third, the stimulus may inhibit ongoing neuronal activity. This could be one mechanism for ERD. In addition, however, ERD could be caused by multiple ERSs occurring at different times in different subgroups of neurons, such that their resultant rhythmic patterns cancel each other out in fields recorded at a distance.

SWEEPS

Calculating a spectrogram can allow us to see how evoked activity changes over a period of time. If we change some parameter of the stimulus during the recording, we might use the spectrogram to watch the response change over time. More simply, we could just calculate the amplitude and phase at a particular frequency and observe how these response characteristics change with the changing stimulus (Regan, 1989, pp. 113–123). This is effectively the same as taking one horizontal line out of the spectrogram. According to its definition, a steady-state response stays constant over time. The response to a changing stimulus changes over time and therefore is no longer truly steady-state. However, if the stimulus changes slowly, the response may be assessed as though it were moving through a sequence of steady-state periods.

The advantage of this "sweep" or "zoom" technique is that our analysis can be facilitated by knowledge about how the response should change with a particular parameter. If we expect the response amplitude to vary with intensity, we should find that the response increases and then decreases as the stimulus intensity increases and then decreases. The expected inverted V shape can then be used to analyze the sweep-response.

A simple approach is to change the intensity of an amplitude-modulated stimulus from low to high and then back again to low (Picton, Van Roon, & John, 2007). This can be repeated many times and the response averaged over the intensity cycles. The spectrogram shows a line at the frequency of modulation. This line should be greater than the averaged EEG background activity at higher and lower frequencies. As the amplitude of the response increases and decreases with the change in stimulus intensity, the response line in the spectrogram changes color. In Figure 3–13, the spectrogam is plotted using a gray scale and the line for the response becomes lighter as its amplitude increases and then darkens as the amplitude decreases.

Figure 3–13 also shows how our knowledge of how the response changes with the swept parameter (the intensity) might facilitate our evaluation of the response. If we assume that the amplitude of the response is linearly related to the intensity of the sound, we can collapse the data over the ascending and descending parts of the sweep and calculate a regression line for the amplitude-intensity function. We then can extrapolate this line to get a threshold for recognizing the response as larger than the background noise, and perhaps an absolute threshold where the response would be zero. This regression approach is illustrated in the upper right diagram of Figure 3–13.

FOURIER ANALYSIS

If we change the frequency of the stimulus over a sweep, the spectrogram derived from multiple short-term FFTs may not accurately represent the response, because the frequency of the stimulus and the response will be changing during each analysis period. The energy of the response thus may be spread over several frequency bins in the FFT. Another approach is to use a Fourier analyzer (Regan, 1977; Regan, 1989, pp. 81–98). In contrast to the discrete Fourier transform, which analyzes the signal over a spectrum of stationary frequencies, the Fourier analyzer relates the recorded response to a reference frequency that need not be stationary. Therefore, the analyzer can follow frequency variations that occur within a single analysis period. This technique thus provides an accurate measure of a response that changes frequency during the recording.

The Fourier analyzer requires orthogonal reference-sinusoids that match the instantaneous frequency of the stimulus. When we are using a sinusoidal amplitude modulation, the references are the sine and cosine of the envelope signal.

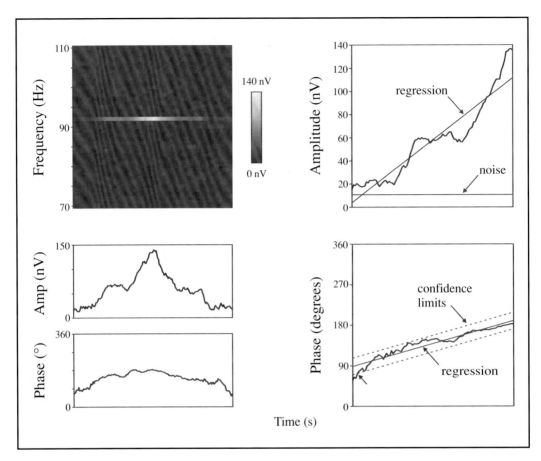

Figure 3–13. *Recording responses to intensity sweeps. The spectrogram in the upper left represents the average amplitudes of one subject to a single tone of 2 kHz amplitude-modulated at a rate of 92 Hz and swept in intensity from 25 dB to 75 dB SPL and then back to 25 dB over 16 seconds. Only the frequencies from 70 to 110 Hz are shown. The response is seen as the light line at 92 Hz. The dark background represents the residual EEG noise in the average response. The lower left of the figure represents the amplitude and phase of the response at 92 Hz in the spectrogram. The amplitude increases to the middle of the sweep and then decreases. The onset phase is largest at the midportion of the sweep and is variable at the beginning and end of the sweep. The right side of the figure shows the amplitude-intensity and phase-intensity functions obtained by collapsing the two halves of the data shown in the lower left. The horizontal line shows the p <0.10 limits of the background EEG noise. The suprathreshold amplitude data have been fitted with a linear function. This would extend to the left of the figure to an intercept at 22 dB SPL. The suprathreshold phase data also have been fitted with a linear function and the dotted lines represent the p <0.05 confidence limits of the regression. The actual phase data begin to exceed these limits at about 27 dB SPL (small arrow).*

Therefore, the analyzer also can be called a "sine-cosine synchronous demodulator" (Regan, 1989). The recorded EEG is mul- tiplied by each of the reference signals. Each multiplication produces a signal with a baseline offset equal to the real or imaginary component of the response, and multiple high-frequency products related to the activity in the recording at frequencies other than the reference signal. These high frequencies are filtered out using a low-pass filter, with the cutoff adjusted to remove most of the noise but still allow the response to change slowly with time. These processes are illustrated in Figure 3–14, which also shows how the system can be set up to evaluate how the ASSR follows sounds that change their rates of modulation (Purcell, John, Schneider, & Picton, 2004). Because the frequency of the stimulus and the amplitude and

phase of the response are continually changing, we are stretching our terms if we call the recorded activity an ASSR—perhaps "envelope-following response" is a more appropriate name in this context.

This approach is helpful in evaluating the brain's response to speech sounds. A vowel will evoke a response from the brain that follows the pitch of the voice. When the vowel is spoken naturally, this pitch will vary from moment to moment. The Fourier analyzer allows us to follow the response more accurately than a simple Fourier transform (Aiken & Picton, 2006, 2008b). Low-frequency variations in

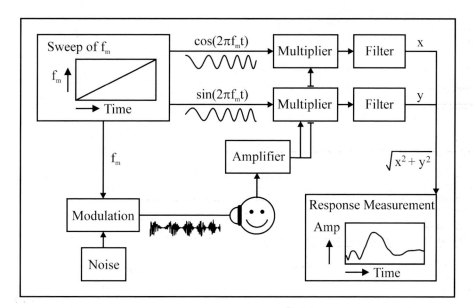

Figure 3–14. *Fourier analyzer. This figure illustrates how a Fourier analyzer evaluates the envelope-following responses to a white noise which is modulated by a frequency that is swept from 10 to 100 Hz. The upper left shows the sweep of the modulation frequency. This then modulates a white noise (lower left) and presents this to the subject. While the stimulus is being presented, the sine and the cosine of the modulating frequency are multiplied with the amplified EEG activity recorded from the subject's scalp. The filtered outputs of the multipliers provide the real and imaginary components (x and y) of the response at the instantaneous frequency of modulation. The amplitude of the response can then be computed (as the square root of the sum of the squares of the real and imaginary values) and plotted against the modulation frequency. The data displayed in the bottom right of the figure demonstrate a peak at 40–45 Hz (the time axis of the graph goes from 10 to 100 Hz).*

the amplitude of ongoing speech—the "speech envelope"—are very important to perception. These rhythms vary in frequency more than can easily be handled by a Fourier analyzer. Correlational techniques may be helpful in seeing how the brain follows this envelope (Aiken & Picton, 2008a). The recorded response is cross-correlated to the envelope signal at different delays. The highest correlation indicates how well the brain is following the speech envelope and the latency where the correlation is highest indicates the timing of this following response.

EVALUATING SIGNALS IN THE FREQUENCY DOMAIN

The frequency domain is a magical kingdom where everything that is in the time domain appears different. We know that being able to move from one domain to the other is helpful when we consider the acoustics of sound. A tone pip can be described in the time domain in terms of its duration and rise and fall times. Other sounds are more easily understood from a frequency perspective. The essential nature of a vowel sound is in its bands of frequency—formants. Nevertheless, the views can complement each other. The spread of frequencies in the tone-pip's spectrum can explain why it does not sound like a pure tone. The temporal periodicity of the vowel shows its vocal pitch. Likewise, auditory EPs often are best viewed in both time and frequency domains. Although the ABR typically is measured in the time domain, the spectrum of the ABR will show us how to set our recording filters. Although the ASSR usually is evaluated in the frequency domain, the time course of ASSR development—how long it takes

to reach a stable value after the onset of the stimulus—can help us to assess the integration time for auditory processing. In recent years, we have begun to use the frequency domain more extensively. This is the home of the brain's rhythms, the complex patterns of activity that follow stimulus changes and that synchronize and desynchronize during information processing. If we want to understand how the brain processes sounds, we need to become fluent in the languages of both time and frequency.

ABBREVIATIONS

AD	Analog-to-digital
ASSR	Auditory steady-state response
EEG	Electroencephalography
EP	Evoked potential
ERD	Event-related desynchronization
ERD	Event-related synchronization
FFT	Fast Fourier Transform
GBR	Gamma-band response
LAEP	Late auditory evoked potential
SNR	Signal-to-noise ratio
SP	Sustained potential

REFERENCES

Aiken, S. J., & Picton, T. W. (2006). Envelope following responses to natural vowels. *Audiology and Neurotology, 11*, 213–232.

Aiken, S. J., & Picton, T. W. (2008a). Human cortical responses to the speech envelope. *Ear and Hearing, 15*, 139–157.

Aiken, S. J., & Picton, T. W. (2008b). Envelope and spectral frequency following responses to vowel sounds. *Hearing Research, 245,* 35–47.

Bijl, G. K., & Veringa, F. (1985). Neural conduction time and steady-state evoked potentials. *Electroencephalography and Clinical Neurophysiology, 62,* 465–467.

Cacace, A. T., & McFarland, D. J. (2003). Spectral dynamics of electroencephalographic activity during auditory information processing. *Hearing Research, 176,* 25–41.

David, O., Kliner, J. M., & Friston, K. J. (2006). Mechanisms of evoked and induced responses in MEG/EEG. *NeuroImage, 31,* 1580–1591.

Diamond, A. L. (1977). Latency of the steady state visual evoked potential. *Electroencephalography and Clinical Neurophysiology, 42,* 125–127.

Elberling, C., Don, M., Cebulla, M., & Stürzebecher, E. (2007). Auditory steady-state responses to chirp stimuli based on cochlear traveling wave delay. *Journal of the Acoustical Society of America, 122,* 2772–2785.

Engel, A. K., & Singer, W. (2001). Temporal binding and the neural correlates of sensory awareness. *Trends in Cognitive Science, 5,* 16–25.

Galambos, R. (1992). A comparison of certain gamma band (40-Hz) brain rhythms in cat and man. In E. Baflar & T. H. Bullock (Eds.), *Induced rhythms in the brain* (pp. 201–216). Boston, MA: Birkhäuser.

Hari, R., Hämäläinen, M., & Joutsiniemi, S. L. (1989). Neuromagnetic steady-state responses to auditory stimuli. *Journal of the Acoustical Society of America, 86,* 1033–1039.

Hari, R., Salmelin, R., Mäkelä, J. P., Salenius, S., & Helle, M. (1997). Magnetoencephalographic cortical rhythms. *International Journal of Psychophysiology, 26,* 51–62.

Jensen, O., Kaiser, J., & Lachaux, J. P. (2007). Human gamma-frequency oscillations associated with attention and memory. *Trends in Neuroscience, 30,* 317–324.

John, M. S., Lins, O. G., Boucher, B. L., & Picton, T. W. (1998). Multiple auditory steady state responses (MASTER): Stimulus and recording parameters. *Audiology, 37,* 59–82.

John, M. S., & Picton, T. W. (2000). Human auditory steady-state responses to amplitude-modulated tones: phase and latency measurements. *Hearing Research, 141,* 57–79.

John, M. S., & Purcell, D. W. (2008). Introduction to technical principles of auditory steady-state response testing. In G. Rance (Ed.), *The auditory steady-state response* (pp. 11–53). San Diego, CA: Plural.

Lyons, R. G. (2004). *Understanding digital signal processing* (2nd ed.). Upper Saddle River, NJ: Prentice-Hall.

Makeig, S., Delorme, A., Westerfield, M., Jung, T.-P., Townsend, J., Courchesne, E., & Sejnowski, T. J. (2004). Electroencephalographic brain dynamics following visual targets requiring manual responses, *PLoS Biology, 2,* 747–762.

Makeig, S., Westerfield, M., Jung, T. P., Enghoff, S., Townsend, J., Courchesne, E., & Sejnowski, T. J. (2002). Dynamic brain sources of visual evoked responses. *Science, 295,* 690–694.

Mäkinen, V., Tiitinen, H., & May, P. (2005). Auditory event-related responses are generated independently of ongoing brain activity. *NeuroImage, 24,* 961–968.

Mazaheri, A., & Jensen, O. (2006). Posterior alpha activity is not phase-reset by visual stimuli. *Proceedings of the National Academy of Sciences (USA), 103,* 2948–2952.

Mazaheri, A., & Picton, T. W. (2005). EEG spectral dynamics during discrimination of auditory and visual targets. *Cognitive Brain Research, 24,* 81–96.

McFarland, D. J, & Cacace, A. T. (2004). Separating stimulus-locked and unlocked components of the auditory event-related potential. *Hearing Research, 193,* 111–120.

Neely, S. T., Norton, S. J., Gorga, M. P., & Jesteadt, W. (1988). Latency of auditory brain-stem responses and otoacoustic emissions using tone-burst stimuli. *Journal of the Acoustical Society of America, 83,* 652–656.

Pantev, C., Elbert, T., Makeig, S., Hampson, S., Eulitz, C., & Hoke, M. (1993). Relationship of transient and steady-state auditory evoked fields. *Electroencephalography and Clinical Neurophysiology, 88,* 389–396.

Pantev, C., Makeig, S., Hoke, M., Galambos, R., Hampson, S., & Gallen, C. (1991). Human auditory evoked gamma-band magnetic fields. *Proceedings of the National Academy of Sciences (USA), 88,* 8996–9000.

Pfurtscheller, G., & Lopes da Silva, F. H. (1999). Event-related EEG/MEG synchronization and desynchronization: Basic principles. *Clinical Neurophysiology, 110,* 1842–1857.

Picton, T. W., John, M. S., Purcell, D. W., & Plourde, G. (2003). Human auditory steady-state responses: Effects of recording technique and state of arousal. *Anesthesia & Analgesia, 97,* 1396–1402.

Picton, T. W., van Roon, P., & John, M. S. (2007). Human auditory steady-state responses during sweeps of intensity. *Ear and Hearing, 28,* 542–557.

Purcell, D. W., John, M. S., Schneider, B. A., & Picton, T. W. (2004). Human temporal auditory acuity as assessed by envelope following responses. *Journal of the Acoustical Society of America, 116,* 3581–3593.

Regan, D. (1977). Evoked potentials in basic and clinical research. In A. Rémond (Ed.), *EEG informatics: A didactic review of methods and applications of EEG data processing.* (pp. 319–346). Amsterdam, The Netherlands: Elsevier.

Regan, D. (1989). *Human brain electrophysiology: Evoked potentials and evoked magnetic fields in science and medicine.* New York, NY: Elsevier.

Rizzuto, D. S., Madsen, J. R., Bromfield, E. B., Schulze-Bonhage, A., Seelig, D., Aschenbrenner-Scheibe, R., & Kahana, M. J. (2003). Reset of human neocortical oscillations during a working memory task. *Proceedings of the National Academy of Sciences (USA), 100,* 7931–7936.

Ross, B., Picton, T. W., & Pantev, C. (2002). Temporal integration in the human auditory cortex as represented by the development of the steady-state magnetic field. *Hearing Research, 165,* 68–84.

Sayers, B. M., & Beagley, H. A (1974). Objective evaluation of auditory evoked EEG responses. *Nature, 251,* 608–609.

Sayers, B. M., Beagley, H. A., & Henshall, W. R. (1974). The mechanism of auditory evoked EEG responses. *Nature, 247,* 481–4833.

Schniter, P. (2005, October 5). *Time-frequency uncertainty principle.* Retrieved from the Connexions Web site: http://cnx.org/content/m10416/2.18/

Schoonhoven, R., Boden, C. J., Verbunt, J. P., & de Munck, J. C. (2003). A whole head MEG study of the amplitude-modulation-following response: Phase coherence, group delay and dipole source analysis. *Clinical Neurophysiology, 114,* 2096–2106.

Shah, A. S. , Bressler, S. L., Knuth, K. H., Ding, M., Mehta, A. D., Ulbert, I., & Schroeder, C. E. (2004). Neural dynamics and the fundamental mechanisms of event-related brain potentials. *Cerebral Cortex, 14,* 476–483.

Tallon-Baudry, C., & Bertrand, O. (1999). Oscillatory gamma activity in humans and its role in object representation. *Trends in Cognitive Science, 3,* 151–162.

Tallon-Baudry, C., Bertrand, O., Delpuech, C., & Permier, J. (1997). Oscillatory gamma-band (30–70 Hz) activity induced by a visual search task in humans. *Journal of Neuroscience, 17,* 722–734.

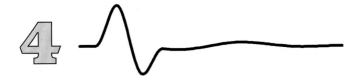

Finding Sources:
Forward and Backward

Wie schwer sind nicht die Mittel zu erwerben
Durch die man zu den Quellen steigt?
Und eh man nur den halben Weg erreicht
Muss wohl ein armer Teufel sterben.

(How hard is it not to find the means
Whereby to reach the sources?
Before reaching only half the way
We poor devils have to die.)

Goethe, *Faust*, Part 1, lines 562–565

Evoked potentials (EPs) are recorded by placing electrodes at different locations in an electric field and recording how this field changes over time in response to a stimulus. Understanding the auditory EPs requires that we know something about the electric fields that are generated by the auditory nervous system as it responds to sounds. Auditory EPs recorded from the human scalp are generated by the separation of charges across membranes in the cells of the ear and the nervous system. To begin this chapter, we review the auditory pathways from the cochlea to the cortex. This sets the stage for the activity that occurs when sounds are processed. Then we consider the physiology of cell membranes and the potentials they can generate. Finally, we look at the relations between what is going on in the brain and what is recorded at the scalp to see if we can derive the intracranial sources from scalp recordings. This entails forward and inverse solutions—the forward and backward of our subtitle. We will find that we can never really define the sources exactly—hence the regret in the quotation from Faust. Nevertheless, we can make reasonable inferences about where in the brain the electrical fields are coming from, particularly if we bring to bear information from other experiments: studying human cerebral blood flow, evaluating the effects of lesions in animal and man, and recording intracranial electric fields. The prognosis for understanding the sources is not as limited as in the days of Goethe.

This chapter is brief and simple, discussing only what is essential for understanding the auditory EPs. More about the cochlea and its potentials is presented in Chapter 7. Møller (2006a) and Pickles (2008) provide more extensive reviews of the anatomy and physiology of the auditory system. Works such as Nicholls, Martin, Wallace, and Fuchs (2001) can be consulted for more details about neuronal physiology, and Nunez and Srinivasan (2005) for the biophysics of electrical and magnetic fields.

ANATOMY OF THE AUDITORY PATHWAYS

Auditory Nerve

The neurons of the auditory nerve are bipolar. Each neuron has a peripheral process that synapses with a hair cell. Most of the afferent neurons connect with only one inner hair cell, and thus the receptive field (or tuning curve) of the neuron is the same as that of the hair cell. In some ways, the peripheral process is like a dendrite in that it receives synaptic input, but in other ways it is like an axon as it generates and conducts action potentials (APs). The cell bodies are located around the central modiolus (axis) of the cochlea, forming a spiral ganglion. The central axons of auditory neurons travel in the auditory nerve through the temporal bone in the internal auditory meatus, which opens into the posterior cranial fossa. In the internal

auditory meatus, the auditory nerve runs together with the vestibular nerve, both being considered part of the eighth cranial nerve, and with the seventh or facial nerve. This is where the acoustic neuroma arises (although the tumor derives from the myelin sheath of the vestibular nerve and is actually a vestibular schwannoma, thus neither auditory nor neuroma). The human auditory nerve then traverses the subarachnoid space—a distance of about 15 mm (Lang, 1985)—to enter the brainstem at the junction of the pons and the medulla. In small mammals, the brainstem is almost directly adjacent to the meatus. The subarachnoid extent of the human auditory nerve (together with the greater conductivity of the cerebrospinal fluid in the subarachnoid space) may be one of the reasons for wave II in the human auditory brainstem response (ABR). ABRs of smaller mammals usually do not have anything clearly homologous to wave II.

Auditory Brainstem and Thalamus

The major auditory regions of the brainstem and their connections are illustrated in Figure 4–1, which views the brainstem from the side, and Figure 4–2, which views the auditory pathways from the back. All fibers from the cochlea synapse in the cochlear nucleus. This nucleus has dorsal and ventral divisions, with the ventral division being further subdivided into anterior and posterior parts. The only place in the brainstem where a lesion can cause a unilateral hearing loss is in the dorsolateral pons (affecting the cochlear nucleus and its axons) as beyond the cochlear nucleus the auditory pathways carry information from both ears. Neurons from all parts of the cochlear nucleus send axons to the

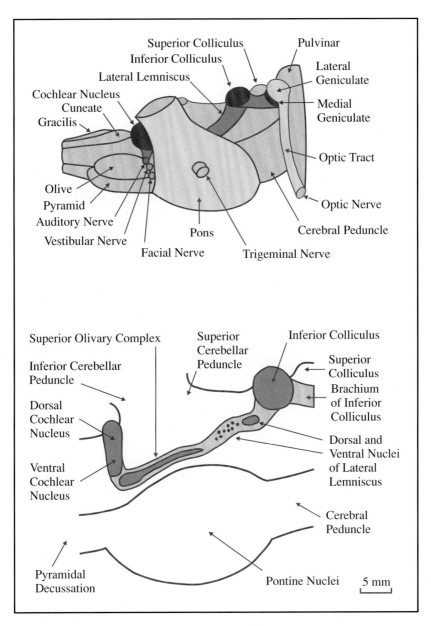

Figure 4–1. *Lateral views of human auditory brainstem pathways.*
The top half of the figure shows a lateral view of the human brainstem with the most important landmarks indicated. The auditory pathway is shown in darker gray with the nuclei indicated in black. The bottom half of the figure uses a see-through brainstem to show the course of the auditory pathways in the pons. This diagram is based on the work of Moore (1987a, 1987b). The human superior olivary complex is mainly composed of medial and lateral superior olivary nuclei and scattered peri-olivary nuclei.

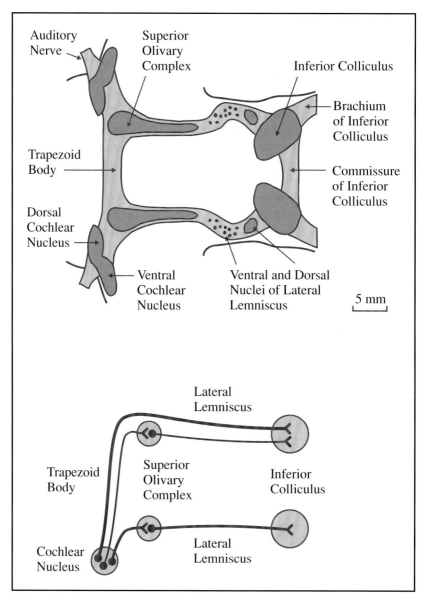

Figure 4–2. *Posterior views of human auditory brainstem pathways. The top half of the figure uses a see-through brainstem to show the course of the ascending auditory pathways. This diagram is similar in scale to the bottom of Figure 4–1. The bottom half of the figure shows a schematic of the three most prominent pathways from the cochlear nucleus to the inferior colliculus. Many other connections occur but most fibers follow one of these three paths. Both diagrams are based on the work of Moore (1987a, 1987b).*

inferior colliculus. The ventral nuclei also send axons to the superior olivary complex, a set of neurons (medial and lateral superior olivary nuclei together with scattered peri-olivary nuclei) in the anterior pons. The superior olive is located above the inferior olive in the medulla, a nucleus in the motor system that has the external shape of an olive. However, the superior olive looks nothing like an olive.

Fibers crossing the midline (from either the cochlear nucleus or the superior olive) travel in the trapezoid body. This band of fibers rests in the anterior pons and is seen in cross sections of the pons as a trapezoid (a quadrilateral with two sides parallel, in this case posterior and anterior). The trapezoid body perhaps is similar to the optic chiasm in the visual system. The optic chiasm takes fibers from the left eye, which are activated from the left side, and transfers them to the right optic tract (and vice versa for the right eye's right-side fibers). This serves to organize visual input on the basis of perceived left or right hemispace rather than left or right eye. The crossing fibers in the trapezoid body may do something similar in the auditory system, although auditory space is much more complicated in its coding than visual space (involving relative timing and intensity of stimulation rather than particular afferent fibers).

The superior olivary complex is the first place in the auditory pathway where information from one ear can be compared to information from the other ear to determine the location of a sound. Fibers from the cochlear nucleus and from both superior olives travel upward and backward to the inferior colliculus (little hill) in the lateral lemniscus (ribbon). The lateral lemniscus is so named because it travels laterally (and later posteriorly) to the medial lemniscus, which carries somato-sensory fibers. Ventral and dorsal nuclei occur in the lateral lemnisci but in human subjects the ventral nuclei are not well organized. The inferior colliculus sends most of its axons to the medial geniculate (little elbow) body in the posterior thalamus through the brachium (arm) of the inferior colliculus.

The auditory pathway in the brainstem is parallel, bilateral, and divergent. The cochlear nucleus sends fibers to all the other nuclei of the brainstem auditory system (Cant & Benson, 2003). Beyond the cochlear nucleus, nothing is activated by just one ear. The number of fibers in the brachium of the inferior colliculus is approximately 10 times more than in the auditory nerve (Møller, 2006a). Auditory information clearly is being repeated in many different ways as it ascends the brainstem. Numerous other auditory connections occur through the reticular formation and bypass the canonical auditory path— these fibers are called extralemniscal.

As well as the ascending pathway, the brainstem also contains multiple descending fibers. These come back down all the way from the cerebral cortex to the cochlea. The final common pathway for the descending system runs from the superior olivary complex to the cochlea in the olivocochlear bundle. The fibers of this bundle synapse mainly on the external hair cells. These cells act like tiny muscles and modulate the tenseness of the connection between their hairs and the tectorial membrane. In this manner, the external hair cells can adjust the tuning and sensitivity of the transduction process.

In the thalamus, the auditory system is represented mainly in the medial geniculate body, which has three main parts: ventral, dorsal, and medial (Hackett, 2007). The ventral division is the main way station of the primary (or lemniscal) auditory pathway and projects to the core area of the primary auditory cortex. The dorsal division receives both lemniscal and extra-lemniscal fibers and projects to the belt area of the auditory cortex. The medial division receives input from other sensory systems as well as the auditory and projects more widely to the cortex.

Auditory Cortices

The human auditory cortex is located mainly on the superior surface of the temporal lobe. The upper part of Figure 4–3 shows its position in the human brain, and the lower part of the figure shows the superior surface of the temporal lobes viewed from above. On this surface, we can usually identify an anterolaterally oriented Heschl's gyrus. However, the gyral patterns in this area are notoriously variable from one individual to another and from one side to another in the same individual (Rademacher et al., 2001). Sometimes there are two or three Heschl's gyri instead of just one (Penhune, Zatorre, MacDonald, & Evans, 1996). The primary auditory cortex is located on the medial half of these gyri. However, the exact location varies greatly (Morosan et al., 2001). In general, the primary auditory cortex is more anterior on the right hemisphere than on the left (Penhune et al., 1996; Rademacher et al., 2001; Warrier et al., 2009).

The primary auditory cortex (also called "core") is surrounded by auditory association areas that are now called "belt" and "parabelt" (Hackett, 2007; Kaas & Hackett, 2000; Wessinger et al., 2001). The parabelt regions extend anteriorly toward the temporal pole, back onto the planum temporale, and out onto the superior temporal gyrus on the lateral surface of the temporal lobe. Information tends to travel outward from the core to the belt and parabelt regions, which then projects to other regions of the cortex. Particular parts of the belt and parabelt may subserve particular auditory processes, but these have not yet been fully identified. Anterolateral regions may be important for processing pitch and posterolateral regions for spatial location (Warren & Griffiths, 2003).

The left and right auditory cortices are asymmetrically activated by different types of auditory information. The left hemisphere is particularly activated by increasing the temporal complexity of a sound, whereas the right is more attuned to spectral complexity (Warrier et al., 2009; Zatorre & Belin, 2001).

Many regions of the auditory cortex are organized tonotopically. Auditory neurons usually are most sensitive to a particular frequency of sound, and there is a progressive change in the characteristic frequency of the neurons as we move in a certain direction across the cortex. Thus, we can construct maps of the cortex according to the frequency preference of its neurons. Recent functional magnetic resonance imaging (fMRI) of the human auditory cortex has shown multiple maps (Talavage et al., 2004; Woods & Alain, 2009). Most of the maps (including those that involve the primary or core cortex) go from high frequencies medially to low frequencies laterally. However, some maps travel in the opposite direction. Different components of the human auditory evoked potential (EP) can show different tonotopic organizations. This is most easily seen using magnetoencephalography (MEG), which localizes dipole sources more precisely than electroencephalography (EEG). The sources of the Pa wave of the middle latency response (MLR) go from low frequencies medially to high frequencies laterally, whereas the sources of the N1 wave of the late auditory evoked

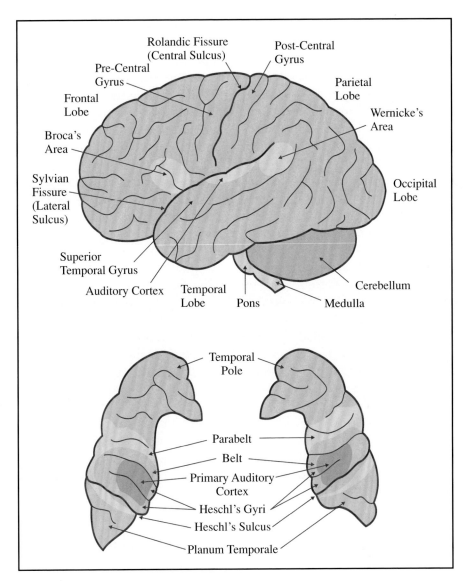

Figure 4–3. Human auditory cortex. *The upper part of the figure shows the human brain viewed from the left. The human auditory cortex is mainly located on the superior surface of the temporal lobe within the Sylvian fissure. The lower diagram shows the top view of both temporal lobes. The primary auditory cortex is located on the medial part of Heschl's gyri although the gyral patterns and the exact location of the cortex vary from subject to subject and from hemisphere to hemisphere. The primary auditory cortex is surrounded by belt and parabelt areas. The right auditory cortex is a little anterior to that on the left. The diagrams derive loosely from the findings of Hackett (2007) and Rademacher et al. (2001).*

potential (LAEP) are organized in the opposite direction (Pantev et al., 1995). The orientations of the dipole sources also change with frequency. The sources for the 40-Hz auditory steady-state response (ASSR) are organized similarly to the N1

(Pantev, Roberts, Elbert, Ross, & Wien-bruch, 1996).

The planum temporale behind Heschl's sulcus receives substantial input from auditory cortex. This region may serve as a "computational hub" for the segregation and matching of spectrotemporal patterns (Griffiths & Warren, 2002; Kumar, Stephan, Warren, Friston, & Griffiths, 2007). The planum temporale is geometrically asymmetric between the two hemispheres, being smaller in area and tilted more superiorly in the right hemisphere (Dorsaint-Pierre et al., 2006).

Recently, several studies have indicated that the auditory system may be similar to the visual system in projecting information into two different streams for the evaluation of the "what?" or the "where?" (Alain, Arnott, Hevenor, Graham, & Grady, 2001; Barrett & Hall, 2006; Wang, Wu, & Li, 2008). Analysis of object identity occurs by projections to the lateral and anterior regions of the temporal lobe and thence to the inferior regions of dorsolateral frontal cortex. Spatial location is analyzed in projections to the parietal lobe and more dorsal regions of the frontal lobe.

MEMBRANE POTENTIALS

Basic Concepts of Electricity

Electricity derives from the properties of subatomic particles—most importantly, electrons and protons, which have an electric charge that is either negative or positive. Like charges repel each other and unlike charges attract. Thus, when unlike charges are separated from each other, a field of force develops that will move a charged probe away from the region with the same charge and toward the region

with the opposite charge. This force or potential is measured in volts. If the regions of positive and negative charge are connected by a conductor, charged particles will move along the conductor as an electric current measured in amps. Current flows from positive toward negative (even though the current flow often is carried by electrons moving in the opposite direction). How poorly or how well the current flows is measured as the resistance (measured in ohms) or conductance (measured in mhos). The unit of conductance—mho—is ohm spelt backwards. Ohm's law states that the voltage is the product of the current and the resistance. Two simple concepts can be derived from this relationship. If the amount of current is the same in conductors of different resistance, the voltage is higher across the conductor with the greater resistance. Second, if the voltage is the same, more current will flow in a conductor of lower resistance. In electric circuits, the flow of current generally is mediated by electrons. In physiological systems, the flow of current most commonly is mediated by charged particles called ions.

Membrane Resting Potential

The concentration of charged ions inside a cell differs from their concentration outside the cell. Specific intracellular concentrations are necessary for the proper function of the enzymes and organelles within the cell. Most importantly, potassium ions are more highly concentrated inside and sodium ions more highly concentrated outside the cell. Ions tend to diffuse from regions of high concentration to regions of low concentration. The transmembrane differences in ionic concentration therefore must be maintained by a molecular pump that moves potassium ions into the cell and sodium ions out. The cell membrane contains channels that are permeable to the different ions. Ions diffuse through these channels (from high to low concentration) until a field is set up across the membrane that exerts an electric force equal and opposite to the diffusion force. In the normal neuron, potassium channels are the most permeable of the ionic channels and the cell membrane becomes polarized near the equilibrium potential determined by the internal and external concentrations of this ion. The resting potential of a normal neuron makes the intracellular fluid about −70 mV relative to the extracellular fluid.

Action Potentials (APs)

Certain cells—muscle cells, neurons—are "excitable" and can undergo dramatic changes in their membrane potential. Figure 4–4 shows a prototypical mammalian neuron. Real neurons come in all shapes and sizes; some have no dendritic tree, others have no myelin, others have a cell body that simply serves to maintain a long axon. The neuron is a communication device. Its three main parts are the dendrites, which receive and integrate information; the axon, which transmits information; and the cell body, which maintains and powers the device. The axon is surrounded by specialized glial cells called Schwann cells. If the axon is myelinated, these cells wrap themselves repeatedly around the axon to form a myelin sheath, which serves to insulate the axon and to make it transmit information more rapidly.

Some regions of the neuronal membrane have special voltage-sensitive sodium channels. In a myelinated neuron, these regions are the axon hillock at the beginning of the axon, and the nodes of Ranvier (small gaps in the myelin sheath). If the membrane potential in these regions reaches a threshold level (about −50 mV), a conformational change in the membrane channels causes them to suddenly and transiently open. This allows free passage of sodium ions from outside to inside the neuron. The membrane loses its potassium-based resting potential (depolarizes) and becomes briefly governed by the sodium equilibrium potential (+55 mV). However, because the change in the channels is transient, the membrane potential never quite reaches the sodium equilibrium potential level, and the membrane quickly changes back to its original level (repolarizes). The membrane actually becomes a little more polarized than it was before (hyperpolarized) and therefore less susceptible to excitation (refractory). This sequence of voltage changes is the AP. It is also known as a neuronal discharge or firing; the nerve cell has been primed by the sodium pump and then is triggered by a stimulus to generate the AP.

The movement of the sodium ions into the neuron causes a transient decrease of positive ions in the extracellular fluid. This is called a current "sink." Positive ions from neighboring regions flow toward this sink. The increased positive ions within the cell diffuse along the axon and exit through the cell membrane into the neighboring extracellular regions. Thus, a current circuit is set up with positive ions flowing into the cell at the point of depolarization and out of the cell at neighboring regions. This current can cause the neuronal membrane further along the axon to decrease its normal transmembrane potential. If this region has voltage-sensitive sodium channels, a new AP will be generated when threshold levels are reached. In this

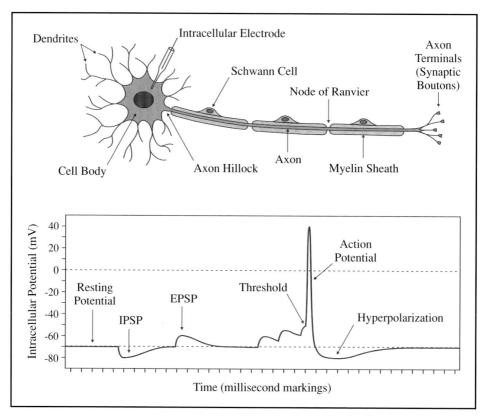

Figure 4–4. *Action potentials (AP) in a neuron. The upper part of the figure shows a prototypical neuron with a myelinated axon. The lower part of the figure shows an intra-cellular recording. Postsynaptic potentials increase (inhibitory) or decrease (excitatory) the polarization of the cell membrane. If the depolarization of the membrane reaches a critical threshold level, voltage-dependent sodium channels undergo a sudden conformational change and allow sodium ions to move through the membrane. The membrane potential abruptly and briefly reverses polarity—the AP. Following the AP there is some hyperpolarization and then the normal resting potential.*

way, the AP regenerates itself and propagates along the axon away from the axon hillock toward the axon terminals.

The transmission of an AP along a myelinated axon differs from that along an unmyelinated axon in two ways. First, the greater resistance between the intracellular fluid and the extracellular fluid caused by the myelin forces the intracellular current to go farther along the axon before exiting the neuron at a point where there is no myelin—the node of Ranvier. Second, the only region of the membrane that is excitable (i.e., contains voltage sensitive sodium channels) is at the node of Ranvier. The AP therefore jumps from one node of Ranvier to the next. This "saltatory" (jumping) conduction is much faster than conduction along an unmyelinated axon.

Synapses

Neurons connect to each other through synapses. At a neuron's axon terminals, where it attaches to the dendrite or cell body of a second neuron, there is a small swelling (the synaptic bouton) containing vesicles of synaptic transmitter. When the AP reaches this nerve ending, it releases the transmitter, which alters the conductance of the ion channels in the postsynaptic membrane of the second neuron. This causes the membrane to change its potential—to depolarize if the synapse is excitatory and to hyperpolarize if it is inhibitory. The various changes in potential over the cell body and dendrites caused by synaptic activation spread toward the axon hillock of the second neuron. If the sum of all the potential changes is sufficient to reach the threshold potential, an AP is generated in the second neuron.

DIPOLE FIELDS

The flow of ions in the extracellular fluid will set up potential fields that can be recorded at a distance. The fields that result from multiple sources and sinks can be very complex. For simplicity, we look first at the field generated from one source and one sink: a dipole. More complicated fields can then be interpreted by converting them into multiple dipoles.

The field set up by a dipole and the currents that it sets up in a volume conductor are shown in Figure 4–5. In a two-dimensional figure (upper left), the voltages can be represented by equipotential lines. These are like the contours on a

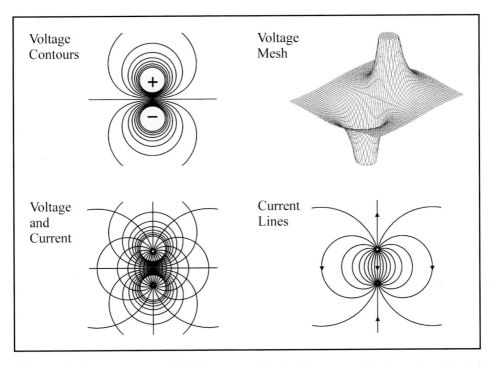

Figure 4–5. Four ways of looking at a dipole. *The upper left shows the potential field; the contours connect points of equal voltage. The upper right shows a view of the field using a mesh to give the semblance of three dimensions. The view is from the lower right a little above the field. The lower left shows the lines of current connecting the source and sink; these lines follow the slope of the field across the voltage contours. The lower right shows the lines of current by themselves.*

topographic map with the positive showing as a mountain and negative as a valley (upper right). Current flows from high potential to low potential—the lines of current run perpendicular to the potential lines (lower left).

When a dipole field is set up in a volume conductor, the extent of the field will depend on the size and shape of the volume conductor and its resistance. Current will flow more readily through regions or layers of low resistance (Ohm's law states that for a given voltage the current is greater when the resistance is lower). A four-sphere model of the head contains a spherical brain surrounded by three shells: cerebrospinal fluid, skull, and scalp (Berg & Scherg, 1994). The resistance of the skull to the passage of current is higher than that of the other tissues and the scalp recorded potential therefore is smaller than would be expected if the conductivity of the head were homogenous. Much of the current generated by intracerebral dipoles will flow through the cerebrospinal fluid on the outside of the brain and only a little will flow through the skull to reach the scalp.

EP FIELDS IN THE EXTRACELLULAR FLUIDS

Compound Action Potentials

When an AP is generated, positive ions enter the neuron. This current sink is associated with a negative potential in the extracellular fluid. Current flows toward this sink from adjacent regions, which act as relative current sources. These currents act to maintain charge equilibrium. The currents thus flow in circles: into the cell at the point where the AP is being gener-

ated and then out of the cell at some distance along the axon (in both directions), and back through the extracellular fluids to the active region.

As an AP is conducted along an axon, an electrode near the axon will record a positive-negative-positive sequence of changes, as the region of the electrode changes from source to sink to source (Schoonhoven & Stegeman, 1991). These changes are illustrated in Figure 4–6.

In the mammalian nervous systems, the axons of many different neurons typ-

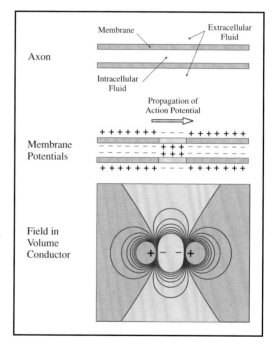

Figure 4–6. Action potential (AP) in a volume conductor. *The upper part of the figure shows a longitudinal section through the axon and the wave of depolarization that occurs in the axonal membrane as the AP propagates along the axon. The fields in the extracellular fluid can be considered as a quadripole, a combination of a leading dipole and a trailing dipole. A quadripole generates the field shown in the bottom half of the figure.*

ically run together in peripheral nerves or in central tracts. The compound action potential (CAP) recorded from a nerve or a tract represents the superimposed potentials of all the active axons. How large a response is recorded is determined by the degree of synchrony among the fibers. If they all discharge at the same time, their fields superimpose and the CAP is large. If there is temporal jitter between the discharges, the positive fields of one fiber will cancel out the negative fields of another and vice versa, so that the CAP becomes small. When the conduction velocities of the fibers differ, the APs of the fibers with slower conduction velocity will arrive later at a particular recording point along the nerve than fibers with faster conduction velocity. This dispersion of the timing will increase with increasing distance traveled. Thus, the CAP decreases in amplitude as it travels farther away from site where the APs were initiated.

The concept of synchrony also explains why a sustained stimulus generates a large CAP at the onset of the stimulus and no further response (even though the individual fibers keep responding during the duration of the stimulus). The fibers all start to discharge at the onset of a stimulus but then continue at different rates. The fiber discharges thus are synchronous at the onset but afterward occur with random timing relative to each other. Thus, a CAP occurs only at the onset of sustained activity in many fibers of a nerve. After the onset, the fields of the randomly firing neurons will cancel each other out.

At a distance away from the nerve, the amplitude of the recorded CAP decreases significantly. The length over which the nerve fiber is depolarized during an AP is of the order of several centimeters; it varies with the conduction velocity. If we are recording at a distance away from the fiber that is significantly greater than that length, the leading and following source regions will contribute almost as much to the field as the sink caused by the AP, and the change caused by the AP will be very small. The extracellular sources and sinks around the region of the axon that is depolarized during the AP can be considered as a quadripole, composed of leading and trailing dipoles with opposite orientation. The field of a quadripole (see Figure 4–6) falls off at a distance much more rapidly than the field of a dipole (by the cube of the distance rather than its square) (Nunez & Srinivasan, 2005). In general, we record very little at the scalp surface from APs within the skull.

However, there are definite exceptions to this generalization. If the volume conductor through which the AP travels changes its characteristics (shape, resistance), or if the AP moves along a curved path, stationary dipole fields can occur and these can be recorded at some distance from their generation. This phenomenon was first described by Stegeman, van Oosterom, and Colon (1987; see also Stegeman, Dumitru, King, & Roeleveld, 1997) in mathematical models of the CAP. Jewett and his colleagues (Deupree & Jewett, 1988; Jewett, Deupree, & Bommannan, 1990) then demonstrated the effects in physiological recordings from nerves. Figure 4–7 illustrates these concepts.

The passage of the CAP of the cochlear nerve from the internal auditory meatus to the cerebrospinal fluid of the cerebellopontine angle represents a significant change in the resistance of the volume conductor. The resultant stationary potential likely contributes to wave II of the

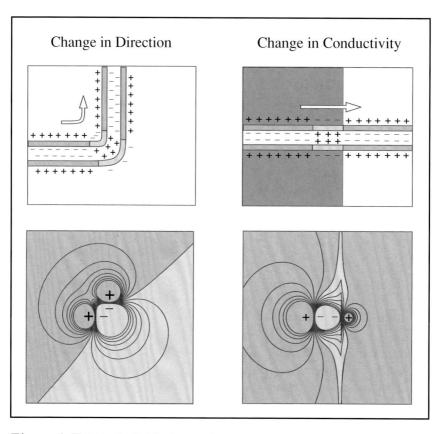

Figure 4–7. *Dipole fields during the propagation of the action potential (AP). Two examples are shown. On the left, the AP moves through a right-angle turn in the axon. At the moment the AP is at the turn, the leading dipole is oriented in one direction and the trailing dipole in another. This leads to a dipolar field pattern oriented at 45° to the two orientations. On the right, the AP leaves a region with low conductivity and enters a region with higher conductivity. The potential fields do not spread as far when the conductivity is high. This causes an imbalance in the fields ahead and behind the AP. At the moment that the AP exits the region of low conductivity, an electrode behind the propagating AP becomes positive relative to an electrode ahead of the AP.*

human scalp recorded ABR. We will return to these conductance phenomena when we consider intracranial recordings from the auditory nerve during surgery in the posterior fossa. The curve of the fibers of the cochlear nucleus and superior olive as they traverse the pons and then continue upward as the lateral lemniscus may contribute to the ABR in the regions of wave IV and V. Nevertheless, the fibers are so short that they are overlapped by the postsynaptic potentials that lead to their initiation and the pre- and postsynaptic potentials that they bring about as the fibers terminate in the nuclei of the lateral lemniscus and the inferior colliculus. All processes may combine to give the electric fields that we record from the scalp.

Another situation in which an AP generates a dipole rather than quadripole occurs when the APs reach the axon terminals. Because the axon does not continue, there is no flow of currents distally to the terminals. An extracellular dipole is thus set up with a negative pole in the region of the terminals and a positive pole in proximal regions of the axon.

These dipolar AP fields are often considered as "far fields" because they can be recorded at larger distance away from their generation than the near fields. A characteristic of a "far field" recording is that, at a large distance from the sources and sinks that are generating the field, the field changes very slowly (Jewett & Williston, 1971). The exact location of the recording electrode therefore does not have a great effect on the recorded potential. Close to the generators (in the near field), the recording changes dramatically as the electrode is moved. The most dramatic change would be the negative to positive polarity reversal as the electrode moves from being close to the sink to close to the sources. However, all fields are generated by sources and sinks, and the generation of far fields is essentially the same as the generation of near fields. Far fields can be considered as dipole fields viewed at a distance. These dipoles may be generated by postsynaptic potentials or by APs traversing a change in the volume conductor.

Postsynaptic Potentials

Changes in ionic conductance at the postsynaptic membrane change the polarization of the neuron's membrane. Postsynaptic potentials typically last several to many milliseconds (an order of magnitude longer than the AP). Most neurons of the central nervous system have an extensive set of dendrites that receive input from multiple synapses. The postsynaptic potentials spread over the dendrites to reach the neuronal body and finally the axon hillock where voltage-sensitive sodium channels can generate an AP.

The current flow that occurs with the postsynaptic potentials is illustrated in the upper part of Figure 4–8 for a cortical pyramidal neuron. If the synapse on the apical dendrite is excitatory, the membrane depolarizes. Current flows into the dendrite and then along the axis of the dendrite and back into the extracellular fluid. Because of the geometry of the dendrite (which increases in diameter as it comes closer to the cell body), more of the intracellular current will flow toward the cell body than toward the tip of the dendrite. Although there will be two extracellular dipoles set up in association with the current flow, the one on the proximal side of the dendrite generally will be greater, and at a distance from the neuron, its dipole field will dominate. Thus, an excitatory synapse will create an extracellular dipole with a current sink (negative) in the region of the dendrite and a current source (positive) in the regions of the neuronal body.

The evoked potentials we record do not come from the fields generated by synaptic activity in a single neuron but from the fields generated by hundreds or thousands of neurons. We have already considered the role of synchrony in determining the amplitude of the CAP. Similar effects occur for synapses. The more synchronously the synapses of a particular

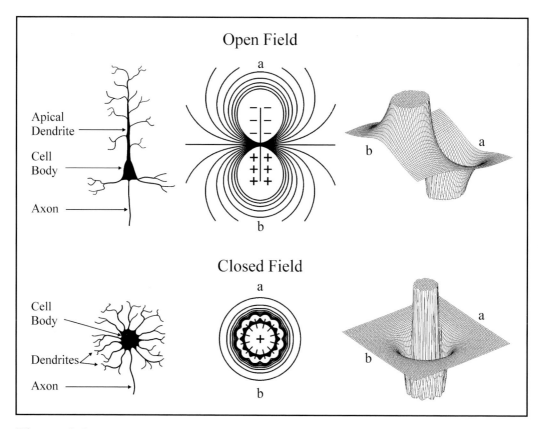

Figure 4–8. Open and closed fields. *The upper half of this figure shows the extracellular potentials that are set up in a cortical pyramidal cell. This neuron has its cell body within the deeper layers of the cortex and has a major dendrite that goes towards the cortical surface. When this apical dendrite is depolarized by excitatory synaptic activity, the extracellular region around the dendrite becomes a sink; positive ions enter the dendrite and the extracellular fluid becomes relatively negative. Currents flow inside the neuron and return to the extracellular fluid in the region of the cell body, causing an extracellular source. Thus, a dipole field is set up with the negative pole near the cortical surface (a) and the positive pole deep in the cortex (b). The right side of the figure shows the dipole viewed in three dimensions (the viewpoint is from the lower right). The field is "open" as it spreads beyond the immediate vicinity of the sources and sinks. Point a is negative and point b positive. The lower half of the figure shows what happens when the dendrites of a stellate neuron are all depolarized. Sinks are set up in the peripheral part of the neuron and sources occur near the cell body. All of the currents flow within the immediate vicinity of the neuron. Because there is no spread to more distant regions of the extracellular fluid, this is a "closed" field. The potential is zero at both point a and point b.*

region of the brain are activated, provided they are activated in the same way (excitatory or inhibitory), the greater the electric fields generated in the extracellular field.

Another major determinant of what might be recorded when neurons are activated is their geometric organization. This geometry involves two things: the arrangement of the dendrites and the arrangement of the neurons within an activated region. If dendrites radiate out in all directions around the cell body (e.g., in "stellate" or star neurons), widespread activation of these dendrites will cause a spherical sink (around the dendrites) surrounding a central source (around the cell body). At any distance away from the neuron, the fields created between the dendrites and the cell body will be randomly oriented with respect to each other and will cancel. Similarly, if neurons are arranged in a nucleus without any clear geometric organization, the various extracellular dipoles from the different neurons will be oriented in random directions and their fields will cancel themselves out at any distance away from the nucleus. These activation patterns create what Lorente de Nó (1947) called "closed fields." Currents do not spread beyond the immediate region of their generation. These are illustrated in the lower half of Figure 4–8.

However, many regions of the brain are organized geometrically. If neurons are set up in a layer and if they are activated so that the sources tend to be on one side of the layer and the sinks on the other, the fields add to each other rather than cancel each other out. Current then flows beyond the immediate vicinity of their generation and an "open field" is created (upper half of Figure 4–8). One example of an open field in the auditory system is in the superior olive. Here many neurons are "bipolar" with dendrites mainly oriented to one side or the other. Even the multipolar cells are asymmetrically activated by left ear or right ear input. The geometry of the neurons and/or their activation patterns set up laterally oriented dipole fields that sum together rather than cancel. Thus, we can record

clear dipole fields in the in the region of waves III to IV of ABR recorded between the two mastoids These dipole fields occur at the same time as other fields caused by the turning of axons into the lateral lemniscus.

The main example of open-field generation in the brain is in the cerebral cortex. Each cortical pyramidal cell has a large apical dendrite oriented toward the cortical surface. Excitation of many pyramidal cells at the level of the cell body, such as might occur with input to the cortex from specific thalamocortical afferents, causes an extracellular sink deep within the cortex. Most of the returning current flow comes from the dendrites; there is very little return through the descending axon as its surface area is minimal compared to that of the dendritic tree. Thus, an extracellular dipole is set up with the dendritic region positive and the region of the cell bodies negative. When multiple adjacent neurons are activated in a similar fashion, their dipole fields overlap to form a "dipole layer." This is illustrated diagrammatically in Figure 4–9.

An activated region of cortex, in which many neurons are synchronously active, generates a dipole layer over the area of its activation. The field generated at a particular location by the dipole layer varies with the solid angle (Ω) that the activated dipole layer subtends at the measuring point as well as by the square of the distance from the layer (discussed further by Gloor, 1985). As shown in Figure 4–9, beyond the immediate vicinity of the dipoles, the field pattern generated by a dipole layer is similar to that of a single dipole source located at the center of the activated region. Thus, we can model the electrical fields from a small region of cortex by means of an equivalent dipole.

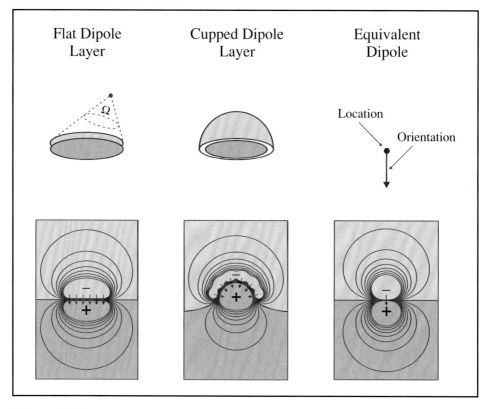

Figure 4–9. Dipole layers. *The left and middle sections of the figure show the electric fields for a flat dipole layer and for a dipole layer in the shape of a cup. The field depends on the solid angle (Ω)—a three-dimensional angle like a cone subtended by the layer at any particular location. Beyond the immediate vicinity, the field of a dipole layer is essentially the same as that of an equivalent dipole, located at the center of the area of the flat dipole or of the rim of a cupped dipole.*

If the dipole layer is curved, the equivalent dipole is localized to the center of the flat virtual surface connecting the edges of the curved surface (Malmivuo & Plonsey, 1995). The middle of Figure 4–9 shows the fields generated by a dipole layer in the shape of an upside-down cup. The equivalent dipole is located at the center of the cup's opening. This explains why cortical equivalent dipoles can be located below the curved surface of the gyri.

Multiple different processes occur in the cortex as it processes incoming information and many different types of cortical neurons are involved (Mitani et al., 1985; Møller, 2006a; Speckmann & Elger, 2005). Figure 4–10 illustrates diagrammatically some of the processes that occur in the cortex and the electrical fields that may result. The initial component of the cortical response is a small negative wave that in the human being peaks near 18 ms following a click. This likely results from the activity in the specific thalamocortical fibers themselves rather than from their synaptic effect on the pyramidal cells (Steinschneider et al., 1992). The wave of depolarization in the axons reaches the

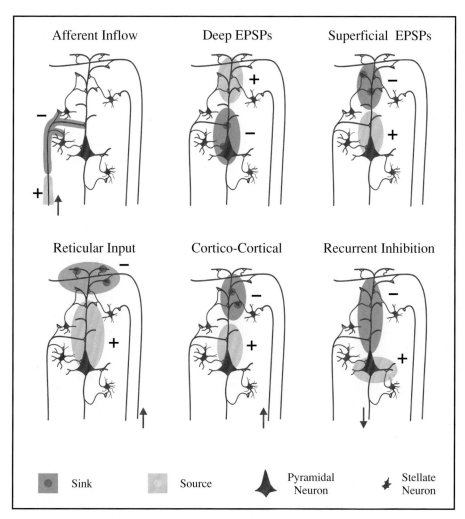

Afferent Inflow **Deep EPSPs** **Superficial EPSPs**

Reticular Input **Cortico-Cortical** **Recurrent Inhibition**

Sink   Source   Pyramidal Neuron   Stellate Neuron

Figure 4–10. *Electrophysiology of the cortex. This figure shows the dipole fields that result as various processes occur in auditory cortex. The cortex is represented by a few cells and connections with the dendrites and synapses accentuated. The cortical model is the same in each section. The upper left shows what occurs with afferent inflow to the cortex from the specific thalamic nucleus. As the action potentials reach the end of the fibers, the source around the distal axon can only get return current from its more proximal regions. The quadripole of Figure 4–6 is replaced by a simple dipole (the leading dipole is no longer), and a negative wave occurs at the cortical surface. The upper middle diagram shows the synaptic activation of the pyramidal cell on and near the cell body deep in the cortex. One of the excitatory synapses is shown by the small dark circle. Return currents are set up in the apical dendrite and a surface positive wave occurs. The upper right diagram shows what happens when the activation occurs in the more apical regions of the dendrite (two synapses are shown with the dark circles), and a surface negative wave occurs. The lower left shows a similar effect from activation of the very superficial dendritic branches (three synapses are indicated) by incoming reticular fibers. The middle diagram at the bottoms shows the effects of cortico-cortical activation of the dendrites. The lower right shows recurrent inhibition; the pyramidal cell activates the adjacent deep stellate cell, which then inhibits the pyramidal cell (at light shaded circle). This causes a source of current in the depth of the cortex.*

nerve endings and then the quadripole associated with an AP becomes just the trailing dipole and a surface negativity occurs (Figure 4–10, upper left). The synaptic effect on the cell bodies and deep dendrites of the pyramidal cells would then show in the subsequent positive wave at 30 ms (Figure 4–10, upper middle). Stellate cells activated by the afferent inflow can cause later depolarization or more apical regions of the dendrite, resulting in a surface negative wave (Figure 4–10, upper right). Thus, the full sequence of afferent input (upper part of Figure 4–10) can be associated with a negative-positive-negative complex of waves at the cortical surface. The more apical regions of the dendrites can also be depolarized from activation of the non-specific thalamocortical afferents or cortico-cortical connections. Then an extracellular current sink occurs in the dendritic region and the returning current comes through the cell bodies (Figure 4–10, lower left and lower middle). An extracellular dipole then is set up such that the surface is negative relative to the depth. A similar surface negativity could be set up by an inhibitory (hyperpolarizing) input to the cell bodies, which would also cause a current source in the depth and a concomitant sink around the surface dendrites (Figure 4–10, lower right).

Studies of the current source density and unit firing in the cortex with multilead electrodes show that the electrophysiology of the cortex is often far more complex than suggested by these simple diagrams (Vaughan & Arezzo, 1988). Sometimes, sources and sinks can occur without representation at the surface. For example, a small area of depolarization on the dendrite could have its return current mediated by regions of the dendrite both above and below the focus of synaptic activity. The opposing fields would cancel themselves out at any distance away from the synapses.

MAGNETO-ENCEPHALOGRAPHY

The flow of current within active neurons generates magnetic fields in addition to extracellular electric fields. This forms the basis of magnetoencephalography or MEG (Hämäläinen, Hari, Ilmoniemi, Knuutila, & Lounasmaa, 1993; Hari, 2005; Williamson & Kaufman, 1987;). When current flows through a conductor, a magnetic field is set up around the conductor according to a right-hand rule. If we imagine grasping the conductor with our right hand such that the thumb points in the direction of current flow, the magnetic field circles the conductor in the direction following the fingers toward the fingertips.

As we considered when describing the electrical fields, a current flows across the neuronal membrane when a synapse is activated. This current then diffuses through the intracellular spaces and returns to the extracellular space some distance away from the synapse. The outgoing and ingoing currents set up sources and sinks in the extracellular space. As discussed in the preceding section of this chapter, these extracellular currents are associated with electric fields. However, extracellular currents do not cause magnetic fields. Because the extracellular currents associated with the sources and sinks are oriented mainly in opposing directions, the magnetic fields created by extracellular currents cancel each other out. However, the intracellular current between the region of synaptic activation and the region where the currents return into or out of the intracellular space is not cancelled, and this generates the magnetic fields that can be recorded at a distance. Thus, the magnetic field is completely determined by the neuronal activity and, unlike the electric potentials, is unaffected by the volume conductor in which the neurons are located. This is illustrated diagrammatically in Figure 4–11.

The magnetic fields generated by the neurons of the brain occur in a volume

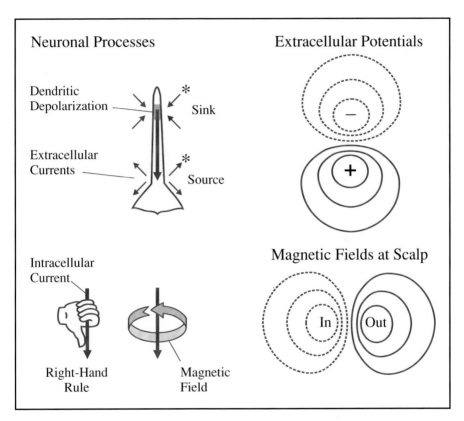

Figure 4–11. Electric and magnetic fields. *The upper half of the figure shows the extracellular fields generated by the depolarization of the apical dendrite of a cortical pyramidal cell. The electric fields are generated by the extracellular currents (thin arrows) that flow from source (around the body) to sink (around the dendrite). The inflow of current at the regions of depolarization returns to the extracellular fluid by means of the intracellular current (thick arrow) that then exits the neuron as an extracellular source at the cell body. The flow of current causes a magnetic field according to the right hand rule illustrated in the lower left of the figure. The extracellular currents from the source and sink are in opposite directions, for example, the two current flows tagged by asterisks. The magnetic fields associated with these currents are in opposite directions and therefore cancel each other out. The intracellular current has no opposing current and therefore is the main source for the recorded magnetic fields. As shown on the right, the electric and magnetic fields recorded from the scalp are oriented orthogonally (at right angles).*

conductor that is roughly spherical. The fields recorded at the surface of this sphere will not change if the intracellular currents are oriented radially, as might occur when the activated neurons are on a gyrus. Basically, the fields circling around the direction of the current flow are equal at all locations on the spherical surface. If, on the other hand, the intracellular currents are oriented tangentially, as occurs when the activated neurons are within a sulcus, a clear dipolar pattern is recorded at the surface. The field exits the head on one side of the dipole and enters on the other side. If the field is created by a single equivalent current dipole, this dipole is located halfway between the maximum and the minimum of the surface field at a depth that is proportional to the distance between these extrema (Williamson & Kaufman, 1987).

Evoked magnetic fields are recorded by special sensors near the scalp. The basic principle of the sensor is that a magnetic field passing through a coil will induce a current in the coil. The magnetic fields generated by the human brain are tiny and the currents they induce can be detected only if the coil is made superconducting by bringing it near to absolute zero by means of liquid helium. Therefore, MEG sensors are placed in a helmet filled with liquid helium and the helmet is brought down over the scalp. Various sensor designs have been used to decrease the magnetic noise in the environment from the earth's magnetic field and nearby electric motors.

Evoked magnetic fields are similar to the evoked potentials as they both ultimately derive from the same neuronal processes. As shown in Figure 4–12, the electrical recordings from a tangential cur-

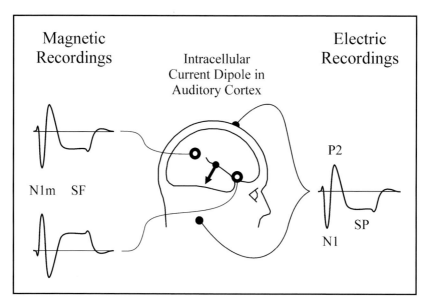

Figure 4–12. Auditory evoked fields. *This figure shows the magnetic fields (left) and the electric potentials (right) that are generated at the scalp by sources in the auditory cortex on the top of the temporal lobe. The magnetic fields are recorded by superconducting coils located near the scalp, whereas the electric potentials are recorded by electrodes attached to the scalp.*

rent dipole are oriented orthogonally to the magnetic field. A major advantage of MEG is that the magnetic fields are not affected by the volume conductor. For example, changes in the thickness of the skull over different regions of the cortex do not affect the measurements. In addition, the component structure of the MEG response usually is simpler than the EEG response because the MEG is blind to radial currents. Both factors make determining the intracerebral sources of scalp-recorded responses more accurate for MEG than for EEG. MEG is easier to record than the EEG as the sensors are simply placed adjacent to the scalp and do not have to be individually applied or electrically connected. The disadvantages of MEG compared to EEG are the high cost of the MEG equipment, its high operating expense, and the inability of MEG to detect radial current sources or deep sources.

INFERENCES ABOUT THE SOURCES OF SCALP-RECORDED POTENTIALS

Intracranial Recordings of the ABR Waves

An obvious way to determine where scalp-recorded potentials come from would be to record from the inside what we normally measure from the outside. This is possible in human subjects undergoing neurosurgical operations in the posterior fossa (Hashimoto, Ishiyama, Yoshimoto, & Nemoto, 1981; Møller, 2006b) or on the temporal lobe (Brugge et al., 2008; Godey, Schwartz, de Graaf, Chauvel, & Liégeois-Chauvel, 2001).

The intracranial portion of the auditory nerve shows N1 and N2 potentials that are later than waves I and II of the ABR and that increase their latency as the location of the recording electrode on the nerve is moved from the internal auditory meatus to the brainstem. Wave I of the ABR thus must relate to the intracochlear portion of the auditory nerve fibers with the posterior fossa portion of the eighth nerve contributing to the ABR near wave II. This might perhaps be related to the changes in the volume conductor as the nerve fibers move from bone to cerebrospinal fluid and then to brainstem. Martin, Pratt, and Schwegler (1995) found that the scalp-recorded ABR in the region of wave II changed dramatically when the auditory nerve was exposed to the air rather than to cerebrospinal fluid during neurosurgical operations. This would be expected as the changes in conductivity then were opposite to what they were with the cerebrospinal fluid. When the nerve is exposed to air, the conductance goes from low (bone) to even lower (air) and then back to moderate (brainstem).

The later waves of the human ABR are recorded widely from electrodes in many locations on and near the brainstem (Hashimoto et al., 1981). Recordings from the fourth ventricle show large potentials near the latency of waves III and IV. Wave III is mainly generated by the cochlear nucleus located in the lateral floor of the fourth ventricle. The superior olivary complex located deeper in the pons may also contribute. Recordings near the midbrain show large waves IV and V.

Recordings from electrodes placed directly within the brainstem nuclei of the auditory pathway are possible in animals. Here, we must be careful to determine which waves are homologous between human and animal ABRs. The ABR in cat and guinea pig typically is measured as a series of positive waves, P1 to P5. As already discussed, the auditory nerve in small mammals has a very short intracranial course, and often no recognizable wave in the animal ABR can be found to correspond to wave II of the human ABR. Sometimes, a small deflection is identified as P2 (e.g., Melcher & Kiang, 1996) but often not (Starr & Don, 1988), and P4 of the animal response then becomes homologous to wave V of the human ABR. Monkey recordings are more similar to those of human subjects, but again the nomenclature (based on Arabic rather than Roman numerals) becomes confusing, with wave 7 of the monkey response the likely homologue of the human wave V (Legatt, Arezzo, & Vaughan, 1986).

One of the main findings of these depth recordings in the auditory nuclei of the brainstem is the absence of any simple wave-to-nucleus correspondence. The ABR is not a sequence of activations with each wave generated at one station in the pathway. The electrical activity recorded from each nucleus or tract is complex, with multiple positive-negative waves, the result of different neuronal populations (such as the basket cells and the spherical cells of the cochlear nucleus) and different neuronal processes (such as synaptic potentials and APs). At any point in time after about 2.5 ms, activities in many different places in the pathway overlap. Adding further complexity to the results is the problem caused by the cochlear delay (to be considered more fully in Chapter 5). In response to a broadband stimulus, neurons from the high-frequency regions of the cochlea fire several milliseconds earlier than those from the low-frequency regions and this temporal dispersion is likely maintained through the brainstem. Thus, wave VI might represent the low-frequency response homologous to the high-frequency response recorded as wave V.

Intracranial Recordings From Cortex

Intracranial recordings from the auditory cortex in human subjects show waves that can be related to the MLR and the LAEP recorded from the human scalp. Godey et al. (2001) recorded from depth electrodes near Heschl's gyrus components that were related to the scalp-recorded magnetic responses Na, Pa, Nb, and Pb. The slow waves (N1 and P2) were more widely recorded, deriving mainly from more lateral and posterior regions of the supra-temporal plane. Brugge et al. (2008) have identified three areas in the human temporal lobe that respond to sounds: the posteromedial region of Heschl's gyrus that shows early responses with latencies near those of the MLR, the anterolateral portion of Heschl's gyrus showing smaller and more variable responses, and a lateral region in the superior temporal gyrus with large late responses (see also Howard et al., 2000). They suggested that these areas may be homologous to the core, belt, and parabelt regions of the primate auditory cortex. Unfortunately, they do not relate these responses to any scalp-recorded magnetic or electrical responses recorded with the same stimuli in the same subjects. Studies of the auditory evoked potentials recorded using depth electrodes by Yvert, Fischer, Bertrand, and Pernier (2005) used a distributed source analysis of the recorded data constrained by the anatomy of the cortex as delineated by structural magnetic resonance imaging (MRI), and then modeled from these sources what scalp potentials might result from the cortical activation. They found that the early MLR components (Po and Na) were specifically localized to the posteromedial portion of Heschl's gyrus. Later components (Pa, Nb, Pb, and N1) were generated over widespread regions of the supratemporal plane, spreading posteriorly to the planum temporale and laterally to the superior temporal gyrus.

Animal studies of the fields generated by the auditory cortex are difficult to interpret. The auditory cortex is different in different species. Even in primates, where we would expect the overall structure to be similar, the geometry—the location and orientation of the different areas —is completely different. The fact that the human cortex has clearly evolved to process speech sounds is another stumbling block in animal-human homology. A final difficulty comes from the fact that even an awake animal may not be attending to the stimuli in the same way as the human subject. The LAEP in the monkey shows an N70 component originating in the region of the auditory cortex that might be homologous to N1 recorded from the human scalp (Arezzo, Pickoff, & Vaughan, 1975), but the wave is much smaller relative to the earlier waves than in the human subject.

Lesions

Lesion studies in animals have indicated that the generation of the scalp ABR results from complex overlapping processes in the brainstem (Legatt et al., 1986; Melcher & Kiang, 1996; Starr & Don, 1988). The findings from these lesion studies are clear about the early waves of the ABR—I coming from the cochlea, II from the intracranial portion of the auditory nerve, and III from the cochlear nucleus— but are more complicated for the later waves. The results have to be tempered by the fact that the human brainstem pathways are not identical to those in animals. For example, the neuronal populations in

the cochlear nucleus are different in different species and the projections from the cochlear nucleus to the trapezoid body and the nuclei of the lateral lemniscus are much less prominent in humans than in cats (Moore, 1987a, 1987b). Despite the complexities of the pathways and the overlapping of the potentials, wave IV and V of the ABR likely mainly represent the activity in the lateral lemniscus, ascending in the midbrain to synapse in the inferior colliculus. Ponton, Moore, and Eggermont (1996; see also Moore, Ponton, Eggermont, Wu, & Huang, 1996) suggest that there are two main pathways from cochlear nucleus to inferior colliculus, one direct and one synapsing in the superior olivary complex (see Figure 4–2, bottom). If the direct pathway causes wave IV and the indirect wave V, then the IV-V interval is equal to the synaptic delay in the superior olive.

Human lesion studies have not been very helpful in identifying ABR generators as human pathology is much less precise than experimental animal lesions. Furthermore, ABR studies of patients usually are limited to measurement of waves I, III, and V. Basically, the effects of eighth nerve lesions on the ABR begin before wave III, the effects of pontine lesions begin at wave III, and the effects of midbrain lesions begin after wave III. These findings are considered more closely in Chapter 14.

In terms of cortical generators, human lesions provide more information than animal lesions because of the difficulty in deciding on homologies between animal and human responses. Lesions to the auditory cortex or to the auditory radiations (involving the thalamocortical pathways) generally reduce the scalp-recorded MLRs. An attenuated scalp response generally remains after a unilateral lesion because of the contribution of the auditory cortex in the other hemisphere, both cortices having dipoles oriented toward the vertex (Kraus, Ozdamar, Hier, & Stein, 1982; Scherg & von Cramon, 1986, 1990). However, all is not simple, and patients with bilateral lesions of the primary auditory cortex sometimes still show some waves of the MLR (Woods, Clayworth, Knight, Simpson, & Naeser, 1987), perhaps because of similar-latency generators in secondary auditory areas.

The LAEPs are not much affected by lesions to the primary auditory cortex if the planum temporale and the posterior portion of the superior temporal gyrus are spared (Knight, Scabini, Woods, & Clayworth, 1988). Lesions to these areas severely attenuate the laterally recorded responses (e.g., N1c) and reduce the vertex responses (N1b). These and other findings can be interpreted by means of tangential and radial dipoles in each temporal lobe (Scherg & von Cramon, 1990). These are discussed further in the next section.

SOURCE ANALYSIS

The various electrical activities that occur within the brain set up sources and sinks that generate the electric fields that we record at the scalp. If we know the sources and sinks (their location, timing, and magnitude) and if we know the electrical characteristics of the head (its geometry and conductance), we can calculate the distribution of the electric fields at the scalp. This is the forward solution (Hallez et al., 2007). To simplify things, we consider the activity of a particular region of the brain in terms of one equivalent dipole rather than the thousands of actual neuronal sources and sinks within the region. The size of these regions may be of the order of centimeters (Brodmann areas) or milli-

meters (facets in a cortical surface modeled from brain images). The activity recorded at a particular electrode on the scalp is the sum of the contributions from each of the sources active during the recording. Figure 4–13 illustrates source- and scalp-waveforms for the auditory MLR.

The contribution of each source to each electrode is the source waveform multiplied by a coefficient that is determined by the location and orientation of the source within the brain and location of the electrode on the scalp. The coefficient depends on the conductance geometry of the head. This conductance geometry can be simple, a sphere (brain) with three shells (cerebrospinal fluid, bone, scalp), or complex, a model of discrete elements based on images of the head (e.g., Neilson, Kovalyov, & Koles, 2005). The array of coefficients and/or the algorithms for calculating them form the "head model."

By recording from multiple scalp locations we can accurately map the surface fields formed by the superposition of the fields generated by all the active intracerebral sources. It would be wonderful if we also could derive the intracerebral distribution of sources (and sinks) from the recorded fields—this is the inverse solution (Grech et al., 2008; Lagerlund & Worrell, 2005; Scherg, 1990; Scherg & Picton, 1991). Unfortunately, more than one intracerebral current distribution can produce the same field topography at the scalp. The inverse solution is not unique. We can make the solution unique by applying constraints. One obvious constraint is not to allow sources outside of the head. Other possible constraints are to restrict locations of sources to grey matter, to limit the number of active sources, and to set rules for the relations between adjacent sources.

Two basic models are used for inverse solutions: discrete and distributed. Dis-

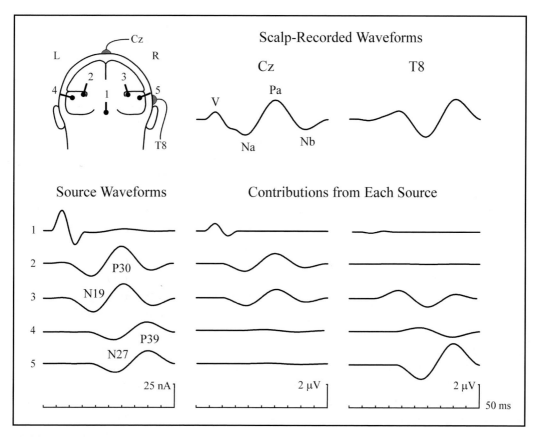

Figure 4–13. **Intracerebral sources for scalp-recorded EPs.** *This figure shows the general concept of source analysis. Each scalp-recorded waveform represents the sum of contributions from each source waveform. The contribution of a source to a particular scalp electrode is the source waveform multiplied by a coefficient that takes into account the distance of the electrode from the source, the orientation of the source relative to the electrode, and the conductance geometry of the head. The waveforms shown in this figure are based on the normative data for the sources of the MLR (Scherg & von Cramon, 1990). The modeling of the sources and their scalp contributions was performed using the DipoleSimulator program of Patrick Berg.*

crete models search for a solution with a small number of focal current dipoles, each representing an active area of the brain. Distributed models allow current dipoles to be present throughout the brain volume, usually represented as a three-dimensional matrix of current dipoles. These different approaches can be considered using a political metaphor. In the discrete models, anything important is done by a small elite group acting independ-

ently (as in a society of the right), whereas in the distributed models, everyone participates but they have to follow strict rules (as in a society of the left).

Brain Electromagnetic Source Analysis (BESA) is an example of the discrete source approach (Scherg, 1990; Scherg & Picton, 1991). BESA uses dipoles with fixed locations and orientations that vary in strength across time. The forward solution for these dipole sources is calculated using a spherical head model and these modeled data are then compared to the actual scalp recordings. The locations and orientations of the dipoles can be fixed a priori on the basis of the known anatomy and connections of the brain, "seeded" from the locations known to be active from fMRI, or determined using iterative fitting protocols that decrease the residual variance between the modeled data and the actual data recorded from the scalp. The analyst has to decide on the number of sources. This can be related to how many principal components are needed to explain the variance in the data, although this will underestimate the number of sources when sources with similar waveforms occur in each of the two hemispheres. Several other criteria also can be applied to the fitting process. For example, the total amount of energy in the sources could be kept low. This removes the tendency for similarly oriented sources to have large and opposite source waveforms.

Examples of the distributed approach to source analysis are the Minimum Norm solution (Hämäläinen et al., 1993), which is constrained to have minimum total current, and Low Resolution Electromagnetic Tomography (LORETA) (Pascual-Marqui, Michel, & Lehmann, 1994), which is constrained to have the spatially smoothest current distribution. Because the constraints are imposed mathematically, the solutions require little or no human input. However, the constraints may not always represent what is happening in the brain. The currents in adjacent regions of the cortex may be quite distinct from each other and may not fit with constraints such as minimum overall current or maximum spatial smoothness.

In addition to the constraints inherent in their mathematics, distributed sources

can be further constrained by anatomic data. Because the main sources of electrical and magnetic activity occur in the grey matter rather than the white matter, possible source locations can be limited to cerebral cortex or to cortex and subcortical gray matter. Initially, this was done by Dale and Sereno (1993) using the minimum norm solution and a representation of the cortical surface derived from MRI. Picton et al. (1999) used a variant of LORETA to constrain auditory source generators to an MRI-based brain model of cerebral gray matter (cortex and subcortical nuclei). Even further constraint can be applied by limiting the analysis to those areas of the brain that show hemodynamic activation on fMRI (Ahveninen et al., 2006; Jääskeläinen et al., 2004).

Some caveats are important to bear in mind when evaluating the results of electric source analysis. Many neuronal processes do not show up in the fields that we can record from the scalp. First, many neuronal activities are not geometrically organized and therefore generate closed fields that cannot be recorded at any distance away from the neurons. Second, some activities that generate open fields can cancel each other out (Ahlfors et al., 2010). For example if there are similar patterns of activation in both walls of a cerebral sulcus or fissure, their oppositely oriented fields will overlap and cancel. Third, many neuronal responses may be insufficiently time locked to the stimulus to generate fields that can be averaged across trials. For these reasons, some centers of activation showing on fMRI may not show any activity when used as seeds for electrical (or magnetic) source analysis. The fact that the electric recordings do not record everything that goes on in the brain does not detract from their ability to distinguish and localize some activities. Activities that can be characterized by source analysis have to be considered in any proposal we put forth to explain how the brain processes sound.

Source Analysis of Auditory EPs

The initial source analyses of the MLR were performed by Scherg and von Cramon (1986, 1990). They proposed that the main generators could be modeled using tangential and radial dipoles in each hemisphere. In response to clicks, the major waves were N17 and P30 for the tangential sources and N27 and P39 for the radial sources. Figure 4–13 is based on their data. In some subjects, a large postauricular muscle reflex occurred; this could be modeled by placing an extra dipole source on the mastoid process. Herdman et al. (2002) combined tangential and radial sources in each temporal lobe with a deep brainstem source to model the 40-Hz steady-state MLR. The sources in the temporal lobe had a phase that differed from that in the brainstem, indicating a delay from brainstem to cortex of 20 to 25 ms. There was a further delay of several milliseconds between tangential and radial sources, although this did not reach significance. The 40-Hz ASSR, which combined brainstem and cortical activities differed from the 80-Hz response, the sources of which were in the brainstem. These brainstem sources for these rapid ASSRs showed overlapping laterally and vertically oriented dipoles, suggesting multiple sources within the brainstem.

The LAEPs show complicated scalp topographies with peaks at different latencies in the temporal and vertex regions. The major finding is that that the N1 peak

in the temporal regions (N1c) occurs about 40 ms after the N1 at the vertex (N1b). There is also an earlier N1 peak in the frontal regions (N1a). These peaks indicate that separate sources with different latencies are generating overlapping fields (Wood & Wolpaw, 1982). Scherg and von Cramon (1986, 1990) modeled the responses with radial and tangential dipole sources in each temporal lobe. The major peaks were N100 and P180 for the tangential dipole source and P100 and N150 for the radial source. Scherg, Vajsar, and Picton (1989) provided a source analysis that evaluated both the N1-P2 onset-response and the SP. Results from this analysis are illustrated in Figure 4–14. In addition to the radial and tangential sources underlying N1-P2, a more anteriorly located and directed source was used to model the sustained potential (SP). Although the dominant sources for the LAEPs are located in the temporal lobe, other sources in the frontal lobes often are simultaneously active as the sounds are processed in relation to attention, memory, or motor response (Picton et al., 1999).

Scherg and von Cramon (1986, 1990) examined the sources of the auditory EPs in neurological patients with lesions to the temporal lobe, describing three patterns of abnormality. In the first, the absence of any clear sources for either MLR or LAEPs in one hemisphere indicated a lesion involving the auditory cortex in that hemisphere. A second type of abnormality that occurred with a lesion to the auditory radiations sparing the auditory cortex showed absent MLR sources in one hemisphere but preserved LAEPs. However, the LAEPs in the affected hemisphere occurred at a longer latency than normal, perhaps because they were activated by commissural fibers from the intact auditory cortex in the other

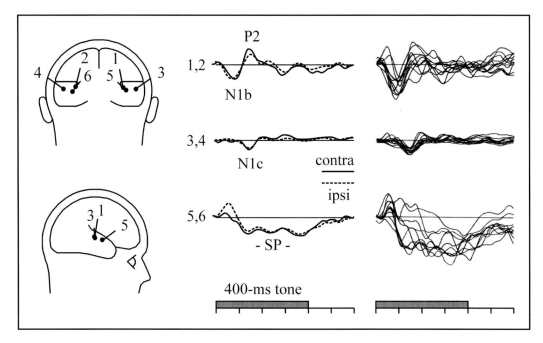

Figure 4–14. *Sources for the slow auditory EPs. This figure shows the source waveforms for scalp-recorded responses to a 400-ms tone of 1 kHz. The left part of the figure shows the source locations and orientations as determined using Brain Electric Source Analysis. The center shows the source waveforms for the average EPs in the hemispheres contralateral and ipsilateral to the stimulated ear. The N1b and P2 waves are generated mainly by tangential dipole sources at the top of the temporal lobe. The N1c wave derives from radially oriented sources, and the sustained potential derives from a tangential source located and oriented a little more anteriorly than the source for the N1b. The source waveforms for individual subjects are shown on the right. The data in this figure are derived from Scherg et al. (1989).*

hemisphere rather than through the usual pathways from the thalamus and primary auditory cortex (Scherg & von Cramon, 1990). A final type of lesion effect was a disconnection between tangential dipole generators on the supratemporal plane (N1b) and the lateral generators on the superior temporal gyrus (N1c); the N100 on the tangential dipole was preserved but the N150 on the radial dipole was absent. This usually was caused by lesions to the auditory association areas on the lateral surface of the temporal lobe or to the thalamic radiations to these areas.

SUMMARY OF SOURCES

Table 4–1 shows probable sources for the different waves of the auditory evoked potential based on the techniques and evidence we reviewed in this chapter. Those listed with a question mark are less definite that the others. Even those without question marks are not completely certain. Much further work is needed.

The subtitle of the chapter presents the idea forward and backward. This is most clearly related to the way in which we estimate the intracranial sources of our

Table 4–1. Probable Sources for Scalp-Recorded Auditory EPs

AEP Wave	Latency (ms)*	Probable Source
I	1.7	Spiral ganglion cells in cochlea
II	2.8	Intracranial portion of auditory nerve
III	3.8	Cochlear nucleus
IV	5.0	? Lateral lemniscus—fibers from cochlear nuclei
V	5.7	? Lateral lemniscus—fibers from superior olivary complexes
VI	7.2	? Lateral lemniscus—fibers activated through apical regions of cochlea, possibly also medial geniculate
No	9	? Unknown—possibly medial geniculate
Po	12	? Unknown
Na	18	? Afferent inflow to cortex from the medial geniculate
Pa	28	Synaptic activation of deep regions of cortex in core and belt regions
Nb	40	? Spread of activation to dendrites in core and belt regions
P1	55	? Unknown
N1a	70	? Unknown
N1b	100	Activation of widespread regions of the auditory cortex especially the posterior parabelt regions on planum temporale and superior temporal gyrus. Other cortical regions (frontal and parietal) probably are also active at this latency.
N1c	140	Activation of parabelt auditory cortex on lateral aspect of superior temporal gyrus
P2	170	? Auditory cortices, together with other cortical areas
SP		? Widespread activation of auditory cortices, with activation extending more anterior than for the N1b

*Typical latency for a rapid-onset stimulus of about 70 dB nHL

scalp-recorded potentials using both forward and inverse solutions. In addition, the phrase suggests the incompleteness of our current state of knowledge. We need to go forward with our research while looking back at what we already know so that we understand more clearly what is yet to be discovered. This idea, stemming from Kierkegaard's proposal that we must live life forward, although we can only understand it backward, has wider application than just to the auditory EPs.

ABBREVIATIONS

ABR	Auditory brainstem response
AP	Action potential
ASSR	Auditory steady-state response
BESA	Brain electric source analysis
CAP	Compound action potential
EEG	Electroencephalography
EP	Evoked potential
EPSP	Excitatory postsynaptic potential
fMRI	Functional magnetic resonance imaging
IPSP	Inhibitory postsynaptic potential
LAEP	Late auditory evoked potential
LORETA	Low-resolution electromagnetic tomography
MEG	Magnetoencephalography
MLR	Middle-latency response
MRI	Magnetic resonance imaging
SP	Sustained potential

REFERENCES

Ahlfors, S. P., Han, J., Lin, F. H., Witzel, T., Belliveau, J. W., Hämäläinen, M. S., & Halgren, E. (2010). Cancellation of EEG and MEG signals generated by extended and distributed sources. *Human Brain Mapping, 31,* 140–149.

Ahveninen, J., Jääskeläinen, I. P., Raij, T., Bonmassar, G., Devore, S., Hämäläinen , M., . . . Belliveau, J. W. (2006). Task-modulated "what" and "where" pathways in human auditory cortex. *Proceedings of the National Academy of Sciences (USA), 103,* 14608–14613.

Alain, C., Arnott, S. R., Hevenor, S., Graham, S., & Grady, C. L. (2001)."What" and "where" in the human auditory system. *Proceedings of the National Academy of Sciences (USA), 98,* 12301–12306.

Arezzo, J., Pickoff, A., & Vaughan, H. G., Jr. (1975). The sources and intracerebral distribution of auditory evoked potentials in the alert rhesus monkey. *Brain Research, 90,* 57–73.

Barrett, D. J., & Hall, D. A. (2006). Response preferences for "what" and "where" in human non-primary auditory cortex. *NeuroImage, 32,* 968–977.

Berg, P., & Scherg, M. (1994). A fast method for forward computation of multiple-shell spherical head models. *Electroencephalography and Clinical Neurophysiology, 90,* 58–64.

Brugge, J. F., Volkov, I. O., Oya, H., Kawasaki, H., Reale, R. A., Fenoy, A., . . . Howard, M. A., 3rd. (2008). Functional localization of auditory cortical fields of human: Click-train stimulation. *Hearing Research, 238,* 12–24.

Cant, N. B., & Benson, C. G. (2003). Parallel auditory pathways: projection patterns of the different neuronal populations in the dorsal and ventral cochlear nuclei. *Brain Research Bulletin, 60,* 457–474.

Dale, A., & Sereno, M. (1993). Improved localization of cortical activity by combining EEG and MEG with MRI cortical surface reconstruction: a linear approach. *Journal of Cognitive Neuroscience, 5,* 162–176.

Deupree, D. L., & Jewett, D. L. (1988). Far-field potentials due to action potentials traversing curved nerves, reaching cut nerve ends, and crossing boundaries between cylindrical volumes. *Electroencephalography and Clinical Neurophysiology, 70,* 355–362.

Dorsaint-Pierre, R., Penhune, V. B., Watkins, K. E., Neelin, P., Lerch, J. P., Bouffard, M., & Zatorre, R. J. (2006). Asymmetries of the planum temporale and Heschl's gyrus: Relationship to language lateralization. *Brain, 129,* 1164–1176.

Gloor, P. (1985). Neuronal generators and the problem of localization in electroencephalography: Application of volume conductor theory to electroencephalography. *Journal of Clinical Neurophysiology, 2,* 327–354.

Godey, B., Schwartz, D., de Graaf, J. B., Chauvel, P., & Liégeois-Chauvel, C. (2001). Neuromagnetic source localization of auditory evoked fields and intracerebral evoked potentials: A comparison of data in the same patients. *Clinical Neurophysiology, 112,* 1850–1859.

Grech, R., Cassar, T., Muscat, J., Camilleri, K. P., Fabri, S. G., Zervakis, M., . . . Vanrumste, B. (2008). Review on solving the inverse problem in EEG source analysis. *Journal of Neuroengineering and Rehabilitation, 5,* 25.

Griffiths, T. D., & Warren, J. D. (2002) The planum temporale as a computational hub. *Trends in Neuroscience, 25,* 348–353.

Hackett, T. A. (2007). Organization of the thalamocortical pathways in man. In R. F. Burkard, M. Don, & J. J. Eggermont (Eds.), *Auditory evoked potentials: Basic principles and clinical application* (pp. 428–440). Philadelphia, PA: Lippincott, Williams & Wilkins.

Hallez, H., Vanrumste, B., Grech, R., Muscat, J., De Clercq, W., Vergult, A., . . . Lemahieu, I. (2007). Review on solving the forward problem in EEG source analysis. *Journal of Neuroengineering and Rehabilitation, 4,* 46.

Hämäläinen, M., Hari, R., Ilmoniemi, R., Knuutila, J., & Lounasmaa, O. V. (1993). Magnetoencephalography: Theory, instrumentation, and applications to noninvasive studies of signal processing in the human brain. *Reviews of Modern Physics, 65,* 413–497.

Hari, R. (2005). Magnetoencephalography in clinical neurophysiological assessment of human cortical functions. In E. Niedermeyer & F. Lopes da Silva (Eds.), *Electroencephalography: Basic principles, clinical applications, and related fields* (5th ed., pp. 1165–1197). Philadelphia, PA: Lippincott, Williams & Wilkins.

Hashimoto, I., Ishiyama, Y., Yoshimoto, T., & Nemoto, S. (1981). Brain-stem auditory-evoked potentials recorded directly from human brain-stem and thalamus. *Brain, 104,* 841–859.

Herdman, A. T., Lins, O., Van Roon, P., Stapells, D. R., Scherg, M., & Picton, T. W. (2002). Intracerebral sources of human auditory steady-state responses. *Brain Topography, 15,* 69–86.

Howard, M. A., Volkov, I. O., Mirsky, R., Garell, P. C., Noh, M. D., Granner, M., . . . Brugge, J. F. (2000). Auditory cortex on the posterior superior temporal gyrus of human cerebral cortex. *Journal of Comparative Neurology, 416,* 76–92.

Jääskeläinen, I. P., Ahveninen, J., Bonmassar, G., Dale, A. M., Ilmoniemi, R. J., Levänen, S., . . . Belliveau, J. W. (2004). Human posterior auditory cortex gates novel sounds to consciousness. *Proceedings of the National Academy of Sciences (USA), 101,* 6809–6814.

Jewett, D. L., Deupree, D. L., & Bommannan, D. (1990). Far-field potentials generated by action potentials of isolated frog sciatic nerves in a spherical volume. *Electroencephalography and Clinical Neurophysiology, 75,* 105–117.

Jewett, D. L., & Williston, J. S. (1971). Auditory-evoked far fields averaged from the scalp of humans. *Brain, 94,* 681–696.

Kaas, J. H., & Hackett, T. A. (2000). Subdivisions of auditory cortex and processing streams in primates. *Proceedings of the National Academy of Sciences (USA), 97,* 11793–11799.

Knight, R. T., Scabini, D., Woods, D. L., & Clayworth, C. (1988). The effects of lesions of superior temporal gyrus and inferior parietal lobe on temporal and vertex components of the human AEP. *Electroencephalography and Clinical Neurophysiology, 70,* 499–509.

Kraus, N., Ozdamar, O., Hier, D., & Stein, L. (1982). Auditory middle latency responses (MLRs) in patients with cortical lesions. *Electroencephalography and Clinical Neurophysiology, 54,* 275–287.

Kumar, S., Stephan, K. E., Warren, J. D., Friston, K. J., & Griffiths, T. D. (2007). Hierarchical processing of auditory objects in humans. *PLoS Computational Biology, 3*(6): e100. doi:10.1371/ journal.pcbi.0030100.

Lagerlund, T. D., & Worrell, G. A. (2005). EEG source localization (model-dependent and model-independent methods). In E. Niedermeyer & F. Lopes da Silva (Eds), *Electroencephalography: Basic principles, clinical applications, and related fields* (5th ed., pp. 829–844). Philadelphia, PA: Lippincott, Williams & Wilkins.

Lang, J. (1985). Anatomy of the brainstem and the lower cranial nerves, vessels, and surrounding structures. *American Journal of Otology, 6*(November Suppl.), 1–19.

Legatt, A. D., Arezzo, J. C., & Vaughan, H. G., Jr. (1986). Short-latency auditory evoked potentials in the monkey. II. Intracranial generators. *Electroencephalography and Clinical Neurophysiology, 64*, 53–73.

Lorente de Nó, R. (1947). Action potential of the motoneurons of the hypoglossus nucleus. *Journal of Cellular and Comparative Physiology, 29*, 207–287.

Malmivuo, J., & Plonsey, R. (1995). *Bioelectromagnetism: Principles and applications of bioelectric and biomagnetic fields.* New York, NY: Oxford University Press.

Martin, W. H., Pratt, H., & Schwegler, J. W. (1995). The origin of the human auditory brain-stem response wave II. *Electroencephalography and Clinical Neurophysiology, 96*, 357–370.

Melcher, J. R., & Kiang, N. Y. (1996). Generators of the brainstem auditory evoked potential in cat. III: Identified cell populations. *Hearing Research, 93*, 52–71.

Mitani, A., Shimokouchi, M., Itoh, K., Nomura, S., Kudo, M., & Mizuno, N. (1985). Morphology and laminar organization of electrophysiologically identified neurons in the primary auditory cortex in the cat. *Journal of Comparative Neurology, 235*, 430–447.

Møller, A. R. (2006a). *Hearing: Anatomy, physiology, and disorders of the auditory system* (2nd ed.). Amsterdam, The Netherlands: Academic Press (Elsevier).

Møller, A. R. (2006b). *Intraoperative neurophysiological monitoring* (2nd ed.). Totowa, NJ: Humana Press.

Moore, J. K. (1987a). The human auditory brain stem: A comparative view. *Hearing Research, 29*, 1–32.

Moore, J. K. (1987b). The human auditory brain stem as a generator of auditory evoked potentials. *Hearing Research, 29*, 33–43.

Moore, J. K., Ponton, C. W., Eggermont, J. J., Wu, B. J., & Huang, J. Q. (1996). Perinatal maturation of the auditory brain stem response: Changes in path length and conduction velocity. *Ear and Hearing, 17*, 411–418.

Morosan, P., Rademacher, J., Schleicher, A., Amunts, K., Schormann, T., & Zilles, K. (2001). Human primary auditory cortex: Cytoarchitectonic subdivisions and mapping into a spatial reference system. *NeuroImage, 13*, 684–701.

Neilson, L. A., Kovalyov, M., & Koles, Z. J. (2005). A computationally efficient method for accurately solving the EEG forward problem in a finely discretized head model. *Clinical Neurophysiology, 116*, 2302–2314.

Nicholls, J. G., Martin, A. R., Wallace, B., & Fuchs, P. A. (2001). *From neuron to brain: A cellular and molecular approach to the function of the nervous system.* Sunderland, MA: Sinauer Associates.

Nunez, P. L. & Srinivasan, R. (2005). *Electric fields of the brain: The neurophysics of EEG* (2nd ed.). New York, NY: Oxford University Press.

Pantev, C., Bertrand, O., Eulitz, C., Verkindt, C., Hampson, S., Schuierer, G., & Elbert, T. (1995). Specific tonotopic organizations of different areas of the human auditory cortex revealed by simultaneous magnetic and electric recordings. *Electroencephalography and Clinical Neurophysiology, 94*, 26–40.

Pantev, C., Roberts, L. E., Elbert, T., Ross, B., & Wienbruch, C. (1996) Tonotopic organization of the sources of human auditory steady-state responses. *Hearing Research, 101*, 62–74.

Pascual-Marqui, R. D., Michel, C. M., & Lehmann, D. (1994). Low resolution electromagnetic tomography: A new method for localizing electrical activity in the brain.

International Journal of Psychophysiology, 18, 49–65.

Penhune, V. B., Zatorre, R. J., MacDonald, J. D., & Evans, A. C. (1996). Interhemispheric anatomical differences in human primary auditory cortex: Probabilistic mapping and volume measurement from magnetic resonance scans. *Cerebral Cortex, 6,* 661–672.

Pickles, J. O. (2008). *An introduction to the physiology of hearing* (3rd ed.). Bingley, UK: Emerald Publishing.

Picton, T. W., Alain, C., Woods, D. L., John, M. S., Scherg, M., Valdes-Sosa, P., . . . Trujillo, N. J. (1999). Intracerebral sources of human auditory-evoked potentials. *Audiology and Neuro-Otology, 4,* 64–79.

Ponton, C. W., Moore, J. K., & Eggermont, J. J. (1996). Auditory brain stem response generation by parallel pathways: Differential maturation of axonal conduction time and synaptic transmission. *Ear and Hearing, 17,* 402–410.

Rademacher, J., Morosan, P., Schormann, T., Schleicher, A., Werner, C., Freund, H. J., & Zilles, K. (2001). Probabilistic mapping and volume measurement of human primary auditory cortex. *NeuroImage, 13,* 669–683.

Scherg, M. (1990). Fundamentals of dipole source potential analysis. In F. Grandori, M. Hoke, & G.L. Romani (Eds.), *Advances in audiology, Vol. 6. Auditory evoked magnetic fields and electric potentials* (pp. 40–69). Basel, Switzerland: Karger.

Scherg, M., & Picton, T. W. (1991). Separation and identification of event-related potential components by brain electric source analysis. *Electroencephalography and Clinical Neurophysiology Supplement 42,* 24–37.

Scherg, M., Vajsar, J., & Picton, T. W. (1989). A source analysis of the late human auditory evoked potentials. *Journal of Cognitive Neuroscience, 1,* 336–355.

Scherg, M, & von Cramon, D. (1986). Evoked dipole source potentials of the human auditory cortex. *Electroencephalography and Clinical Neurophysiology, 65,* 344–360.

Scherg, M., & von Cramon, D. (1990). Dipole source potentials of the auditory cortex in normal subjects and in patients with temporal lobe lesions. In F. Grandori, M. Hoke, & G. L. Romani (Eds.), *Advances in audiology, Vol. 6. Auditory evoked magnetic fields and electric potentials* (pp. 165–193). Basel, Switzerland: Karger,.

Schoonhoven, R., & Stegeman, D. F. (1991). Models and analysis of compound nerve action potentials. *Critical Reviews in Biomedical Engineering, 19,* 47–111.

Speckmann, E. J., & Elger, C. E. (2005). Introduction to the neurophysiological basis of the EEG and DC potentials. In E. Niedermeyer & F. Lopes da Silva (Eds.), *Electroencephalography: Basic principles, clinical applications, and related fields* (5th ed., pp. 17–29). Philadelphia, PA: Lippincott, Williams & Wilkins.

Starr, A., & Don, M. (1988). Brain potentials evoked by acoustic stimuli. In T. W. Picton (Ed.), *Handbook of electroencephalography and clinical neurophysiology. (Revised series): Vol. 3. Human event-related potentials* (pp. 97–155). Amsterdam, The Netherlands: Elsevier.

Stegeman, D. F., Dumitru, D., King, J. C., & Roeleveld, K. (1997). Near- and far-fields: Source characteristics and the conducting medium in neurophysiology. *Journal of Clinical Neurophysiology, 14,* 429–442.

Stegeman, D. F., van Oosterom, A., & Colon, E. J. (1987). Far-field evoked potential components induced by a propagating generator: Computational evidence. *Electroencephalography and Clinical Neurophysiology, 67,* 176–187.

Steinschneider, M., Tenke, C. E., Schroeder, C. E., Javitt, D. C., Simpson, G. V., Arezzo, J. C., & Vaughan, H. G., Jr. (1992). Cellular generators of the cortical auditory evoked potential initial component. *Electroencephalography and Clinical Neurophysiology, 84,* 196–200.

Talavage, T. M., Sereno, M. I., Melcher, J. R., Ledden, P. J., Rosen, B. R., & Dale, A. M. (2004). Tonotopic organization in human auditory cortex revealed by progressions of frequency sensitivity. *Journal of Neurophysiology, 91,* 1282–1296.

Vaughan, H. G. Jr., & Arezzo, J. C. (1988). The neural basis of event-related potentials. In T. W. Picton (Ed.), *Handbook of electroencephalography and clinical neurophysiology. (Revised series): Vol. 3. Human event-related potentials* (pp. 45–96). Amsterdam, The Netherlands: Elsevier.

Wang, W-J., Wu, X-H., & Li, L. (2008). The dual-pathway model of auditory signal processing *Neuroscience Bulletin, 24,* 173–182.

Warren, J. D., & Griffiths, T. D. (2003). Distinct mechanisms for processing spatial sequences and pitch sequences in the human auditory brain. *Journal of Neuroscience, 23,* 5799–5804.

Warrier, C., Wong, P., Penhune, V., Zatorre, R., Parrish, T., Abrams, D., & Kraus, N. (2009). Relating structure to function: Heschl's gyrus and acoustic processing. *Journal of Neuroscience, 29,* 61–69.

Wessinger, C. M., VanMeter, J., Tian, B., Van Lare, J., Pekar, J., & Rauschecker, J. P. (2001). Hierarchical organization of the human auditory cortex revealed by functional magnetic resonance imaging. *Journal of Cognitive Neuroscience, 13,* 1–7.

Williamson, S. J., & Kaufman, L. (1987). Analysis of neuromagnetic signals. In A. S. Gevins & A. Rémond (Eds.), *Handbook of electroencephalography and clinical neurophysiology:* *Vol. 1. Method of analysis of brain electrical and magnetic signals* (pp. 405–448). New York, NY: Elsevier.

Wood, C. C., & Wolpaw, J. R. (1982). Scalp distribution of human auditory evoked potentials. II. Evidence for overlapping sources and involvement of auditory cortex. *Electroencephalography and Clinical Neurophysiology, 54,* 25–38.

Woods,. D. L., & Alain, C. (2009). Functional imaging of human auditory cortex. *Current Opinion in Otolaryngology-Head and Neck Surgery, 17,* 407–411.

Woods, D. L., Clayworth, C. C., Knight, R. T., Simpson, G. V., & Naeser, M. A. (1987). Generators of middle- and long-latency auditory evoked potentials: Implications from studies of patients with bitemporal lesions. *Electroencephalography and Clinical Neurophysiology, 68,* 132–148.

Yvert, B., Fischer, C., Bertrand, O., & Pernier, J. (2005). Localization of human supratemporal auditory areas from intracerebral auditory evoked potentials using distributed source models. *NeuroImage, 28,* 140–153.

Zatorre, R. J., & Belin, P. (2001). Spectral and temporal processing in human auditory cortex. *Cerebral Cortex, 11,* 946–953.

5

Acoustic Stimuli:
Sounds to Charm the Brain

> Be not afear'd; the isle is full of noises,
> Sounds and sweet airs, that give delight and hurt not.
> Sometimes a thousand twangling instruments
> Will hum about mine ears; and sometimes voices,
> That if I then had waked after long sleep,
> Will make me sleep again.
>
> Shakespeare, *Tempest*, Act III, Scene 2, lines 146–151

Our world is full of sounds. The subject whose auditory evoked potentials (EPs) are being recorded will hear many different types of sounds presented in many different ways. Almost always these sounds are repeated, sometimes many thousand times. The subject often comes to the end of the recording session feeling much like Caliban in the epigraph.

This chapter describes the main stimuli used to elicit auditory EPs, and some of the paradigms in which they are presented. A "paradigm" is a pattern or model for how things are done. The term originally was used in the context of grammar to define templates for the conjugation of verbs or the declension of nouns. In the field of EPs, it describes how a stimulus or set of stimuli are organized and presented to the subject, what instructions are given to the subject, and what behavioral responses are recorded in addition to the EPs. As well as the stimulus features (intensity, duration, frequency, etc.), the paradigm outlines the timing of the stimuli and their probabilities. An essential feature is the rate at which stimuli are presented. This often is described in terms of the interstimulus interval, but this is ambiguous because we are never sure whether the interval is between the offset of one stimulus and the onset of the next (the basic meaning of the term) or between the onsets of the two stimuli (essentially interstimulus-onset interval). In this book, we use the term "stimulus onset asynchrony"

(SOA), which clearly means the interval between the onsets of the stimuli.

Each sound we hear comes from a source (an auditory object). The source usually is located somewhere in space and typically has a defining spectrotemporal pattern—the song of the blackbird on a branch, or the voice of one's mother on the phone. The main physical parameters of a sound are its frequency and intensity; generally, these are represented in a spectrum where the amplitude is plotted against frequency. Usually, we hear intensity as loudness and frequency as pitch. However, loudness varies with many things in addition to the amplitude of the sound; the duration of the sound and the bandwidth of its energy are the most important. Furthermore, the relations between pitch and frequency are particularly complex. Pitch often is determined mainly by the rate or periodicity of a sound. The pattern of the spectral frequencies present in a sound make up its "timbre." One feature of timbre is harmonicity. Many sounds are composed of a fundamental frequency and its harmonics. A violin and a flute playing the same note have the same fundamental frequency but the relative intensities of the harmonics are different. One can produce the vowel /i/ and the vowel /u/ with the same vocal pitch. Distinguishing between them depends on our ability to recognize which harmonics are accentuated by resonances in the vocal tract to make up the particular "formants" of each vowel.

This chapter reviews some of the different stimuli that have been used to evoke responses from the human cochlea and brain. Our main focus is on the acoustic properties of these stimuli and how these properties are measured. However, we will also be interested in how the different stimuli are perceived, as we use them to study how we hear.

TRANSDUCERS

The easiest way to begin our evaluation of the stimuli used in auditory EP studies is to consider clicks. The universe may have begun with a big bang but auditory EPs often begin with a little bang. A click is produced by passing a sudden voltage change through a speaker—an electrical to acoustic transducer. The most commonly used click is caused by a brief pulse lasting 0.1 ms (100 µs). This stimulus has a spectrum that contains all frequencies except for nulls at a frequency equal to the reciprocal of the click's duration (i.e., 10,000 Hz and harmonics of that frequency). However, the speakers that present clicks to the ear have transfer functions that pass some frequencies and not others. Speakers used in audiometry are designed to pass frequencies from 125 to 8000 Hz but typically do not pass frequencies much above 8000 Hz. Special transducers can be used to present higher frequencies (e.g., Fausti, Frey, Henry, Olson, & Schaffer, 1992).

Free-Field Speakers and Earphones

Free-field speakers can be used to present sounds for auditory EP studies, and are important in evaluating hearing aids or the localization of sounds in space rather than the lateralization of sounds between the ears. Most commonly, however, we use earphones so that we can test one ear relative to another and so that we do not have to worry about the reverberation of sounds in the testing environment. The most common types of audiometric earphones have supra-aural cushions. This allows them to be calibrated using an artificial ear with a 6-cc coupler, the average volume in the adult ear's concha and external auditory meatus. Earphones with circumaural cushions can provide better attenuation of external sounds. Recently lightweight see-through circumaural transducers have been used in babies. These allow the examiner to see that the ear canal remains patent, which may be a problem with the heavier circumaural earphones designed for adults. Circumaural earphones are more difficult to calibrate because of the variability in the volume of air between the transducer and the tympanic membrane (Durrant, Sabo, & Delgado, 2007).

Ear Inserts

Ear inserts often are used to present the sound. These have three main advantages over earphones (Beauchaine, Kaminski, & Gorga, 1987; Clemis, Ballad, & Killion, 1986). First, they prevent sounds other than those specifically presented through the tube from entering the external ear canal. This is very helpful when testing in noisy environments such as an intensive care unit or an operating room. It also is helpful when trying to test one ear independently of the other. When compared to supra- or circumaural earphones, inserts show significantly greater interaural attenuation—the amount that the intensity of a sound presented to one ear is decreased when heard by the other. When the foam plug is pushed deeply into the external auditory canal, inserts generally show an interaural attenuation greater than 70 dB (Killion, Wilber, & Gudmundsen, 1985).

A second advantage is that the insert ensures that the sound reaches the tympanic membrane. In infants (and some other patients), the external ear canal is not as rigid as in adults, and a supra-aural earphone may cause the canal to collapse, causing a conductive hearing loss.

A final advantage—specific to electrophysiologic recordings—is that the electrical artifact occurs before the sound reaches the ear. The main time difference is the length of the tube divided by the velocity of sound in air. Typical tubes are 24 cm long, which translates to a delay of 0.7 ms (as the velocity of sound in air at 20° C is 343 m/s.). There also is a filtering delay in the transducer, making the total delay between the electrical pulse reaching the microphone and the sound reaching the ear about 0.9 ms.

Figure 5–1 shows the time waveforms and spectra for a click stimulus presented through a supra-aural earphone and a transducer connected to an ear insert.

Bone Conduction

Auditory stimuli can be presented by bone conduction as well as the more usual air conduction. Conductive loss is definitively diagnosed when bone conduction thresholds are lower than air conduction thresholds. Bone vibrators cause the skull to vibrate. This sets up traveling waves in the basilar membrane in the same way as vibration of the stapes, although much less efficiently. Bone conduction can occur when the stimulator is placed anywhere on the skull. Typically, the vibrator is applied to one mastoid but, in an adult or older child, this will also stimulate the contralateral ear with little interaural attenuation.

Normative hearing levels for bone conduction vary with the location of the vibrator on the skull and with the occlusion of the external ear canal. Occluding the ear canal makes bone-conducted sound easier to hear, particularly at lower frequencies (Small & Stapells, 2003). Bone vibrators are effective for stimuli of both high and low frequency (Durrant & Hyre,

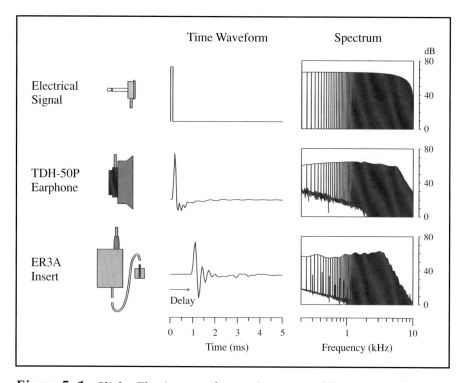

Figure 5–1. **Clicks.** *The time waveform and spectrum of the electrical click stimulus—a 100-μs pulse—is shown in the upper part of the figure. The spectrum was based on an average of the stimuli presented over 1 s at a rate of 40 Hz. The lines in the spectrum (plotted logarithmically from 200 to 10,000 Hz) therefore recur every 40 Hz. The spectrum continues out until a nul region at 10,000 Hz (the reciprocal of the pulse duration). The middle row of diagrams shows the acoustic click as transduced by an earphone and measured using a 6-cc coupler. The lower row shows the acoustic click, as transduced through an ER3A system, presented to the ear through an insert, and measured in a 2-cc coupler. There is a delay caused by the transmission of the click down the tube connecting the transducer to the insert. Furthermore, the frequency response of this system does not extend as far to the high frequencies as the TDH-50P earphone.*

1993) and can present the same stimuli we use to elicit auditory EPs by air conduction. Bone vibrators do not show the same intensity range as ear phones; therefore the maximum hearing levels for brief stimuli are low. Stimulus artifact is a major problem when recording auditory EPs to bone-conducted stimuli. Because this can interfere with the detection of early auditory EPs, we typically use stimuli that alternate in polarity to cancel the electrical artifact (e.g., Foxe & Stapells, 1993).

MEASUREMENT OF STIMULUS INTENSITY

The intensity of a stimulus is measured in terms of sound pressure level (SPL), the amount of force exerted by the stimulus over a particular area. The unit is the Pascal (Pa), which is defined as 1 Newton/m^2 (or 10 dynes/cm^2). Sound levels typically are expressed in logarithmic units, as decibels (dB) relative to a reference level. For measurements of SPL, the reference is set to 20 µPa, an arbitrary level considered to be the lowest level of normal human hearing: 1 Pa is then 94 dB SPL.

An acoustic stimulus will vary in the amount of instantaneous force it exerts as its waveform varies from condensation to rarefaction. Therefore, we typically use a root-mean-square (rms) measurement to characterize the intensity level. Sound level meters can calculate this rms measurement over different times—from 35 ms ("impulse") to several hundred milliseconds. For short duration sounds, more information is provided by measuring the peak SPL (pSPL), or "peak-to-peak equivalent SPL" (peSPL). When the stimulus is asymmetrical about the baseline (e.g., a click), the peSPL is a better measurement because subtle changes in the transducer to ear connection will alter the peak measurement more than the peak-to-peak measurement. The peSPL is the rms SPL of a pure tone that has the same peak-to-peak amplitude as the stimulus being calibrated. This is the current usage of the term (e.g., Durrant & Boston, 2007; Haughton, Lightfoot, & Stevens, 2003; Richter & Fedtke, 2005). Earlier procedures where the tone was made to equal the peak-amplitude of the transient ("peak equivalent" rather than "peak-to-peak equivalent") were confusing and uninformative (as the peak equivalent measurement is always exactly 3 dB less than the peak measurement) and should no longer be used. Figure 5–2 shows how peSPL is measured. Table 5–1 provides the normal thresholds for clicks and brief tones

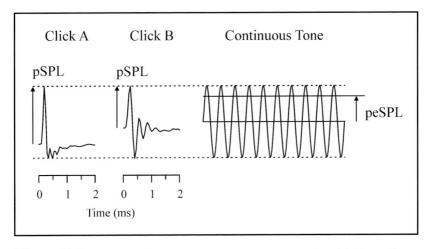

Figure 5–2. Measuring the intensity of brief stimuli. *This figure shows the time waveforms of two clicks with the same peak-to-peak equivalent SPL (peSPL) but different peak SPL (pSPL). The pSPL is measured at the maximum deflection of the waveform from baseline. Click A is much more asymmetric around the baseline than click B and has a larger pSPL. The peSPL is the root-mean-square intensity of a pure tone that has the same peak-to-peak amplitude as the click. This requires that the time waveforms of the sounds being measured by the sound level meter are observed on an oscilloscope. The peak-to-peak amplitude of the click is measured on the oscilloscope (dashed lines). Then a tone is presented instead of the click. The amplitude of the tone is increased until it reaches the peak-to-peak amplitude of the click and then the tone's root-mean-square intensity (thin line) is read from the meter.*

Table 5–1. Normal Behavioral Thresholds (peSPL) for Brief Stimuli*

Stimulus	*Frequency (Hz)*	*TDH-39 Phone with Supra-Aural Cushion*	*ER-3A Transducer with Foam Insert*
Clicks (100 μs)		31.0	35.5
2-1-2 Tones	500	23.0	23.5
	1000	20.0	21.5
	2000	25.0	30.5
	4000	27.5	33.0

*Table presents the mean values from ISO 389-6 (2007). Values (to closest 0.5 dB) were derived from Richter and Fedtke (2005) for clicks and Fedtke and Richter (2007) for tone. Stimuli were presented at a rate of 20 Hz for a duration of 1 s. Stimuli were calibrated using an artificial ear for the TDH-39 for the supra-aural phones and an occluded ear simulator for the inserts. A 6-cc coupler provides similar results to the artificial ear. However, there are significant differences between the occluded ear simulator and the more commonly used 2-cc coupler used to calibrate inserts (see Haughton, 2006 for compensation factors).

A second way the intensity of a sound can be measured is relative to normal human hearing. This hearing level (HL) varies with the frequency of the sound. Human beings normally hear best at frequencies between 1000 and 4000 Hz, with the thresholds at higher and lower frequencies rising significantly above these minimum levels. HL calibrations delineate the zero line of the audiogram. Various standards have provided HL calibrations for the different audiometric frequencies using different acoustic transducers (e.g., ISO, 1994, 1998a, 1998b).

CONCEPTS OF THRESHOLD

When scientists began to evaluate hearing using the auditory EPs, they found that the thresholds for detecting the electrophysiologic responses to brief tones were significantly elevated above HL. An important reason for this was the brevity of the stimuli—the behavioral thresholds were also elevated for these brief stimuli. Because of temporal integration, a sound that is shorter than about 500 ms will not be detected at as low a level as a longer sound (ISO, 2007). The relationship between threshold and signal duration is not simple, with different slopes occurring for durations 200 to 10 ms and durations less than 10 ms. Brief stimuli presented at different rates also are integrated over an observation interval, but this does not follow the same relationship as duration (two stimuli are not heard as well as one stimulus of twice the duration). Different neuronal systems might be integrating the stimulus energy at shorter and longer durations, or there might be a "leaky" integrator that stores stimulus energy over time but is subject to a continuing attenuation. Furthermore, the system that checks to see if there was a sound must operate according to some schedule and may combine the information from "multiple looks" (Viemeister & Wakefield, 1991). Whether the integration systems underlying stimulus detection are similar to those underlying stimulus discrimination or loudness assessment remains unclear. Another issue in the use of brief stimuli is that the temporal integration functions may be different in patients with hearing loss (Olsen, 1987).

To compensate for the brevity of the stimuli, a new calibration standard began to be used—nHL or the average threshold level for any given stimulus in young normal-hearing adults. Effectively, nHL or normal hearing level was HL "normalized" for the specific characteristics (particularly duration and rate) of the stimulus being used. The term came into use in the 1970s, and was perhaps first noted in Picton, Woods, Baribeau-Braun, and Healey (1977), who used a lower case "n" to distinguish the abbreviation from that of the National Hockey League. Other scientists continued to use HL as meaning relative to normal human hearing for whatever stimulus was being used. However, because HL is most widely defined and standardized only on the basis of frequency (and not rate or duration), this becomes confusing.

When the auditory brainstem response (ABR) was being used to assess threshold, we compared the ABR threshold to the behavioral thresholds for the same stimuli (clicks or brief tones) that were used to evoke the ABR. Because there was a 5-dB difference in threshold between stimuli presented at 5/s and those presented at 80/s (Stapells, Picton, & Durieux-Smith, 1982), most settled on 10/s or 20/s as the rate at which the stimulus should be calibrated. The ABR thresholds then began to fit reasonably well with those recorded behaviorally, with average electrophysiologic-behavioral threshold differences around 10 dB. If averaging was prolonged and care was taken to reduce the amount of physiologic background noise, this difference for the click ABR became only a few decibels (Elberling & Don, 1987).

Forgotten in the move toward nHL was the fact that much of the difference

between the physiologic and the behavioral thresholds was not really related to either the duration or rate of the stimuli. The click ABR is evoked within several milliseconds. Clearly, it is evoked or not, regardless of whether the next stimulus occurs 10 ms later or 1000 ms later. Transient EPs are responses to stimulus change. In the case of stimuli used to measure hearing thresholds, the change is the "onset," the increase in stimulus intensity from below to above threshold. The ABR is evoked by the onset of a stimulus and does not vary with its duration beyond about 3 ms (Brinkmann & Scherg, 1979; Suzuki & Horiuchi, 1981). Thus, even though there is a significant 7-dB difference in hearing threshold between 1-kHz tones lasting 5 and 14 ms (Davis, Hirsh, Popelka, & Formby, 1984), we should not expect different thresholds for recognizing the ABR evoked by the onsets of these stimuli.

Confusion can occur with nHL when we present brief stimuli at different rates —should nHL change with the stimulus rate? Behavioral thresholds decrease at more rapid rates. The human brain integrates over several hundred milliseconds before deciding whether a response is present or not. However, we should not make compensatory changes in the intensity of the click or brief tone when assessing the ABR, as whatever physiology determines the presence or absence of an ABR will not be affected by changing the SOAs if they are longer than the latency of the response (Lightfoot, Sininger, Burkard, & Lodwig, 2007). The relation between physiologic and behavioral thresholds is further muddied when we consider the effects of adaptation. Physiologic responses are smaller at more rapid rates and thus more difficult to distinguish from the residual background electroencephalogram (EEG). Wave V of the ABR is resistant to these effects but even this wave gets smaller when the rates become very rapid. Thus, increasing the rate of stimulation can cause the thresholds for the physiologic response to increase even as the perceptual thresholds decrease.

The approximately 20-dB elevation of ABR thresholds to brief tones over what would be expected from HL thresholds for long-duration tones is caused by several physiologic factors. One is the background electrical noise in the recording—there is always some residual EEG noise. Elberling and Don (1987) have shown how the ABR threshold can be significantly reduced by decreasing the background EEG noise. A second factor is the degree of synchronization among the multiple responses elicited by the repeating stimuli. When the response approaches threshold, it can become variable in its occurrence and in its timing. This variability may be caused by the background acoustic noise. This noise can be both environmental (in the testing chamber) and physiologic (the noise generated by such processes as blood flow and breathing). Thus, at 10 dB above threshold, the response may only be evoked by about half of the stimuli and may occur at latencies that vary over several milliseconds. The physiologic responses may not average together to give a reliable response, although they would be sufficient to be "heard" at higher centers of the nervous system that integrate input (regardless of its latency) over time.

The problems of nHL become obvious when we compare transient responses to brief tones with auditory steady-state responses (ASSRs) to amplitude-modulated tones. The steady-state responses are evoked by periodic increases in the level of the ongoing tone and therefore are similar to those evoked by the periodic onsets of the tones that evoke the ABRs. How-

ever, threshold levels for the tone-ABRs generally Are related to nHL calibrations (usually based on stimuli presented at rates of 10 or 20 Hz), whereas ASSR threshold levels are determined by the HL thresholds for tones of long duration.

Rance, Tomlin, and Rickards (2006) and Van Maanen and Stapells (2008) both reported that the thresholds in infants for the ABRs evoked by brief tones and for ASSRs evoked by amplitude-modulated tones were similar in terms of peSPL (although quite different in terms of nHL or HL). In adults and older children, the HL thresholds for the ASSR are lower than the peSPL thresholds for brief tones. It is possible that there is some integration period in the ASSR (that combines the responses over several cycles to give a larger response) in older subjects but not in infants. This could explain the fact that the 40-Hz ASSR has a threshold that is very close to the behavioral threshold for the continuous tone, as the integration time constant of the 40-Hz response is close to 200 ms (Ross, Picton, & Pantev, 2002). We might predict that the integration time constant for the 80-Hz response is shorter than for the 40-Hz response, and that this time constant might be even shorter in the newborn and get longer as the infant matures.

Perhaps we should move away from nHL and use a reference such as physiologic threshold level (PTL). This would be the mean threshold for detecting a physiologic response to a given stimulus in young adults. Then we would not need to remember how much to compensate the nHL measurements to determine an estimated behavioral threshold from a physiologic threshold. Right now we use two values: the nHL determined by the behavioral thresholds for the stimuli and the physiologic-behavioral difference.

PTL would provide only one value. We would need some provisos about the signal-to-noise ratios and/or the levels of residual EEG noise in the recordings. Clearly, the PTL would decrease as the duration of the analysis increases and the EEG noise levels decrease (Picton, Dimitrijevic, Perez-Abalo, & van Roon, 2005). However, these are necessary requirements for using the physiologic-behavioral difference as well.

BRIEF TONES AND FREQUENCY SPECIFICITY

The most commonly used stimulus in behavioral audiometry is a pure tone. Auditory EPs typically are evoked by much briefer stimuli than those used in behavioral audiometry, stimuli lasting a few rather than several hundred milliseconds. Even if long-duration tones are used, the EP is initiated by the onset of the tone. Brief tones and the onsets of longer tones do not have the same frequency specificity as a pure tone. The spectrum of a brief tone has a maximum at the nominal frequency of the tone, but stimulus energy also spreads to other frequencies. This spread is often described in terms of "skirts," and like the skirt of a dress, it can have various patterns, depending on the duration and waveform of the tone's "envelope." Figure 5–3 shows the spectra of some brief tones that have been used in EP audiometry.

If the stimulus contains energy at multiple frequencies, we never can be sure which frequency is eliciting the response. This lack of frequency specificity is a particular problem when there is a steep high-frequency hearing loss. A brief tone presented at a frequency where there is little or no hearing can activate a response by means of the low frequencies present in its spectrum. This response will occur later than expected because of the longer latency of the responses from the low-frequency regions.

Several studies have compared the frequency specificity of brief tones with different envelopes (e.g., Oates & Stapells, 1997a, 1997b; Purdy & Abbas, 2002). No difference could be found between the different envelopes. This is likely because the bandpass of the cochlear filter is wider than the acoustic spectra of the different brief tones.

The most commonly used brief tone in EP studies uses linear rise and fall times that each last 2 cycles and a plateau that lasts 1 cycle – the "2-1-2" tone (Davis et al., 1984; Fedtke & Richter, 2007). The duration of the tone decreases with increasing frequency but the spectrum shows a similar width when expressed on a logarithmic frequency scale. Behavioral thresholds for such tones are given in Table 5–1.

When considering frequency specificity, we also should consider the differentiation between acoustic specificity (also known as frequency specificity) and place specificity (Burkard & Don, 2007). The basilar membrane is set up so that the regions close to the stapes respond best to high frequencies and regions close to the apex to low frequencies. Because of the asymmetry of the traveling wave, a continuous pure tone, which has energy only at the frequency of the tone, also activates regions of the basilar membrane that respond best to higher frequencies. To get to the low-frequency regions, the sound has to travel through (and inadvertently activate) these high-frequency regions. Thus a long-duration tone is acoustically quite specific, having energy only at its nominal frequency. However, at moderate or high intensity, the tone is not place specific,

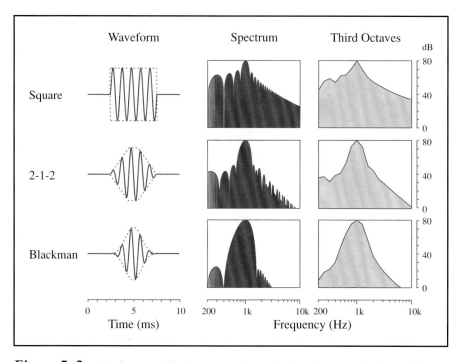

Figure 5–3. Brief tones. The time waveforms for brief tones with three different envelopes (dashed lines) are shown on the left. Each tone has a frequency of 1 kHz and a total duration of 5 ms. The spectra are shown on the right using a full FFT evaluation (center) and third-octave filters (right). The FFT was based on averages of waveforms presented at 10 Hz and therefore the lines in the spectrum are much closer than in Figure 5–1. The spectra have been adjusted to have equal maximum amplitudes of 80 dB. The square envelope causes a large spread of energy to frequencies other than 1 kHz. The energy of tones with 2-1-2 or Blackman envelopes is more concentrated near 1 kHz and the energy one octave away is reduced by 30 to 40 dB from the peak at 1 kHz.

activating the basilar membrane both at the location specific to the frequency of the tone and also, to a lesser extent, at locations specific to higher frequencies. When we try to evaluate an isolated severe low-frequency hearing loss during routine audiometry, we are unable to register a threshold higher than about 40 or 50 dB HL because louder tones activate the normal high-frequency regions. This also happens when we use brief tones, although the effect is compounded by the spread of energy in the spectrum of the brief tone.

MASKING

These problems with frequency specificity —our sometime inability to know where on the basilar membranes our EP is coming from—lead to the concept of masking. Masking is what prevents recognition— enjoyable during carnival but frustrating in real life. In hearing, masking typically occurs when we are listening to someone speak in the presence of background noise (from traffic, air conditioners, or other speakers). Masking can be measured behaviorally by the decrement in perception that occurs when a masking sound is presented together with the sound that the subject is detecting, discriminating, or otherwise evaluating. The classic masking experiment is to detect a tone of one frequency in the presence of a tone of another frequency ("tone on tone" masking). The main finding is that tones have a greater masking effect (an increase in the threshold for detection) on tones of higher frequency than on tones of lower frequency.

The physiologic processes underlying masking are complex and likely involve at least three different processes. The first involves "busy line" effects—neurons responding to one frequency (the masking tone) cannot respond additionally to another frequency (the probe tone). Because of the traveling wave and the hair cell filter, a tone causes maximal movement of the basilar membrane at a particular place on the basilar membrane. However, it also activates regions of the basilar membrane closer to the stapes. The activation pattern caused by a 1-kHz pure tone is shown in Figure 5–4. Although the maximal activation of the basilar membrane by this tone occurs in the middle turn of the cochlea, significant activation occurs at regions of the basilar membrane in the basal turn that respond best to higher frequencies. These regions of the cochlea may not be able to respond any more when high-frequency tones are presented because they are already busy responding to the 1-kHz tone. There is an asymmetry to the masking pattern of a tone—masking spreads more to higher frequencies than to lower. From the activation pattern shown in Figure 5–4, one can calculate the tuning curve of a single auditory neuron located on the basilar membrane (Figure 5–5). The tip of the tuning curve is related to the hair cell filter and the tail is caused by the traveling wave.

Once a neuron has been activated by one sound, it can also be "suppressed" by another sound. This is a second process that can cause masking. "Suppression" is measured physiologically when a neuron responding to a tone at its characteristic frequency is inhibited by a tone of another frequency. Suppression probably occurs at the level of the hair cells. It has effects in both frequency directions—high on low and low on high.

Once auditory information reaches the central nervous system, inhibitory interactions can occur between neurons. Common to all neural networks is the phenomenon of lateral inhibition, whereby activity in one neuron inhibits the activity of adjacent neurons. This plays a role in central masking, typically evaluated by the effects of stimuli presented in one ear on the responses to stimuli in the other ear. These effects can be seen in middle and later auditory EPs but are largely absent when studying the ABR. The monaural ABR generally is not affected by stimuli in the contralateral ear unless they are presented at levels that can be cross-heard in the ipsilateral ear. Central masking also occurs between sounds in one ear, but this is very difficult to distinguish from the cochlear causes of masking.

Notched Noise

A stimulus has its major masking effect on stimuli with the same or similar frequency. Thus, we might be able to use masking to limit the region of the basilar membrane that can respond to a stimulus. If we are concerned that a brief tone may be activating regions of the basilar membrane that are actually place-specific to frequencies other than the nominal frequency of the tone, we can use masking noise in the same

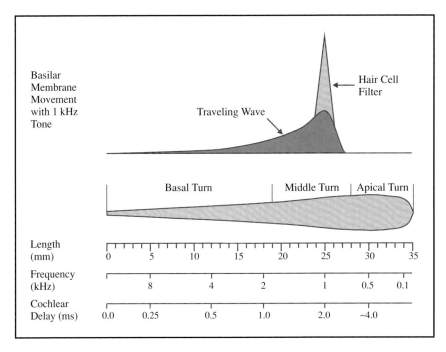

Figure 5–4. *Activation of the human basilar membrane. This figure illustrates how the basilar membrane is activated by a pure tone of 1 kHz. As the traveling wave moves along the basilar membrane from the stapes to the apex, it causes maximum movement at a region specific to 1 kHz in the middle turn of the cochlea. The movement pattern of the traveling wave is such that the regions of the basilar membrane closer to the stapes* (on the left in the diagram) *are also activated, although to a lesser extent than at the 1-kHz region. There is little spread of activation to lower frequency regions. When the hair cells are functioning normally, the 1-kHz region shows an additional enhancement of the activation—this is considered the result of the cochlear amplifier or "hair cell filter." The combined effect of the traveling wave and the filter causes a delay in the response that we have called the "cochlear delay." For the 1-kHz region, this is about 2 ms. The representation of the basilar membrane* (from the stapes on the left to the apex on the right) *shows its width as well as length. It is based on typical adult male measurements; female measurements are slightly smaller. This representation of derives from a slide made by Curtis Ponton.*

ear to prevent those regions from responding. Notched noise—broadband noise with a small range of frequencies removed—should fulfill these needs (Picton, Ouellette, Hamel, & Durieux-Smith, 1979; Stapells, Picton, & Durieux-Smith, 1993). Brief tones are presented mixed with broadband noise that is notched at the frequency of the tone. The noise should allow the tone to activate the regions of the basilar membrane that are place-specific for the tone's frequency and prevent any spread of activation to other regions. The effect of notched noise on the responses to brief tones is shown in Figure 5–6. In the upper part of this figure, the responses were evoked

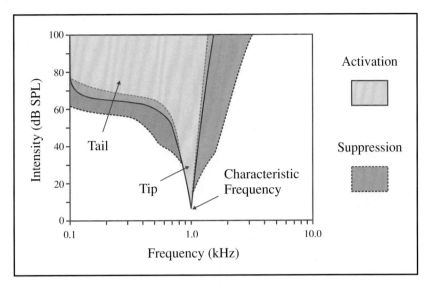

Figure 5–5. *Tuning curves. This diagram shows how a single auditory afferent fiber coming from hair cells in the 1-kHz region of the basilar membrane responds to sound. The light-shaded area shows the frequency and intensity regions where the fiber responds to sound. The continuous line is the "tuning curve," above which the fiber responds. At the lowest level, it responds only at its "characteristic frequency." The tuning curve has a shape that is related to the activation pattern shown in Figure 5–4, with the "tip" caused by the hair cell filter and the tail caused by the asymmetry of the traveling wave. The diagram also shows darker regions where stimulation suppresses the response of a fiber to a sound presented at its characteristic frequency.*

by tones presented without any masking noise. The 4-kHz tone presented by itself evokes responses at 75 dB pSPL, an intensity significantly below the patient's behavioral thresholds (for long duration tones) at 4 kHz. This is because the response is mediated by the low-frequency energy present in the spectrum of the brief tone. Indeed, the latency and morphology of the response is similar to the response to a tone at 1 kHz. With notched noise, the response can only come from the frequencies in the stimulus that are passed through the notch. Here the response is visible only at 125 dB pSPL, which is compatible with the behavioral audiogram.

Notched noise is not as good as we might hope because of the asymmetry of the masking function. Masking spreads from the low edge of the notch to interfere with the perception of frequencies within the notch. This spread of masking makes it difficult to detect responses to clicks in notched noise because the masking noise has to be at the same level as the click. However, the procedure works well with brief tones, where the masking noise can be presented at an SPL about 20 dB below the peak intensity of the tone. This level is sufficient to mask any response to the brief tone's spectral skirts, and low enough to let the energy at the nominal frequency of the brief tone elicit a response of reasonable amplitude.

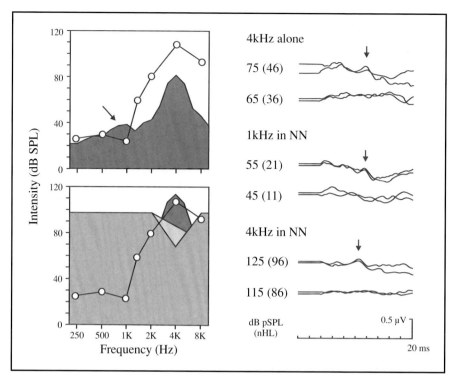

Figure 5–6. *Frequency specificity and notched noise. This upper part of this figure illustrates how a brief tone can activate areas of the basilar membrane that respond optimally to frequencies other than the nominal frequency of the tone. The diagram in the upper left of the figure shows the spectrum of a brief 4-kHz tone* (dark shading) *superimposed on the audiogram of a patient with a high-frequency hearing loss, plotted* (connected circles) *in terms of SPL rather than HL and upside-down from the usual audiogram. At a peak-intensity of 80 dB, the brief tone is below threshold at 4 kHz. However, the skirts of the spectrum can activate a response through the 1-kHz region of the basilar membrane where the threshold is close to normal* (arrow). *The lower left of the figure shows the how notched noise* (NN, medium shading) *can prevent the brief tone from activating a response through the skirts of the spectrum. The diagram also shows the spread of masking from the low-frequency edge of the notch into the notch* (light shading). *The tone in NN can activate a response in this patient only when the peak intensity exceeds the threshold at 4 kHz. The left side of the figure shows the actual ABR recordings in this patient. Intensities are presented in both pSPL and nHL* (in brackets). *When the brief 4-kHz tone is presented alone* (upper two recordings), *a response can be seen at 75 dB pSPL, below the behavioral threshold at that frequency. The latency of wave V in this response is similar to the latency of wave V in the response to a 1-kHz tone* (middle two recordings), *suggesting that the response is mediated through the 1-kHz region of the basilar membrane. The bottom two recordings show the response to the 4-kHz tone presented in NN. Now, we can only obtain a response at 125 dB pSPL, which fits with the elevated behavioral threshold at 4 kHz. The latency of this response is shorter than that at 1 kHz, in part because the response is elicited through the 4-kHz region of the basilar membrane (which is activated earlier than the more apical 1-kHz region). These data derive from Picton et al. (1979).*

Derived Responses

Low-frequency sounds interfere with the processing of high frequency sounds, but there is little spread of masking from high to low frequency. Using this asymmetry, Teas, Eldridge, and Davis (1962) developed a method of using high-pass noise to derive the components of the compound action potential recorded from the cochlear nerve in response to a click. This technique later was used to evaluate the compound action potential recorded in the human electrocochleogram (Eggermont, 1976; Elberling, 1974), and then the ABR (Don & Eggermont, 1978; Don, Eggermont, & Brackmann, 1979; Parker & Thornton, 1978a, 1978b).

The process of deriving narrow-band ABRs is illustrated in Figure 5–7. As we

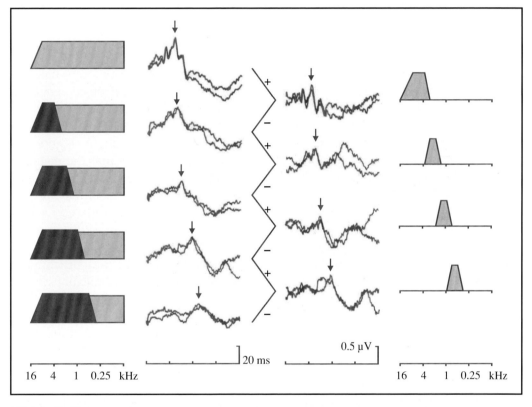

Figure 5–7. Derived responses. The first column of the figure diagrammatically represents the activation of the basilar membrane by 39/s 70 dB nHL clicks (gray) presented alone and then together with high-pass noise masking (black) with decreasing cutoff settings. The second column shows the ABRs to each of these click presentations. Sequential subtraction of one response from the response with a higher cutoff yields the derived response shown in the third column. Because of the subtraction process, the residual EEG noise level in these derived responses is higher than in the original high-pass noise responses. This can be seen in the reduced replicability of the two superimposed responses. The latency of wave V (arrows) in both the high-pass responses and the derived responses increases as the cutoff frequencies decrease. The column on the right shows the narrow band regions which evoke the derived responses. Because the slopes of the high-pass noise filters are not infinitely steep, the center of the derived bands is close to the lower of the two cutoff frequencies. Data derived from Stapells et al. (1993).

have seen, the click contains a broad band of frequencies and activates all regions of the cochlea. The click is mixed with broadband noise at an intensity that masks both the perception of the click and the generation of any recognizable ABR. Then the broadband noise is high-pass filtered using a filter with a steep cutoff slope (96 dB/octave or more). This high-frequency noise masks the responses of neurons with characteristic frequencies higher than the cutoff. The activation pattern of the high-pass noise on the basilar membrane does not spread to the low-frequency regions, which still responds to the click. The response to the click in high-pass noise thus represents the response coming from neurons with characteristic frequencies below the cutoff frequency. If we then decrease the cutoff frequency of the high-pass noise, we can record the response of a smaller group of neurons with lower characteristic frequencies. This response can be subtracted from the previous response to get the "derived narrow-band response"—effectively the response of the neurons that have characteristic frequencies between the two high-pass filter settings. Because the filters do not have infinite slopes, the center of the actual derived narrow band is closer to the lower of the two filter cutoffs. A rough estimate of the center frequency of the derived band is the square root of the product of the two cutoff frequencies (Parker & Thornton, 1978b).

The derived ABR changes dramatically as the center frequency of the narrow band decreases. Wave V increases in latency by 3 to 4 ms as the center frequency decreases from near 4000 to near 500 Hz (arrows on the right of Figure 5–7), and it becomes broader in its morphology. The delay is caused by a combination of the traveling wave delay and an additional delay in the hair cell filter, which combine to give a

"cochlear response time" (Don, Ponton, Eggermont, & Masuda, 1993, 1994). The broader morphology of the response at lower frequencies likely is caused by the summation of responses over a region of the basilar membrane with more variable latencies. The traveling wave slows down as it progresses and the latencies included within an octave-band span a greater range as the frequencies get lower (see Figure 5–5).

Stacked ABR

If we sum together the different narrowband derived responses, we can get back the original click response. However, this combination of responses causes much cancellation. For example, in Figure 5–8 (middle panel), we see that the negative peak (trough) of the derived 2.8-kHz narrowband response occurs at the same time as the positive peak of the derived 1.4-kHz narrowband response, resulting in much cancellation of these activities in the sum. Don Masuda, Nelson, and Brackmann (1997) showed that this cancellation caused both the latency and amplitude of wave V of the response to a click stimulus to be dominated by the activity coming from the high-frequency regions. If only the top two derived narrowband responses (11.3 and 5.7 kHz bands) are summed, the resultant waveform is similar both in amplitude and latency to that of the response to the click alone. Thus, any changes to the response coming from the middle and lower frequency regions of the basilar membrane may not be visible in the combined response. The predominance of the contributions from the high-frequency regions to the click-ABR has severe drawbacks in assessing the presence of pathologies such as acoustic tumors. Unless the tumor affects the con-

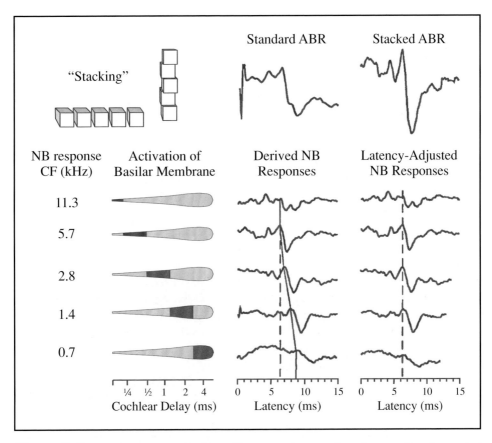

Figure 5–8. ***Stacked ABR.*** *This figure illustrates the procedure for recording the stacked ABR (Don et al., 1997). Basically, the standard ABR is broken down into its building blocks—the derived narrow band responses—using the high-pass noise technique illustrated in Figure 5–7, and then these blocks are adjusted so that they have the same latency and then recombined into the stacked ABR. For each narrowband center frequency, there is an ABR with peak latencies that increase as the center frequency decreases (center column). As represented on the left, this is caused by the increasing cochlear delay as the area of activation (black) isolated by the derived response technique moves along the basilar membrane from the stapes to the apex. We can adjust the latencies of the derived responses so that all the wave V peaks occur at the same time (right column). This prevents the waveforms from canceling each other out in the summed response (e.g., the derived responses for the 2.8- and 1.4-kHz responses). The latency-adjusted responses can then be recombined to give the stacked ABR in the upper right. This is between 1.5 and 2 times larger than the standard ABR.*

tributions from the high-frequency regions, the click-ABR will appear normal. Since small (<1 cm) acoustic tumors often do not affect the high-frequency fibers, ABR latency measures may not be adequate for detecting these small lesions.

Don et al. (1997) and Don, Kwong, Tanaka, Brackmann, and Nelson (2005) therefore developed the "stacked ABR" technique to provide a better evaluation of all the responses coming from all regions of the basilar membrane. The click-ABR is decomposed into derived narrowband responses, the latencies of these responses are adjusted to the wave V latency of each derived response ("stacking process"), and the responses then are recombined. Essentially the response is decomposed into its building blocks and then these are restacked one atop the other. This gives an ABR in which the wave V amplitude measurement more accurately portrays the number of fibers responding to the click. If a small tumor compromises a significant number of fibers, there will be a reduction in the amplitude of the stacked ABR. This reduction does not depend solely on only the high-frequency fibers being affected as all fibers are contributing to the total activity in the stacked ABR. Thus, this procedure (illustrated in Figure 5–8), can provide a more accurate detection of small acoustic neuromas than simply measuring the click ABR latency.

CHIRPS

A click activates the whole basilar membrane but each region of the membrane responds at a different time, the low-frequency regions responding later than the high frequency regions. Several researchers (Elberling, Callø, & Don, 2010; Elberling & Don, 2008; Elberling, Don, Cebulla, & Stürzebecher, 2007; Fobel & Dau, 2004) have constructed transient stimuli composed of different frequencies that begin at different times. The timing of these "chirps" can be adjusted according to the cochlear response times for the different frequencies. Such stimuli are illustrated in Figure 5–9. The idea is to make the different regions of the cochlea respond simultaneously. Thus, low-frequency components of the stimulus begin earlier than high-frequency components. Chirps evoke larger responses than clicks. Because large

responses can be recognized more quickly, chirps may become helpful in rapid tests of hearing, or in tests to evaluate abnormal response amplitudes. The response to a broadband chirp should be similar to the stacked ABR to a click. In the chirp response, the latency adjustment is done in the stimulus whereas in the stacked ABR the latency adjustment is done on the basis of the derived narrow-band responses.

The chirp illustrated in Figure 5–9 is composed of a broad band of frequencies. We can also construct chirps composed of a limited band of frequencies (Elberling, Cebulla, & Stürzebecher, 2007). In this way, we can separately test high- and low-frequency regions of the cochlea, or use narrowband chirp stimuli instead of brief tones as frequency-specific stimuli.

MODULATION OF CONTINUOUS STIMULI

Auditory EPs can be evoked by continuous as well as transient stimuli. As discussed in Chapter 1, a continuing auditory stimulus may evoke a sustained potential that lasts through the duration of the stimulus. If the continuing stimulus is periodically modulated in some way, we can also evoke ASSRs.

ASSRs can be evoked by many different types of modulation. Figure 5–10 shows some of these stimuli, together with their acoustic spectra. Amplitude modulation (AM) is the most common stimulus, and the most common type of AM is the sinusoidal amplitude-modulation (SAM) of a continuous tone (top left of the figure). This stimulus is much more frequency-specific than repeating brief tones because the SAM tone contains energy only at the carrier frequency and at two side bands separated from the carrier by the modulation frequency. Despite this acoustic speci-

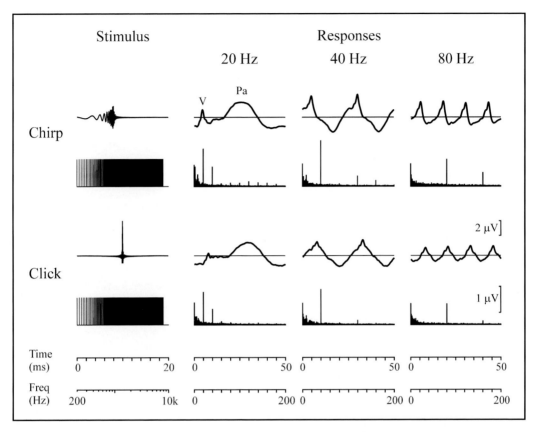

Figure 5–9. *Chirps. Like clicks, chirps contain frequencies across the audible frequency range, but the relative timing (or phase) of the frequencies within the stimulus can be adjusted to compensate for the normal cochlear delay. This allows activation to occur simultaneously at the different regions of the cochlea. The chirp shown in the upper left was constructed according to the procedures of Elberling et al. (2007). The click shown at the lower right was actually a chirp without any timing difference between the frequencies. The amplitude spectra for the stimuli plotted below the waveforms are identical. Responses were recorded using stimulus rates of 20, 40, or 80 Hz. At 20 Hz, wave V of the response is larger for the chirp, and this gives a larger ASSR at both 40 and 80 Hz. The responses are shown, like the stimuli, in both time and frequency domains.*

ficity, the stimulus is not better than brief tones in terms of place specificity (Herdman, Picton, & Stapells, 2002), probably because the bandpass of the cochlear filter is wider than the spectrum of either brief tones or SAM tones.

Exponential amplitude modulation —using an envelope that is a function of the square or cube of the sine function— causes more rapidly rising envelopes than simple sinusoidal modulation and evokes larger ASSRs (John, Dimitrijevic, & Picton, 2002). Similar stimuli can be constructed in other ways (Stürzebecher, Cebulla, & Pschirrer, 2001).

Frequency-modulation (FM) also can evoke a response, perhaps because the stimulus moves in and out of different regions of the basilar membrane. Mixed modulation (MM), combining both AM and FM, evokes a response that approximates the sum of the responses to the two

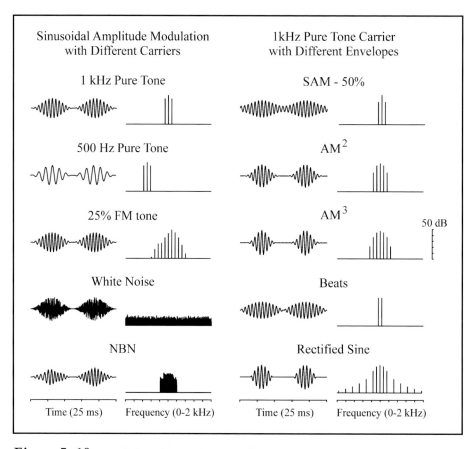

Figure 5–10. ***Modulated stimuli.*** *Ten different modulated stimuli are presented in both time and frequency domains. All stimuli have been adjusted to have the same root-mean-square amplitude. On the left side, five different carrier signals are modulated by the same 80-Hz sinusoidal envelope. The third of these, which combines both amplitude- and frequency-modulation, also has been called "mixed modulation" (John et al., 2001). Various amplitude modulated noise stimuli are described in John, Dimitrijevic, and Picton (2003). The amplitude modulated narrowband noise (NBN) is one-third octave in width. In the spectrum, the narrowband noise carrier and both sidebands are all one-third octave in width. Each cycle of the NBN varies in amplitude and waveform within the constraints of the noise bandwidth. On the right, different envelopes (all at 80 Hz) are applied to the same 1-kHz carrier. The two exponential envelopes (AM² and AM³) are described in more detail in John et al. (2002). The rectified sine wave envelope shown at the bottom right was used by Riquelme, Kuwada, Filipovic, Hartung, and Leonard (2006).*

modulations. The phases of the FM and AM responses are similar (and the MM response larger) when the highest frequency occurs at approximately the same time as the highest amplitude (Cohen, Rickards, & Clark, 1991; John, Dimitrijevic, van Roon, & Picton, 2001). Because the optimal relative phase between AM and FM can vary with the subject and with the carrier frequency, we have come to prefer exponential AM to MM.

Beats formed by presenting two tones with carrier frequencies differing by the beat frequency are even more frequency-specific than SAM tones as they contain acoustic energy at only two points in the spectrum. However, they evoke responses with only 70% of the amplitude of the SAM response (Picton et al., 2005).

AM broadband noise evokes a large ASSR that can be quickly recognized and may become helpful in hearing screening procedures (John, Dimitrijevic, & Picton, 2003).

BINAURAL STIMULI

Binaural Interaction Component

Sounds from the two ears begin to interact in the brainstem at the level of the superior olive. The physiologic demonstration of binaural interaction thus is a simple measurement of central auditory processing. An easy way to evaluate binaural processing is to compare responses to the same stimuli presented monaurally and binaurally. The simplest paradigm records responses to clicks presented to the left ear, right ear, and to both ears. Any difference between the binaural response and the sum of the two monaural responses represents binaural interaction. Formally calculating the difference yields a "binaural interaction component" (Dobie & Norton, 1980; Levine, 1981; McPherson & Starr, 1993; Picton, Rodriguez, Linden, & Maiste, 1985). This is illustrated in Figure 5–11. The binaural interaction component in the ABR is much smaller than the raw ABR, and often is difficult to demonstrate because the subtraction process increases the background noise levels in the recording. Even when clearly demonstrated, the ABR binaural interaction component remains difficult to interpret. Brainstem neurons often are characterized by whether they are excited or inhibited by ipsilateral or contralateral input. Although some of the neurons are excited by input from one ear and inhibited by input from the other, many neurons are excited by either ear. If so, their initial response to binaural stimulation will be less than the sum of their responses to each ear. Basically, the neuron will discharge in the same way to left, right, or binaural stimuli. The subtraction process then will give the responses of these particular neurons in inverted form. What this means in terms of binaural interaction is not known.

The binaural interaction components for the middle latency response (MLR) and late auditory EP (LAEP) are much larger than for the ABR, but again it is not clear what they might represent. Basically, the response to a binaural stimulus evokes an EP that is only a little larger than the response to either monaural stimulus. There is either inhibition between the responses to each ear or a process of occlusion; the system responds to either or both ears in the same way (Picton et al., 1985). The subtraction then gives a binaural interaction component that is about the same size as the monaural response but inverted in polarity. One interpretation is that the information coming to the auditory cortex from the brainstem is already tagged by its spatial location. Auditory objects from one or other side or from straight ahead are treated equally (Picton & Ross, 2010).

Changes in Interaural Timing and Correlation

When we use noise as a stimulus, we can change the relative timing between the ears and cause the perceived sound to shift its lateralization. Because the noise is unpredictable from moment to moment, such a change is not perceptible in either

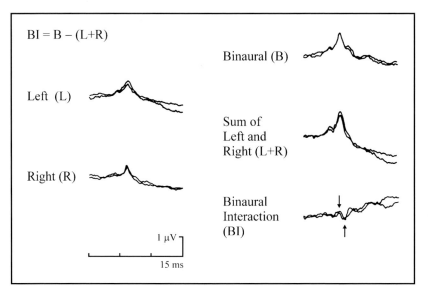

Figure 5–11. Binaural interaction components. *ABRs were recorded from vertex to larynx in response to 50 dB nHL rarefaction clicks presented at 21 Hz to the left ear, right ear, and binaurally. The binaural response (upper right) is almost twice the size of either monaural response. Subtracting the sum of the monaural responses from the binaural response provides the binaural interaction component (lower left). Two main components are present (arrows), a vertex positive wave just before the peak latency of wave V and a negative wave just after. In addition, there is a large negative shift in the binaural interaction waveform at the end of the recording; this is the binaural interaction component for the Na wave of the middle latency response. Data derived from Picton et al. (1985).*

ear alone. This type of stimulus was first used by Halliday and Callaway (1978) and more recently by McEvoy, Picton, Champagne, Kellett, and Kelly (1990) and Jones, Pitman, and Halliday (1991). The change in lateralization evokes an N1-P2-like component with a latency that is 20 to 50 ms later than the response to the simple onset of a stimulus. The stimuli and the responses are illustrated in the left section of Figure 5–12. The increased latency of the response to the change in lateralization has caused some discussion about whether the response is more similar to a mismatch negativity than the onset N1. The idea is that the response might reflect the change in the stimulus rather than its onset (Jones et al., 1991). As we will see in

Chapter 11, the mismatch negativity and the N1 component of the LAEP may represent similar processes.

An even simpler binaural noise stimulus is the change between stimuli that are identical (or to some extent correlated) in the two ears and stimuli that are uncorrelated. The change from correlated to uncorrelated noise is heard as a change from a sound that is focal in its location to one that is diffusely located—from right here to everywhere. Responses to changes in binaural correlation have been studied using the LAEPs (Jones et al., 1991; Lüddemann, Riedel & Kollmeier,) and the ASSRs (Dajani & Picton, 2006). The stimuli and responses are illustrated in right section of Figure 5–12.

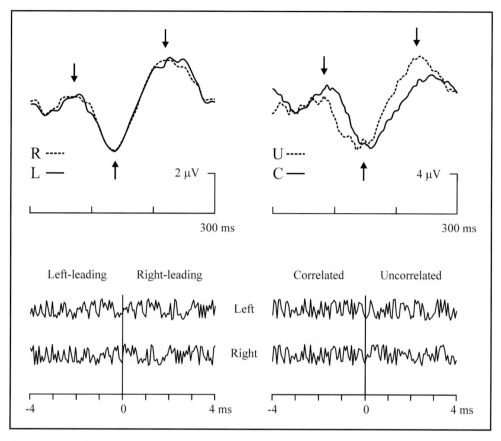

Figure 5–12. **Binaural stimuli.** *White noise stimuli were presented to the two ears at an intensity of 60 dB SL. The responses on the left were elicited by a transition from left-leading to right-leading (R), or vice versa (L). Periods of 4 ms before and after the R transition are illustrated below. In the first 4 ms, the waveform of the noise is the same in the two ears but it occurs 1 ms later in the right ear; in the second 4 ms, the left ear is 1 ms later. The transition was heard as a white noise in the left ear suddenly switching to the right. The auditory EPs in the upper left are from McEvoy et al. (1990). The responses on the right were elicited by a change from correlated to uncorrelated noise (U) or vice versa (C). The U transition illustrated below shows the acoustic waveforms, which were the same in both ears before the transition and different afterward. The responses at the upper right are from Jones et al. (1991). These responses were recorded at a longer SOA (3 rather than 2 seconds) and over fewer trials than the responses on the left. These differences may partially explain the amplitude differences. Both sets of EPs show a positive-negative-positive waveform (arrows) at the vertex.*

Changing the Interaural Phase Differences

When we use tones rather than noise or clicks, localization is often based on the interaural phase. This is equivalent to interaural timing. Abruptly changing the phase of a pure tone would generate an audible click and we would not be able to distinguish binaural processing from click detection. However, Ross and his colleagues (Ross, Fujioka, Tremblay & Picton, 2007; Ross, Tremblay, & Picton, 2007) designed a stimulus that allows the phase of a continuous tone to be changed without any audible transient. The tone is amplitude-modulated at 40 Hz with a 100% depth of modulation. The change in phase is set to occur at the point in the modulation when the instantaneous amplitude is zero. Figure 5–13 shows how the stimulus can be used to change the interaural phase difference. This change in interaural phase evoked a P1-N1-P2 response with a latency that was 10 to 40 ms later than for the response to sound onset. It could be recognized with carrier frequencies up to 1250 Hz in young subjects. In elderly subjects, it could only be recorded up to 760 Hz, suggesting that

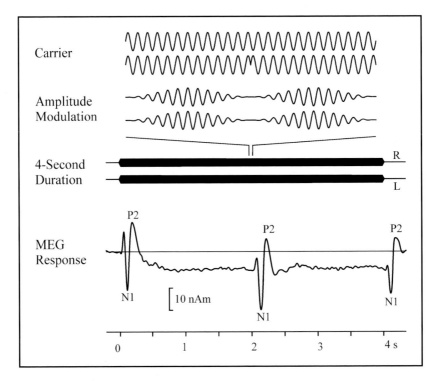

Figure 5–13. Changing the interaural phase difference. *This stimulus was created by changing the interaural phase of a 500-Hz tone from 0 degrees (the stimuli in the left and right ears are the same) to 180 degrees (the stimulus in the left ear is inverted in relation to that in the right ear). Because this change would be heard as a click, the stimulus was amplitude modulated so that the phase change occurred at zero amplitude. The upper part of the figure shows the carrier frequency in the two ears and the modulated stimulus from 25 ms before to 25 ms after the phase change. This change occurred at the middle of a 4-second amplitude-modulated tone* (shown in the middle of the figure)*. In addition to onset and offset responses, the MEG recording showed a P1-N1-P2 complex in response to the interaural phase change. This response has been filtered to remove the 40-Hz steady-state response and thus make the transient responses more visible (see Picton & Ross, in press). The data in this figure were derived from Ross, Fujioka, Tremblay, and Picton (2007).*

elderly subjects could not process the phase of the carrier frequency as precisely as younger subjects.

SPEECH STIMULI

Speech is the most important stimulus that we listen to. It is the primary way by which we communicate with one another. Speech is a complicated stimulus with many different parameters. Auditory EPs have been studied in relation to many of these parameters. In this chapter, we introduce some concepts underlying speech through the stimulus "da."

Figure 5–14 shows how speech sounds are produced. "Voiced" sounds are generated by vibrations of the vocal folds. In these sounds, periodic bursts of air come through the larynx and resonate in the different regions of the vocal tract—throat, mouth, and nose. Adjustments of the tongue can alter the volumes of these regions and cause different frequency bands to resonate—"formants." Vowels

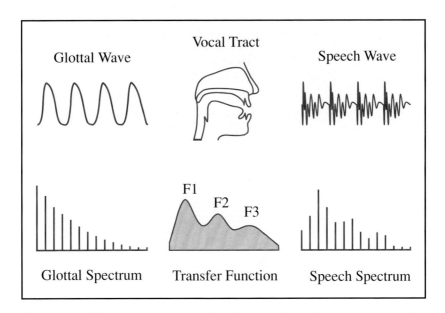

Figure 5–14. ***Speech sounds.*** *This diagram shows how a vowel sound is produced. Air passes through the larynx and is made pulsatile by the vibrations of the vocal folds. The spectrum of the glottal wave contains its greatest energy at the rate of vocal-fold vibration—the pitch of the voice—but also contains energy at the harmonics of this rate. The air coming out of the glottis then enters the vocal tract. Volumes in the vocal tract—particularly the pharynx, mouth, and nose—resonate at certain frequencies to accentuate the energy at various regions in the glottal spectrum called formants (F1, F2, F3). The relative frequencies of these formants are adjusted by the shape of the mouth and the position of the tongue. The speech wave is periodic at the frequency of the vocal-fold vibration and each pulse of sound contains the frequencies of the formants. The speech spectrum shows harmonics of the vocal pitch with enhancement of the harmonics within the formant bands. This diagram derives from the work of Fant (1960).*

are characterized by the relative frequencies of these formants. Consonants generally are much briefer than vowels and often are associated with rapid changes in the vocal tract.

As an illustration, Figure 5–15 gives the onset of the syllable "da" as used by Johnson, Nicol, and Kraus (2005). There is an onset as the tongue moves away from the teeth to allow the passage of sound.

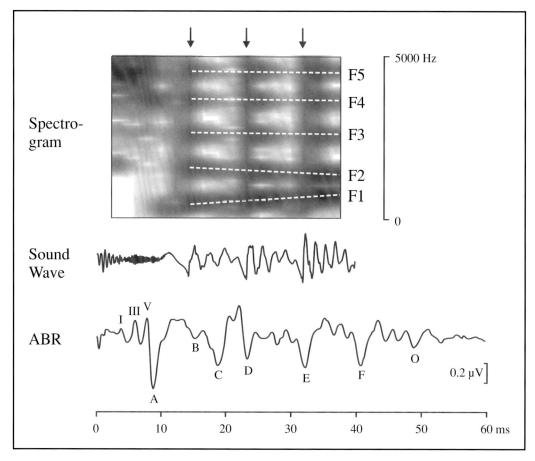

Figure 5–15. *Brainstem response to "da."* This stimulus is described more fully in Johnson et al. (2005), from which this figure has been adapted. The sound is the onset of the "da" sound. The upper part of the figure shows the spectrogram of the sound wave obtained using the program PRAAT (Boersma & Weenink, 2005). The spectrogram begins 2.5 ms after the onset (and finishes 2.5 ms before the offset) of the sound shown in the time domain in the middle of the figure. The spectrogram is plotted so that darker areas represent higher levels of energy, and there is some pre-emphasis to compensate for the decreasing energy levels at higher frequencies. The voicing with the glottal pulses of sound are indicated by the arrows. The formants are indicated by the dotted white lines. The formants activated at the beginning of the sound show the characteristic frequency changes (F2 decreasing and F1 increasing) that are heard as the transition of the "d" consonant to the "a" vowel. At the bottom is shown the ABR elicited by this brief speech stimulus. It contains an ABR evoked by the initial onset of the sound (mainly high-frequency). This is followed by a transition period (A, B, C), a frequency-following response (D, E, F) that follows the envelope of the glottal pulses, and a small offset response (O).

The resonance characteristics of the vocal tract change as the tongue moves to the position that will generate the vowel. At about the same time, we start to hear the periodic bursts of sound that represent the voicing. This sound activates a complex set of responses in the brainstem. Most important are an ABR-like response to the onset and a later periodic response to the voicing.

CONCLUSIONS

We have only touched on some of the simpler sounds that fill our world. More complex sounds—fine words and sweet music —also may be used to elicit auditory EPs. Creativity is needed to set up stimuli and paradigms so that we can measure the brain's response to these sounds and learn how it is that we hear and understand them.

ABBREVIATIONS

ABR	Auditory brainstem response
AM	Amplitude modulation
ASSR	Auditory steady-state response
EEG	Electroencephalography
EP	Evoked potential
FM	Frequency modulation
HL	Hearing level
LAEP	Late auditory evoked potential
MEG	Magnetoencephalography
MLR	Middle-latency response
MM	Mixed modulation
NBN	Narrowband noise
nHL	Normal hearing level
NN	Notched noise
peSPL	Peak-to-peak equivalent sound pressure level
pSPL	Peak sound pressure level
PTL	Physiologic threshold level
rms	Root-mean-square
SAM	Sinusoidal amplitude modulation
SOA	Stimulus onset asynchrony
SPL	Sound pressure level

REFERENCES

Beauchaine, K. A., Kaminski, J. R., & Gorga M. P. (1987). Comparison of Beyer DT48 and Etymotic insert earphones: Auditory brain stem response measurements. *Ear and Hearing, 8,* 292–297.

Boersma, P., & Weenink, D. (2005): PRAAT: Doing phonetics by computer. Available from: http://www.praat.org/

Brinkmann, R. D., & Scherg, M. (1979). Human auditory on- and off-potentials of the brainstem. *Scandinavian Audiology, 8,* 27–32.

Burkard, R. F., & Don, M. (2007). The auditory brainstem response. In R. F. Burkard, M. Don, & J. J. Eggermont (Eds.), *Auditory evoked potentials: Basic principles and clinical application* (pp. 229–253). Philadelphia, PA: Lippincott Williams & Wilkins.

Clemis, J. D , Ballad, W. J., & Killion, M. C. (1986). Clinical use of an insert earphone. *Annals of Otology, Rhinology and Laryngology, 95,* 520–524.

Cohen, L. T., Rickards, F. W., & Clark, G. M. (1991). A comparison of steady-state evoked potentials to modulated tones in awake and sleeping humans. *Journal of the Acoustical Society of America, 90,* 2467–2479.

Dajani, H. R., & Picton, T. W. (2006). Human auditory steady-state responses to changes in interaural correlation. *Hearing Research, 219,* 85–100,

Davis, H., Hirsh, S. K., Popelka, G. R., & Formby, C. (1984). Frequency selectivity and thresholds of brief stimuli suitable for electric response audiometry. *Audiology, 23,* 59–74.

Dobie, R. A., & Norton, S. J. (1980). Binaural interaction in human auditory evoked potentials. *Electroencephalography and Clinical Neurophysiology, 49,* 303–313.

Don, M., & Eggermont, J. J. (1978). Analysis of the click-evoked brainstem potentials in humans using high-pass noise masking. *Journal of the Acoustical Society of America, 63,* 1084–1092.

Don, M., Eggermont, J. J., & Brackmann, D. E. (1979). Reconstruction of the audiogram using brain stem responses and high-pass noise masking. *Annals of Otology, Rhinology and Laryngology Supplement, 57,* 1–20.

Don, M., Kwong, B., Tanaka, C., Brackmann, D., & Nelson, R. (2005). The stacked ABR: A sensitive and specific screening tool for detecting small acoustic tumors. *Audiology and Neurotology, 10,* 274–290.

Don, M., Masuda, A., Nelson, R., & Brackmann, D. (1997). Successful detection of small acoustic tumors using the stacked derived-band auditory brain stem response amplitude. *American Journal of Otology, 18,* 608–621.

Don, M., Ponton, C. W., Eggermont, J. J., & Masuda, A. (1993). Gender differences in cochlear response time: An explanation for gender amplitude differences in the unmasked auditory brain-stem response. *Journal of the Acoustical Society of America, 94,* 2135–2148.

Don, M., Ponton, C. W., Eggermont, J. J., & Masuda, A. (1994). Auditory brainstem response (ABR) peak amplitude variability reflects individual differences in cochlear response times. *Journal of the Acoustical Society of America, 96,* 3476–3491.

Durrant, J. D., & Boston, J. R. (2007) Stimuli for auditory evoked potential assessment. In R. F. Burkard, M. Don, & J. J. Eggermont (Eds.), *Auditory evoked potentials: Basic principles and clinical applications* (pp. 42–72). Baltimore, MD: Lippincott Williams & Wilkins.

Durrant, J. D., & Hyre, R. (1993). Relative effective frequency response of bone versus air conduction stimulation examined via masking. *Audiology, 32,* 175–184.

Durrant, J. D., Sabo, D. L., & Delgado, R. E. (2007). Call for calibration standard for newborn screening using auditory brainstem responses. *International Journal of Audiology, 46,* 686–691.

Eggermont, J. J. (1976). Electrocochleography. In W. D. Keidel & W. D. Neff (Eds.), *Handbook of sensory physiology. Vol. V/3 Auditory system. Clinical and special topics* (pp. 625–705). Berlin, Germany: Springer-Verlag.

Elberling, C. (1974). Action potentials along the cochlear partition recorded from the ear canal in man. *Scandinavian Audiology, 3,* 13–19.

Elberling, C., Callø, J., & Don, M. (2010). Evaluating auditory brainstem responses to different chirp stimuli at three levels of stimulation. *Journal of the Acoustical Society of America, 128,* 215–223.

Elberling, C., Cebulla, M., & Stürzebecher, E. (2007). Simultaneous multiple stimulation of the auditory steady-state response (ASSR) In T. Dau, J. M. Buchholz, J. M. Harte, T. U. Christiansen (Eds.), *Auditory signal processing in hearing-impaired listeners* (ISAAR 2007) (pp. 201–209). Copenhagen, Denmark: Centertryk (GN ReSound Audiological Library).

Elberling, C., & Don, M. (1987). Threshold characteristics of the human auditory brain stem response *Journal of the Acoustical Society of America, 81,* 115–121.

Elberling, C., & Don, M. (2008). Auditory brainstem responses to a chirp stimulus designed from derived-band latencies in normal-hearing subjects. *Journal of the Acoustical Society of America, 124,* 3022–3037.

Elberling, C., Don, M., Cebulla, M., & Stürzebecher, E. (2007). Auditory steady-state responses to chirp stimuli based on cochlear traveling wave delay. *Journal of the Acoustical Society of America, 122,* 2772–2785.

Fant, G. (1960). *Acoustic theory of speech production.* The Hague, The Netherlands: Mouton.

Fausti, S. A., Frey, R. H., Henry, J. A., Olson, D. J., & Schaffer, H. I. (1992). Early detection of ototoxicity using high-frequency, tone-burst-evoked auditory brainstem responses. *Journal of the American Academy of Audiology, 3,* 397–404.

Fedtke, T., & Richter, U. (2007). Reference zero for the calibration of air-conduction audiometric equipment using "tone bursts" as test signals. *International Journal of Audiology, 4,* 1–10.

Fobel, O., & Dau, T. (2004). Searching for the optimal stimulus eliciting auditory brainstem responses in humans. *Journal of the Acoustical Society of America, 116,* 2213–2222.

Foxe, J. J., & Stapells, D.R. (1993). Normal infant and adult auditory brainstem responses to bone-conducted tones. *Audiology, 32,* 95–109.

Halliday, R., & Callaway, E., (1978). Time shift evoked potentials (TSEPs): Methods and basic results. *Electroencephalography and Clinical Neurophysiology, 45,* 118–121.

Haughton, P. (2006). Insert earphones—a comparison of short-duration signals measured with an occluded ear simulator and a 2cc coupler. *International Journal of Audiology, 45,* 60–65.

Haughton, P. M., Lightfoot, G. R., & Stevens, J. C. (2003). Peak-to-peak equivalent sound pressure level. *International Journal of Audiology, 42,* 494–495.

Herdman, A. T., Picton, T. W., & Stapells, D. R. (2002). Place specificity of auditory steady state responses. *Journal of the Acoustical Society of America, 112,* 1569–1582.

ISO 389-1. (1998a). Acoustics—Reference zero for the calibration of audiometric equipment—Part 1: Reference equivalent threshold sound pressure levels for pure tones and supra-aural earphones. Geneva, Switzerland: International Standards Association.

ISO 389-2. (1994). Acoustics—Reference zero for the calibration of audiometric equipment—Part 2: Reference equivalent threshold sound pressure levels for pure tones and insert earphones. Geneva, Switzerland: International Standards Association.

ISO 389-3. (1998b). Acoustics—Reference zero for the calibration of audiometric equipment—Part 3: Reference equivalent threshold force levels for pure tones and bone vibrators. Geneva, Switzerland: International Standards Association.

ISO 389-6. (2007). Acoustics—Reference zero for the calibration of audiometric equipment—Part 6: Reference threshold of hearing for test signals of short duration. Geneva, Switzerland: International Standards Association.

John, M. S., Dimitrijevic, A., & Picton, T. W. (2002). Auditory steady-state responses to exponential modulation envelopes. *Ear and Hearing, 23,* 106–117.

John, M. S., Dimitrijevic, A., & Picton, T. W. (2003). Efficient stimuli for evoking auditory steady-state responses. *Ear and Hearing, 24,* 406–423.

John, M. S., Dimitrijevic, A., van Roon, P., & Picton, T. W. (2001). Multiple auditory steady-state responses to AM and FM stimuli. *Audiology and Neuro-Otology, 6,* 12–27.

Johnson, K. L., Nicol, T. G., & Kraus, N. (2005). Brain stem response to speech: A biological marker of auditory processing. *Ear and Hearing, 26,* 424–434.

Jones, S. J., Pitman, J. R., & Halliday, A. M. (1991). Scalp potentials following sudden coherence and discoherence of binaural noise and change in the inter-aural time difference: A specific binaural evoked potential or a "mismatch" response? *Electroencephalography and Clinical Neurophysiology, 80,* 146–154.

Killion, M. C., Wilber, L. A., & Gudmundsen, G. I. (1985). Insert earphones for more interaural attenuation. *Hearing Instruments, 36(2),* 34–35.

Levine, R. A. (1981). Binaural interaction in brainstem potentials of human subjects. *Annals of Neurology, 9,* 384–393.

Lightfoot, G., Sininger, Y., Burkard, R., & Lodwig, A. (2007). Stimulus repetition rate and the reference levels for clicks and short tone bursts: A warning to audiologists, researchers, calibration laboratories, and equipment manufacturers. *American Journal of Audiology, 16,* 94–95.

Lüddemann, H., Riedel, H., & Kollmeier, B. (2009). Electrophysiological and psychophysical asymmetries in sensitivity to interaural correlation steps. *Hearing Research, 256,* 39–57.

McEvoy, L. K., Picton, T. W., Champagne, S. C., Kellett, A. J. C. ,& Kelly, J. B. (1990). Human evoked potentials to shifts in the lateralization of a noise. *Audiology, 29,* 163–180.

McPherson, D. L., & Starr, A., (1993). Binaural interaction in auditory evoked potentials: Brainstem, middle- and long-latency components. *Hearing Research, 66,* 91–98.

Oates, P., & Stapells, D. R. (1997a). Frequency specificity of the human auditory brainstem and middle latency responses to brief tones. I. High-pass noise masking. *Journal of the Acoustical Society of America, 102,* 3597–3608.

Oates, P., & Stapells, D. R. (1997b). Frequency specificity of the human auditory brainstem and middle latency responses to brief tones. II. Derived response analyses. *Journal of the Acoustical Society of America, 102,* 3609–3619.

Olsen, W. O. (1987). Brief tone audiometry: A review. *Ear and Hearing, 8*(Suppl. 4), 13S–18S.

Parker, D. J., & Thornton, A. R. D. (1978a). Frequency specific components of the cochlear nerve and brainstem evoked responses of the human auditory system. *Scandinavian Audiology, 7,* 53–60

Parker, D. J., & Thornton, A. R. D. (1978b). Cochlear travelling wave velocities calculated from the derived components of the cochlear nerve and brainstem evoked responses of the human auditory system. *Scandinavian Audiology, 7,* 67–70.

Picton, T. W., Dimitrijevic, A., Perez-Abalo, M. C., & van Roon, P. (2005). Estimating audiometric thresholds using auditory steady-state responses. *Journal of the American Academy of Audiology, 16,* 143–156.

Picton, T. W., Ouellette, J., Hamel, G., & Durieux-Smith, A. (1979). Brainstem evoked potentials to tone pips in notched noise. *Journal of Otolaryngology, 8,* 289–314.

Picton, T. W., Rodriguez, R. T., Linden, R. D., & Maiste, A. C. (1985). The neurophysiology of human hearing. *Human Communication Canada, 9,* 127–136.

Picton, T. W., & Ross, B. (in press). Physiological measurements of human binaural processing. In J. Buchholz, J. C. Dalsgaard, T. Dau, & T. Poulsen (Eds.), *Binaural processing and spatial hearing: Proceedings of the Second International Symposium on Audiological and Auditory Research (ISAAR 2009).* Helsingør, Denmark: Danavox Jubilee Foundation.

Picton, T. W., Woods, D. L., Baribeau-Braun, J., & Healey, T. M. (1977). Evoked potential audiometry. *Journal of Otolaryngology, 6,* 90–119.

Purdy, S. C., & Abbas, P. J. (2002). ABR thresholds to tonebursts gated with Blackman and linear windows in adults with high-frequency sensorineural hearing loss. *Ear and Hearing, 23,* 358–368.

Rance, G., Tomlin, D., & Rickards, F. W. (2006). Comparison of auditory steady-state responses and tone-burst auditory brainstem responses in normal babies. *Ear and Hearing, 27,* 751–762.

Richter, U., & Fedtke, T. (2005). Reference zero for the calibration of audiometric equipment using "clicks" as test signals. *International Journal of Audiology, 44,* 478–487.

Riquelme, R., Kuwada, S., Filipovic, B., Hartung, K., & Leonard, G. (2006). Optimizing the stimuli to evoke the amplitude modulation following response (AMFR) in neonates. *Ear and Hearing, 27,* 104–119.

Ross, B., Fujioka, T., Tremblay, K. L., & Picton, T. W. (2007). Aging in binaural hearing begins in mid-life: Evidence from cortical auditory evoked responses to changes in interaural phase. *Journal of Neuroscience, 27,* 11172–11178.

Ross, B., Picton, T. W., & Pantev, C. (2002). Temporal integration in the human auditory cortex as represented by the development of the steady-state magnetic field. *Hearing Research, 165,* 68–84.

Ross, B., Tremblay, K., & Picton, T. (2007). Physiological detection of interaural phase differences. *Journal of the Acoustical Society of America*, 121, 1017–1027.

Small, S. A., & Stapells, D. R. (2003). Normal brief-tone bone-conduction behavioral thresholds using the B-71 transducer: Three occlusion conditions. *Journal of the American Academy of Audiology*, 14, 556–562.

Stapells, D. R., Picton, T. W., & Durieux-Smith, A. (1982). Normal hearing thresholds for clicks. *Journal of the Acoustical Society of America*, 72, 74–79.

Stapells, D., Picton, T., & Durieux-Smith, A. (1993). Electrophysiologic measures of frequency-specific auditory function. In J. T. Jacobson (Ed.), *Principles and applications of auditory evoked potentials* (pp. 251–283). New York, NY: Allyn & Bacon.

Stürzebecher, E., Cebullam, M., & Pschirrer, U. (2001). Efficient stimuli for recording of the amplitude modulation following response. *Audiology*, 40, 63–68.

Suzuki, T., & Horiuchi, K. (1981). Rise time of pure-tone stimuli in brain stem response audiometry. *Audiology*, 20, 101–112.

Teas, D. C., Eldridge, D. H., & Davis, H. (1962). Cochlear responses to acoustic transients: an interpretation of whole-nerve action potentials. *Journal of the Acoustical Society of America*, 34, 1438–1459.

Van Maanen, A., & Stapells, D. R. (2009). Normal multiple-ASSR thresholds to air-conducted stimuli in infants. *Journal of the American Academy of Audiology*, 20, 196–207.

Viemeister, N. F., & Wakefield G. H. (1991). Temporal integration and multiple looks. *Journal of the Acoustical Society of America*, 90, 858–865.

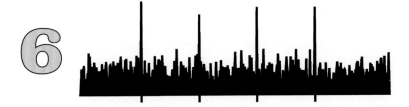

Interpreting the Waveforms: Time and Uncertainty

> But all the clocks in the city
> Began to whirr and chime:
> "O let not Time deceive you,
> You cannot conquer Time.
>
> "In the burrows of the Nightmare
> Where Justice naked is,
> Time watches from the shadow
> And coughs when you would kiss."
>
> W. H Auden, *As I Walked Out One Evening*, 1937

This chapter reviews some principles that enable us to be reasonably certain when interpreting the auditory evoked potentials (EPs). Faced with our recordings, we must decide whether a response is present, if that response is normal, how the threshold for eliciting the response relates to hearing, and if some response parameter relates to normal or abnormal neurologic function. Unfortunately, nothing is fully certain about these decisions. We must always be aware of the limits of our interpretations.

One of the most important principles in interpretation is that we cannot conquer time. The best decisions are based on the best data and the best data require time. Nevertheless, we should not be time's slaves. Rather, we must set up our recording protocols to use time optimally.

Although every decision we take could be wrong, we can get some feeling for our uncertainty by estimating the chances of being wrong. If the chances are low, we can act on our decision. Typically, we use a criterion of at least one in 20 before coming to a conclusion. This is generally expressed as $p < 0.05$. If a tossed coin is coming up heads repeatedly, we start to worry that there might be something wrong with the coin—perhaps the coin has heads on both sides—after the fourth or fifth head in a row. For a normal coin, the chances are 1 in sixteen for four heads in a row, and 1 in 32 for five. When the chances of something are near 1 in 20, most people start to doubt.

Two main decisions are made when interpreting EPs (Hyde, Sininger, & Don, 1998). The first—"detection"—is that a recording shows an EP and not just the residual background electroencephalogram (EEG) that has not been averaged away. The second—"analysis"—is that a particular EP measurement is different from what might be expected in a group of normal subjects. We would like to qualify these decisions with some assessment of certainty or uncertainty. If possible, this should be the probability that we are wrong, that there is no EP present in the recording or that the EP is not significantly different from normal. Often, we can only estimate this probability rather than measure it exactly.

SIGNALS IN NOISE

The EPs recorded from the scalp, the "signals" we want to identify or measure, are recorded simultaneously with the EEG from the brain and the electromyogram (EMG) from the muscles of the head and scalp, the "noise" that interferes with our evaluation of the signal. Evaluating the EPs electrically is similar to listening to auditory signals in background noise (tones in white noise or words in multitalker babble). As discussed in Chapters 2 and 3, we can use techniques such as averaging to

reduce the background noise and allow us to measure the signal. One measurement of how reliable our recordings are (and how confident our interpretations can be) is the signal-to-noise ratio (SNR). This ratio is often expressed in terms of a power or variance ratio using logarithmic units. Because EPs typically are considered in terms of amplitudes, we are sometimes more comfortable using amplitude rather than power. An SNR of 6 dB means that the signal has twice the amplitude of the noise, and 20 dB means 10 times the amplitude. Table 6–1 gives some relations between the different SNR ratios. When we determine the SNR, the measurement of the EP signal usually is clear as it is the result of our recording. The noise is more difficult to measure. Several different approaches can be used to measure the residual noise in a recording. To begin, we consider the transient evoked potentials as measured in the time domain, and then move to the auditory steady-state responses (ASSRs) as measured in the frequency domain.

Table 6–1. Signal-to-Noise Ratios*

Amplitude Ratio	Variance Ratio	Decibels
10.00	100.0	20
5.00	25.0	14
3.16	10.0	10
2.00	4.0	6
1.41	2.0	3

*The variance ratio is the square of the amplitude ratio. Decibels are calculated as 10 times the log of the variance ratio or 20 times the log of the amplitude ratio. The relationship between variance and amplitude is similar to that between pressure and power when measuring sound levels.

Time Domain SNR Measurements

The simplest way to assess the SNR of an EP recording is to consider how well replicated EP waveforms superimpose. Two independent averages are obtained and the waveforms are superimposed, moving one up or down relative to the other to get the least overall separation. The initial question is whether the recorded waveform is significantly different from what might be expected if no EP were present. Is the recording just residual noise? A simple way to assess whether a response is present is to unfocus the eyes until the two replicate tracings become one and decide whether we can still see the waveform (Figure 6–1). Another rule of thumb is that if the size of the response is more than four times the average distance between the replications, the response is likely not background EEG noise (Picton & Hink, 1974).

This approach can be made more formal by considering the (±) reference (Schimmel, 1967; Wong & Bickford, 1980). Averaging EPs consists of adding single-trial waveforms together and then dividing by the number of waveforms. If, instead of just adding, we alternately add and subtract the waveforms, we cancel

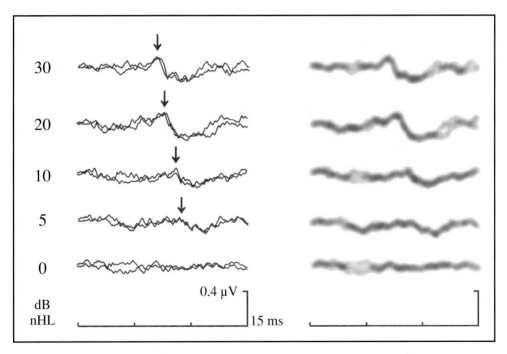

Figure 6–1. Replications. This figure demonstrates how replications can be used to demonstrate the presence of an ABR as distinct from residual background noise. Responses on the left are the ABRs evoked by clicks at intensities near normal threshold. The clicks were presented at 11/s and each tracing represents the average of 2000 single responses. We can check the reliability of the responses by unfocusing our eyes so that the replicate tracings blur into each other (as demonstrated on the right). If wave V remains recognizable in the blurred tracings, we can conclude that it differs from what might be expected from residual noise.

out the effect of any EP in the tracings. Each time the EP is added in, it is then subtracted out. The background EEG noise, however, is similar whether it is right side up or upside down, and thus the resultant (±) reference represents what might be expected if the recordings contained only background EEG noise. A simple SNR measurement then would be the ratio of the average waveform to the (±) reference. This ratio could be expressed as a ratio of the variances or the standard deviations (SDs) of the two recordings (Picton, Linden, Hamel, & Maru, 1983). The standard deviation ratio (SDR) is essentially an SNR expressed in terms of amplitude rather than variance (the SD is the square root of the variance). This ratio increases as averaging progresses. Unfortunately, the significance level of such a ratio (when is it large enough to be sure that the EP is bigger than the noise?) is difficult to determine because we cannot be sure of the degrees of freedom of either the response or the noise (Picton, Hink, Perez-Abalo, Linden, & Wiens, 1984). The number of points in each waveform does not represent the degrees of freedom because the points are not independent; adjacent points are highly correlated. We can estimate the degrees of freedom by the number of independent frequencies present in the spectrum of the response, but it is only an estimate. Generally, a variance ratio greater than 4 (or a SDR ratio greater than 2) means that a response is present. Figure 6–2 illustrates the use of the (±) reference in evaluating the auditory brainstem response (ABR). The right section of the figure shows how the SDR increases as the number of individual waveforms in the average increases for five different subjects.

The (±) reference approach does not distinguish physiologic response from artifact. It will identify a consistent stim-ulus artifact in the same way as a response coming from the brain. Therefore, we usually limit our evaluation to regions of the recording where there is little or no stimulus artifact. If we are using stimuli with a single polarity, we do not begin the (±) reference calculation until after 1 ms for the click ABR and after the end of the tone for tone ABR. Furthermore, the overall variance (or SD) ratio will be attenuated if it includes regions of the waveform where there is little response (or where the response becomes variable). Thus, for the ABR to high-intensity clicks, we might limit the analysis to between 1 and 11 ms.

Measuring the correlation between replications is another way of assessing the reliability of an average waveform (Coppola, Tabor & Buchsbaum, 1978; Picton et al., 1983). The main problem with this method is the same as with the (±) reference. Because we do not know the degrees of freedom of the measurements, it is difficult to give a probability to any conclusion that the response is present or not, although general confidence limits can be obtained for each type of EP recording.

A more efficient approach to tracking the SNR of a recording is the Fsp, the F-ratio at a single point (Don, Elberling, & Waring, 1984; Elberling & Don, 1984). The trial-to-trial variance of a single point in the recorded waveform is calculated. This variance estimate can be based on all trials or a selected portion of them. If we can assume that the background EEG noise is constant across the recording sweep, the variance of this single point can be considered representative of the variance of the whole recorded waveform. We can divide that variance by the number of single-point measurements to estimate what variance should be present in the average waveform. We then can divide this into the variance of the average waveform to get

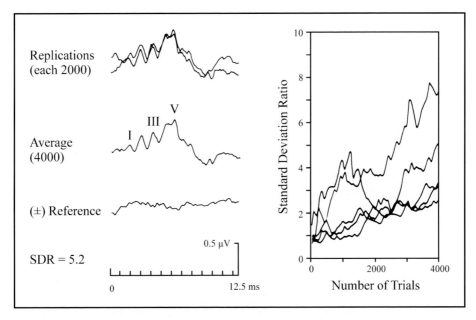

Figure 6–2. *Evaluation of residual noise by the (±) reference. On the left are shown ABRs to 70 dB nHL clicks presented at a rate of 11/s. Two replicate responses (each the average of 2000 responses) are superimposed to show the reliability of the recording. Averaging the replicate waveforms together gives the average response, whereas the difference between the recordings gives the (±) reference. The SNR can be calculated as the ratio between the standard deviation of the average divided by the standard deviation of the (±) reference (both measures calculated between 1 and 11 ms) —the standard deviation ratio (SDR). The graph on the right shows how the SDR increases as the averaging proceeds for five different subjects. Note that the SDR is actually the ratio between the signal+noise and the noise and thus begins near 1 rather than at 0. Figure based on data reported in Picton et al. (1983).*

the SNR. The degrees of freedom of the noise measurement is exactly equal to the number of trials in the single-point calculation; there is no correlation between these points, separated as they are by the stimulus onset asynchrony (SOA). We still need to estimate the degrees of freedom of the average EP—perhaps about 5 for a near-threshold ABR where the waveform is quite simple. Using 250 single-point estimates, this gives an F value of 3.1 for a criterion of $p < 0.01$.

The development of digital signal processing techniques has made possible the online calculation of the variance of the recording at all time points rather than just a single point. In this manner a multiple-point F-ratio can be calculated— the Fmp (Özdamar & Delgado, 1996).

Detecting Difference Waveforms

Sometimes we need to detect whether one response is different from another. The most common example of occurs when we study the mismatch negativity (MMN).

Here we need to show that the response to an improbable deviant is significantly different from the response to a standard stimulus. The difference usually is demonstrated by subtracting the standard response from the deviant response and determining whether the difference waveform is significantly larger than what might be expected from the variability of the recordings.

The SNR of MMN recordings generally is low (Cacace & McFarland, 2003). The difference waveform typically is smaller than the waveforms of the standard response. Furthermore, the subtraction process itself increases the residual noise in the recording—the residual noise recorded with the standard response is added to the residual noise recorded with the less probable deviant response. Therefore, we need to average responses over many more deviants than we usually record standard responses to individual stimuli because the difference waveform is smaller than the onset response and because the subtraction process itself creates additional noise. We should use all standard responses when creating the standard response to be subtracted from the deviant. Randomly choosing an equivalent number of standards as deviants is inappropriate; this just increases the residual noise in the difference waveform.

These SNR issues often make it difficult to determine that a recorded MMN is significantly different from what might be expected if the standards and deviants evoked the same responses. The MMN can occur at different latencies in different subjects and lasts about the same duration as a typical wave in the residual noise. There almost always will be a negative wave in the residual noise with a latency somewhere between 100 and 300 ms. Simply picking this peak and identifying it as the MMN is unjustified, and can lead to many false positive measurements.

Several techniques can be used to support the interpretation that an MMN exists. A simple approach uses multiple *t*-tests (at each point in the waveform) to determine whether the difference waveform is larger than what should be expected by the confidence limits of the *t*-test (e.g., McGee, Kraus & Nicol, 1997; Petermann et al., 2009). To compensate for the multiple tests (some of which would be significant by chance alone), the criterion for recognizing significant differences should be adjusted (Hochberg & Tamhane, 1987). A conservative approach (Bonferroni) is to divide the original criterion by the number of points in the waveform. Another approach is to require that the *t*-tests remain significant over a several adjacent points in the waveform. This requires some assessment of how often this occurs in similar data where there is no MMN (see Blair & Karniski, 1993).

Ponton, Don, Eggermont, and Kwong (1997) proposed a new method based on the integrated difference waveform. They integrated the difference between the deviant and standard waveforms over time, measured this integrated difference on multiple subaverages of the recorded deviant and standard waveforms, and assessed the confidence limits of the integrated difference. An MMN would be identified as soon as the integral was significantly different from zero. The latency at which the integrated activity is assessed should be determined a priori. In choosing this latency, we have to allow the MMN to integrate and make sure that the integral is not depleted by a subsequent positive wave such as the P3a.

Picton, Alain, Otten, Ritter, and Achim (2000) proposed a technique deriving from Achim (1995) to identify a consistent difference waveform. Multiple difference waveforms were computed (based on sub-averages) and the first component of these waveforms was determined using a principal component analysis. Each separate difference waveform was then related to the principal component waveform and given a component score based on point-by-point multiplication. A *t*-test on these multiple component scores could then determine whether the scores differed significantly from zero. The advantage of this approach is that it does not depend on the difference waveform having a set latency or polarity—it just has to be similar from trial to trial.

Frequency Domain SNR Measurements

In the frequency domain, the distinction between signal and noise is easier. Each measurement in the spectrum is independent of the other measurements. Thus, we can compare the amount of activity measured at the frequency of stimulation to the activity measured at adjacent frequencies in the spectrum. We assume that the activity in these adjacent frequencies does not vary with frequency, that the residual background noise in a tracing is "white." For the ASSRs that we measure at 40 and 80 Hz, this assumption is not far from reality. The amount of background activity decreases with increasing frequency but this change is not large and it is not necessary to compensate for it prior to testing. We calculate a ratio of the power at the stimulus frequency to the power at N adjacent frequencies. If there is no response, the ratio is distributed as F with degrees of freedom 2 and $2N$. The

factor 2 stems from the spectral measurements being two dimensional—real and imaginary. Thus, we can give a probability that an identified response is significantly different from the background EEG activity. Figure 6–3 illustrates this approach to evaluating ASSRs.

Several other measurements can be used to assess the SNR of the ASSR. These are based on multiple measurements of the response rather than comparing the response at one frequency to the noise in adjacent frequencies. Single-trial recordings or multiple subaverages of the response are examined. The intertrial or interaverage replicability of the amplitudes and/or phases are assessed. One of the simplest approaches is to measure the phase coherence—how similar the phases are between different measurements (Fisher, 1993). When the recording does not contain any response locked to the frequency of the stimulus, the phase of the recorded activity will vary randomly. Graphed on a polar plot, the phases will look like a starburst. When there is a response in the recordings, the phases will tend to cluster around the phase of the response, and the plot will look more like a comet. Magnitude squared coherence considers amplitude as well as phase. Hotelling's T^2 test estimates the distribution of the responses in two dimensions (real and imaginary) and determines whether zero is within the confidence limits of the mean (Picton, Vajsar, Rodriguez, & Campbell, 1987; Valdes et al., 1997). A revised version of Hotelling's T^2 test, called the circular T^2 test, assumes that the real and imaginary components have equal variance, and that the confidence limits therefore plot a circle rather than an ellipse (Victor & Mast, 1991). Although computationally different, the magnitude squared coherence and the

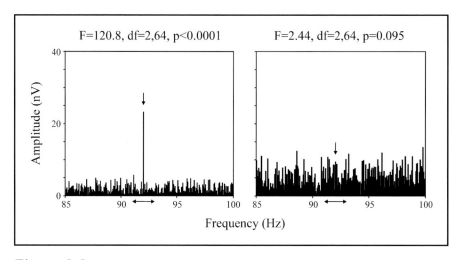

F=120.8, df=2,64, p<0.0001   F=2.44, df=2,64, p=0.095

Figure 6–3. Detecting ASSRs in the spectrum using F-test. These results show the spectrum of the ASSR to a 25 dB SPL 2 kHz tone amplitude-modulated at 92 Hz and presented to the left ear for a period of 11 minutes in two different subjects. The graphs show only the 85-100 Hz region of the spectrum. The amplitude of the response at the frequency of modulation can be compared to the amplitude of the recording in 32 adjacent bins (16 on either side of the response frequency) to determine the probability that the response might be within the expected range of amplitudes in the rest of the spectrum. The extent of the comparison bins is shown by the double headed arrows. The response shown on the left is significantly different from the background EEG noise, but the response on the right, which is smaller and recorded in higher levels of noise, is not significant at a criterion of p *<0.05.*

circular T^2 test are essentially equivalent, and both give results similar to the F-test based on the spectrum (Dobie & Wilson, 1996). Figure 6–4 illustrates how these different tests can be used to distinguish the ASSR from background EEG noise.

Transient EPs also can be evaluated using frequency-domain techniques. Ross, Lütkenhöner, Pantev, and Hoke (1999) measured the trial-to-trial phase coherence of the late auditory EPs (LAEPs) over different latency periods and different frequency bands and assessed the probability that the phases were randomly related in each frequency-latency region. Figure 6–5 shows sample results using this technique. Because the test involves multiple tests of significance, a $p < 0.0001$ criterion was used to identify responses.

Unbiased Estimates of Amplitude

The recorded EP always contains residual noise as well as signal. The numerator of the SNR that we have been estimating is actually the sum of the signal and the noise rather than just the noise. When the EP becomes small relative to the noise, such a measurement will tend toward 1 rather than 0. This is illustrated in Figure 6–2 where the SDR begins near 1 and then increases as the averaging proceeds.

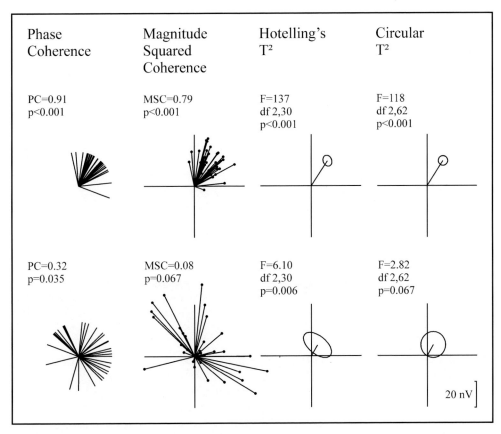

Phase Coherence	Magnitude Squared Coherence	Hotelling's T^2	Circular T^2
PC=0.91 p<0.001	MSC=0.79 p<0.001	F=137 df 2,30 p<0.001	F=118 df 2,62 p<0.001
PC=0.32 p=0.035	MSC=0.08 p=0.067	F=6.10 df 2,30 p=0.006	F=2.82 df 2,62 p=0.067

20 nV

Figure 6–4. Detecting ASSRs using replications. *These graphs show the same data as represented in Figure 6–4, but viewed through the replicability of 32 subaverages rather than through the spectrum of the final average. The same two subjects are examined. In this figure the first subject is in the upper set of data and the second subject below. Each column shows a different evaluation. The data are graphed using polar plots. The first subject's response is clearly significant on all tests. The second subject is just significant at* p *<0.05 on phase coherence and Hotelling's* T^2 *but not significant on the magnitude squared coherence or the circular* T^2 *(which are statistically equivalent).*

Figure 6–6 illustrates the effect of noise on the measurement of amplitude in the frequency domain. The signal is represented as a vector and the noise as a circle of values added to the signal. What we measure in the spectrum is the sum of the signal and the noise. Depending on the relative phases between the signal and the noise, the sum may be smaller or larger than the signal. However, there will be a tendency for it to be larger—the dark shaded area is larger than the light shaded area. In the frequency domain, we can estimate the true (or unbiased) amplitude of the signal by subtracting the estimated noise power (at the frequencies adjacent to the stimulus frequency) from the power recorded at the signal frequency (which is a combination of signal and noise). Ménard, Gallégo, Berger-Vachon, Collet,

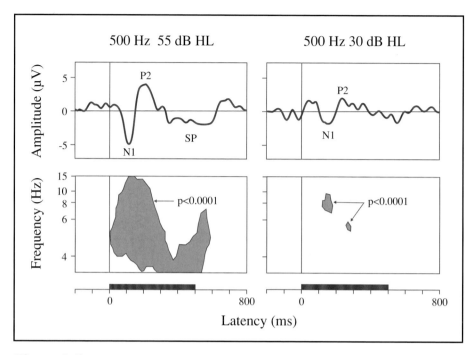

Figure 6–5. **Use of phase coherence to identify responses.** *The upper half of this figure shows LAEPs in response to 500 Hz tones at two intensities. The responses were recognized as significantly different from what might be expected from the background EEG by calculating the inter-trial phase coherence at frequencies between 3 and 15 Hz and at each of the latencies. The lower half of the figures shows the coherence measurements, which were calculated for different frequencies (y-axis) at different latencies (x-axis). The shaded regions show where the coherence was significantly different from zero. Because of the multiple statistical tests (at each frequency and latency), a very stringent criterion (p <0.0001) is used. At 55 dB HL the test identifies the N1 and P2 waves of the onset response and the sustained potential (SP) whereas at 30 dB, only the N1 and the peak of the P2 wave are identified. Figure adapted from Ross et al. (1999).*

and Thai-Van (2008) used this approach to study the effects of stimulus intensity on the amplitude of the 80-Hz ASSR and the relationship between response amplitude and loudness perception.

Biasing the Detection Process

If we know what the response is supposed to look like, we can bias our detection procedures to look only for responses similar to those expected. We could, for example,

correlate the recorded waveform to a normal template of the response and use the resultant correlation as a means to detect the presence of a response or as a factor to bias another detection procedure. This is sometimes difficult for the transient EPs as subtle changes in latency can cause large changes in any correlation measurement.

A simple example of using a priori knowledge to help us recognize a response depends on the usual latency increase of an EP wave with decreasing intensity. Thus, if we are sure of a wave at one inten-

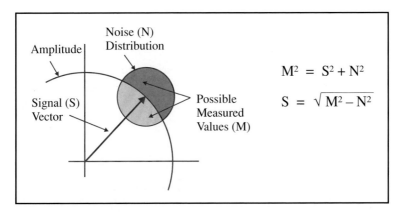

Figure 6–6. Unbiased estimate of spectral amplitude. *This diagram shows a sample signal recorded in noise. The actual signal is represented by the arrow. The noise is represented by the shaded circle, which plots the standard deviation of the noise. The measured signal falls within this circle. The phase of the measured signal varies around the actual phase but is not biased to either side of the vector. The measured amplitude, however, overestimates the actual amplitude—the dark-shaded portion of the noise circle is larger than the light-shaded portion. The equations on the right show how an unbiased estimate of the signal can be obtained.*

sity, we would not normally recognize it at a shorter latency when the intensity was reduced. As well as helping to recognize a small response at low intensities, latency also can help to distinguish stimulus artifact from physiologic response; the artifact does not change its latency with decreasing intensity.

Sininger, Hyde, and Don (2001) proposed an extension of the Fsp measurement to take into account the expected waveform of the response. Instead of over the whole waveform, the response variance is calculated at several latencies—the points when the expected waveform has maximum and minimum values and other peaks and troughs separated from each other by a latency at which the autocorrelation becomes insignificant. This provides a "point-optimized variance ratio," which is distributed as F with M and N-1 degrees of freedom where M is

the number of points selected and N is the number of trials over which the variance is computed. This technique works well for the ABR to screening-level clicks in newborn infants, where the expected waveform is simple and does not change greatly in latency between individual subjects. The points need to be selected on the basis of normative data for each application and subject group; the process depends on how well the responses of different subjects fit to the template. A similar, although less formal, template-based algorithm was used in the automatic ABR screening of infants (Herrmann, Thornton, & Joseph, 1995).

For ASSRs, the expected phase of the response can be used to improve the detection of the responses. Dobie and Wilson (1994) initially used a phase-weighting algorithm to improve the detection of ASSRs. Their approach was to weight the recorded response according to the cosine function of the difference in phase between the recorded response and the expected response. A similar approach was used by Lins et al. (1996). Dobie (personal communication) also suggested a simpler approach, which projected the two-dimensional recorded data onto a line oriented at the expected phase gives a one-dimensioned set of data that can be evaluated using a *t*-test. Figure 6–7 shows how the technique can be applied to detecting the ASSR when multiple measurements of the response are available (see also Picton,

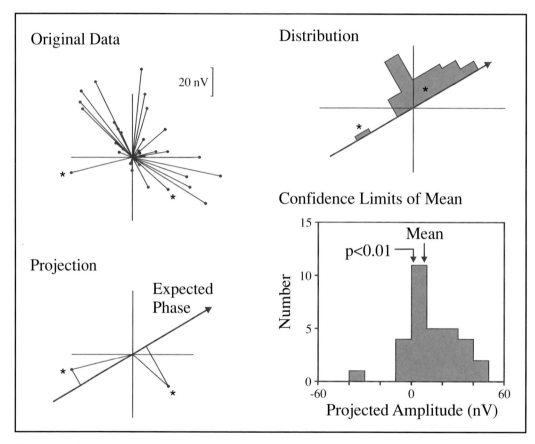

Figure 6–7. *Phase-weighting in detecting ASSRs. This figure shows a technique suggested by Robert Dobie and described more fully in Picton et al. (2003) that allows us to consider how close the phase of the response is to an expected phase. The replicated measurements from the second subject in Figure 6–4 are shown in the upper left polar plot. The expected phase of this response is 30 degrees. The lower left shows how the data are projected onto the line of the expected phase. For clarity, the projections, of only two data points (asterisks) are illustrated. From these projections, we obtain a distribution of the data along the expected phase (upper right). We can calculate the mean and standard error of this distribution and from these measurements determine the* p <0.01 *confidence limits of the mean. The data show that the lower confidence limit is just above zero. The actual probability that the mean is different from zero in this case is* p = 0.0064. *Thus a response that is not significant on initial testing (Figures 6–3 and some of the tests in Figure 6–4) can be considered significant because its phase is similar to that expected.*

John, Dimitrijevic, & Purcell, 2003). Picton, Dimitrijevic, John, and van Roon (2001) showed that a variant of this approach (based on spectral measurements rather than replications) could improve the detection of ASSRs.

DECISIONS AND ERRORS

When we record auditory EPs, we must decide whether what we have recorded represents a real response generated in the ear or brain or just fluctuations in the residual background noise. To make this decision, we set up a null hypothesis that the recorded activity is actually noise and perform a statistical test to give us some idea of the chances that such a null hypothesis is true. If the chances are low, we decide that the response is real.

Statistical tests generally work with null hypotheses. This is the opposite of how we make hypotheses in everyday life. Statistical tests usually cannot prove something is the same as expected, only that something is different. Thus, we cannot use a test to prove that the recording contains no response—that what we recorded is the same as what we might have expected from the background noise. Therefore, we are less certain about saying that a response is absent than that a response is present. Because of this, we usually use additional rules for the no-response decision. Most importantly, we should make such a decision only if the background noise level in the recording has been reduced to a level that would normally allow us to recognize a response if it were there.

The efficient detection of EPs uses four main stopping rules. First, a minimum recording time must have passed: decisions are not made until at least several responses have been averaged or otherwise analyzed. Second, the recording can stop once a response has been recognized in terms of the SNR attaining a set criterion. Third, if the criterion is not reached, the recording continues until the background noise is reduced below a criterion level, at which time we can decide that a response is not present (and in audiometric terms that we are below the physiological threshold). Fourth, if the background noise level cannot be reduced to the criterion level within a set maximum recording time, we conclude that no decision can be made about the presence or absence of the response. Stopping has four parameters—minimum and maximum recording time, a probability level for the SNR decision, and a minimum level for the residual background noise (given that the probability criterion has not been reached).

Applying such decision rules means that most of the recording time will be required to decide when responses are not present. Detecting a suprathreshold response can occur quickly but deciding there is no response at subthreshold levels takes a longer time.

Making decisions when we are not certain can lead to errors. In statistics, errors are classified as false positives (type I errors or false alarms)—rejecting a null hypothesis when we should not—and false negatives (type II errors or misses)—not rejecting a null hypotheses we should have. These errors always occur. The probability criterion of the test gives us the frequency with which type I errors occur; it is often not possible to assess the probability of type II errors. We should not be surprised if every once in a while our algorithms identify an EP when the sound level is below threshold or fail to identify an EP when the sound is above physiologic threshold.

Sensitivity and Specificity

Because of these statistical errors, our interpretation of the results of a test may or may not be correct. This has led to measurements of sensitivity and specificity that can tell us the probability that our interpretation is wrong. These concepts, illustrated in Figure 6–8, typically are explained in terms of a test for a particular disease. In a particular patient, the test is either positive for the disease or negative, and the patient either has the disease or not. Sensitivity is the proportion of sick patients who test positively. Specificity is the proportion of well patients who test negatively. As shown in Figure 6–8, we can adjust the criterion at

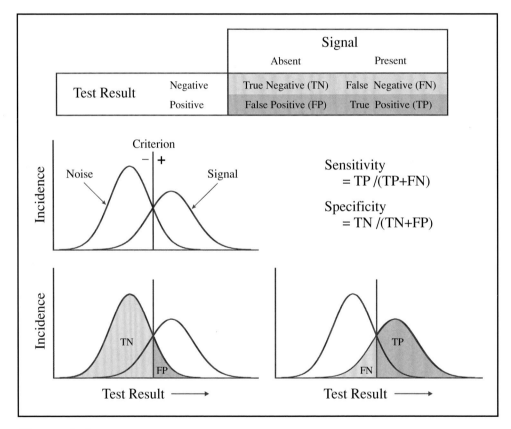

Figure 6–8. Sensitivity and specificity. This figure illustrates how test results are related to the actual presence or absence of a signal. Here we are considering the detection of a signal in noise, for example, an auditory EP in the background EEG. The diagram also relates to the detection of pathology in a population of patients—this would require substituting "pathology" for "signal." The upper part of the figure shows the relations between test result and reality. The middle left shows the overlapping distributions of the signal and noise. A criterion level is selected, above which the signal is interpreted as present. The lower left shows the possible results with this criterion when there is no signal and the lower right when there is a signal.

which a test becomes positive. Increasing the criterion decreases the sensitivity of the test (fewer sick patients are identified) but increases the specificity of the test (more well patients are identified as well). As shown in the figure, these measurements usually are calculated using the values true positive (TP), true negative (TN), false positive (FP), and false negative (FN). The criterion for a clinical test typically is adjusted so that the incidence of FP (the chance of a well person giving a positive test result) is 5%. However, this level may be adjusted if the cost of missing a person with a disease is high and the cost of treating a person without the disease is low.

We use sensitivity and specificity in later chapters of this book when we consider how well an EP test identifies a patient with a particular pathology: How well does an abnormal ABR latency identify patients with an acoustic neuroma? How well does screening with the ABR to a click presented at 35 dB nHL (normal hearing level) identify an infant with a hearing-impairment?

Sensitivity and specificity also are applicable to identifying the auditory EP in residual background noise. In this regard, the test is positive if it identifies the EP and negative if it considers the recording noise. Averaging an EP over a larger number of trials generally increases both the sensitivity and specificity of the test.

When we evaluate the sensitivity and specificity of our decisions, we must always remember what null hypothesis is being tested. When identifying an EP as different from background noise, the null hypothesis is that there is no EP. However, when identifying an infant with hearing impairment using a physiologic screening test, the null hypothesis is that the child

has normal hearing. Thus, the false-positive identification of an EP when none was present leads to the false-negative detection (miss) of a hearing-impairment.

Receiver Operating Characteristics

The concepts of sensitivity and specificity also can be considered in terms of receiver operating characteristics (ROC). This approach comes from communication theory and the idea that a receiver may or may not correctly interpret the transmitted signal because of noise. Figure 6–9 shows how we move from sensitivity and specificity to the ROC. The left column illustrates the probabilities that a particular measurement of a signal comes from either the distribution of the noise or from the distribution of the signal. Typically, we set our decision criterion at the level (arrow) where 5% of noise measurements (dark shading) would be interpreted as signal (type I error). Depending on the distribution of the signal measurements, there would be either a moderate (upper row) or high (lower row) probability of detecting the signals (light shading). In addition, the probability of missing some of the signals (type II error) would be high (upper row) or low (lower row)—the unshaded area of the dashed line distribution. As well as illustrating how signals are distinguished from noise, these diagrams also indicate how well pathologic measurements can be distinguished from normal.

How do we compare the different techniques for measuring the SNR of a recording? The basic intent of the SNR is to decide whether a response is present. However, the number of responses detected will vary with the criterion used,

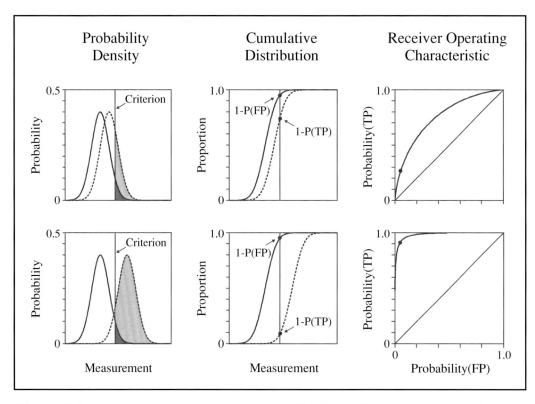

Figure 6–9. *Receiver operating characteristics. This figure illustrates how we can determine the differences between two sets of measurements. In the context of detecting signals in noise, these measurements could represent the noise (*continuous line*) and the signal (*dashed line*). In the context of deciding between normal and abnormal waveforms, these could represent normative data (*continuous*) and pathologic findings (*dashed*). The upper section shows measurements whose distributions overlap extensively. The lower section shows measurements with little overlap. The first column shows the probability density of the measurements. A criterion measurement has been selected such that only 5% of the noise/normal measurements exceed this criterion (*dark shading*). These would be false positive (FP) results if we based our decision on this criterion. The light shading indicates the portion of the signal/pathologic measurements that are detected by the criterion (correct detections); the unshaded area of this distribution shows the false negatives. The middle column shows the probability density data plotted cumulatively. 95% of the noise/normal data are below the criterion measurement and 5% above the FP. The false negatives (FN) represent those data from the signal/pathologic distributions that are missed: 72% in the upper illustration and 8% in the lower. The remaining proportion of the data would be correctly detected—true positives (TP). On the right are plotted the receiver operating characteristic (ROC) curves for these comparisons. As the criterion is varied, the curve tracks the relative probabilities of TP and FP. An ROC curve that extends more to the upper left of these graphs indicates a comparison where the distributions have less overlap.*

and, when we adjust this so that more responses are detected (the criterion in Figure 6–9 is moved to the left), more false positives also occur. This is illustrated more extensively in Figure 6–9. Determining the optimal setting for a particular method and deciding whether this is better or worse than another method can be done by plotting ROC curves (e.g., Dobie & Wilson, 1996; Picton et al., 2001; Swets, 1988; Valdes et al., 1997). As illustrated in the right section of Figure 6–9, receiver-operating characteristic curves plot the proportion of responses detected when there was a true response by the proportion of false alarms when there was not. Different points on the graph can be determined by varying the test criterion, or by altering some parameter of the test such as the relative probabilities of signal and nonsignal trials. If the test could not discriminate between signal and noise, the curve runs along the diagonal from lower left to upper right. The test works better if the ROC curve moves toward the upper left of the graph (and the area under the curve becomes larger).

Figure 6–10 compares several protocols for detecting the steady-state responses using ROC curves. On the left, the curves

are plotted based on 1 minute of recording and on the right the curves are plotted for 6 minutes. Within each graph, the effects of phase-weighting (as described in the preceding section of this chapter) are compared to using the routine F-test. Phase-weighting is better than not (especially if the recording time is short). The most striking effect, however, is related to the time spent in recording. Increased recording time greatly improves the distinction between signal and noise, giving an ROC curve that is much farther from the diagonal than when the recording time is short.

TIME AND EFFICIENCY

This is where the epigraph to the chapter becomes relevant: we cannot conquer time. We cannot record reliable EPs without

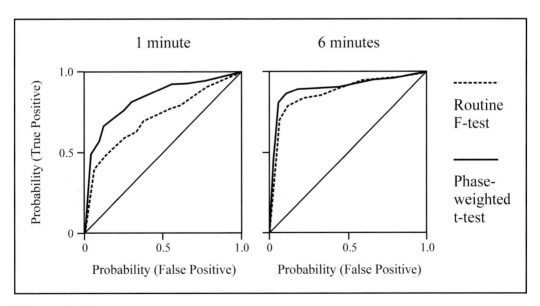

Figure 6–10. *Phase-weighting evaluated by ROC curves. These ROC curves show the improvement in the detection of ASSRs when using a phase-weighted t-test (cf. Figure 6–6) instead of a routine F-test. Measurements were compared after 1 minute (left) and after 6 minutes (right) of recording. The longer recording allows better distinction of signal from background noise. Data from Picton et al. (2001).*

devoting time to reducing the background EEG/EMG noise so that the waveforms can be confidently recognized or measured. Our intent in recording the EPs is to increase the SNR as quickly as possible. The faster we can recognize the EPs, the more information we obtain in the time available for the test. Several approaches have been used to increase test efficiency.

Optimum Stimulus Rates

The faster we present stimuli when recording the transient EPs, the more EPs we can average in a given amount of time. If the amplitude of the response is unaffected by the rate of stimulation, the SNR increases more rapidly for faster rates. However, many EPs decrease their amplitude at fast rates, causing a tradeoff between the decreasing amplitude of the response (related to the refractory period) and the decreasing amplitude of the noise (related to the averaging). The N1-P2 components of the LAEP decrease in size as the interval between the stimuli decreases below 10 seconds (reviewed in Picton, Woods, Baribeau-Braun, & Healey, 1977). We can calculate an efficiency index from this function by dividing the amplitude by the square root of the SOA. This index evaluates the change in the SNR when averaging more trials at faster rates. As shown in the left section of Figure 6–11, this gives maximum values when the SOA is near 3

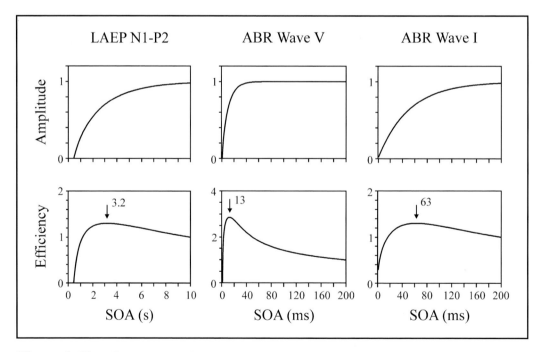

Figure 6–11. *Efficiency. This figure illustrates how we can determine the optimal rate for recording different transient auditory EPs. The upper section of the figure shows the amplitude of the response plotted against the stimulus-onset asynchrony (SOA). These plots are derived from the amplitude-SOA functions in the papers quoted in the text. The lower section of the figure plots an efficiency index showing how much faster the response can be recognized compared to when recordings are made using the maximum SOA plotted. The arrows indicate the SOAs where the efficiency is maximal.*

seconds. If the amplitude of the response at twice the rate is more than 70.7% ($1/\sqrt{2}$) the original amplitude, it is more efficient to record at the faster rate.

Different components of the auditory EP will have different amplitude-SOA functions. Wave V of the click ABR does not decrease in amplitude significantly until rates of the stimulation reach 70/s or more (see Figure 8 of Picton, Stapells, & Campbell, 1981). Therefore, it is more efficient to record at rates near 80/s than at lower rates (see middle section of Figure 6–11). This is not true for wave I of the ABR (or the N1 wave of the electrocochleogram), which decreases regularly in amplitude at rates greater than 5/s (Eggermont, 1976), and which can be optimally recorded at rates near 15/s (right section of Figure 6–11). We can use different stimulus rates depending on which components of the ABR are being measured: 10 or 20/s if we are recording the click ABR for neurologic purposes and are interested in both wave I and wave V, and more than 50/s if we are interested in hearing thresholds and just wish to recognize wave V. Wave V continues to be recognizable even at rates that cause the response to one stimulus to overlap with the responses to following stimuli. Disentangling the separate responses requires special techniques, which we discuss next.

Maximum Length Sequences

In the preceding section, we considered the possibility of increasing the efficiency of response detection by increasing the stimulus rate. However, as the SOA approaches the latency of the response, the response to the preceding stimulus can overlap the present response and distort the recorded waveform or even occasion-

ally cancel out its presence. This is not a problem for the late transient EPs as they become vanishingly small when the SOA approaches the several-hundred-millisecond latency of their slowest components. However, it is an issue for the ABR and the MLR, both of which are robustly present at rapid stimulus rates.

Some powerful mathematical (some say "mathemagical") techniques can be used to disentangle the responses to stimuli presented at very rapid rates. One of these is to present the stimuli at intervals determined by a "maximum length sequence" (MLS). This technique was initially applied to recording the ABR by Eysholdt and Schreiner (1982). A brief minimum SOA interval is selected and the stimuli are presented according to a special pseudorandom sequence of 1 and –1 that repeats itself for the duration of the recording. For recording EPs, the 1 triggers a stimulus and the –1 triggers no stimulus. A full sequence has a length (L) equal to 2^N-1 intervals, with N being the "order" of the sequence. Stimuli occur at $2^N/2$ of the possible positions in the sequence, so that the average SOA is almost twice the minimum interval. The sequence is set up specially so that, if we add together L responses to the whole sequence with each response shifted backward by one interval relative to the preceding response, we obtain the response to a single stimulus—any overlapping responses have canceled themselves out. This process is best understood by working through the graphic illustrations in Figure 6–12. This figure also indicates how the procedure is even more efficient when the 1 and –1 codes can trigger stimuli of opposite polarity that evoke responses of opposite polarity such as otoacoustic emissions (Picton, Kellett, Vezsenyi, & Rabinovitch, 1993).

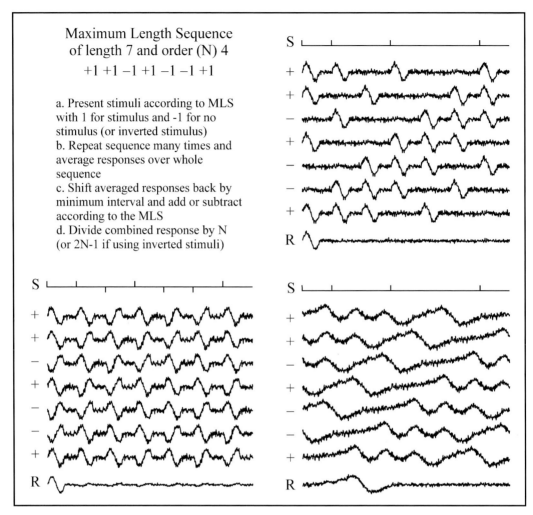

Figure 6–12. Maximum length sequences (MLS). *The upper half of this figure illustrates how MLS procedures can evaluate the EP, using a brief sinusoid as an example. For simplicity, the illustration is based on an MLS with a length (7) much shorter than typically used. The upper right tracing shows where stimuli occur according to the sequence (S). The next tracing is the actual average response to the sequence. The subsequent six tracings represent this response shifted back by one interval. In order to see how a single response comes out of the sequence of multiple responses when the shifting and adding/subtracting is performed, we should determine what happens at each position in the sequence. In the first position, the response is added at the four +1 positions and subtracted at the three −1 positions (where there is no response to subtract). The final combination gives the sum of four responses which is divided by the number of stimuli (4) to give the final response (R). In the second position the response is added, then nothing is added, then the response is subtracted, then nothing is subtracted and then added, then the response is subtracted and then added. Ultimately the responses have been canceled out, so there is no response to overlap that occurring in the first position. Similar cancellations occur at the other positions. The data in the lower right illustrate how MLS can be used to evaluate responses that change in polarity with changing polarity of the stimulus (e.g., acoustic signals or otoacoustic emissions). The lower right shows data to illustrate responses that last longer than the minimum interval and therefore overlap. In all three illustrations, the responses have been combined with a small amount of noise. The noise is reduced more by the MLS analysis in the lower left than in the other two analyses.*

The MLS technique allows us to record auditory EPs at very rapid rates (Burkard, Shi, & Hecox, 1990; Lasky, Shi, & Hecox, 1993; Picton, Champagne, & Kellett (1992). This approach can be used to stress the auditory system in order to determine how rapidly it can respond. For example, Jiang, Brosi, Shao, and Wikinson (2008) found that infants who had suffered perinatal asphyxia showed greater abnormalities in their click-ABR when very rapid rates were used (455 or 910/s). These rates were based on the minimum SOA, the overall rate of stimulus presentation would be approximately half the listed rates. The technique also can be used to distinguish different components of the auditory EP by showing that they are differentially sensitive to rate. For example, Picton et al. (1992) showed that the Pa wave of the MLR is less sensitive to rapid rates than the later components.

The MLS technique is one of many different deconvolution approaches to disentangle overlapping responses (Delgado & Özdamar, 2004; Jewett et al., 2004). Using several different techniques together can help explain the generation of the 40-Hz ASSR from the overlapping of MLR and ABR (Bohórquez & Özdamar, 2008).

Simultaneous Stimuli

If there is little interaction between stimuli, it may be possible to record responses to multiple stimuli simultaneously. Multiple transient responses can be recorded, provided the stimulus sequences are set up so that one response does not interfere with the others (Plourde, Picton, & Kellett, 1988). For example, a visual EP may be recorded simultaneously with an auditory EP if the rates of stimulation are sufficiently unrelated that one response can be considered random noise with respect to the other ("overlapping"). Another approach is to record one response in the interval between the recording of other responses, provided that there are no late responses in that interval that can interfere with the interpretation ("interweaving"). For example, the ABR to right-ear and left-ear stimuli can be recorded simultaneously if the stimuli are alternated.

Responses to multiple stimuli with different tonal frequencies can be recorded more rapidly if they are randomly interwoven (Ross et al., 1999). The refractory period of the EP usually shows frequency-specificity; this is particularly true for the N1-P2 components of the LAEP. This means that the response is larger if the tonal frequency changes from one stimulus to the next. When stimuli have different tonal frequencies, they can be presented at faster rates than if they all have the same tonal frequency. Thus, if we record LAEPs to four different tones occurring randomly we can use a faster overall rate than if we record each of them in separate blocks.

Multiple stimulus paradigms are easier to set up when recording steady-state responses. Several stimuli are presented simultaneously with each stimulus modulated at a unique rate. Responses then can be recorded at each of the different modulation frequencies. Regan and Heron (1969) initially used this approach to record responses to visual stimuli presented simultaneously at four different locations in the visual fields (see Regan, 1989, pp. 123–126 for discussion). Lins and Picton (1995) recorded responses to auditory stimuli presented simultaneously at four different carrier frequencies. The modulation frequency of the stimulus serves as the signature for finding the response in the spectrum. Figure 6–13 illustrates how the response to one stimulus (right) is

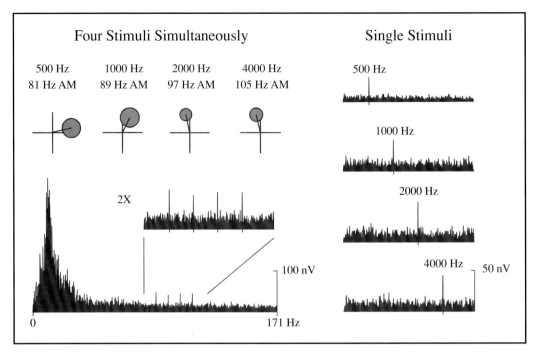

Figure 6–13. **Multiple stimuli.** *This figure compares the ASSRs recorded to four stimuli presented singly and presented simultaneously at 60 dB SPL. The upper left shows the responses (of a single subject) graphed using polar plots for the stimuli presented simultaneously. The shaded circles represent the 95% confidence limits of the response; when zero is not included in these circles the response is significantly different from what might be expected from the residual noise at $p < 0.05$. The lower left shows the spectrum for the responses, with a large amount of slow EEG/EMG activity high-pass filtered at 10 Hz. The region of the spectrum between 72 and 116 Hz has been magnified and inset to show the four responses more clearly. The responses to each stimulus when presented by itself are shown on the right. There is little change from when the stimuli were presented simultaneously. In this particular subject, there is a slight increase in the 500 Hz response in the simultaneous condition. This figure has been adapted from Lins and Picton (1995). In particular, the phases of the responses have been adjusted to compensate for the 90° difference between stimulus modulation and response measurements in the original figure.*

not reduced when three other stimuli are presented simultaneously (inset).

Recording several responses simultaneously is more efficient than recording each one singly in separate recording sessions, provided the presence of the other stimuli does not decrease the amplitude of the response more than the benefit from using multiple simultaneous stimuli. It is more efficient to record K responses simultaneously if the amplitude of each response does not decrease below $1/\sqrt{K}$ between single and simultaneous stimulation (John, Purcell, Dimitrijevic, & Picton, 2002). The 80-Hz ASSRs do not change significantly when stimuli are presented simultaneously, provided the intensity is not greater than 60 dB SPL, the carrier-frequencies are separated by at least a half octave, and the modulation frequencies are separated by at least 2 Hz (John, Lins, Boucher, & Picton, 1998). Nevertheless, it is not four times faster to record four stimuli simultaneously when assessing thresholds, because we wind up recording for the time required to detect the smallest of the four responses (or to decide that this particular response is not present). We can handle this problem by changing the intensity of each stimulus "on the fly" as soon as a decision is made about whether a response to that particular stimulus is present or absent (John et al., 2002; Van Dun et al., 2008).

Probability Issues

Some of the techniques we have been considering in the preceding paragraphs raise probability concerns. If we conduct multiple tests using a criterion set for one test, the chances of one of the tests becoming significant is higher than the criterion. If we conduct 20 tests to determine whether a response is present, we should not be surprised if one of these turns out significant at $p < 0.05$ even when there is no response and we are just evaluating residual noise. A simple way to compensate for this is to use a Bonferroni correction, to divide the criterion probability by the number of tests. This may be too stringent. A recent approach to this problem is to adjust the "false discovery rate" on the basis of the actual experimental findings (Benjamini & Hochberg, 1995). If we are evaluating M simultaneous stimuli and using a criterion value of p, the probabilities determined for each of the M responses are sorted in ascending order $k = 1, 2 \ldots M$, and we reject any hypothesis where the probability is less than or equal to $(k/M)p$. At least one of the

responses must have attained the Bonferroni criterion but the others may use less stringent criteria.

This issue of multiple testing also applies when we monitor whether the response has attained a criterion SNR as the recording progresses. Figure 6–14 shows the results of evaluating responses at multiple times for the ASSR to an amplitude-modulated tone. Each look at the response is an application of a statistical test, and therefore more stringent criteria should apply than when the responses are recorded for a set period of time and the test applied only after the recording is complete. One approach is to require that the responses attain significance (at normal levels such as $p < 0.05$) and remain significant as the recording progresses for some minimum extra time (Luts, Van Dun, Alaerts, & Wouters, 2008). For example, we can continue the recording after the response first become significant and ensure the response remains significant on the next eight consecutive tests. At present, these are rules of thumb rather than theoretically based principles.

Another approach is to adjust the criterion to a lower level to compensate for the multiple looks. Applying the Bonferroni adjustment to testing performed every few seconds is likely too stringent. Exactly how to adjust the significance criterion and how often to apply the testing can be examined with Monte Carlo simulations—using models based on random data instead of actual recordings (Stürzebecher, Cebulla, & Elberling, 2005). John and Purcell (2008) have suggested using some of the statistical principles used to determine endpoints when evaluating clinical trials (Sankoh, Huque, & Dubey, 1997). For example, the criterion can be reduced less when the results are more

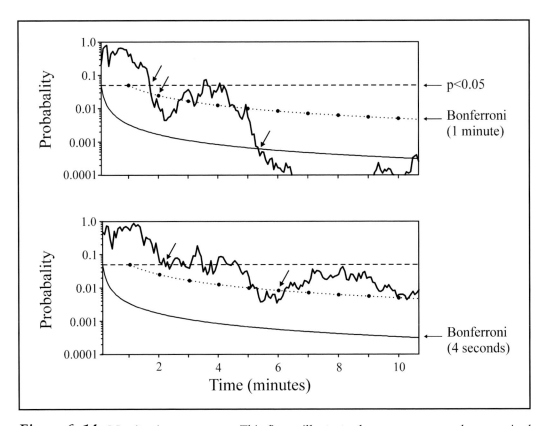

Figure 6–14. **Monitoring responses.** *This figure illustrates how responses can be recognized during a recording, thus allowing the recording to be abbreviated. ASSRs evoked by 25 dB SPL 1-kHz tones amplitude-modulated at 85 Hz were evaluated every 4 seconds using an F-test. The probability that the response could have been explained by the residual EEG noise is plotted on a logarithmic scale. At the beginning of the recording, this probability is near 50%; as the noise is decreased by the averaging process, the probability decreases. The decrease is not regular because the background EEG/EMG fluctuates during the recording. If we wish to stop the recording as soon as a response is detected, we must beware of false detections, which would occur frequently if we simply used a criterion of p <0.05 for each test. We therefore need to compensate for the multiple tests being performed. The Bonferroni criterion divides the probability by the number of tests. The continuous line shows the Bonferroni criterion when monitoring occurs every 4 seconds and the dotted line when monitoring occurs every minute (i.e., at every large dot). The diagonal arrows indicate when the response is judged present according to the different criteria. For the second subject, illustrated in the lower half of the figure, the response never becomes significant when we use the 4-second Bonferroni criterion. However, the response would be significant if we used some of the less stringent approaches described in the text. For example, the response stays significant at p <0.05 after about 5 minutes of recording.*

correlated from evaluation to evaluation. The correlations between consecutive estimates of the amplitude and phase of the signal can be calculated easily from eval-uation to evaluation and the significance criterion adjusted for each time the testing is performed. This approach certainly deserves further investigation.

Optimal Paradigms for Recording MMN

The principles whereby we have tried to optimize the recording efficiency for simple auditory responses also can be applied to recording the MMN. The MMN paradigm involves both standard and deviant stimuli, with the deviants occurring less probably than the standards. The typical probability for the deviant is between 0.1 and 0.2. Because the SNR of the recording depends on the number of deviants, and the MMN is very small, it can take a long time to record the MMN at the normal 1/s stimulus rate used for the LAEPs. How can the paradigm be improved?

First, we present the stimuli as quickly as possible without losing MMN amplitude. The MMN only becomes small when the interval between the deviants becomes less than a second or two; the refractory period of the MMN is very similar to that of the N1 wave to stimulus onset (see Picton et al., 2000). If we present the stimuli at a rate of one every 400 ms, the deviants will occur on average at a rate of once every 2 seconds, given a probability of 0.2. The responses to the standard may become quite small but there will be no great decline in MMN amplitude. Even faster rates can be used—stimuli can be presented at rates of 3 or 4/s.

Second, we can record several different MMNs concomitantly. Näätänen, Pakarinen, Rinne, and Takegata (2004) proposed a paradigm with five different deviants. The deviants differed from the standards in terms of frequency, intensity, location (of perceived sound source), duration, or envelope (whether there was a gap in the middle of the tone). Stimuli occurred every 500 ms with a probability of 0.5 for the standard stimulus and 0.1 for each deviant. Although a deviant of one kind or another occurred on average once a second, each particular deviant occurred on average once every 5 seconds. The MMNs recorded in this multideviant paradigm were not significantly different from the MMNs recorded when single deviants were presented with a probability of 0.1 in separate recording sessions (one for each type of deviant). Therefore, five different MMNs could be recorded in the same time that it would take to record one. We return to this paradigm in Chapter 11.

PHYSIOLOGIC AND BEHAVIORAL THRESHOLDS

An important application of the auditory EPs is to assess audiometric thresholds in subjects who cannot respond reliably during normal behavioral testing. Auditory EPs do not require the subject to make a decision about whether a sound can be heard; they simply indicate that the sound has been received by the auditory system. Thus, they can provide an "objective" test of hearing. As pointed out by Dobie (1993), a truly objective test of hearing would also remove from the procedure any subjective interpretation of the waveforms. The previous sections of this chapter reviewed the ways whereby responses can be confidently recognized. Now we need to determine how to measure thresholds and, ultimately, how to estimate a subject's audiogram from the EPs.

The general approach is to record the auditory EPs to sounds at lower and lower intensities until we no longer can recognize a response. The physiologic threshold is then the lowest intensity at which a response is recognized. This is similar to behavioral testing although, because it takes longer to record the EP than to recognize a button press, we usually do not repeat the tests. Furthermore, rather than using a "down 10 dB, up 5 dB" strategy, we typically do not use steps smaller than 10 dB. Once we have a physiologic threshold, we can estimate the behavioral threshold on the basis of normative data relating physiologic and behavioral thresholds. For example, we may have measured the physiologic threshold as 30 dB HL and estimated the behavioral threshold as 20 dB HL because our normative data show a mean physiologic-behavioral dif-

ference of 10 dB. When reporting thresholds, we always must indicate clearly whether the threshold is "physiologic" or "estimated behavioral."

The process of estimating behavioral thresholds is illustrated in the left half of Figure 6–15. The average threshold for an auditory EP (the physiologic threshold) is generally 5 to 20 dB higher than the behavioral threshold. Although it is important to be within about 20 dB of threshold, the mean difference between physiologic and

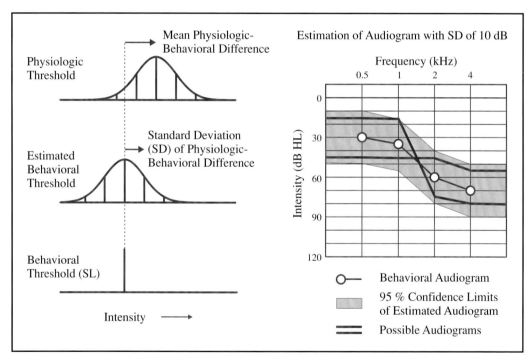

Figure 6–15. Estimating behavioral thresholds. *The thresholds for detecting a physiologic response to a sound typically are higher than the behavioral thresholds, and there is some intersubject variability in the physiologic-behavioral difference* (upper left). *To estimate the behavioral thresholds from the physiologic responses, we subtract the mean physiologic-behavioral difference. The estimated thresholds then vary around the actual behavioral threshold with a standard deviation (SD) equal to that of the physiologic-behavioral difference. The 95 % confidence limits for where the actual behavioral threshold of an individual subject then occurs at ±2 SD. The right side of the figure demonstrates how accurately the behavioral audiogram might be estimated when the SD is 10 dB at each audiometric frequency. Very different audiometric patterns could be possible. However, because a particular individual's physiologic-behavioral difference tends to be similar across the frequencies, the audiometric pattern may be better estimated than suggested in this illustration.*

behavioral thresholds is less important than the variability of this difference. Basically, we can subtract the expected difference from the physiologic threshold to give an estimated behavioral threshold. The mean physiologic-behavioral difference can limit the range over which thresholds are estimated. If the maximum level at which the stimulus can be presented is 110 dB and the average behavioral-physiologic difference is 20 dB, one cannot estimate thresholds above 90 dB.

Once we have removed the mean physiologic-behavioral difference, we are left with the intersubject variability of this difference—the main determinant of the accuracy of the estimation. The variability of this measurement usually is measured by the SD. If the data are normally distributed (and they typically are), 19 out of 20 subjects will have estimated thresholds that are less than two SDs away from the real behavioral threshold. A commonly reported SD for EP thresholds is 10 dB. This means that the actual thresholds for a particular individual will be between 20 dB below and 20 dB above the estimated threshold. As illustrated in the right half of Figure 6–15, this means that we may not be sure of the audiometric pattern, as well as not know the exact degree of hearing loss. However, results such as those of Perez-Abalo et al. (2001) suggest that within an individual the difference between estimated and actual thresholds varies little with frequency. Thus, the audiometric pattern is reasonably well preserved in the estimated thresholds.

The variability of the threshold estimation will be smaller when the background EEG noise is less and the SNR consequently higher. If the response is relatively unaffected by sleep (e.g., the ABR or the 80-Hz ASSR), the background EEG noise in the frequency region of the response can be attenuated by having the subject sleep. Most importantly, the residual background EEG noise can be reduced by increasing the amount of time for the recording. In normal subjects, 80-Hz thresholds can be estimated with an accuracy (as measured by the SD) of 7 dB with recordings that last up to 10 minutes, but only 12 dB with recordings of about 100 seconds (Picton, Dimitrijevic, Perez-Abalo, & van Roon, 2005).

The amount of hearing loss also can affect the physiologic-behavioral difference. Physiologic thresholds in subjects with cochlear hearing loss on average will tend to be closer to the behavioral thresholds than in normally hearing subjects. Because of physiologic recruitment, the response is larger just above threshold and therefore easier to distinguish from the background EEG noise (Picton et al., 2005). When estimating thresholds, the amount that we should take away from the physiologic threshold therefore can vary with the amount of hearing loss. This is the basis for the regression equations used to estimate the behavioral thresholds in some ASSR systems (e.g., Rance & Rickards, 2002; Rance, Rickards, Cohen, De Vidi, & Clark, 1995). The effect is less if one averages for longer periods of time (and can therefore recognize smaller responses).

Temporal integration is another variable that can affect the physiologic-behavioral difference. Many of the physiologic responses that we use for objective audiometry are evoked by either a brief stimulus or the onset of a longer stimulus. The behavioral thresholds normally are measured using tones of much longer duration. Because the subject can integrate perception over several hundred milliseconds, the thresholds for these tones will be lower than for brief tones. The normal difference is part of the physiologic-behavioral difference estimated in normal subjects. However, the amount of temporal integration may be less than normal in patients with a sensorineural hearing loss. This would mean that we should use a smaller physiologic-behavioral difference when estimating the behavioral thresholds. This issue is discussed at greater length in Schoonhoven, Prijs, and Grote (1996). The final effect on our estimation procedures is similar to that for recruitment, although the mechanism is different.

NORMAL AND ABNORMAL WAVEFORMS

As well as providing audiometric information by being an objective indicator of the brain's response to sound, auditory EPs can demonstrate neurologic abnormalities. Neurologic interpretation depends on demonstrating an abnormal rather than absent waveform. Components of the response are identified and the amplitudes and latencies of these components are compared to what is expected for normal subjects of the same age and gender.

Many EP measurements are normally distributed, and the limits of normal can be derived reasonably well from SDs. The confidence limits for a normally distributed variable are ±1.96 SDs for $p < 0.05$ and ±2.58 SDs $p < 0.01$ from the mean. This means that 1 out of 20 subjects will normal show values that are more than 1.96 SDs from the mean (either above or below), and 1 out of 100 subjects will show values more than 2.58 SDs from the mean. However, as we usually do not look for a wave that is too early, we can consider just the probability of exceeding upper confidence limits for latency measurements at 1.65 ($p < 0.05$) and 2.33 ($p < 0.01$) SDs above the mean. Most clinical laboratory tests give the normal values as ±2 SDs. The normal values for EP measurements have been set at various levels from 2 to 3 SDs above the mean of a group of normal subjects. The American Electroencephalographic Society (1994) recommended that upper limits of normal be set at 2.5 or 3 SDs above the normal mean to minimize false positive results and to compensate for the fact that the normative data were often based on smaller samples than usually collected to assess confidence limits.

Some EP measurements are not normally distributed. Amplitudes tend not to be normally distributed as they have a lower limit of zero and no upper limit. Confidence limits for these measurements can be estimated in two ways. We can use some transformation to "normalize" the data (e.g., we can take the logarithm or the square root of the measurement), calculate the limits from the SDs of the normalized data, and then convert these limits back to the units that we measure. Or we can collect sufficient normative data that we can directly locate the $p = 0.05$ or 0.01 level in the distribution, the level above and/or below which only 5 or 1% of the data occur.

In order to detect an abnormal waveform, the SNR must be higher than when just detecting the presence or absence of a response. Residual background noise in the recording can make it difficult to recognize particular peaks and can alter the measurement of their latency and amplitude. There has not been much in the way of quantifying the reliability of a peak measurement. A rule-of-thumb recommendation would be that replicate traces be recorded and that the distance between the replicate measurements be no more than the SD of the normal measurements. The American Clinical Neurophysiology

Society (2006) recommends that the inter-replication measurement be within 1% of the sweep duration for latency and within 15% of each other for the amplitude.

Abnormal Patterns

Recent years have seen many developments in pattern recognition. Pattern analysis uses multiple measurements to discriminate between different groups or to identify different individuals. Several studies have used pattern recognition techniques to detect a response in noise (e.g., Davey, McCullagh, Lightbody, & McAllister, 2007) or to provide prognostic information (e.g., Wilson et al., 2006). Unfortunately little has been done to discriminate normal from abnormal waveforms or to classify different types of EP abnormality.

Dynamic time warping is a technique whereby one waveform is stretched or compressed in time to fit another. Initially used in speech recognition algorithms to fit an individual utterance to a known template, the procedure also can be used to evaluate abnormal EPs (Picton, Hunt, Mowrey, Rodriguez, & Maru, 1988). The two waveforms are compared according to selected parameters, such as amplitude and slope, with each latency in the recorded waveform compared to each latency in the template. This gives a dissimilarity matrix that shows how different the measurement at each time-point in one waveform is from all measurements in the other waveform. An optimum path then is traced through the matrix to give the lowest total dissimilarity between the waveforms, and the recorded waveform is adjusted according to this path. The technique then gives the amount of latency adjustment necessary for optimal warping, the timing of this latency adjustment, and the ampli-tude differences between that adjusted waveform and the template. Figure 6–16 illustrates how a template ABR has to be stretched to best fit the ABR recorded in a patient with multiple sclerosis.

In addition to warping individual waveforms to a template, dynamic time warping also can be used to construct a more representative template than simple averaging. Waveforms in the normative data set are warped to each other using parameters such as amplitude and slope. The template obtained by warping is not distorted by the latency jitter between individual subjects which tends to smear the average waveform.

CONCLUSIONS

The interpretation of EP recordings requires a series of decisions. Initially, responses must be recognized as different from the background EEG noise. This requires us to assess the SNR of our recordings. The presence or absence of a response at different intensities then can be used to determine physiologic thresholds. From these, we can estimate the behavioral thresholds. Once a response has been recognized as present, the latencies and amplitudes of its components can be measured and compared to normative data. These measurements require a higher SNR than the simple decision as to whether the response is real or not. Two factors run throughout the procedures of detection and analysis: time and uncertainty. It takes time to get good results, and the more time we spend, the more certain we can be about our interpretations. Even with the best of recordings, however, we cannot be completely certain. A wise interpretation always will be qualified by an estimate of the chances that it may be wrong.

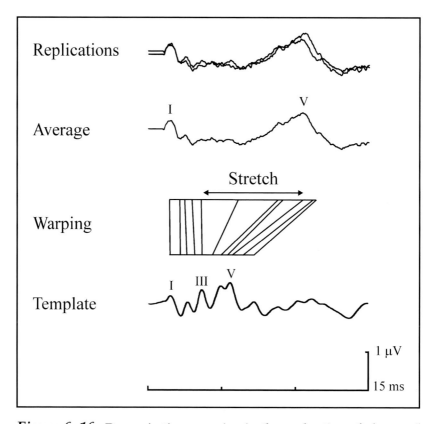

Figure 6–16. **Dynamic time warping in the evaluation of abnormal EP waveforms.** *The ABR waveforms in the upper part of the figure come from a patient with multiple sclerosis. The first two waves of the ABR are recognizable but then the waveform is distorted and delayed with what appears to be a wave V at a latency near 10 ms. If we warp the normal template ABR to fit this patient's ABR, we need to stretch the waveform in the region of the template between wave III and wave V. The warping diagram connects the peak and trough latencies of the template waveform to the latencies in the abnormal ABR to which they best correspond. The template was itself formed by warping together a set of normal waveforms. Warping preserved the morphology of the response (e.g., the IV–V peaks) better than simple averaging. Data from Picton et al. (1988).*

ABBREVIATIONS

ABR	Auditory brainstem response
AM	Amplitude modulation
ASSR	Auditory steady-state response

EEG	Electroencephalogram
EP	Evoked potential
EMG	Electromyogram
Fsp	F-ratio at a single point
Fmp	F-ratio at multiple points

FN	False negative
FP	False positive
nHL	Normal hearing level
LAEP	Late auditory evoked potential
MLR	Middle-latency response
MLS	Maximum length sequence
MMN	Mismatch negativity
ROC	Receiver operating characteristic
SD	Standard deviation
SDR	Standard deviation ratio
SNR	Signal-to-noise ratio
SOA	Stimulus onset asynchrony
TN	True negative
TP	True positive

REFERENCES

American Clinical Neurophysiology Society. (2006). Guidelines on evoked potentials. *Journal of Clinical Neurophysiology, 23*, 125–137.

American Electroencephalographic Society. (1994). Guidelines on evoked potentials. *Journal of Clinical Neurophysiology, 11*, 40–73.

Achim, A. (1995). Signal detection in averaged evoked potentials: Monte Carlo comparison of the sensitivity of different methods. *Electroencephalography and Clinical Neurophysiology, 96*, 574–584.

Benjamini, Y., & Hochberg, Y. (1995) Controlling the false discovery rate: A practical and powerful approach to multiple testing. *Journal of the Royal Statistical Society, Series B (Methodological), 57*, 125–133.

Blair, R. C., & Karniski, W. (1993). An alternative method for significance testing of waveform difference potentials. *Psychophysiology, 30*, 518–524.

Bohórquez, J., & Özdamar, O. (2008). Generation of the 40-Hz auditory steady-state response (ASSR) explained using convolution. *Clinical Neurophysiology, 119*, 2598–2607.

Burkard, R., Shi, Y., & Hecox, K. E. (1990). A comparison of maximum length and Legendre sequences for the derivation of brain-stem auditory-evoked responses at rapid rates of stimulation. *Journal of the Acoustical Society of America, 87*, 1656–1664.

Cacace, A. T., & McFarland, D. J. (2003). Quantifying signal-to-noise ratio of mismatch negativity in humans. *Neuroscience Letters, 341*, 251–255.

Coppola, R., Tabor, R., & Buchsbaum, M. S. (1978). Signal to noise ratio and response variability measurements in single trial evoked potentials. *Electroencephalography and Clinical Neurophysiology, 44*, 214–222.

Davey, R., McCullagh, P., Lightbody, G., & McAllister, G. (2007). Auditory brainstem response classification: A hybrid model using time and frequency features. *Artificial Intelligence in Medicine, 40*, 1–14.

Delgado, R. E., & Özdamar, O. (2004). Deconvolution of evoked responses obtained at high stimulus rates. *Journal of the Acoustical Society of America, 115*, 1242–1251.

Dobie, R. A. (1993). Objective response detection. *Ear and Hearing, 14*, 31–35.

Dobie, R. A., & Wilson, M. J. (1994). Phase weighting: a method to improve objective detection of steady-state evoked potentials. *Hearing Research, 79*, 94–98.

Dobie, R. A., & Wilson, M. J. (1996). A comparison of t test, F test, and coherence methods of detecting steady-state auditory-evoked potentials, distortion-product otoacoustic emissions, or other sinusoids. *Journal of the Acoustical Society of America, 100*, 2236–2246.

Don, M., Elberling, C., & Waring, M. (1984). Objective detection of averaged auditory brainstem responses. *Scandinavian Audiology, 13*, 219–228.

Eggermont, J. J. (1976). Electrocochleography. In W. D. Keidel & W. D. Neff (Eds.), *Handbook of sensory physiology Vol. 3. Auditory system. Clinical and special topics* (pp. 625–705). Berlin, Germany: Springer-Verlag.

Elberling, C., & Don, M. (1984). Quality estimation of averaged auditory brainstem responses. *Scandinavian Audiology, 13,* 187–197.

Eysholdt, U., & Schreiner, C. (1982). Maximum length sequences—a fast method for measuring brain-stem-evoked responses. *Audiology, 21,* 242–250.

Fisher, N. I. (1993). *Statistical analysis of circular data.* Cambridge, UK: Cambridge University Press.

Herrmann, B. S., Thornton, A. R., & Joseph, J. M. (1995). Automated infant hearing screening using the ABR: Development and validation. *American Journal of Audiology. 4,* 6–14.

Hochberg, Y., & Tamhane, A.C. (1987). *Multiple comparison procedures.* New York, NY: Wiley.

Hyde, M. L., Sininger, Y. S., & Don, M. (1998). Objective detection and analysis of ABR: An historical perspective. *Seminars in Hearing, 19,* 97–113.

Jewett, D. L., Caplovitz, G., Baird, B., Trumpis, M., Olson, M. P., & Larson-Prior, L. J. (2004). The use of QSD (q-sequence deconvolution) to recover superposed, transient evoked-responses. *Clinical Neurophysiology, 115,* 2754–2775.

Jiang, Z. D., Brosi, D. M., Shao, X. M., & Wilkinson, A. R. (2008). Sustained depression of brainstem auditory electrophysiology during the first months in term infants after perinatal asphyxia. *Clinical Neurophysiology, 119,* 1496–1505.

John, M. S., Lins, O. G., Boucher, B. L., & Picton, T. W. (1998). Multiple auditory steady state responses (MASTER): Stimulus and recording parameters. *Audiology, 37,* 59–82.

John, M. S., & Purcell, D. W. (2008). Introduction to technical principles of auditory steady-state response testing. In G. Rance (Ed.), *Auditory steady-state response: Generation, recording, and clinical applications* (pp. 11–53). San Diego, CA: Plural.

John, M. S., Purcell, D. W., Dimitrijevic, A., & Picton, T. W. (2002). Advantages and caveats when recording steady-state responses to multiple simultaneous stimuli. *Journal of the American Academy of Audiology, 13,* 246–259.

Lasky, R. E., Shi, Y., & Hecox, K. E. (1993). Binaural maximum length sequence auditory-evoked brain-stem responses in human adults. *Journal of the Acoustical Society of America, 93,* 2077–2087.

Lins, O. G., & Picton, T. W. (1995). Auditory steady-state responses to multiple simultaneous stimuli. *Electroencephalography and Clinical Neurophysiology, 96,* 420–432.

Lins, O. G., Picton, T. W., Boucher, B. L., Durieux-Smith, A., Champagne, S. C., Moran, L. M., . . . Savio, G. (1996). Frequency-specific audiometry using steady-state responses. *Ear and Hearing, 17,* 81–96.

Luts, H., Van Dun, B., Alaerts, J., & Wouters, J. (2008). The influence of the detection paradigm in recording auditory steady-state responses. *Ear and Hearing, 29,* 638–650.

McGee, T., Kraus, N., & Nicol, T. (1997). Is it really a mismatch negativity? An assessment of methods for determining response validity in individual subjects. *Electroencephalography and Clinical Neurophysiology, 104,* 359–368.

Ménard, M., Gallégo, S., Berger-Vachon, C., Collet, L, & Thai-Van, H. (2008). Relationship between loudness growth function and auditory steady-state response in normal-hearing subjects. *Hearing Research, 235,* 105–113.

Näätänen, R., Pakarinen, S., Rinne, T., & Takegata, R. (2004). The mismatch negativity (MMN): Towards the optimal paradigm. *Clinical Neurophysiology, 115,* 140–144.

Özdamar, Ö., & Delgado, R. E. (1996) Measurement of signal and noise characteristics in ongoing auditory brainstem response averaging. *Annals of Biomedical Engineering, 24,* 702–715.

Perez-Abalo, M. C., Savio, G., Torres, A., Martín, V., Rodríguez, E., & Galán, L. (2001). Steady state responses to multiple amplitude-modulated tones: An optimized method to test frequency-specific thresholds in hearing-impaired children and normal-hearing subjects. *Ear and Hearing, 22,* 200–211.

Petermann, M., Kummer, P., Burger, M., Lohscheller, J., Eysholdt, U., & Döllinger, M. (2009). Statistical detection and analysis of mismatch negativity derived by a multi-deviant design from normal hearing children. *Hearing Research, 247,* 128–136.

Picton, T. W., Alain, C., Otten, L., Ritter, W., & Achim, A. (2000). Mismatch negativity: Different water in the same river. *Audiology and Neuro-Otology, 5,* 111–139.

Picton, T. W., Champagne, S. C., & Kellett, A. J. C. (1992). Auditory evoked potentials recorded using maximum length sequences *Electroencephalography and Clinical Neurophysiology, 84,* 90–100.

Picton, T. W., Dimitrijevic, A., John, M. S., & van Roon, P. (2001). The use of phase in the detection of auditory steady-state responses. *Clinical Neurophysiology, 112,* 1692–1711.

Picton, T. W., Dimitrijevic, A., Perez-Abalo, M. C., & van Roon, P. (2005). Estimating audiometric thresholds using auditory steady-state responses. *Journal of the American Academy of Audiology, 16,* 143–156.

Picton, T. W., & Hink, R. F. (1974). Evoked potentials: How? What? and Why? *American Journal of EEG Technology, 14,* 9–44.

Picton, T. W., Hink, R. F., Perez-Abalo, M., Linden, R. D., & Wiens, A. S. (1984). Evoked potentials: How now? *Journal of Electrophysiological Technology, 10,* 177–221.

Picton, T., Hunt, M., Mowrey, R., Rodriguez, R., & Maru, J. (1988). Evaluation of brainstem auditory evoked potentials using dynamic time warping. *Electroencephalography and Clinical Neurophysiology, 71,* 212–225.

Picton, T. W., John, M. S., Dimitrijevic, A., & Purcell, D. W. (2003). Human auditory steady-state responses. *International Journal of Audiology, 42,* 177–219.

Picton, T. W., Kellett, A. J. C., Vezsenyi, M., & Rabinovitch, D. E. (1993). Otoacoustic emissions recorded at rapid stimulus rates. *Ear and Hearing, 14,* 299–314.

Picton, T. W., Linden, R. D., Hamel, G., & Maru, J. T. (1983). Aspects of averaging. *Seminars in Hearing, 4,* 327–341.

Picton, T. W., Stapells, D. R., & Campbell, K. B. (1981). Auditory evoked potentials from the human cochlea and brainstem. *Journal of Otolaryngology, 10*(Suppl. 9), 1–41.

Picton T. W., Vajsar, J., Rodriguez, R., & Campbell, K. B. (1987). Reliability estimates for steady state evoked potentials. *Electroencephalography and Clinical Neurophysiology, 68,* 119–131.

Picton, T. W., Woods, D. L., Baribeau-Braun, J., & Healey, T. M. G. (1977). Evoked potential audiometry. *Journal of Otolaryngology, 6,* 90–119.

Plourde, G., Picton, T., & Kellett, A. (1988). The interweaving and overlapping of evoked potentials. *Electroencephalography and Clinical Neurophysiology, 71,* 405–414.

Ponton, C. W., Don, M., Eggermont, J. J., & Kwong, B. (1997). Integrated mismatch negativity (MMNi): A noise-free representation of evoked responses allowing single-point distribution-free statistical tests. *Electroencephalography and Clinical Neurophysiology, 104,* 143–150. Erratum (1997) *Electroencephalography and Clinical Neurophysiology, 104,* 381–382.

Rance, G., & Rickards, F. (2002). Prediction of hearing threshold in infants using auditory steady-state evoked potentials. *Journal of the American Academy of Audiology, 13,* 236–245.

Rance, G., Rickards, F. W., Cohen, L. T., De Vidi, S., & Clark, G. M. (1995) The automated prediction of hearing thresholds in sleeping subjects using auditory steady state evoked potentials. *Ear and Hearing, 16,* 499–507.

Regan, D. (1989). *Human brain electrophysiology: Evoked potentials and evoked magnetic fields in science and medicine.* Amsterdam, The Netherlands: Elsevier.

Regan, D., & Heron, J. R. (1969). Clinical investigation of lesions of the visual pathway: A new objective technique. *Journal of Neurology, Neurosurgery and Psychiatry, 32,* 479–483.

Ross, B., Lütkenhöner, B., Pantev, C., & Hoke, M. (1999). Frequency-specific threshold determination with the CERAgram method: Basic principle and retrospective evaluation of data. *Audiology and Neuro-Otology, 4,* 12–27.

Sankoh, A. J., Huque, M. F., & Dubey, S. D. (1997). Some comments on frequently used multiple endpoint adjustment methods in clinical trials. *Statistics in Medicine, 16,* 2529–2542.

Schimmel, H. (1967). The (±) reference: Accuracy of estimated mean components in average response studies. *Science. 157,* 92–94.

Schoonhoven, R., Prijs, V. F., & Grote, J. J. (1996). Response thresholds in electrocochleography and their relation to the pure tone audiogram. *Ear and Hearing, 17,* 266–275.

Sininger, Y., Hyde, M., & Don, M. (2001). Method for detection of auditory evoked potentials using a point optimized variance ratio. U.S. Patent No.6,200,273.

Stürzebecher, E., Cebulla, M., & Elberling, C. (2005). Automated auditory response detection: Statistical problems with repeated testing. *International Journal of Audiology, 44,* 110–117.

Swets, J. A. (1988). Measuring the accuracy of diagnostic systems. *Science, 240,* 1285–1293.

Valdes, J. L., Perez-Abalo, M. C., Martin, V., Savio, G., Sierra, C., Rodriguéz, E., & Lins, O. (1997). Comparison of statistical indicators for the automatic detection of 80 Hz auditory steady state responses. *Ear and Hearing, 18,* 420–429.

Van Dun, B., Verstraeten, S., Alaerts, J., Luts, H., Moonen, M., & Wouters, J. (2008). A flexible research platform for multi-channel auditory steady-state response measurements. *Journal of Neuroscience Methods, 169,* 239–248.

Victor, J. D., & Mast, J. (1991). A new statistic for steady-state evoked potentials. *Electroencephalography and Clinical Neurophysiology, 78,* 378–388. Erratum (1992) in: *Electroencephalography and Clinical Neurophysiology, 83,* 270.

Wilson, W. J., Chapple, J. A., Phillips, K. M., Snell, K. T., Bradley, A. P., & Darnell, R. (2006). Over-complete discrete wavelet transformation of the normal auditory brainstem response improves prediction of outcome following severe acute closed head injury. *Audiology and Neurotology, 11,* 249–258.

Wong, P. K., & Bickford, R. G. (1980). Brain stem auditory evoked potentials: the use of noise estimate. *Electroencephalography and Clinical Neurophysiology, 50,* 25–34.

7

Electrocochleography: From Song to Synapse

> The shaking air rattled Lord Edward's membrana tympani; the interlocked malleus, incus and stirrup bones were set in motion so as to agitate the membrane of the oval window and raise an infinitesimal storm in the fluid of the labyrinth. The hairy endings of the auditory nerve shuddered like weeds in a rough sea: a vast number of obscure miracles were performed in the brain, and Lord Edward ecstatically whispered "Bach!"
>
> Aldous Huxley, *Point Counter Point*, Chap. 3, 1928

The human ear is the product of long evolution. The first cleft between the gills of fishes became the external auditory canal, leftover bones from the lower jaw formed the ossicles of the middle ear, and the rudimentary auditory epithelium invaginated and coiled itself into the present cochlea. These changes allowed us to hear sounds transmitted through the air rather than through the water where our ancestors dwelled. The range and sensitivity of our hearing is exquisite; we can hear movements of air molecules that are much smaller than their own size. This chapter begins with a brief review of the ear and its physiology. Geisler (1998) provides a more extensive evaluation, and the subtitle

of this chapter pays homage to his work. The physiology of the ear is also covered in Møller (2006) and Pickles (2008). After the basic physiology we consider in more detail the findings of human electrocochleography (ECochG), the electrical activity we can record from the ear as it converts incoming sounds to neuronal impulses.

ANATOMY AND PHYSIOLOGY

Anatomy of the Ear

The general structure of the ear is shown in Figure 7–1. The external ear, which consists of the pinna and the external auditory

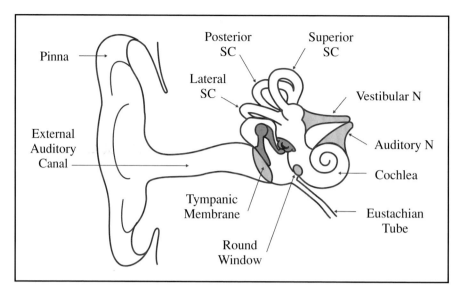

Figure 7–1. *Anatomy of the ear. This diagram shows the right ear viewed from the front. The tympanic membrane* (light shading) *separates the external ear from the middle ear. The bones of the middle ear—malleus, incus, and stapes—are darkly shaded. The stapes is attached to the oval window in the medial wall of the middle ear. The oval window leads into the cochlear duct (scala media). The round window* (light shading) *is between the middle ear and the scala tympani. Within the inner ear are the vestibular end organs—the vestibule, the saccule, and the semicircular canals (SC)—and the cochlea.*

canal, funnels sound to the tympanic membrane or eardrum. The ossicles of the middle ear—malleus (hammer), incus (anvil), and stapes (stirrups)—convert the large-amplitude low-force movements of the air into the small-amplitude high-force movements of the footplate of the stapes. This impedance-matching process became necessary when we evolved into land animals; without it, most of the air-borne sound energy would be reflected back from the tympanic membrane and not transmitted into the cochlea. As well as three ossicles, the middle ear contains two muscles—the tensor tympani attaching to the handle of the malleus and the stapedius muscle attaching to the neck of the stapes. When activated by loud sounds, these muscles decrease the mobility of the ossicles and decrease the energy being

transmitted into the cochlea. The inner ear consists of the auditory sense organ—the cochlear duct—and the vestibular sense organs—the semicircular canals, utricle, and saccule. These organs, which contain a special fluid called endolymph, float within a supporting fluid called peri-lymph, which is itself encased in the temporal bone.

The cochlear duct begins in the bony labyrinth near the oval window and then spirals into the cochlea, finally reaching its apex. A cross section of the cochlea contains three "rooms": scala vestibuli, scala media (cochlear duct), and scala tympani (Figure 7–2). The scala vestibuli is separated from the scala media by Reissner's membrane, a thin partition that isolates the endolymph from the perilymph. The basilar membrane separates scala media

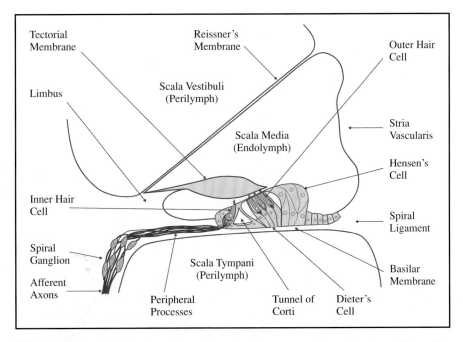

Figure 7–2. *Cochlea. This diagram shows a section through the cochlear. The organ of Corti is composed of the hair cells (dark shading), supporting cells, and tectorial membrane. It sits on the basilar membrane that separates the scala media from scale tympani. The oval window (with the footplate of the stapes) connects to the scala vestibuli and the round window with the scala tympani.*

from scala tympani. This membrane connects the modiolus (central axis of the cochlea) to the spiral ligament on the outer wall. The basilar membrane becomes wider and less tense with increasing distance away from the oval window. These physical characteristics causes sound to travel from near the oval window toward the apex, and to distribute different frequencies to different parts of the basilar membrane. As discussed in Chapter 5, high frequencies activate the basilar membrane close to the stapes and low frequencies activate its apical regions.

Organ of Corti

On the basilar membrane is the organ of Corti, which is composed of inner and outer hair cells, supporting cells (Hensen's), and a tectorial membrane. This is where sound becomes electric. The inner hair cells, arranged in a single row, are the main afferent receptors. Each inner hair cell is in synaptic contact with about 20 afferent nerve endings, with each afferent nerve contacting only a single internal hair cell. This precision—each afferent nerve fiber coming from only one hair cell—allows the labeled line or place coding of frequency. As the traveling wave distributes the frequencies of a sound along the basilar membrane, the brain can interpret which frequencies are present in the sound by determining which afferent fibers are firing. Each fiber indicates activation at a precise place on the basilar membrane.

The presynaptic region in the hair cell is highly specialized with a ribbon organelle (or synaptic bar) that anchors synaptic vesicles, and likely makes it possible for the synapse to transfer information very rapidly and precisely (Nouvian, Beutner, Parsons, & Moser, 2006). The speed of the synaptic processing allows the afferent fibers to synchronize with sounds of low frequency, thereby providing a temporal coding for frequency. Thus, frequency can be coded in two ways: by the place on the basilar membrane and by the rate of firing of the neurons.

Three rows of outer hair cells have hairs that are tightly fixed to the tectorial membrane. These cells display motility. In a way, they are like little muscles. Prestin is their main contractile molecule (Ashmore, 2008; Dallos, Zheng, & Cheatham, 2006). In Chapter 5, we described the tuning curve of an auditory nerve fiber and suggested that it represents two components: a rather coarse tuning brought about by the traveling wave and a much more precise tuning caused by activity of the external hair cells. In response to sound, the outer hair cells move, adding energy to the incoming sounds, and making the transduction process more efficient and more specific. They provide the tip for the tuning curve and the energy for the otoacoustic emissions. This motility of the outer hair cells is the basis for the "cochlear amplifier" that makes hearing an active rather than passive process (Hudspeth, 2008).

The outer hair cells receive synaptic input from efferent fibers in the olivocochlear bundle. Activity in these fibers can alter the general contractility of the hair cells. Figure 7–3 shows the inner and outer hair cells and their innervation. The main function of the outer hair cells is to control the tuning and sensitivity of the transduction processes, leaving the inner hair cells as the main afferent transducers.

The footplate of the stapes moves the perilymph in the region near the junction of the saccule and the cochlear duct. An inward deflection of the footplate moves the basilar membrane toward the scala tympani. The scala tympani connects to the middle ear at the round window. The elasticity of the membrane covering the round window allows the basilar membrane to move freely with the movements impinging on it from the scala vestibuli. As the basilar membrane moves up and down, the tectorial membrane moves the stereocilia (hairs) on the top of the hair cells. As the basilar membrane moves upward (e.g., from a rarefaction sound causing the stapes to move outward), the tectorial membrane pushes the tips of the stereocilia outward (away from the modiolus). Then a miracle occurs. What was acoustic now becomes electric.

Acoustic Transduction

The miracle is set up by the special electrical characteristics of the endolymph (Wangemann, 2006). The perilymph is a typical extracellular fluid, with a composition similar to that of the cerebrospinal fluid. However, the endolymph differs from any other extracellular fluid in the body by having a high concentration of potassium ions and a low concentration of sodium ions. These concentrations are maintained by ionic pumps in the stria vascularis, the highly metabolic (and highly vascular) external wall of the scala media. The endolymph is electrically positive compared to the perilymph (and other extracellular fluids) by about 80 mV. Normal intracellular fluids are high in potassium but electrically negative relative to extracellular fluids—the electric potential across the cell membrane is deter-

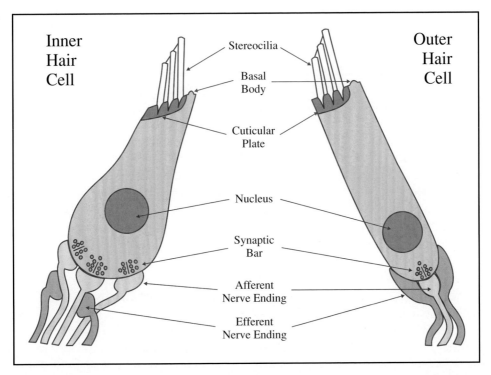

Figure 7–3. **Hair cells.** *The structure and connections of the two different kinds of hair cells are shown diagrammatically. Most of the efferent fibers* (dark gray) *to the inner hair cells synapse on the afferent fibers* (light gray) *rather than the hair cells. The efferent fibers to the outer hair cells synapse directly on the hair cells.*

mined by the membrane's permeability to potassium ions. The endolymph's positivity is determined by the permeability of the surrounding membranes to sodium ions. Because hair cells have a normal intracellular potential of about –50 mV, a potential difference of 130 mV is set up over the top of the hair cells—this is the battery that powers the process of transduction.

When the stereocilia are moved away from the modiolus, highly specialized channels in the tips of the stereocilia are opened mechanically (Vollrath, Kwan, & Corey, 2007). These allow the passage of positively charged ions (mainly potassium) to enter the stereocilia under the electrical gradient established by the endolymphatic potential. These ions enter the hair

cell body through the bases of the stereocilia, depolarizing the membrane potential of the hair cell. As the back-and-forth movement of the hairs is determined by the in-and-out movement of the stapes, the membrane potential of the hair cell faithfully reproduces the acoustic waveform. The fields generated by all the hair cells activated by a sound sum to produce the cochlear microphonic (CM). This is the receptor potential of the cochlea, representing the change from acoustic energy to electric energy.

Depolarization of the hair-cell membrane causes release of transmitter (probably glutamate) from the specialized synaptic ribbon region at the base of the cell (Nouvian et al., 2006). This in turn causes depolarization of the peripheral process of the spiral ganglion cells and the initiation of action potentials. During these processes, a summating potential (SP) is generated. The exact origin of this potential is not known. As its name suggests, several processes likely combine to give the potential: an asymmetry in the CM, depolarization of the synaptic region of the hair cell and depolarization of the afferent nerve endings.

As the afferent nerve endings are depolarized beyond their threshold level, action potentials (APs) are generated and these propagate along the auditory nerve fibers into the brain. The rate at which these action potentials are generated depends on two factors. First is the intensity of the sound which, by means of the amplitude of the CM and SP, causes more or less release of transmitter at the synapse between hair cell and afferent fiber. Second is the frequency of the sound, with the discharges tending to synchronize with the rarefaction movements of the stimuli, at least for the lower frequencies. This allows a temporal coding of frequency, which combines with a place coding (based on where the basilar membrane is activated) to provide our brains with two different mechanisms for the perception of frequency. The APs in the afferent nerve fibers represent the conversion of the analog electrical signals of the cochlear microphonic into a digital signal. The summed fields generated by all the afferent nerve fibers give the compound action potential (CAP) of the auditory nerve, a large negative wave (N1) followed by a smaller positive wave. As discussed in Chapter 4, this depends on the synchronization between the discharges in the different fibers, and will occur at the beginning of a sound when all the fibers tend to fire simultaneously. A smaller second wave (N2) can

occur (if there is some degree of synchrony among some of the fibers when they fire a second time). However, if the sound continues and evokes sustained activity in the fibers, this firing will occur asynchronously in different nerve fibers and their different fields will cancel each other out, leaving us with only the onset response.

The ECochG records the CAP of the auditory nerve rather than a single AP from a single fiber. Therefore, although using the initials AP to denote the compound action potential has become common, we use the abbreviation CAP.

Otoacoustic Emissions

The active processes of the cochlea can be directly measured by the evoked otoacoustic emissions (OAEs: Kemp, 2002; Probst, Lonsbury-Martin, & Martin 1991; Robinette & Glattke, 2007; Shera, 2004). Spontaneous OAEs can occur in the absence of sound, but these are not as important as the evoked OAEs. The sounds generated by the hair cells in response to incoming sounds are measured by a tiny microphone connected to a probe in the external ear canal. The probe also contains one or two tubes for the presentation of sounds to the ear. Two main types of OAEs are measured: the transient evoked OAE following a click or brief tone, and the distortion product OAE that occurs in response to a combination of tones. The distortion product OAE typically is evoked by two tones (f1 and f2) and measured at the 2f1-f2 frequency (the quadratic distortion product). Other distortion product OAEs can be measured but these are less reliable than the 2f1-f2 emission. Stimulus frequency OAEs also can be recorded but these are very difficult to disentangle from the simultaneous stimuli. The presence of OAEs indicates that the hair cells are working and that the hearing threshold is therefore below about 35 dB HL at the frequency where the OAEs are generated (near the frequency measured in the transient OAE and near f2 in the distortion product OAE). The demonstration of hair-cell function is important in screening of infants for hearing loss and in monitoring hair cell function during ototoxic medication.

The olivocochlear bundle sends efferent fibers to the hair cells. Activation of these fibers using contralateral noise can decrease the amplitude of the OAEs (Berlin, Hood, Hurley, & Wen, 1994; Collet, Veuillet, Bene, & Morgon, 1992; Purcell, Butler, Saunders, & Allen, 2008). The change is small—of the order of one to several dB—but can be reliably demonstrated. We have to be careful to use a stimulus that is not loud enough to cause middle ear muscle reflexes or interaural masking, both of which would reduce the OAEs. Once stimulus levels have been appropriately chosen, contralateral suppression of the OAEs indicates normal functioning of the medial olivocochlear system. This procedure is a useful addition to our clinical battery for evaluating disorders of the auditory nerve and brainstem.

COCHLEAR EVOKED POTENTIALS

Recording Electrodes

The electrical responses of the cochlea to sounds can be recorded from electrodes placed near the cochlea. The closer the electrode is to the generators, the larger the response that is recorded. Electrodes usually are placed in the middle ear or in the external auditory canal (Figure 7–4).

Cochlear potentials can be recorded from the mastoid or earlobe but these are very small and extensive averaging is required to obtain a reasonable signal-to-noise ratio.

The transtympanic electrode usually is inserted through the posterior inferior quadrant of the tympanic membrane. Prior to insertion, the tympanic membrane is anesthetized (Bath, Beynon, Moffat, & Baguley, 1998; Sass, Densert, & Arlinger, 1998). The electrode comes to rest on the promontory of the cochlea. Some laboratories have had more success (particularly for recording responses to low-frequency stimuli) using a "golf-club" electrode placed in the round window niche (Aso & Gibson, 1994), but this requires general anesthesia and a myringotomy to allow direct visualization of the middle ear. The original promontory procedure used a long rigid electrode held in place outside the pinna (upper right of Figure 7–4). Schwaber and Hall (1990) demonstrated that similar recordings can be obtained with a short needle (e.g., 12 mm) passed through the tympanic membrane using forceps under the operating microscope. The flexible electrode cable then is held in place by the foam insert used to deliver the stimuli.

Many techniques are available for recording from the external auditory canal. Coats (1974) designed a butterfly electrode that opens within the canal to hold the electrode in place. Another approach uses a foil electrode wrapped around the foam insert used to present the stimuli. Probably the best procedure is to place an electrode with a cotton tip impregnated with electrode jelly lightly against the tympanic membrane and to hold it in place using a foam insert (Ferraro & Durrant, 2006; Stypulkowski & Staller, 1987). This is illustrated in the upper left of Figure 7–4. Recordings with this tympanic

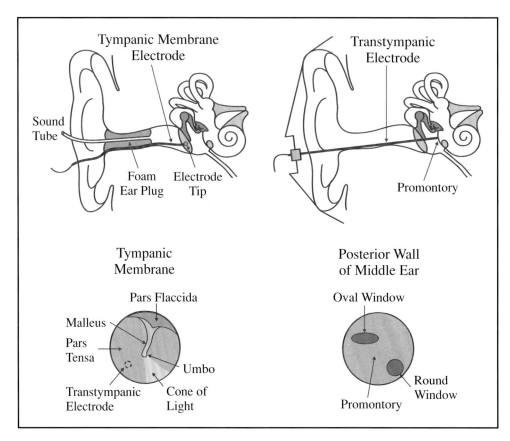

Figure 7–4. Electrodes for electrocochleography. The upper left shows the placement of an electrode on the eardrum (adapted from Ferraro & Durrant, 2006). The upper right shows the placement of a transtympanic electrode on the promontory (adapted from Eggermont, 1976a). At the bottom left is a view of the tympanic membrane (for the right ear, anterior is to the right), indicating where the transtympanic electrode passes through the membrane. The bottom right shows of the medial wall of the middle ear (viewed from within the middle ear).

membrane electrode (or "tymptrode") generally give larger and less variable recordings than those obtained with electrodes placed in the ear canal at some distance away from the tympanic membrane.

Transtympanic recordings give responses that are between 2 and 10 times larger than those recorded from the tympanic membrane (Ferraro, Thedinger, Mediavilla, & Blackwell, 1994; Schoonhoven, Fabius, & Grote, 1995). Recordings from more external regions of the canal

are about half the amplitude of those recorded from the eardrum, with the relative size depending on the distance from the eardrum (Coats, 1986). Recordings from the mastoid or earlobe are smaller still. As a rule of thumb, we would expect the typical CAP for a very loud click to be about 15 µV on the promontory, 3 µV on the eardrum, 1.5 µV in the canal and 0.5 µV on the mastoid.

Although there are subtle differences in the input-output functions between the different recording sites, the general morphology of the click-responses remains the same. However, there are differences in the SP when using tonal stimuli. Although always negative in tympanic membrane and ear-canal recordings, the SP can be positive in transtympanic recordings when using high-frequency tones (Eggermont, 1976a; Sass et al., 1998). This may be caused by the closeness of the promontory electrode to the high-frequency region of the basilar membrane.

Both transtympanic and extratympanic electrodes have a higher electrical impedance than scalp electrodes, perhaps 50 to 100 kOhms for the transtympanic needles (with a very low surface area) and 10 to 20 kOhms for the extratympanic electrodes (Schoonhoven, Prijs, & Grote, 1996). This can lead to high noise levels, particularly for the transtympanic recordings. Furthermore, the amplifiers need to have high input impedance so that differences between the impedances of active and reference electrodes do not distort the recording. Reference electrodes commonly are placed on the ipsilateral or contralateral mastoid. If the contralateral mastoid is used, there may be contamination from the auditory brainstem response (ABR), particularly when stimulus rates are rapid (and the ABR to one stimulus can occur during the CAP to the next). Many investigators use an additional channel, recording between the ECochG electrode and a vertex reference, to examine the ABR as well as the ECochG.

Disentangling the Different Potentials

Three different evoked potentials are recorded from the cochlea in response to sound: the CM, the SP and the auditory nerve CAP. These overlap in time and can obscure each other. A simple technique to distinguish the CM from the other components requires recording separate responses to stimuli of opposite polarity. Averaging the two responses together will cancel out the CM and leave the SP and CAP. Subtracting one response from the other (and dividing by 2) gives the CM by itself. These procedures are illustrated in Figure 7–5.

At rapid stimulus rates, the amplitude of the CAP decreases substantially and its latency increases slightly. Auditory fibers have difficulty in firing consistently and synchronously at stimulus rates of 100/s or more. Because the amplitude of the SP is not affected by increasing stimulus rate, recording responses at both slow and fast rates can help distinguish between the SP and the CAP (see the left side of Figure 7–6). This can be particularly helpful when the notch at the junction between the SP and CAP is difficult to identify. The response recorded at the rapid rate can be subtracted from that recorded at the slower rate to give the CAP without the SP. This subtraction process is not perfect as there are small latency changes in the SP at rapid rates between the rates and a small (and delayed) CAP can remain even at the rapid rates.

Another possible way to distinguish between the CAP and the SP might be to present the stimuli in broadband noise of sufficient intensity to prevent the time-locked generation of the CAP and yet insufficient to alter the receptor potentials (Figure 2 of Starr, Picton, Sininger, Hood, & Berlin, 1996). The masking noise should then remove the CAP and leave the CM and the SP. However, it can be difficult to select a masking intensity that removes the CAP without also attenuating the receptor potentials.

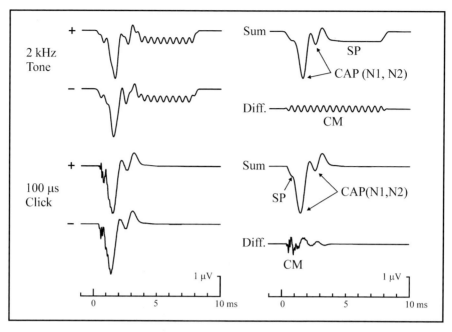

Figure 7–5. Component structure of the ECochG. In the right column are shown the responses to either tones or clicks presented with the stimulus beginning with either a condensation (+) or rarefaction (–) movement. If the two waveforms are added together and divided by 2, we can recognize the CAP and SP in the "Sum" waveform on the right. If the difference between the two waveforms is divided by 2 to get the "Diff." waveforms, only the CM remains. Since the +CAP is slightly later than the –CAP for clicks, the later part of the click Diff waveform is as much the difference between +CAP and –CAP as it is CM. All waveforms are computer-modeled.

Cochlear Microphonic (CM)

Although the CM provides a direct measurement of hair cell function, it has not been used extensively in human recordings. One difficulty is that it represents the sum of the fields generated by all the hair cells activated by a sound. At more than moderate intensities, the high-frequency spread of activation by the traveling wave makes the CM quite nonspecific in terms of where on the basilar membrane it is generated. Masking techniques can make it possible to examine place-specific hair-cell responses to different frequencies (Ponton, Don, & Eggermont, 1992). However, such information is more easily available from measurements of the CAP.

The main use of the CM has been in evaluating residual hair-cell function in patients with auditory neuropathy. For the diagnosis of auditory neuropathy, we need to demonstrate an absent or abnormal auditory nerve response despite preservation of hair cell function. Hair cell function typically is demonstrated with the OAEs, but if these are absent we can show some preservation of the hair cells by recordings a CM. Some subjects with auditory neuropathy may have a CM that is larger than in normal subjects. This possibly may relate to some disorder in the

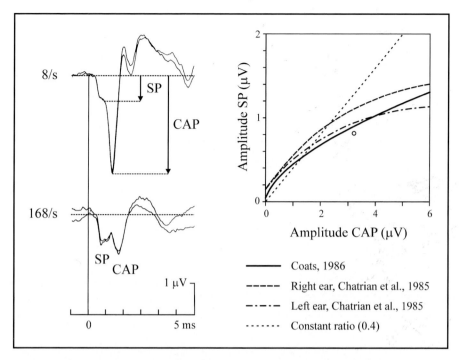

Figure 7–6. *Measurements of the summating potential (SP). On the left are shown the responses to clicks presented with alternating polarity at an intensity of 90 dB nHL at two different rates. At the faster rate, the amplitude of the CAP is markedly reduced and its latency increased. This makes it easier to measure the SP, which is little affected by rate. The waveforms are derived from Chatrian, Wirch, Lettich, Turella, and Snyder (1982) but plotted using a positive-up convention. The graph on the right plots the p <0.05 limits of normal for SP amplitude as a function of the CAP amplitude. Three different curves are plotted: two from Chatrian et al. (1985) and one from Coats (1986). Anything above the curves would be considered abnormal according to the data in these studies. The upper normal limits of the SP/CAP ratio decrease with increasing CAP amplitude. The dotted straight line represents what would be considered abnormal using a constant ratio (0.4) for all CAP amplitudes. The data point (o) represents the SP and CAP amplitudes for the waveforms at the upper left of the figure.*

efferent control of the CM by the olivo-cochlear bundle. These phenomena are reviewed in Chapter 15.

Summating Potential (SP)

The SP has been extensively studied in human subjects in relation to Ménière's disease. The underlying pathophysiology of this disorder is endolymphatic hydrops, a swelling of the membranous labyrinth because of increased production or decreased resorption of the endolymph. In the cochlea, this causes increased pressure in the scala media or cochlear duct. Reissner's membrane balloons out and the basilar membrane becomes tense. Hair-cell function becomes distorted and inefficient. The SP becomes larger than normal, and as the disorder progresses, the CAP decreases in size. Therefore, a critical measurement is the SP/CAP ratio, which was first suggested by Eggermont (1976b). Although this can be measured using brief tones, it has become customary to measure the ratio in the response to loud clicks. The SP to tones is more variable, and, as we have mentioned, may actually become positive at high frequencies in transtympanic recordings. In transtympanic recordings, the SP to a click may initially start positively and then go negative (Mori, Asai, Sakagami, & Matsunaga, 1987). Because the click contains all frequencies and the traveling wave distributes the excitation to the higher frequencies before the middle and low frequencies, an initial high-frequency positive SP leads to a negative SP for middle frequencies.

Many studies have measured the normal SP/CAP ratio to clicks. Responses are recorded separately for condensation and rarefaction clicks and measurements are made on the average of the two waveforms. Although we can simply record a response to clicks that alternate in polarity from click to click, making separate recordings allows us to evaluate the CM and to measure the latency difference between condensation and rarefaction clicks. The clicks are presented at high intensity—typically 80 to 90 dB nHL (normal hearing level)—because the transition between the SP and the CAP is difficult to identify at lower intensities. Click rate is usually between 5 and 15/s. Averaging is continued until the waveforms are clear enough to allow reliable measurement. This will require several hundred to a thousand trials for the transtympanic recordings and several thousand trials for ear canal recordings.

The measurement requires identifying an inflection point in the waveform as the SP plateaus (or even begins to return to baseline) and is overtaken by the CAP. The most common approach to measurement is illustrated in Figure 7–6, and the results from several studies using this measurement are given in Table 7–1. Other results are summarized by Schoonhoven (2007) and Abbas and Brown (2009). The results are reasonably consistent among the different studies—SP/CAP ratios greater than 0.5 should not occur in normal subjects and ratios of greater than 0.4 are unusual. The ratio changes little with the different electrode placements. Several studies have directly compared promontory to ear canal recordings and found no significant differences in the ratio, although the absolute amplitudes were much larger in the promontory recordings (Ferraro et al., 1994; Levine, Margolis, Fournier, & Winzenburg, 1992; Ruth & Lambert 1989). In a meta-analysis of many papers, Wuyts, van de Heyning, van Spaendonck, and Molenberghs (1997) found that the upper limits of normal were slightly higher for extratympanic recordings than transtympanic recordings (0.42 vs. 0.36). Coats (1986) reported that the SP/CAP ratio became larger with increasing distance from the eardrum. The SP/CAP ratio is not significantly different between left and right ears or between female and male subjects (Chatrian et al., 1985). The ratio decreases when the CAP measurement increases (Chatrian et al., 1985; Coats, 1986). Because of this relationship graphing the upper limits of SP versus the amplitude of the CAP (as shown on the right of Figure 7–6) might allow us to discriminate abnormal measurements better than simply measuring the SP/CAP ratio. If this ratio were constant, the SP versus CAP graph would show a linear relationship (with the slope of the line being the upper limits of the ratio). In actuality, the graph

Table 7–1. SP/CAP Ratio for Clicks in Normal Subjects

Study	Electrode Location*	Intensity (dB nHL)	Rate (Clicks/s)	Amp CAP (μV)	SP/CAP Ratio (Mean±SD)	Upper Limit**
Roland et al., 1995	TT	95	9.7	11.8	0.29±0.10	0.49
Sass et al., 1998	TT	95	10	18.4	0.26±0.11	0.48
Ohashi et al. 2009	TT	82	nr	nr	0.24±0.06	0.35
Campbell et al., 1992	TM	90	11.7	1.8	0.27±0.15	0.50
Margolis et al., 1995	TM	88	13	3.2	0.26±0.09	0.42
Wilson et al., 2002	TM	90	7.1	0.5	0.32±0.14	0.60
Coats, 1986	EC	85	8	2.7	0.20±0.08	0.36
Roland et al., 1995	EC	95	9.7	1.1	0.27±0.13	0.53
Chung et al., 2004	EC	90	8.1	nr	0.23±0.06	0.34

nr = not reported.

*TT = transtympanic, TM = tympanic membrane, EC = ear canal.

**Upper limit determined as mean +2 SD unless a 95% limit estimated in the paper.

is curvilinear, and although it is close to the straight line for low values of the CAP, it falls away as the CAP gets larger. When we obtain the SP and CAP measurements from a patient, we can plot them on the graph and determine whether they are abnormal (above the line) or normal (below the line).

Other measurements relating the SP to the CAP are possible (Abbas & Brown, 2009; Ferraro & Durrant, 2006). We could measure the CAP amplitude from the inflection point between the SP and the CAP to the peak of the CAP, or we could measure the area of a wave rather than simply its peak (Ferraro & Tibbils, 1999). However, these measurements are not any more specific than the usual SP/CAP ratio (Baba et al., 2009).

Several studies have proposed that the absolute amplitude of the SP to a brief tone may be a better measurement of endocochlear function than the SP/CAP ratio for the click response (e.g., Conlon & Gibson, 2000; Dauman, Aran, Charlet de Sauvage, & Portmann, 1988; Iseli & Gibson, 2009). Responses are evoked by brief (e.g., 10 ms) tones of high intensity (e.g., 110 dB SPL) using frequencies of 1 or 2 kHz. Because the CAP evoked by the onset of the tone is not important (and will vary with rise time and tonal frequency), the tones are presented at more rapid rates than for clicks (e.g., 30/s). The SP amplitude is measured after combining responses to tones of opposite polarity (to cancel the CM) and taking a mean amplitude measurement after the onset response is completed (e.g., from 3–10 ms). Unfortunately, the absolute amplitudes vary with the details of the ECochG technique. Even among studies using a transtympanic approach the mean normal amplitudes may vary from 2 to 10 μV for a 1-kHz tone (Sass et al., 1998). Therefore, laboratory-specific normative data must be collected before assessing these absolute SP measurements in patients.

The SP to a click or brief tone can be "biased" if the stimulus is presented together with a high-intensity tone of very low frequency (Durrant & Dallos, 1974). The low-frequency tone (e.g., 30 Hz) moves the whole basilar membrane slowly up and down. Responses to clicks or high-frequency tones simultaneously presented with such a continuous low-frequency tone are then averaged separately based on the phase of this biasing tone. Depending on whether the basilar membrane is up (rarefaction part of the low-frequency tone) or down (condensation), the amplitude of the CM and SP evoked by the simultaneously presented stimulus will change. The exact mechanism (mechanical or electrical) is unknown but the phenomenon can be reliably recorded in normal subjects (Iseli & Gibson, 2009). Endolymphatic hydrops reduces the effects of biasing, probably because tension from the swollen cochlear duct makes it difficult to move the basilar membrane. We return to this phenomenon in Chapter 14.

COMPOUND ACTION POTENTIAL (CAP) OF THE AUDITORY NERVE

Subject Variables

Chatrian et al. (1985) described several subject variables that affect the measurement of the ear canal CAP. The amplitude of the CAP is significantly larger for female (mean 1.6 μV) than for male subjects (mean 1.1 μV) in ear-canal recordings. The CAP also is slightly larger for clicks presented to the right ear (mean 1.5 μV) compared to left (mean 1.2 μV). The CAP amplitude also gets smaller with increasing age, mainly in relation to the increasing thresholds for 4- and 8-kHz tones. Similar ear and gender effects were found by Coats (1986), although his overall amplitudes were larger.

Intensity Effects

The main N1 wave of the CAP is larger in amplitude and shorter in latency at higher intensity. The N2 is clearly present only at high intensities. It has become common to plot CAP amplitudes and latencies logarithmically as this gives plots that approximate straight lines (Eggermont, 1976a). A linear scale for the amplitude curve would make it more difficult to assess the low-level responses when plotting responses over a large range of intensities. However, the linear scale works well for responses to low and moderate intensities (as in Figure 7–7). A small plateau region occurs in the normal amplitude curve at intensities of 30 to 50 dB above threshold.

When recruitment is present, the slope of the amplitude-intensity function for the

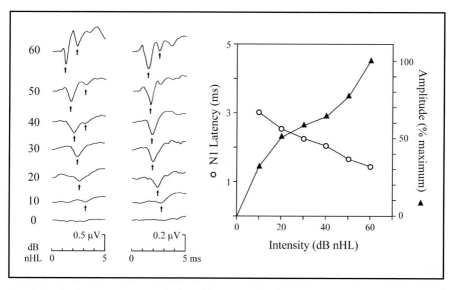

Figure 7–7. AP intensity effects. *The left side of the figures shows CAPs recorded using a tympanic membrane electrode in two subjects. The stimulus was a 10-μs click presented at a rate of 5/s using alternating polarity. At the higher intensities two different negative peaks (N1 and N2) are clearly visible (arrows) but only N1 remains at lower intensities. On the right are plotted the average amplitudes (triangles) and latencies (circles) for the N1 component plotted against stimulus intensity.*

cochlear nerve CAP increases (Eggermont & Odenthal, 1974; Schoonhoven, 2007). In a cochlear hearing loss, the CAP therefore shows both an elevated threshold and a greater slope of the amplitude-intensity function. In Ménière's disease, the SP is larger than normal, whereas in cochlear hearing losses related primarily to hair-cell damage the SP is reduced.

The threshold for recognizing the CAP is very close to the behavioral threshold. Indeed, the mean physiologic-behavioral difference varies from –7.5 to +1.5 dB for tones with 2-cycle rise- and fall-times and a 4-ms plateau (Schoonhoven et al., 1996). The standard deviations (SD) are close to 11 dB. Because of temporal integration (which is less in patients with hearing loss), the physiologic-behavioral difference is larger in subjects with normal

hearing than in patients with hearing loss. Provided the averaging is sufficient to obtain reliable recordings, transtympanic and extratympanic recordings are not significantly different (Schoonhoven et al., 1996). The CAP therefore can provide accurate objective auditory thresholds. However, the variability of the results (as shown by the SD) is similar to that of other techniques such as the tone-ABR and the auditory steady-state response (ASSR). One advantage of ECochG is the small mean physiologic-behavioral difference (near 0 dB compared to 10 or 15 dB for tone ABRs and 80 Hz ASSRs). This may make is easier to assess very high thresholds. Another advantage is that ECochG provides information about hair-cell function through the SP and CM measurements. The SP can be helpful in evaluating patients with possible Ménière's disease (see Chapter 14), and the CM can be important in evaluating patients with auditory neuropathy (see Chapter 15).

Rate Effects

The CAP decreases its amplitude and increases its latency at rapid stimulus rates. As we have seen, this effect is useful in distinguishing the CAP from the SP. Normative data for different rates are available (e.g., Eggermont, 1976a, for transtympanic recordings; Wilson, Bowker, & Wilson, 2002, for tympanic membrane recordings). At rapid rates, it may become difficult to distinguish the CAP from the SP, especially if we are using a simple peak to baseline measurement. We also should be careful to determine possible overlapping effects of wave V of the ABR when rates are more than 150/s. The CAP amplitude may show an increased susceptibility to increasing rate in auditory neuropathy.

Stimulus Polarity

The peak latency of the N1 wave is longer for condensation than for rarefaction clicks, usually by an average of between 0.06 and 0.12 ms (Coats & Martin, 1977; Levine et al., 1992; Orchik, Ge, & Shea, 1998; Ohashi, Nishino, Arai, Hyodo, & Takatsu, 2009). The upper limits of normal have been variably reported between 0.13 and 0.30 ms. The mechanism for this latency difference is that the APs in the auditory nerve fibers tend to synchronize with upward movement of the basilar membrane. A rarefaction click causes an initial upward movement followed by a downward movement at a latency determined by the resonance frequency of each region of the basilar membrane (i.e., one half-cycle later). The opposite occurs for the condensation click. The initial activation of the nerve fibers (through the rarefaction movement) is one half cycle later for the condensation click. Thus, we can presume that the click-evoked CAP is predominantly generated by the region of the basilar membrane specific to frequencies equal to $1/(2d)$ where d is the condensation-rarefaction latency difference. The 0.06- to 0.12-ms range of d gives frequencies between 8 and 4 kHz. As we will see when we examine the ABR in the next chapter, this logic may not work for stimuli of low to moderate intensity.

Frequency Effects

The latency of the CAP response to brief tones is longer for tones of lower frequency (Eggermont, 1976c). It is important to consider the effects of rise-time as well as the frequency, as a longer rise time will lead to longer latencies. At high intensities, the responses to low-frequency tones will activate the high-frequency regions of the cochlea and will have an earlier latency than that predicted by their frequency. Derived response techniques, as reviewed in Chapter 5, can demonstrate these effects. Derived responses also can be used to analyze the click-evoked CAP and provide estimates of the cochlear delay, composed of both the traveling wave latency and the filter buildup time (Eggermont, 1976a; Elberling, 1974).

Tuning Curves

Some estimate of the frequency selectivity of the auditory nerve fibers can be obtained from the CAP using procedures similar to those used to obtain psychophysical tuning curves. The CAP is elicited by a brief probe tone that is close to threshold but sufficiently above threshold to give a reliable response. CAP tuning curves then can be constructed by measuring the intensities at which masking tones (or narrow band noises) of frequencies higher and lower than the probe reduce the amplitude of the probe response by some proportion such as 25 or 50% (Eggermont, 1976a; Harrison, Aran, & Erre, 1981; Rutten, 1986). The effects can be measured by presenting a continuous masking tone ("simultaneous masking") or by presenting a brief masking tone immediately before the probe ("forward masking"). As shown in the left section of Figure 7–8, these CAP tuning curves are similar to those obtained by mapping the response area of a single auditory nerve fiber. Frequency selectivity can be measured by dividing the frequency of the probe by the width of the tuning curve 10 dB above its lowest point to give a "quality factor measured at 10 dB" or Q_{10dB}. The tuning curves of patients with hair-cell damage show a broadening of the tuning curve (and a lower Q_{10dB}). Figure 7–8 shows two examples.

The CAP tuning curve is not really the same as the response area of a single nerve fiber, because the probe tone is activating many fibers rather than one. If the

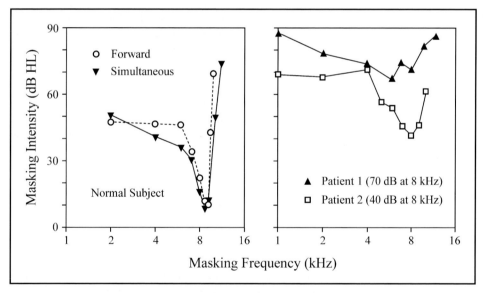

Figure 7–8. **CAP tuning curves.** *This figure shows CAP tuning curves from a normal subject (left) and from two patients with cochlear hearing loss (right). All tuning curves were obtained using a probe tone of 8 kHz. For the normal subject, the tuning curves were obtained using both simultaneous and forward masking paradigms. For the patients, only simultaneous masking was used. The normal tuning curve shows a tip with its most sensitive point just above the test frequency. Forward masking gives a narrower tip than simultaneous masking, perhaps because of suppression effects with simultaneous masking. The patients show tuning curves that are wider and shallower than normal. The threshold elevations at 8 kHz are in brackets. These figures were derived from data presented in Figures 12, 13, and 14 of Harrison et al. (1981).*

probe tone is of higher intensity (as may be necessary when there is a hearing loss), it will activate a broad region of the basilar membrane and thus combine the response areas of individual fibers with different characteristic frequencies. In addition, simultaneous masking will cause suppression, which is not present when the response area of a single nerve fiber is measured. These issues also are present for psychophysical tuning curves (Moore, 1978).

Constructing CAP tuning curves requires multiple threshold estimations even when only one probe tone is used. At each frequency of the masker, several recordings must be obtained to estimate the level at which the masker causes the criterion decrease in the CAP. Although the technique provides a measure of the frequency selectivity of the auditory nerve fibers, it is so time consuming that it has not been widely used.

Electrically Evoked CAPs

When a patient has a cochlear implant, it is possible to evoke the auditory nerve CAP by passing an electrical stimulus through one of the electrode contacts in the multicontact electrode implanted in the cochlea. The response—the electrical CAP or ECAP—can be recorded from another electrode contact. With the appropriate programs and interface to the implant, stimulation and recording can both be accomplished with telemetry. The stimulus information is conveyed from the interface to the implant and the recorded data are conveyed from the implant to the interface using radio-frequency transmission.

Recording the ECAP directly from within the cochlea gives a very large response and this can be recognized much more quickly than when it is recorded from an electrode external to the cochlea.

However, the electrical stimulus-artifact also is very large and this typically overwhelms the recorded ECAP. Several methods have been developed to remove or reduce the artifact (Franck & Norton, 2001; Miller, Abbas, & Brown, 2000). These are illustrated in Figure 7–9. A simple way to remove the artifact would be to use brief (e.g., 10 μs) electrical stimuli of alternating polarity. Both stimuli would evoke the ECAP and the latency difference between the two would be minimal. However, the artifact would be of opposite polarity for the two types of stimuli and would cancel during the averaging process. A second approach would model the suprathreshold artifact from subthreshold recordings and then subtract this away from the suprathreshold recording. The electrical artifact, however, may not be perfectly linear and the cancellation may not be complete. A third technique is based on masking. The response (and the artifact) is evoked in the first recording. In the second recording a masking electrical stimulus is presented a short interval (e.g., 0.6 ms) before the probe stimulus that evokes the ECAP. This masking pulse puts the nerve into a refractory state and there is little or no response to the probe. The recording contains a clear probe-stimulus artifact. Subtracting this away from the simple response leaves the response to the probe without the probe artifact. However, there remains the problem of the masker artifact and the masker response. Our difference waveform now contains an inverted copy of the later parts of the response to the masker pulse. Therefore, we must also record the response to the masker presented alone and add this to the difference waveform. Other techniques based on masking also can be used (Miller et al, 2000).

One possible use of the ECAP is to help set the stimulus levels for patients who are unable to respond behaviorally to

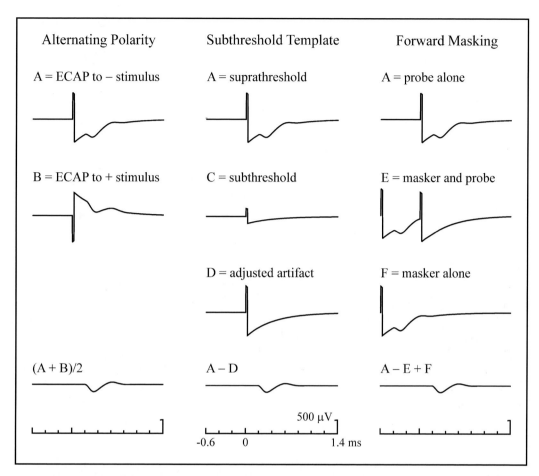

Alternating Polarity

A = ECAP to − stimulus

B = ECAP to + stimulus

(A + B)/2

Subthreshold Template

A = suprathreshold

C = subthreshold

D = adjusted artifact

A − D

Forward Masking

A = probe alone

E = masker and probe

F = masker alone

A − E + F

500 µV

-0.6   0   1.4 ms

Figure 7–9. *Recording the electrical compound AP (ECAP). This figure shows three different ways to remove the artifact when recording the ECAP. The first column shows the approach of alternating polarity. This may not work perfectly as the response may change in latency and amplitude when the stimulus polarity is changed. The middle column shows how we can record the artifact at a stimulus level that is subthreshold, adjust the amplitude of the recorded artifact until it matches the amplitude used for suprathreshold stimulation, and then subtract it away from the suprathreshold recording. The right column shows the masking approach. Any response is prevented by preceding the stimulus by a masking stimulus (at a typical interval of 0.5–1.0 ms, here 0.6 ms). The masking stimulus puts the afferent fibers into a refractory state and they are unable to respond to the probe stimulus. Subtracting the masked probe response from the unmasked probe response removes the probe artifact but leaves the ECAP with an inverted waveform of the artifact and response for the masker. These contributions can be removed by adding back in the response to the masker alone. This figure derives from Figure 1 of Miller et al. (2000).*

the stimuli (Miller, Brown, Abbas, & Chi, 2008). Each electrode of the cochlear implant is adjusted so that its stimulation occurs between a threshold level and a maximal comfort level. The threshold for recording an electrical AP occurs between these two levels. It represents a level at which a stimulus is clearly audible but not uncomfortable. Algorithms might be able to fit the implant levels based on the ECAP threshold but exactly where the ECAP threshold lies between the threshold and comfort levels varies from subject to subject. Some behavioral data therefore are necessary in addition to the ECAP threshold. ECAP thresholds do indicate levels at which conditioning can be initiated in young children in order to obtain the necessary behavioral thresholds. We return to these issues in Chapter 16.

CONCLUSION

Many different potentials can be recorded from the human cochlea. These potentials can tell us about the different processes that convert the acoustic energy of sound into the firing patterns of the auditory nerve fibers. In the past, transtympanic ECochG was used to assess auditory thresholds. In that respect, its role has been superseded by other less invasive tests like the ABR and the ASSR. Even with extratympanic ECochG, the time and technical expertise required to place the electrode on or near the tympanic membrane still makes the ABR and ASSR more efficient in terms of objective audiometry. However, ECochG recordings have several other uses. First is the identification of the auditory nerve CAP when wave I of the ABR is too small to measure. Second is the measurement of the SP when evaluating patients for endolymphatic hydrops. Third is the monitoring of cochlear function during operations in the posterior fossa, in conjunction with other recordings such as the ABR or direct recordings from the intracranial auditory nerve. These three uses are considered in Chapter 14. A fourth application is in the adjustment of the electrode stimulus levels for a cochlear implant. This is discussed further in Chapter 16. A final use is in the evaluation and differential diagnosis of auditory neuropathy (Chapter 15). Just as Lord Edward could not do without the cochlea when listening to the music of Bach, the audiologist cannot do without the ECochG when evaluating a patient's hearing loss or fitting a cochlear implant.

ABBREVIATIONS

ABR	Auditory brainstem response
AP	Action potential
ASSR	Auditory steady-state response
CAP	Compound action potential
CM	Cochlear microphonic
ECAP	Electrical compound action potential
ECochG	Electrocochleography
HL	Hearing level
nHL	Normal hearing level
OAE	Otoacoustic emission
Q_{10dB}	Quality factor measured at 10 dB
SC	Semicircular canal
SD	Standard deviation
SP	Summating potential

REFERENCES

Abbas, P. J., & Brown, C. J. (2009). Electrocochleography. In J. Katz (Ed.), *Handbook of clinical audiology* (6th ed., pp. 242–264). Baltimore, MD: Lippincott Williams & Wilkins.

Ashmore, J. (2008). Cochlear outer hair cell motility. *Physiological Review, 88*, 173–210.

Aso, S., & Gibson, W. P. (1994). Electrocochleography in profoundly deaf children: comparison of promontory and round window techniques. *American Journal of Otology, 15,* 376–379.

Baba, A., Takasaki., Tanaka, F., Tsukasaki, N., Kumagami, H., & Takahashi, H. (2009). Amplitude and area ratios of summating potential/action potential (SP/AP) in Meniere's disease. *Acta Oto-Laryngologica, 129,* 25–29.

Bath, A., Beynon, G., Moffat, D., & Baguley, D. (1998). Effective anaesthesia for transtympanic electrocochleography. *Auris Nasus Larynx, 25,* 137–141.

Berlin, C. I., Hood, L. J., Hurley, A., & Wen, H. (1994). Contralateral suppression of otoacoustic emissions: An index of the function of the medial olivocochlear system. *Otolaryngology-Head and Neck Surgery, 110,* 3–21.

Campbell, K. C., Harker, L. A., & Abbas, P. J. (1992). Interpretation of electrocochleography in Meniere's disease and normal subjects. *Annals of Otology, Rhinology and Laryngology, 101,* 496–500.

Chatrian, G. E., Wirch, A. L., Edwards, K. H., Turella, G. S., Kaufman, M. A., & Snyder, J. M. (1985). Cochlear summating potential to broadband clicks detected from the human external auditory meatus: A study of subjects with normal hearing for age. *Ear and Hearing, 6,* 130–138.

Chatrian, G. E., Wirch, A. L., Lettich, E., Turella, G., & Snyder, J. M. (1982). Click-evoked human electrocochleogram. Noninvasive recording method, origin and physiologic significance. *American Journal of EEG Technology, 22,* 151–174.

Chung, W.-H., Cho, D.-Y., Choi, J.-Y., & Hong. S. H. (2004). Clinical usefulness of extratympanic electrocochleography in the diagnosis of Ménière's disease. *Otology and Neuro-Otology, 25,* 144–149.

Coats, A. C. (1974) On electrocochleographic electrode design. *Journal of the Acoustical Society of America, 56,* 708–711.

Coats, A. C. (1986). The normal summating potential recorded from external ear canal.

Archives of Otolaryngology-Head and Neck Surgery, 112, 759–768.

Coats, A. C., & Martin, J. L. (1977). Human auditory nerve action potentials and brainstem evoked responses: effects of audiogram shape and lesion location. *Archives of Otolaryngology, 103,* 605–622.

Collet, L., Veuillet, E., Bene, J., & Morgon, A. (1992). Effects of contralateral white noise on click-evoked emissions in normal and sensorineural ears: Towards an exploration of the medial olivocochlear system. *Audiology, 31,* 1–7

Conlon, B. J., & Gibson, W. P. (2000). Electrocochleography in the diagnosis of Meniere's disease. *Acta Otolaryngologica, 120,* 480–483.

Dallos, P., Zheng, J., & Cheatham, M. A. (2006). Prestin and the cochlear amplifier. *Journal of Physiology, 576,* 37–42.

Dauman, R., Aran, J. M., Charlet de Sauvage, R., & Portmann, M. (1988). Clinical significance of the summating potential in Ménière's disease. *American Journal of Audiology, 9,* 31–38.

Durrant, J. D., & Dallos, P. (1974). Modification of DIF summating potential components by stimulus biasing. *Journal of the Acoustical Society of America, 56,* 562–570.

Eggermont, J. J. (1976a). Electrocochleography. In W. D. Keidel & W. D. Neff (Eds.), *Handbook of sensory physiology. Vol. V/3 Auditory system. Clinical and special topics* (pp. 625–705). Berlin, Germany: Springer-Verlag.

Eggermont, J. J. (1976b). Summating potentials in electrocochleography: Relation to hearing disorders. In R. J. Ruben, C. Elberling, & G. Salomon (Eds.), *Electrocochleography* (pp. 67–87). Baltimore, MD: University Park Press.

Eggermont, J. J. (1976c). Analysis of compound action potential responses to tone bursts in the human and guinea pig cochlea. *Journal of the Acoustical Society of America, 60,* 1132–1139.

Eggermont, J. J., & Odenthal, D. W. (1974). Electrophysiological investigation of the human cochlea. Recruitment, masking and adaptation. *Audiology, 13,* 1–22.

Elberling, C. (1974). Action potentials along the cochlear partition recorded from the ear canal in man. *Scandinavian Audiology, 3*, 13–19.

Ferraro, J. A., & Durrant, J. D. (2006). Electrocochleography in the evaluation of patients with Ménière's disease/endolymphatic hydrops. *Journal of the American Academy of Audiology, 17*, 45–68.

Ferraro, J. A., Thedinger, B., Mediavilla, S. J., & Blackwell, W. (1994) Human summating potential to tonebursts: Observations on TM versus promontory recordings in the same patient. *Journal of the American Academy of Audiology, 5*, 24–29.

Ferraro, J. A., & Tibbils, R. P. (1999). SP/AP area ratio in the diagnosis of Ménière's disease. *American Journal of Audiology, 8*, 21–28.

Franck, K. H., & Norton, S. J. (2001). Estimation of psychophysical levels using the electrically evoked compound action potential measured with the neural response telemetry capabilities of Cochlear Corporation's CI24M device. *Ear and Hearing, 22*, 289–299.

Geisler, C. D. (1998). *From sound to synapse. Physiology of the mammalian ear.* New York, NY: Oxford University Press.

Harrison, R. V., Aran, J. M., & Erre, J. P. (1981). AP tuning curves from normal and pathological human and guinea pig cochleas. *Journal of the Acoustical Society of America, 69*, 1374–1385.

Hudspeth, A. J. (2008). Making an effort to listen: Mechanical amplification in the ear. *Neuron, 59*, 530–545.

Iseli, C., & Gibson, W. (2009). A comparison of three methods of using transtympanic electrocochleography for the diagnosis of Meniere's disease: Click summating potential measurements, tone burst summating potential amplitude measurements, and biasing of the summating potential using a low frequency tone. *Acta Oto-Laryngologica, 26*, 1–8.

Kemp, D. T. (2002). Otoacoustic emissions, their origin in cochlear function, and use. *British Medical Bulletin, 63*, 223–241

Levine, S. E., Margolis, R. H., Fournier, E. M., & Winzenburg, S. M. (1992). Tympanic electrocochleography for evaluation of endolymphatic hydrops. *Laryngoscope, 102*, 614–622.

Margolis, R. H., Rieks, D., Fournier, E. M., & Levine SE. (l995). Tympanic electrocochleography for diagnosis of Ménière's disease. *Archives of Otolaryngology-Head and Neck Surgery, l21*, 44–45.

Miller, C. A., Abbas, P. J., & Brown, C. J. (2000). An improved method of reducing stimulus artifact in the electrically evoked whole-nerve potential. *Ear and Hearing, 21*, 280–290.

Miller, C. A., Brown, C. J., Abbas, P. J., & Chi, S. L (2008). The clinical application of potentials evoked from the peripheral auditory system. *Hearing Research, 242*, 184–197.

Møller, A. R. (2006). *Hearing: Anatomy, physiology, and disorders of the auditory system* (2nd ed.). Amsterdam, The Netherlands: Academic Press (Elsevier).

Moore, B. C. (1978) Psychophysical tuning curves measured in simultaneous and forward masking. *Journal of the Acoustical Society of America, 63*, 524–532.

Mori, N., Asai, H., Sakagami, M. & Matsunaga, T. (1987) Comparison of summating potential in Ménière's disease between trans- and extratympanic electrocochleography. *International Journal of Audiology, 26*, 348–355.

Nouvian, R., Beutner, D., Parsons, T. D., & Moser, T. (2006). Structure and function of the hair cell ribbon synapse. *Journal of Membrane Biology, 209*, 153–165.

Ohashi, T., Nishino, H., Arai, Y., Hyodo, M., & Takatsu, M. (2009). Clinical significance of the summating potential-action potential ratio and the action potential latency difference for condensation and rarefaction clicks in Meniere's disease. *Annals of Otology, Rhinology and Laryngology, 118*, 307–312.

Orchik, D. J., Ge, N. N., & Shea, J. J., Jr. (1998). Action potential latency shift by rarefaction and condensation clicks in Ménière's disease. *Journal of the American Academy of Audiology, 9*, 121–126.

Pickles, J. O. (2008). *An introduction to the physiology of hearing* (3rd ed.). Bingley, West Yorkshire, UK: Emerald Publishing.

Ponton, C. W., Don, M., & Eggermont, J. J. (1992). Place-specific derived cochlear microphonics from human ears. *Scandinavian Audiology, 21*, 131–141.

Probst, R., Lonsbury-Martin, B. L., & Martin, G. K. (1991). A review of otoacoustic emissions. *Journal of the Acoustical Society of America, 89*, 2027–2067.

Purcell, D. W., Butler, B. E., Saunders, T. J., & Allen, P. (2008). Distortion product otoacoustic emission contralateral suppression functions obtained with ramped stimuli. *Journal of the Acoustical Society of America, 124*, 2133–2148.

Robinette, M. S., & Glattke, T. J. (2007) *Otoacoustic emissions. Clinical applications* (3rd ed.). New York, NY: Thieme.

Roland, P. S., Yellin, M. W., Meyerhoff, W. L. & Frank, T. (1995). Simultaneous comparison between transtympanic and extratympanic electrocochleography. *American Journal of Otology, 16*, 444–450.

Ruth, R. A., & Lambert, P. R. (1989). Comparison of tympanic membrane to promontory electrode recordings of electrocochleographic responses in patients with Menière's disease. *Otolaryngology-Head and Neck Surgery, 100*, 546–552.

Rutten, W. L. (1986). The influence of cochlear hearing loss and probe tone level on compound action potential tuning curves in humans. *Hearing Research, 21*, 195–204.

Sass, K., Densert, B., & Arlinger, S. (1998). Recording techniques for transtympanic electrocochleography in clinical practice. *Acta Otolaryngologica (Stockholm), 118*, 17–25.

Schoonhoven, R. (2007). Responses from the cochlea: cochlear microphonic, summating potential and compound action potential. In R. F. Burkard, M. Don, & J. J. Eggermont (Eds.), *Auditory evoked potentials: Basic principles and clinical application* (pp. 180–198). Philadelphia, PA: Lippincott Williams & Wilkins.

Schoonhoven, R., Fabius M. A., & Grote J. J. (1995). Input/output curves to tone bursts and clicks in extratympanic and transtympanic electrocochleography. *Ear and Hearing, 16*, 619–630.

Schoonhoven, R., Prijs, V. F., & Grote J. J. (1996). Response thresholds in electrocochleography and their relation to the pure tone audiogram. *Ear and Hearing, 17*, 266–275.

Schwaber, M. K., & Hall, J. W., 3rd (1990). A simplified technique for transtympanic electrocochleography. *American Journal of Otology, 11*, 260–265.

Shera, C. A. (2004). Mechanisms of mammalian otoacoustic emission and their implications for the clinical utility of otoacoustic emissions. *Ear and Hearing, 25*, 86–97.

Starr, A., Picton T. W., Sininger, Y. S., Hood, L. J., & Berlin, C. I. (1996). Auditory neuropathy. *Brain, 119*, 741–753.

Stypulkowski, P. H., & Staller, S. J. (1987). Clinical evaluation of a new ECoG recording electrode. *Ear and Hearing, 8*, 304–310.

Wangemann, P. (2006). Supporting sensory transduction: cochlear fluid homeostasis and the endocochlear potential. *Journal of Physiology, 576*, 11–21.

Wilson, W. J., & Bowker, C. A. (2002). The effects of high stimulus rate on the electrocochleogram in normal-hearing subjects. *International Journal of Audiology, 41*, 509–517.

Wuyts, F. L., van de Heyning, P. H., van Spaendonck, M. P., & Molenberghs, G. (1997). A review of electrocochleography: Instrumentation settings and meta-analysis of criteria for diagnosis of endolymphatic hydrops. *Acta Otolaryngologica Supplement, 526*, 14–20.

Vollrath, M. A., Kwan, K. Y., & Corey, D. P. (2007). The micromachinery of mechanotransduction in hair cells. *Annual Review of Neuroscience, 30*, 339–365.

8

Auditory Brainstem Responses: Peaks Along the Way

L'unica gioia al mondo è cominciare. È bello vivere perché vivere è cominciare, sempre, ad ogni istante. Quando manca questo senso— prigione, malattia, abitudine, stupidità—si vorrebbe morire.

(The sole joy in the world is to begin. It is beautiful to be alive, because living is always beginning, at every moment. When this feeling is lacking—because of prison, sickness, convention or stupidity—one might as well die.)

C. Pavese, *Il Mestiere di Vivere* (This Business of Living)
Diary entry for November 23, 1937

The analysis of sound by the central nervous system begins in the brainstem. Information from the cochlea concerning the spectral content of the sounds and their time structure is preserved and relayed to the cortex. The brainstem nuclei carry out additional analyses of the auditory information, most importantly dealing with the location of the sound source, the periodicity of the sound, and its harmonic structure. The hallmarks of brainstem auditory function are its rapidity and its consistency. Sounds are quickly and reliably analyzed and the results are provided to the cortex so that the meaning of the sounds can be evaluated.

As the auditory brainstem pathways are activated, they generate electrical fields that are recorded from the scalp as the auditory brainstem response (ABR), a series of 6 or 7 positive waves recorded between the vertex and the earlobe or mastoid. The peaks of these waves are usually numbered with Roman numerals I to VII according to the convention of Jewett and Williston (1971). The negative troughs following the peaks are often named as I', II', etc. The largest of the positive waves is V, which has a typical peak-latency of 5.6 ms when evoked by a click at 70 dB nHL (normal hearing level). Wave V is followed by a rapid falloff in potential, usually passing below the baseline. This positive-negative transition is perhaps the most striking visual feature of the waveform. Wave I of the response is basically the N1 wave of the electrocochleogram (ECochG) recorded at a distance. Between waves I and V, the most prominent deflection is wave III. Wave II is a small peak in the valley between waves I and III, and waves IV and VI ride on the beginning and end of wave V. The sequence of waves has a very characteristic morphology, similar in some ways to the famous Eiger (Ogre), Mönch (Monk), and Jungfrau (Maiden) peaks of the Bernese Alps in Switzerland. Figure 8–1 shows the archetypical morphology of the human ABR: an adult's response to a 70 dB nHL click presented at a rate of 11/s.

We begin with this archetypical ABR, detailing how and where it is recorded, describing how it is measured, and con-

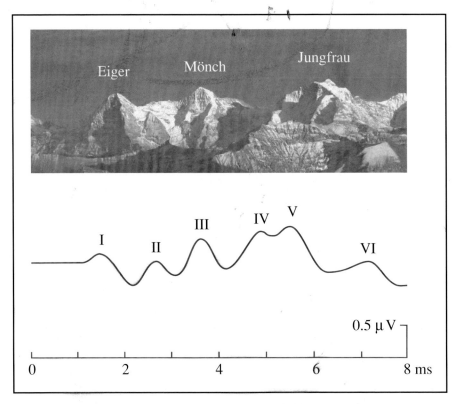

Figure 8–1. Morphology of human ABR. The middle of this figure shows the typical morphology of the human ABR evoked by a 70 dB nHL click presented at a rate of 11/s and recorded between the vertex and the mastoid ipsilateral to stimulation. The waveform was obtained by warping together the ABRs from 16 normal subjects (Picton, Hunt, Mowrey, Rodriguez, & Maru, 1988). Warping preserves the micromorphology of the response—such as the separation of waves IV and V—that is often lost when the responses are simply averaged together (see Chapter 6). The upper part of the figure shows a view of the Bernese Alps from the northwest, a sequence of peaks similar in some ways to the ABR.

sidering the normal limits of these measurements. Having grown familiar with the basic ABR pattern, we then see how it is changed by manipulation of stimulus parameters and how it varies with subject factors.

BASIC PRINCIPLES

Recording Parameters

The spectrum of frequencies present in the ABR was reviewed in Chapter 2. This spectrum determines the optimal frequency bandpass of the amplifiers. The response typically is recorded using a low-pass filter of between 2000 and 3000 Hz and a high-pass filter between 5 and 30 Hz (e.g., American Clinical Neurophysiology Society, 2006). However, many earlier studies used a high-pass cutoff frequency of 100 Hz. This setting, especially if the cutoff slope is gradual (6 or 12 dB/octave), filters out the low-frequency noise very efficiently. In a way, it acts like an optimum filter (see Chapter 2) as the signal-to-noise ratio (SNR) of the response decreases as the frequency decreases. However, the 100-Hz cutoff also can decrease the amplitude of wave V, particularly if this occurs later than in the archetypical response—when the stimulus is near threshold, when the subject very young, or when the response is affected by pathology. The ABR generally is averaged over 2000 trials and the recording replicated to show that the measurements are reliable.

The stimulus is a click (made by passing a 100-μs square wave through a supra-aural earphone) presented at an intensity of 70 dB nHL and at a rate close to 10/s. Some laboratories use a click of alternating polarity, some use a monopolar rarefaction click, and some separately record responses to rarefaction and condensation clicks. The alternating click protocol cancels out most of the stimulus artifact and the cochlear microphonic (CM). However, as we will see later, the ABR waveforms evoked by condensation and rarefaction clicks are different, and the combined response can sometimes be difficult to interpret.

The response usually is recorded between an electrode at the vertex and an electrode on the earlobe or mastoid ipsilateral to stimulation. Recording between the vertex and the neck will show a slightly different waveform wave I is decreased in size and wave V increased (Terkildsen & Osterhammel, 1981). Because it is generated within the cochlea, wave I becomes larger when the electrode is placed in the external auditory meatus (ear canal) rather than on the mastoid or earlobe. This is illustrated in Figure 8–2. Electrodes can be placed in the ear canal using one of the several techniques described in the preceding chapter.

The scalp topography of the ABR varies with the different waves of the response (McPherson, Hirasugi, & Starr, 1985; Starr & Squires, 1982). If we use a noncephalic reference, wave I is maximally recorded near the ear being stimulated, and wave V is maximally recorded at the vertex and midfrontal regions. The waveform near wave III and wave III' is more complex—it often reverses polarity between the mastoids, though the wave measured between the mastoids may have a slightly different latency from that measured on the vertex to mastoid recording (Picton, Hillyard, Krausz, & Galambos, 1974; Starr & Squires, 1982). These findings suggest that at least two different processes underlie this region of the ABR, one generating a vertically oriented dipole and the other a more laterally oriented dipole. The nature of these two sources is

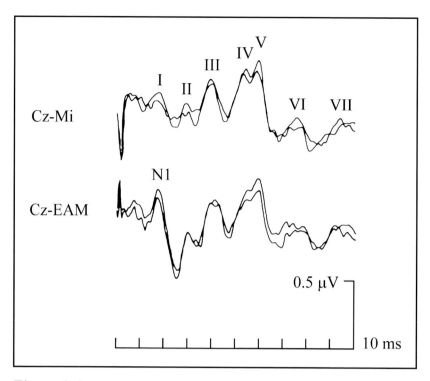

Figure 8–2. Human ABR components. These responses were evoked by 80 dB nHL clicks of alternating polarity presented at a rate of 11/s. The response recorded between the vertex and the ipsilateral mastoid (Cz-Mi) shows six positive peaks, labeled with Roman numerals. The first peak is equivalent to the N1 wave of the ECochG and is recorded with much greater amplitude when the reference electrode is a needle in the posterior wall of the external auditory meatus (EAM).

not fully understood. There may be two brainstem dipoles, one in the cochlear nucleus and one in the superior olive. It also is possible that there is a vertically oriented brainstem dipole to the high-frequency part of the broadband click and a late cochlear wave I evoked by the low-frequency part of the broadband click. We consider this later when we describe the ABR waveforms derived for the different regions of the basilar membrane (see also Chapter 5).

The ABR to a monaural click usually is recorded simultaneously from two electrode derivations: vertex to left mastoid and vertex to right mastoid. Figure 8–3 shows

the typical morphology of the response in these two channels. This two-channel recording means that the electrodes do not need to be changed when the ears are changed—we just pay attention to whatever channel is using the ipsilateral reference. Although the main measurements are taken from the ispilateral channel, the contralateral channel can help in the identification of the ispilateral peaks. Wave I is seldom visible on the contralateral recording, although wave I' is present (upgoing arrows in Figure 8–3) and can be used as a latency marker to identify wave I in the ipsilateral recording, which must occur before wave I'. On the contralateral record-

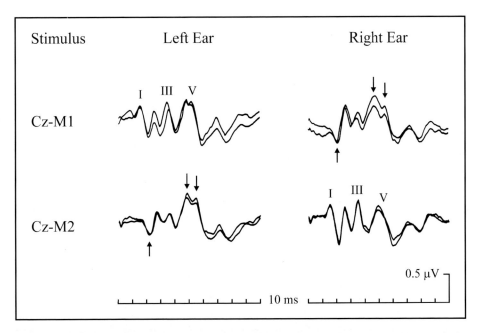

Figure 8–3. Ipsilateral and contralateral recordings. *ABRs to 70 dB nHL clicks presented at a rate of 11/s were recorded simultaneously from the vertex to left mastoid (Cz-M1) and from the vertex to right mastoid (Cz-M2). Waves I and III are much larger in the recording made using the mastoid ipsilateral to the stimulus ear. Although wave I is not visible on the contralateral recording, the negative wave following wave I is quite distinct* (upward arrow). *Waves IV and V often are more easily distinguished on the contralateral recording* (downward arrows) *than on the ipsilateral recording.*

ing, wave III is smaller and waves IV and V tend to be more separate (downgoing arrows in Figure 8–3).

The generators of the ABR recorded from the scalp can be considered as equivalent dipoles near the center of the brain, or as one dipole that changes its orientation and amplitude over time. This concept led to the procedure of tracking how the dipole changes over time using a three-channel Lissajous trajectory (Ino & Mizoi, 1980; Pratt, Har'el, & Golos, 1984; Sininger, Gardi, Morris, Martin, & Jewett, 1987). The ABR is simultaneously recorded using three orthogonal electrode derivations: vertex to neck (typically, the seventh cervical vertebra, the prominent bump at the base of the neck), mastoid to mastoid, and nasion to inion. The voltage recorded in each of these derivations is considered as the location of the trajectory in a three-dimensional space. Since the trajectory has three dimensions, it is difficult to represent in a simple two-dimensional figure; we would need at least two views to get the full trajectory. Furthermore, because the different latency regions of the response overlap, it is sometimes advantageous to plot different figures for different latencies. Figure 8–4 presents frontal views of the trajectory for the ABR to a 70 dB nHL click presented at 10/s (Picton, Stapells, & Campbell, 1981). Such trajectories are called Lissajous figures after a 19th-century French mathematician who analyzed harmonic motion. The lateral view (not illustrated) shows a complex trajectory through the region of wave III and then the

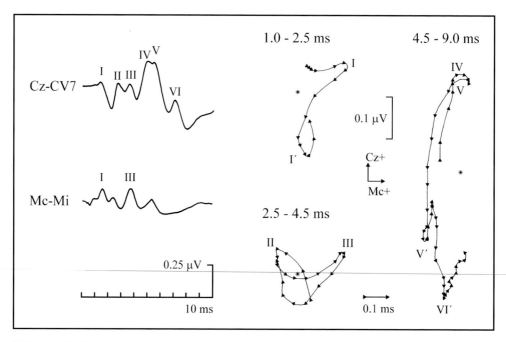

Figure 8–4. Lissajous trajectory for ABR. *ABRs were recorded in response to 70 dB nHL rarefaction clicks presented at a rate of 11/s to either the left or right ear, using three electrode derivations—vertex to the seventh cervical vertebra (Cz-CV7), contralateral to ipsilateral mastoid (Mc-Mi), and nasion to inion (not shown). The waveforms shown on the left represent the average waveforms of eight subjects. The left- and right-ear responses were combined. Lissajous trajectories for the frontal plane are shown on the right. The time course of the plot is indicated by the direction of the arrows with the interval from one arrowhead to the next representing a latency shift of 0.1 ms. To simplify its visualization, the Lissajous figure is separated into three latency regions. Wave I is indicated by the vector pointing upward and toward the contralateral mastoid. Waves IV and V have a vector pointing upward toward the vertex.*

main IV–V region tilts frontally. The interpretation of the trajectory is complicated (Jewett, 1987): a straight line represents a single stationary dipole that fluctuates in amplitude, whereas a planar segment can represent either a dipole that rotates or the concomitant activation of two dipoles. The trajectory shows planar segments near wave III, but tends toward the straight line near wave V.

These Lissajous representations of the ABR show the complexity of the recorded waveform. They are helpful in determining which two electrodes might

best show each wave of the response; the line between the electrodes should parallels the direction of the trajectory. Thus wave I might be recorded equally well between the ipsilateral mastoid and the vertex and between the two mastoids, whereas wave V is best recorded from vertex to neck. In infants, the ABR trajectory generally is more laterally than vertically oriented (Hafner, Pratt, Joachims, Feinsod, & Blazer, 1991). Unlike in adults, wave V of the infant ABR is often smaller when recorded between the vertex and contralateral mastoid than between the vertex and ipsilateral mastoid. We consider this more fully in Chapter 13 (compare Figure 8–3 to Figure 13–9).

The trajectory traces out the orientation of the ABR dipole at the latencies of the different peaks. The trajectory plotted in Figure 8–4 shows the different latencies by means of the triangles and the direction of the plot (increasing latency) by the orientation of the triangle. Wave I is oriented up and toward the contralateral side. It usually is equally large on vertex to ipsilateral mastoid or on mastoid to mastoid recordings. Over the region of wave III and III', the trajectory maps a circular path, which might fit with two underlying dipoles.

Lissajous trajectories have not been used extensively in clinical studies of brainstem function. The measurement and interpretation of the trajectories are difficult, and the available normative data are far less extensive than for single-channel measurements.

Normative Data

Tables 8–1, 8–2, and 8–3 present normative data from a group of young adults (age 17–35 years) with normal hearing—38 male and 38 female (Campbell et al., 1981). The stimulus was a click that alternated in polarity and was presented at 11/s. For the tabulated values, the measurements were collapsed across left and right ears. We found no overall difference between the ears and the interear differences for individual subjects were limited: the latency of wave V differed by no more than 0.32 ms between left and right ears, and wave I–V interpeak latency differed by no more than 0.45 ms. The smaller wave V was always greater than 33% of the larger; for wave III this limit was 32%. Similar data are available for other normative studies: Table 8–2 includes the studies of Chiappa, Gladstone, and Young (1979, reviewed in Chiappa, 1997) and Stockard, Stockard, and Sharbrough (1978) who used clicks presented at 60 dB SL (above the individual subject's threshold), which in the usual acoustic conditions of the laboratory is likely close to 70 dB nHL. The interpeak latencies are the most important measurements. These tend to be constant for different intensities. The amplitude ratios are very sensitive to the intensity of the stimulus and to how the amplitudes are measured. The amplitude of wave V is generally taken from the maximum positive amplitude in the IV–V complex

Table 8–1. Normal Latencies and Amplitudes of Human Click-ABR*

	I	II	III	IV	V	VI
Latency Mean	1.69	2.78	3.77	4.97	5.63	7.23
Standard Deviation	0.13	0.19	0.20	0.24	0.24	0.31
Amplitude Mean	0.30	0.17	0.34	0.06	0.61	0.25
Standard Deviation	0.13	0.11	0.16	0.02	0.22	0.23

*Data for 70 dB nHL click presented with alternating polarity at rate of 11/s and recorded with 100–3000 Hz bandpass (Campbell et al., 1981). Latencies measured in ms from onset of click in supra-aural earphone. Amplitudes measured in µV between peak and subsequent trough.

Table 8–2. Normal Interpeak Latencies of Human Click-ABR

	I–III	*III–V*	*I–V*
Mean Both Genders	2.07	1.86	3.95
Standard Deviation	0.19	0.19	0.23
Mean Female	2.02		3.87
Standard Deviation	0.15		0.23
Mean Male	2.13		4.01
Standard Deviation	0.22		0.21
Upper Limits ($p <0.01$)	2.56	2.39	4.52
Stockard et al., 1978	2.63	2.31	4.59
Chiappa et al., 1979	2.48	2.35	4.58

Sources: Upper three entries are data for 70 dB nHL alternating clicks presented at rate of 11/s and recorded with 100–3000 Hz bandpass (Campbell et al., 1981). The data from Stockard et al. and Chiappa et al. are the upper limits of normal for 60 dB SL rarefaction clicks. For the Chiappa et al. data we have used the mean +2.5 SD rather than their tabulated +3 SD.

Table 8–3. Relative Amplitudes of Waves in Normal Human Click-ABR

	III/I	*V/I*
Mean	1.33	2.51
Standard Deviation	1.01	2.06
Lower Limits ($p <0.01$)	0.29	0.69

Source: Data for 70 dB nHL click presented at rate of 11/s and recorded with 100–3000 Hz bandpass (Campbell et al., 1981). These ratios are highly susceptible to the intensity of the click and to the setting of the high-pass filter.

to the maximum negative amplitude in the succeeding 3 ms (i.e., to the most negative of V' or VI').

Picking the peaks is usually a simple process. Figure 8–5 illustrates a general approach to identifying the peaks of the ABR. We start with waves I and V. Wave I is the most positive peak before the waveform crosses baseline in a negative-going direction after 1 ms. Wave V is the positive peak or deflection immediately before the main negative-going baseline-crossing occurring after 5 ms. As shown by the arrows in the diagram, the eye starts at the left of the tracing, goes to the baseline-crossing and returns to wave I. The eye then starts from the right of the tracing, reaches the major baseline crossing and ascends to wave V—either a peak or a deflection on the up-going slope. The movement from the left should occur at a level halfway from baseline to the maximum positivity. These approaches are appropriate only when the high-pass cutoff is no more than 100 Hz—we do not want to attenuate the slow wave underlying the change from V to V'. Even then, the techniques may not always work, and we often must use supplementary record-

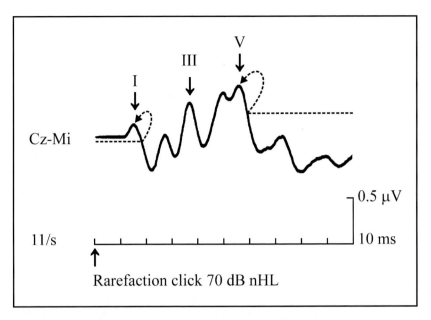

Figure 8–5. Identification of ABR peaks. *The ABR waveform was obtained by warp-averaging together the responses of 16 normal subjects. The dashed-line arrows indicate the movements of the eyes in finding peaks I and V. Wave I is the positive peak preceding the negative-going baseline crossing after 1 ms, and wave V is the positive peak preceding the major negative-going baseline crossing between 10 and 5 ms. Wave III is the most distinct positive peak between I and V.*

ings to distinguish the waves or to confirm our choice (Table 8–4). We have already considered changing the electrode locations. We describe the effects of intensity and rate later in this chapter. Once waves I and V are identified, we can find wave III as the most prominent peak between waves I and V.

The waveform of the ABR has several normal variations that can make the interpretation difficult. This variability is caused by small interindividual differences in either the cochlear response times at different regions of the basilar membrane (Don, Ponton, Eggermont, & Masuda, 1994) or the anatomy of the brainstem pathways. In approximately 5% of cases, wave III has two peaks (Chiappa et al., 1979). We

generally measure the largest of these peaks. However, when comparing the response for one ear to that for the other, we should pick the peaks that have the closest latencies. The wave IV–V complex has several morphologies, as illustrated in Figure 8–6 (Chiappa et al., 1979). When there is no clear distinction between the peaks, we measure a simple wave V. However, if we are comparing a response in one ear containing distinct IV and V waves with a response in the other ear containing only one wave V, we probably should use the average of the two latencies in the ear with the distinct components. In general, the rule is to make comparisons that tend to give normal results rather than to seek abnormality.

Table 8–4. Recognizing Waves I and V of the Click-ABR

Procedure	Wave I	Wave V
Recording Electrodes	Use a reference electrode in the external auditory meatus; consider using a recording between ipsilateral mastoid or meatus and contralateral mastoid	Use a reference electrode on the low neck; sometimes wave V can be distinguished from wave IV more clearly on the vertex to contralateral recording
Intensity	Use a higher intensity; wave I is always larger at higher click intensity	Use a lower intensity; wave V does not decrease with decreasing click intensity as much as wave IV and wave VI
Rate	Use a slower rate; wave I gets larger at slower click rates—try 5/s instead of 11/s.	Use a faster rate; wave V does not decrease with increasing click rate as much as other ABR waves
Stimulus Polarity	Use rarefaction clicks; wave I tends to be bigger with rarefaction clicks	Try using a different polarity; wave V may be larger with either condensation or rarefaction clicks

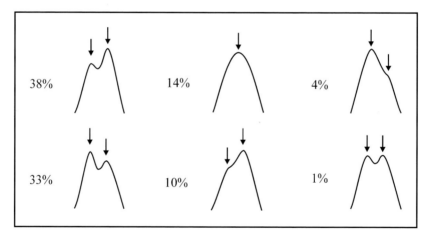

Figure 8–6. *Variability of the IV-V complex in the ABR. This figure gives the different patterns of the ABR in the IV–V latency region as seen in normal subjects, and the relative frequency of their occurrence. Data derived from Chiappa et al., 1979).*

Narrowband-Derived Responses

Crucial to the interpretation of the click-evoked ABR is its deconstruction into a set of narrowband-derived responses using high-pass masking (Don & Eggermont, 1978; Eggermont & Don, 1980; Parker & Thornton, 1978a, 1978b). The click is a broadband stimulus that activates all regions of the cochlea. As discussed in Chapter 5, each region of the cochlea responds best to a particular frequency with the lower frequencies located more apically along the basilar membrane. The latency before the activation of the nerve fibers (or cochlear delay) depends on a combination of the travel time along the basilar membrane and the filter buildup time in the hair cell transduction process. High-pass filtered noise prevents stimulus-locked activation of the regions of the cochlea that respond to frequencies higher than the filter cutoff. Sequential subtraction of the response in high-pass masking with the filter at one setting from the response with the filter at a higher setting gives the narrow band derived response of the cochlea for frequencies between the two filter settings (see Figure 5–7 for a more detailed illustration).

Figure 8–7 illustrates how wave V in the narrowband-derived responses of the human click-ABR changes with intensity (Eggermont & Don, 1980; Picton et al., 1981). The latency of the response depends on two main parameters: the frequency of the sound (which is equivalent to the place on the basilar membrane where the response is initiated), and the intensity of the sound. Although smaller than wave V, the other waves of the ABR show similar relations in to the frequency and intensity of the sound.

The findings from derived response studies of the ABR are intriguing and not what we initially would assume. Although there is little or no interaction between the different regions of the cochlea in the ECochG, we could easily hypothesize interactions between frequencies in the brainstem that would have completely confounded the recordings from the brainstem pathways. The ABR thus appears to derive from brainstem systems that do not interact between frequencies. Once initiated in one region of the cochlea, the sequence of waves from I to V occurs regardless of what happens in other regions.

This leads to the concept that the scalp-recorded ABR represents the convolution of the post-stimulus-time histogram of the responding auditory nerve fibers with a basic ABR response (Dau, 2003). The post-stimulus-time histogram, derived from multiple responses of an afferent auditory fiber, shows how the fiber discharges are distributed in time after the stimulus. Figure 8–8 shows post-stimulus-time histograms for various auditory nerve fibers. The plots are diagrammatic and are derived from the data presented by Kiang, Watanabe, Thomas, and Clark (1965). The characteristic frequencies of the fibers were measured using tuning curves (as in Figure 5–5), and then their discharge patterns in response to a click were assessed. These discharge patterns show that the response starts later (measurement L) for fibers that have a lower characteristic frequency. Fibers that respond best to mid- and low-frequency tones show a periodic discharge pattern. The fiber discharges at a rate that is equivalent to its characteristic frequency (measurement P). These results provide strong evidence for both the traveling wave and the resonance characteristics of the hair-cell filter. Unfortunately, we do not know the actual distribution of fibers contributing to the human ABR, the exact post-stimulus-time histograms of these fibers, or the basic ABR response waveform. However, if we use the human click-ABR as the basic waveform and convolve this with post-stimulus-time histograms from animal studies, we can predict responses to clicks and to brief tones (Dau, 2003).

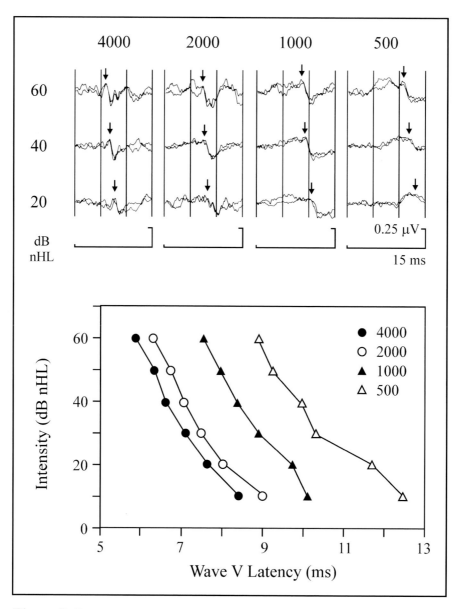

Figure 8–7. Narrowband-derived ABRs. *The upper section of the figure shows sample derived band responses from a single subject (data from Picton et al., 1981). Responses were obtained by presenting clicks in high-pass masking and sequentially subtracting responses with lower high-pass settings from those with higher (see Figure 5–7 for a further illustration of the procedure). Because the clicks were presented at a rate of 50/s, waves I–IV of the response are not as recognizable as wave V, which is indicated by the arrows. The bottom section of the figures plots average wave V latencies from Eggermont and Don (1980), who used a click rate of 13/s. The graph is plotted with the latency on the x-axis to make it visually compatible with the waveforms in the upper section of the figure.*

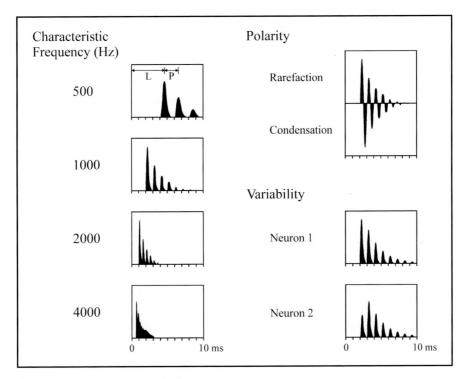

Figure 8–8. Post-stimulus-time histograms for auditory nerve fibers. These *diagrams show the firing patterns for auditory nerve fibers for repeated presentations of a click. The vertical scale is the number of fiber discharges at a particular time after the onset of the click. Two main parameters are shown in the upper left diagram: the latency to the first peak (L) and the interval between the peaks (P). The diagrams on the left show how the latency decreases as the characteristic frequency of the fiber (the frequency at which it responds at the lowest intensity as shown in Figure 5–6) increases. This latency represents the cochlear delay: low-frequency fibers begin to respond later than high-frequency fibers. The interval between peaks is equal to one cycle of the characteristic frequency (e.g., 2 ms for the 500-Hz fiber). The upper right section of the figure shows the effects of click polarity on a fiber with a 1-kHz characteristic frequency. The histogram for the condensation click is plotted upside down to better demonstrate the relationship. Responses to rarefaction clicks typically begin earlier by one half cycle (0.5 ms). The lower right section of the figure shows the variability of the histograms. Sometimes the second peak in the response is larger than the first. This often occurs when the click decreases in intensity but it also may occur for two different neurons of similar characteristic frequencies for a click of the same intensity. These diagrams are derived from the work of Kiang et al. (1965).*

STIMULUS PARAMETERS

Click Polarity

The click-ABR usually is evoked by a rarefaction click or by clicks of alternating polarity. The alternating polarity approach will cancel out the artifact and the CM. The response to a rarefaction click tends to show responses that are, on average, slightly earlier and slightly larger than the response to a condensation click (e.g., Schwartz et al., 1990). The general explanation for the mean result has been that the movement of the basilar membrane toward the scala media during the rarefaction part of a sound causes excitation of the afferent fibers. Simple monopolar rarefaction clicks will change to a bipolar rarefaction-condensation movement as the click is transmitted into the ear (see Figure 5–2), and condensation clicks will become condensation-rarefaction movements. These bipolar waves spread out as the traveling wave moves along the cochlea —basically each region of the cochlea resonates at its characteristic frequency (see the left side of Figure 8–8). A rarefaction click generally will initiate earlier discharges in the afferent auditory nerve fibers than a condensation click as the rarefaction movement (and excitation of the hair cells) occurs first. This is shown in the upper right of Figure 8–8. The response to the condensation click will be delayed until the initial condensation movement is followed by a rarefaction. However, the post-stimulus-time histogram of the afferent nerve discharges can show complex effects for stimulus polarity (see lower right of Figure 8–8) and these effects can change with stimulus intensity. Individual subjects may show differences that are much greater than shown in the mean waveforms from many subjects. Some subjects can show large differences in the

ABR between condensation and rarefaction clicks, and these can change dramatically with intensity. Figure 8–9 shows an example of such changes.

Early studies (Coats & Martin, 1977; Borg & Löfqvist, 1982) showed large differences in the latency of wave V in patients with steep high-frequency hearing losses. The basic idea was that the condensation-ABR would be initiated later than the rarefaction-ABR by one half cycle of the resonant frequency in the main responding area. When, for example, the main responding area was near 500 Hz, the difference in latency would be about 1 ms. Because the main peaks (I, III, and V) of the ABR tend to be separated by about 2 ms, this latency shift could effectively invert the ABR waveform—the peak of the condensation response occurring near the trough of the rarefaction response. This would severely attenuate the response to alternating clicks. This was one of the reasons for recommending a single-polarity click.

If these results were consistent, we should expect that wave V in the narrow-band-derived response would show clear latency differences between condensation and rarefaction clicks—equal to one half cycle of their center-frequency. However, this is not the case. Don, Vermiglio, Ponton, Eggermont, and Masuda (1996) found that the latency difference between condensation and rarefaction derived responses averaged close to zero and did not vary with the center frequency of the narrowbands. They attributed this to the intersubject variability of the post-stimulus-time histograms, which often spread out over several cycles of the fiber's characteristic frequency. This is illustrated in the lower right tracings of Figure 8–8.

Given these findings, we should be aware of the possible changes with stimulus polarity when we record ABRs. One approach might be to record separate

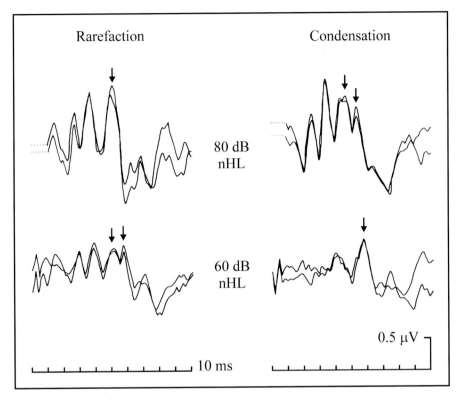

Figure 8–9. ***Effects of click polarity on the ABR.*** *Clicks of different polarity can cause dramatic alterations in the morphology of the response. Often wave V is larger with condensation clicks and wave I larger with rarefaction clicks. Usually, wave V separates itself more from wave IV with rarefaction clicks. However, as illustrated in these recordings from one subject, these polarity effects can vary with the intensity of the click.*

average ABRs to condensation and rarefaction clicks. Combining the two recordings gives an ABR equivalent to that evoked by alternating clicks. However, we then still have the ABRs to each polarity, something that would not be available if we had originally alternated the polarity and averaged all responses.

Brief Tones

To eliminate the electrical artifact associated with the stimulus, the tone-ABR is most commonly recorded using stimuli that either alternate in polarity or that have random phase in relation to the stimulus envelope. As discussed in Chapter 5, the most common envelope for the tone has linear rise- and fall-times of 2 cycles each, and a plateau of 1 cycle.

The ABR to a brief tone (or to the onset of a longer one) is determined by its rise-time, intensity, and frequency. For high-frequency tones—4 or 2 kHz—the ABR shows a waveform that is similar to that evoked by a click, although the latencies will be delayed by some factor of the rise time (Brinkmann & Scherg, 1979; Suzuki & Horiuchi, 1981). For tones of lower frequency, the latencies of the ABR peaks are longer as they are mainly initiated through the apical low-frequency regions of the basilar membrane. They also become less clearly defined, likely because the tones activate a broader region of the basilar membrane, spanning a larger range of latencies. This latency variability makes the response smoother.

If the response to the brief tone were initiated only from the regions of the basilar membrane specific to the frequency of the tone, the latency of the response should vary with the frequency of the tone in the same way as the narrowband-derived response. However, this is not true for low-frequency tones presented at high intensity. Because of the spread of energy in the acoustic spectrum of a brief tone, the high-intensity stimulus will activate more basal regions of the basilar membrane and initiate an earlier and better-synchronized response from that region as well as the response from the specific apical region of the cochlea. At high intensities, measurements of the peak latency are dominated by the response coming from the basal regions and therefore are earlier than expected from the derived narrowband response. If notched noise is used to limit the spread of energy in the spectrum (Picton, Ouellette, Hamel, & Durieux-Smith, 1979), the basal response no longer occurs and the latencies fit with those of the narrowband-derived response (with an additional delay due to the rise time of the tone). This is illustrated in Figure 8–10.

If we use tones of a single polarity and phase, we can see a frequency-following response (FFR) beginning at about the same latency as wave V. The FFR waveform repeats at the frequency of the tone and lasts the duration of the tone; it is like a brainstem microphonic. The FFR occurs only for frequencies below 1500 Hz where it is possible for afferent fibers to phase-lock to each cycle of the stimulus (see Figure 1–10). Furthermore, the FFR occurs only at intensities greater than 40 dB above threshold. At lower levels, there is likely insufficient phase-locking to generate the response. If we separately record the responses to tones of opposite polarity, we can average the two responses together to get the transient response to the onset of the tone and take the difference between the waveforms to get the FFR waveform uncontaminated by the transient response (Yamada, Yamane, & Kodera, 1977). There appear to be two distinct components of the human FFR: the typical FFR recorded from the vertex-to-ear montage and beginning at about the latency of wave V and an earlier one that is best recorded from a mastoid-to-mastoid recording and occurs 1.5 to 2.0 ms earlier (Stillman, Crow, & Moushegian, 1978). The recording is further complicated by the possibility of a stimulus artifact and a small CM recorded from electrodes near the cochlea. The artifact can be distinguished from the CM by using an acoustic delay line. At low intensities, the CM might be distinguished from later brainstem FFRs by recording the response in masking noise, which will eliminate any phase-locked neural response but may still leave the CM. However, if the noise is too intense, it also may mask the CM.

Intensity and Threshold

As the intensity of the click is decreased, the waves of the ABR become longer in latency, with similar latency changes occurring for all the waves. Because the individual peak latencies change in parallel, the interpeak latencies remain constant regardless of the intensity (Chiappa, 1997); Stockard, Stockard, & Sharbrough,

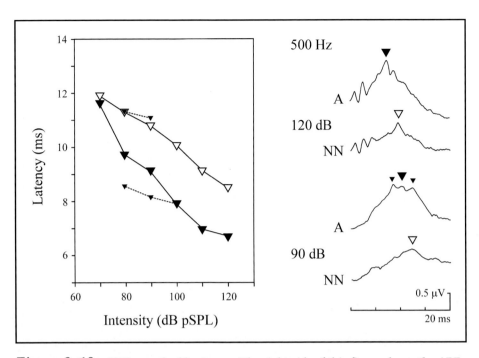

Figure 8–10. *ABRs evoked by tones. The right side of this figure shows the ABRs of a single subject in response to a brief 500-Hz tone (1 ms each for rise- and fall-times and 1 ms plateau) presented at a rate of 40/s. The normal behavioral threshold for the stimulus was 44 dB pSPL. The ABRs were recorded in two conditions, alone or in notched noise. At 120 dB, the ABR is dominated by a large early peak (filled triangle) when the tone is presented alone, but has a much later peak (open triangle) when the tone is presented in notched noise. At 90 dB, the ABR has multiple peaks when the tone is presented alone. The graph on the left shows the mean data for eight normal subjects. At 100 to 120 dB pSPL the responses are completely different in the two recording conditions. Between 90 and 80 dB pSPL, a transition occurs, and at 70 dB, pSPL wave V has a similar latency for both the tone alone and the tone in notched noise. Because the responses were recorded using a rate of 40 tones per second, a 40-Hz steady-state response occurs with the ABR. This is shown as a large slow positive wave underlying wave V. Data derived from Picton et al. (1979).*

1978. This means that we do not need to be too concerned about the stimulus intensity when using interpeak measurements as our main clinical tool; we just need to present the click at an intensity that provides clearly recognizable waves I, III, and V.

The peak latencies of the ABR increase by approximately 3.5 ms as the click decreases from 80 to 10 dB nHL, with the relationship showing less change over the higher intensities than the lower. Figure 8–11 shows normal ABR waveforms at different click intensities and Figure 8–12 shows the normal latency-intensity function for Wave V. This type of graph, initially plotted by Hecox and Galambos (1974), has become a mainstay in clinical ABR studies (Starr & Achor, 1975; Yamada, Yagi, Yamane, & Suzuki, 1975).

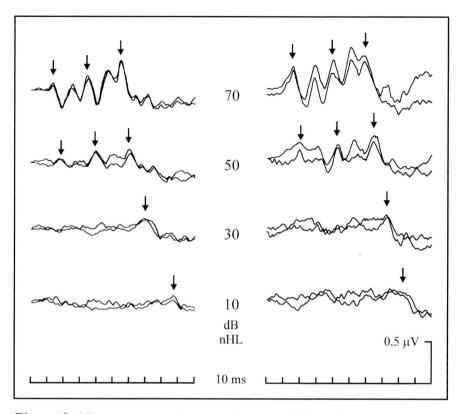

Figure 8–11. *Effects of intensity on the click ABR. ABRs are shown for two subjects: on the left to clicks presented at a rate of 11/s and on the right to clicks presented at 20/s. Waves I, III, and V are recognizable down to 50 dB nHL but only wave V is clearly visible at lower intensities.*

The latency change for the click ABR is a little larger than the intensity-related latency change that occurs for a narrow-band-derived response (see Figure 8–7). From 60 to 10 dB nHL, there is an average of 2.5 ms change for the narrowband response and about 3.0 ms for the unmasked click response. The intensity change within the narrowband is likely caused by the decreased rise time at the hair-cell synapse with lower intensity, and the resultant delay of the initial fiber discharge. Once the nerve fiber is activated, there are no further delays in the brainstem, as the interpeak latencies do not change. The

additional half millisecond of latency change seen in the unmasked click ABR probably is due to a shift in the location on the basilar membrane that is predominantly contributing to the response—from the high-frequency 2- to 4-kHz region at 60 dB to the 1 kHz region near 10 dB nHL.

As the intensity decreases, the amplitude of the click-ABR decreases. However, wave V decreases less than the other waves of the response and remains recognizable down to intensities near the behavioral threshold. Below about 40 dB nHL, the waves of the response other than

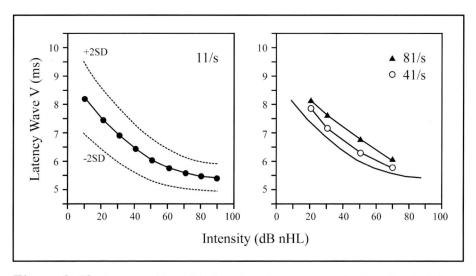

Figure 8–12. *Latency intensity function for wave V of ABR. On the left are plotted the values for alternating clicks presented at a rate of 11/s. Means are plotted with the circles and the limits of normal are plotted as ±2 SD. These data derive from Picton et al. (1981). The right side shows the effects of increasing the rate of stimulation to 41 or 81/s, with the mean data at 11/s replotted from the left graph. These data derive from Campbell et al. (1981).*

V are small and often cannot be reliably identified in the usual levels of residual background EEG.

The threshold at which wave V becomes recognizable depends mainly on the level of background EEG noise in the recording. If we average for a long time—say 10,000 trials—and if we attenuate the effect of trials contaminated by muscle artifact (by using weighted averaging), we can detect wave V down to 5 dB above behavioral threshold (Elberling & Don, 1987). Because the behavioral thresholds involve some integration over many stimuli and the ABR is evoked by only a single stimulus, it is likely that wave V is elicited whenever a stimulus exceeds threshold.

However, averaging over 10,000 trials is not usual in clinical testing. When averaging over 2000 trials in adults with normal hearing, we generally find that the click ABR is recognizable at intensities at least as low as 20 dB nHL. Another factor that affects the threshold is the electrode derivation. Moving the reference electrode lower down on the neck, away from the mastoid, will result in a larger wave V and a lower threshold (Sininger & Don, 1989).

Plotting the latency-intensity function for wave V in a patient with a hearing impairment can give us some idea of type of hearing loss (Picton, 1990; Yamada et al., 1975). Figure 8–13 shows the different types of abnormal latency-intensity function. There are two main patterns. In one, the response latency is within normal limits at high intensity. As we reach threshold, either wave V continues to have normal latencies but then ceases to be present at an abnormally elevated threshold or it jumps out to a longer latency than normal

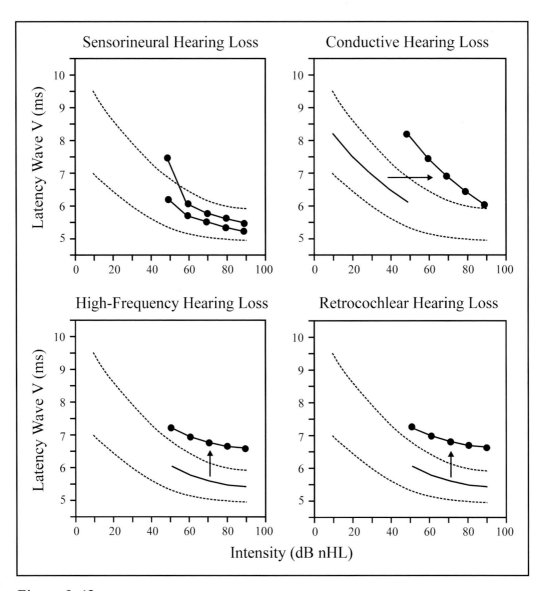

Figure 8–13. Abnormal latency-intensity functions. In a patient with a recruiting sensorineural hearing loss (upper left), wave V latency is normal but the threshold is elevated. In a patient with a conductive hearing loss (upper right), the function is shifted to the right by that amount of conductive loss. In a patient with a high-frequency hearing loss (lower left), the latency is shifted upward by an amount equal to the traveling-wave delay. In a patient with a retrocochlear hearing loss (lower right) the latency is shifted upward by the increased transmission time between the cochlea and the brainstem.

for that intensity and then vanishes. This type of pattern typically is found in patients with a sensorineural hearing loss and recruitment. In the second pattern of abnormal latency-intensity function, wave V is delayed. This can be caused in three different ways. A conductive hearing loss simply attenuates the intensity of the click before it reaches the cochlea. The function is shifted to the right by the amount of the conductive loss. This type of loss can be confirmed objectively by obtaining ABRs to bone-conducted clicks. In a patient with a steep high frequency hearing loss and relatively preserved hearing at the low frequencies, wave V is delayed by the increased time taken by the traveling wave to reach a functioning region of the cochlea. The function is shifted upward by the amount of delay. This type of hearing-impairment can be confirmed by obtaining tone-ABR thresholds at different frequencies and demonstrating the high-frequency loss. In a patient with a retrocochlear hearing loss, wave V is delayed by the increased time taken between the cochlea and the brainstem generator of wave V. This diagnosis requires recording at a sufficiently slow rate to recognize wave I and demonstrating an abnormally long I-V interval.

When brief tones are used as stimuli, the latency-intensity functions change with the frequency of the tone. The intensity-related latency shift is greater for lower frequency tones than for higher (e.g., Gorga, Kaminski, Beauchaine, & Jesteadt, 1988). This frequency effect is almost completely removed if the tone-ABR is recorded using notched noise to limit the spread of activation on the basilar membrane specific to the frequency of the tone (Picton, Ouellette, Hamel, & Durieux-Smith, 1979; Stapells, Picton, & Durieux-Smith, 1993). As already discussed, at high intensities the lower frequencies activate the basal regions of the cochlea as well as the apical regions specific to their frequency; these regions respond earlier and as they are more synchronized their response is more prominent in the ABR.

Determining the thresholds for the tone-ABR at different tonal frequencies has become an important way to estimate the audiogram in subjects who cannot cooperate reliably with behavioral testing. This is particularly useful in the assessment of hearing impairment in infants (Stapells et al., 1993; Stapells, 2010). The thresholds at which a tone-ABR can be recognized depend on the age of the subject and the type of hearing loss. Table 8–5 presents the results of a meta-analysis of many studies by Stapells (2000). As discussed in

Table 8–5. Thresholds for Recognizing the Tone ABR

Group	Frequency (Hz)			
	500	1000	2000	4000
Normal Adults	20±13	16±10	13±7	12±8
Hearing-Impaired Adults	13±10	10±6	8±7	5±10
Normal Children	20±11	17±12	13±10	15±13
Hearing-Impaired Children	6±15	5±14	1±12	-8±12

Source: Data from the meta-analysis by Stapells (2000). Thresholds are in dB nHL for the normal subjects and in dB nHL relative to the elevation in threshold above HL for the hearing-impaired subjects. The standard deviations were calculated from the standard errors of the mean in the original paper. The negative value in the data at 4000 Hz for the hearing-impaired children may be caused by the spread of energy in the skirts of the brief tone to activate lower frequency regions of the cochlea.

Chapter 6, the physiologic thresholds are closer to behavioral thresholds in subjects with a sensorineural hearing loss. This likely is caused by recruitment making the response grow in amplitude more rapidly just above threshold. We discuss the audiometric use of the tone-ABRs in infancy in more detail in Chapter 13.

Stimulus Rate

When clicks or tones are presented at more rapid rates that the original 10 to 20/s, all waves except wave V become smaller. Figure 8–14 shows the effects of rate on the ABRs of two normal-hearing subjects. Wave V does not decrease in amplitude until the rate exceeds 70/s. Because the thresholds for recognizing wave V are not affected by presenting the stimuli at rapid rates, it is much more efficient to record wave V at rates of 50 to 80/s than at rates of 10 to 20/s (as discussed in Chapter 6). Wave V increases its peak latency by a small amount with increasing stimulus rate. This latency change is consistent across different inten-

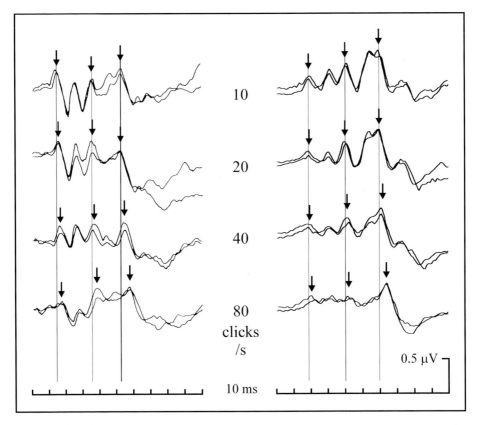

Figure 8–14. *Effects of stimulus rate on click-ABR. Responses are shown for two different subjects: on the left to clicks presented at an intensity of 70 dB nHL, and on the right at an intensity of 60 dB nHL. Waves I, III, and V are identified. Waves I and III decrease in size and show small latency increases at the more rapid rates. Wave V does not decrease its amplitude significantly but shows a larger latency increase than the earlier waves.*

sities, suggesting that it is caused by a process different from that which causes the latency change with intensity (Don, Allen, & Starr, 1977). The right side of Figure 8–12 shows the effects of click rate on the latency-intensity function. The effects of rate on the latency are less for waves I and III than for wave V. The latency changes with rate are probably related to synaptic adaptation, there being one more synapse in the pathways subserving wave V than wave III (see Chapter 4). The effects of rate on the ABR have wide normal limits. The amplitude of wave V at 81/s should not be smaller than 28% its amplitude at 11/s; the latency change of wave V from 11 to 81/s has a mean of 0.43 ms and should not exceed 0.83 ms (Campbell et al. 1981).

Techniques such as maximum length sequences (MLS, reviewed in Chapter 6) take advantage of the resilience of wave V to increasing click rate (Leung, Slaven, Thornton, & Brickley, 1998). Using such procedures, the ABR can be recorded at stimulus rates of several hundred per second. However, it is not clear how this might increase recording efficiency (discussed by Burkard & Don, 2007). Although the amplitude of wave V remains stable at rates of up to 70 Hz, at very rapid rates wave V does get smaller. In addition, the enhancement of the SNR by MLS is not as good as by normal averaging, and there is some latency-jitter in the responses due to the different intervals in the MLS. Finally, at very high rates, we run the risk of adaptation and, if the intensity is greater than 60 dB nHL, of temporary threshold shift. In general, audiometric uses of the ABR probably are most efficient at regular rates of 50 to 80/s.

The ABR recorded at rapid rates can sometimes be contaminated by strange overlapping effects from later components of the auditory EP. Using rates near 40 Hz can cause the ABR to be superimposed upon the 40-Hz steady-state response. For 500-Hz tones, this can lead to a larger overall response. However, for 4000- or 2000-Hz tones, the ABR and the 40 Hz response may move in opposite directions and the ABR part of the response can be distorted. Postauricular muscle (PAM) responses also can follow at rapid rates of stimulation. Figure 8–15 shows how the PAM reflex (recorded on left side and not the right) can distort the ABR recording (Campbell et al., 1981). The solution for this problem is to move the reference electrode away from the mid-mastoid location—either to the earlobe or to a lower part of the mastoid. The muscle is very small and its field potential decreases dramatically when the electrode is not directly over the muscle. We consider this reflex more extensively in Chapter 9.

SUBJECT FACTORS

Gender

Despite largely overlapping distributions for individual data, the mean latencies and amplitudes of the ABR show clear and significant differences between male and female subjects (Allison, Wood, & Goff, 1983; Kjaer, 1979; McClelland & McCrea, 1979; Stockard, Stockard, & Sharbrough, 1978). Campbell et al. (1981) found no difference in wave I latency but all subsequent waves were on average later in male than female subjects. Wave V is between 0.1 and 0.2 ms later in male than in female subjects. Table 8–3 shows the interpeak latency results. In addition, the female ABR shows, on average, significantly larger amplitudes.

Much research has tried to determine the main cause for these gender effects. The differences are either absent or very

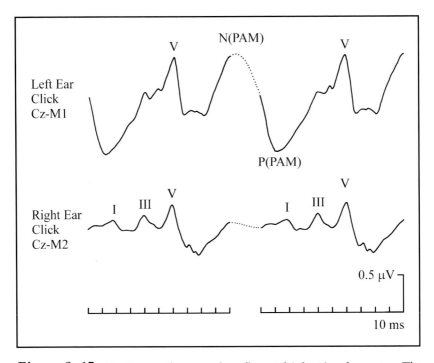

Figure 8–15. *Postauricular muscle reflex at high stimulus rates. The ABRs recorded in this subject at a click rate of 81/s and an intensity of 70 dB nHL showed a very distorted pattern for the left ear, and a normal ABR for the right ear. This distortion was due to a postauricular muscle (PAM) reflex recorded on the left mastoid but not on the right. To demonstrate how this overlaps with the ABR, the recordings are repeated in the right side of the figure and separated from the tracings on the left by the 2.3 ms before the next click occurs at a rate of 81/s. The dotted lines trace out the hypothetical muscle reflex response. This consists of a negative-positive complex with peak latencies near 10 and 14 ms. As this is recorded from the second electrode of the pair, the negative-positive complex shows as an upward and then downward deflection. The asymmetry of the reflex may be related to eye gaze, to some normal asymmetry in the muscle, or to some asymmetry in the placement of the mastoid electrodes (M1 and M2).*

small in infancy and become apparent in mid-childhood (O'Donovan, Beagley, & Shaw, 1980; Thivierge & Côté, 1990). Head size is one possibility: the greater head size in male subjects could increase the latencies due to longer brainstem pathways, and could decrease the amplitudes because of the greater attenuation caused by the larger volume and the thicker skull. However, the relationship between head size and ABR measurements is not that striking (e.g., Durrant, Sabo, & Hyre, 1990).

The possible role of body temperature can be discounted since, although there are changes in female body temperature through the menstrual period, there is little, if any, overall gender difference in temperature (e.g., Mackowiak, Wasserman, & Levine, 1992).

The main cause of the gender differences appears to be the length of the basilar membrane. Using derived narrowband responses, Don, Ponton, Eggermont, and Masuda (1993, 1994) found that female subjects showed smaller latency-shifts between the high- and low-frequency responses than male subjects. The shorter cochlea results in earlier latencies. Because each frequency band would be distributed over a shorter length of the basilar membrane, the resultant greater synchronization in the nerve fiber discharges also would result in larger female amplitudes.

Temperature

Some early studies showed that the click-ABR latencies increased during induced hypothermia for cardiopulmonary bypass (e.g., Stockard, Sharbrough, & Tinker, 1978). Marshall and Donchin (1981) reported changes in ABR latency with normal circadian changes in body temperature, the latency of wave V increasing about 0.2 ms with a decrease of 1°C. Picton et al. (1981) showed that the circadian change in temperature and in ABR latency persisted even if the subjects stayed awake for 24 hours. This result removed any possible confounding effect of sleep. Campbell et al. (1981) found a variation in the wave I–V latency across the menstrual cycle in female subjects, with the latency being 3.8 ms on days 12 through 26 and 3.9 ms on other days. This small effect was likely related to body temperature.

Arousal and Attention

Extensive studies have shown that the ABR does not change significantly during sleep (e.g., Campbell & Bartoli, 1986; Deacon-Elliot, Bell, & Campbell, 1987). Neither the morphology of the response nor the threshold for detecting it is affected by any stage of sleep. Sleep decreases the background noise in the recording—EEG slow waves may get larger during sleep, but the activity that obscures the ABR recording is mainly muscular in origin and this is dramatically decreased during sleep. Therefore, ABRs are most efficiently recorded during sleep. Sometimes it is necessary to sedate a very active patient in order to obtain a measureable ABR. In this regard, we can rest assured that the ABR is unaffected by any of the common medications used to put patients to sleep for testing. Even anesthetics have little or no effect on the ABR (e.g., Hall, 2006, pp. 237–240; Nuwer, 1986, pp. 158–161). The small changes that do occur are more likely related to concomitant changes in the body temperature or mild conductive hearing losses caused either by the use of inhalational agents (which can increase the middle ear pressure) or intubation (which can decrease the function of the Eustachian tube).

Although several studies have noted changes in the ABR with changes in attention, the general consensus has been that the ABR remains the same regardless of whether the evoking stimulus is attended to or ignored (Connolly, Aubry, McGillivary, & Scott, 1989; Hirschhorn & Michie, 1990; Picton & Hillyard, 1974; Picton, Hillyard, Galambos, & Schiff, 1971; Woldorff, Hansen, & Hillyard, 1987). This insensitivity of the ABR to fluctuations in attention makes sense with the fact that the ABR does not change significantly from wakefulness (where there must be some level of attention) to sleep or anesthesia. Nevertheless, two provisos might be considered. First, the ABR represents only a small part of the brainstem response to sounds. Brainstem processing that does not contribute to the transient ABR might be affected by attention. For example, Galbraith, Olfman, and Huffman (2003) have reported effects of attention on the FFR. Second, in complex stimulus conditions, attention may alter the interactions between stimuli and this might show at the brainstem level. For example, Ikeda, Seki-guchi, and Hayashi (2008) have shown small changes in the ABR with attention when attended stimuli are presented together with contralateral masking noise.

Infancy

The ABR of the normal newborn is about one half the size of the adult ABR and the latencies of the different waves are signif-icantly longer than in the adult (Starr, Amlie, Martin, & Sanders, 1977). We pro-vide more detail about this response in Chapter 13, which considers the use of click- and tone-ABRs in the identification and assessment of neonatal hearing loss. In this chapter, we briefly consider the development of the ABR from prematu-rity to adulthood. Figure 8–16 shows ABRs recorded from infants at different ages. Table 8–6 presents some normative data for the responses. More extensive data are

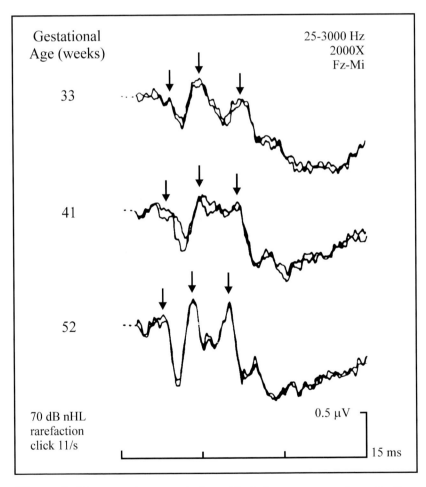

Figure 8–16. *ABRs in young infants. Typical responses are shown for three age-groups: premature newborn, full-term newborn, and 3-month old infant. The stimulus characteristics are shown at the lower left and the recording parameters at the upper right. Data derived from Durieux-Smith et al. (1985).*

Table 8–6. Normal ABR Latencies in Infants*

Age	I	III	V	I–V
Premature (36 weeks GA)	2.1±0.3	5.0±0.4	7.4±0.4	5.3±0.3
Full-term neonate	2.0±0.3	4.8±0.3	7.0±0.3	5.0±0.3
3 months	1.7±0.2	4.3±0.3	6.4±0.3	4.7±0.3
2 years	1.7±0.2	3.8±0.2	5.7±0.2	4.0±0.2

*Latencies in ms for the ABRs elicited by 70 dB nHL rarefaction clicks presented at a rate of 11/s. Means and standard deviations. GA is gestational age.

available (e.g., Durieux-Smith, Edwards, Picton, & McMurray, 1985; Jiang, Zheng, Sun, & Xiang, 1991; Jiang, Zhang, Wu & Liu, 1993; Picton, Taylor, & Durieux-Smith, 2005). The main findings are that wave I attains normal adult latency values by age 6 months but that wave V does not reach adult values until age 2 years. The most important latencies to remember are those of the newborn: the I–V latency of 5 ms and the wave V latency of 7 ms at 70 dB nHL.

The ABR can be recorded at rapid rates in normal term infants. The latency changes with rate may be greater than those seen with adults, but wave V is still recognizable (Durieux-Smith et al., 1985; Fujikawa & Weber, 1977; Lasky, 1984). ABRs also can be recorded in infants using MLS techniques (Jiang, Brosi, & Wilkinson, 1999).

The scalp distribution of the neonatal ABR is very different from that of the adult response (Edwards, Durieux-Smith, & Picton, 1985; McPherson et al., 1985). The difference probably is caused by the incomplete myelination of much of the neonatal auditory pathway. In the neonate, wave I often is larger on a mastoid-to-mastoid recording than on a vertex-to-mastoid recording. The dipoles underlying waves III and V also are more laterally oriented. On a recording between the vertex and the contralateral mastoid, waves III and V are small and appear to have opposite polarity to those recorded on the ipsilateral montage. In Chapter 13, we stress the importance of recording the infant ABR from the vertex (or midfrontal region) to the mastoid ispsilateral to the stimulus.

Click-ABRs can be recorded in premature infants as early as 26 weeks' gestational age (Cox, Martin, Carlo, & Hack, 1993: Schulman-Galambos & Galambos, 1975). In the very premature infants, they are evoked only by stimuli presented at high intensity and slow rates. The amplitude of the response, particularly wave V, is smaller than that in full-term neonates. The latencies of all the components of the response decrease with increasing gestational age. Responses can be reliably recorded in moderately premature infants at rates as fast as 91/s (Jiang & Wilkinson, 2008)

The threshold for detecting the click-ABR in a normal newborn infant is below 30 dB nHL provided the infant is quiet and averaging is sufficient to make the response recognizable (Galambos, Wilson, & Silva, 1994). This threshold decreases by about 10 dB in the first 3 months of life and by a further 5 dB by the end of the first year (Kaga & Tanaka 1980; Mochizuki, Go, Ohkubo, & Motomura, 1983).

These changes probably are related to several factors, including the resolution of neonatal conductive hearing loss and maturation of the cochlea and brainstem. Studies of the tone-ABR in infants are reviewed in Chapter 13.

The most important determinants of latency are the conduction-velocity in the pathway from the cochlea to the generator of the ABR wave and the length of this pathway (Picton & Taylor, 2007). Conduction-velocity depends mainly on the degree of myelination of the axons in the pathway. Latency also may be affected by synaptic efficiency, but this is less important than myelination. Both conduction-velocity and pathway length change during development. An example of how these factors interact derives from measurements of the wave III-IV interpeak latency of the click-evoked auditory brainstem response (ABR). This latency, which indicates the time taken to travel along axons directly connecting the cochlear nucleus to the inferior colliculus (Moore, Ponton, Eggermont, Wu, & Huang, 1996; Ponton, Moore, & Eggermont, 1996), decreases from birth until it reaches the normal adult value at 1 year of age. Because the length of the pathway continues to increase until the age of 3 years, myelination must continue until age 3 so that the conduction velocity can keep pace with the increase in pathway length.

Old Age

The ABR of the elderly adult typically shows latencies that are slightly longer and slightly more variable than those observed in young adults (Allison, Wood, & Goff, 1983; Rowe, 1978). When interpreting click-ABR interpeak latencies, we should increase the upper limits of normal by about 0.1 ms for elderly adults.

Because most elderly adults suffer from some degree of hearing loss, it is difficult to determine how much of this latency-change is related to peripheral hearing loss and how much to central dysfunction (discussed by Boettcher, 2002). Ottaviani, Maurizi, D'Alatri, and Almadori (1990) suggested that the causes were mainly peripheral, in terms of a mild high-frequency cochlear loss causing a delay before the response is initiated. However, an increased susceptibility to higher rates of stimulation in the elderly (e.g., Fujikawa & Weber, 1977) may indicate additional central dysfunction. Poth, Boettcher, Mills, and Dubno (2001) found decreased responsiveness to the second of two noise bursts separated by a short gap (4 or 8 ms) in elderly subjects. Not all studies show an interaction between age and rate. In an extensive study of the interactions between age and stimulus rate on the ABR, Burkard and Sims (2001) found that the absolute latencies of wave I and V were slightly longer in elderly than in young subjects. However, they found that the I–V latency was not different between young and old subjects, although it increased in both groups at increasing stimulus rates. The amplitude of wave V was smaller in the elderly and decreased in both groups with increasing rate. Presbycusis often combines a peripheral high-frequency hearing loss (causing latency delays and elevated ABR thresholds at the high frequencies) with a central dysfunction of temporal processing (causing increased rate effects and decreased gap-ABRs).

CONCLUDING COMMENTS

Although this chapter comes midway through the book, students probably will begin their studies of the human auditory EPs by recording the ABR. This response is the most reliably recorded auditory EP. We can attach electrodes on the scalp, turn on the clicks, and within a minute or two watch wave V and its friends appear on the screen. The response has more precision in its measurements than other EPs; we know when it occurs and what it is supposed to look like. Furthermore, we know more about its relation to different experimental parameters than any other component of the human auditory EP. It is a comfortable place to begin. However, we do not know everything, and further study of the ABR will still be rewarding— it has not yet lost its sense of beginning.

ABBREVIATIONS

ABR	Auditory brainstem response
CM	Cochlear microphonic
EAM	External auditory meatus
ECochG	Electrocochleogram
FFR	Frequency-following response
GA	Gestational age
MLS	Maximum length sequence
nHL	Normal hearing level
PAM	Postauricular muscle
SD	Standard deviation
SL	Sensation level
SNR	Signal-to-noise ratio
SP	Summating potential

REFERENCES

Allison, T., Wood, C. C., & Goff, W. R. (1983). Brain stem auditory, pattern-reversal visual, and short-latency somatosensory evoked potentials: Latencies in relation to age, sex, and brain and body size. *Electroencephalography and Clinical Neurophysiology, 55,* 619–636.

American Clinical Neurophysiology Society. (2006). Guidelines on short-latency auditory evoked potentials. *Journal of Clinical Neurophysiology, 23,* 157–167.

Borg, E., & Löfqvist, L. (1982). Auditory brainstem response (ABR) to rarefaction and condensation clicks in normal and abnormal ears. *Scandinavian Audiology, 11,* 227–235.

Boettcher, F. A. (2002). Presbyacusis and the auditory brainstem response. *Journal of Speech, Language, and Hearing Research, 45,* 1249–1261.

Brinkmann, R. D., & Scherg, M. (1979). Human auditory on- and off-potentials of the brainstem. *Scandinavian Audiology, 8,* 27–32.

Burkard, R. F., & Don, M. (2007). The auditory brainstem response. In R. F. Burkard, M. Don, & J. J. Eggermont (Eds.), *Auditory evoked potentials: Basic principles and clinical application* (pp. 229–253). Philadelphia, PA: Lippincott Williams & Wilkins.

Burkard, R. F., & Sims, D. (2001). The human auditory brainstem response to high click rates: Aging effects. *American Journal of Audiology, 10,* 53–61.

Campbell, K. B., & Bartoli, E. A. (1986). Human auditory evoked potentials during natural sleep: The early components. *Electroencephalography and Clinical Neurophysiology, 65,* 142–149.

Campbell, K. B., Picton, T. W., Wolfe, R. G., Maru, J., Baribeau-Braun, J., & Braun, C. (1981). Auditory potentials. *Sensus, 1,* 21–31.

Chiappa, K. H. (1997). *Evoked potentials in clinical medicine.* Philadelphia, PA: Lippincott Williams & Wilkins.

Chiappa, K. H., Gladstone, K. J., & Young, R. R. (1979). Brain stem auditory evoked responses: Studies of waveform variations in 50 normal human subjects. *Archives of Neurology, 36,* 81–87.

Coats, A. C., & Martin, J. L. (1977). Human auditory nerve action potentials and brain stem evoked responses: Effects of audiogram shape and lesion location. *Archives of Otolaryngology, 103,* 605–622.

Connolly, J. F., Aubry, K., McGillivary, N., & Scott, D. W. (1989). Human brainstem auditory evoked potentials fail to provide evidence of efferent modulation of auditory input during attentional tasks. *Psychophysiology, 26,* 292–303.

Cox, L. C., Martin, R. J., Carlo, W. A., & Hack, M. (1993). Early ABRs in infants undergoing assisted ventilation. *Journal of the American Academy of Audiology, 4,* 13–17.

Dau, T. (2003). The importance of cochlear processing for the formation of auditory brainstem and frequency following responses. *Journal of the Acoustical Society of America, 113,* 936–950.

Deacon-Elliott, D., Bell, I., & Campbell, K. B. (1987). Estimation of auditory threshold during sleep using brainstem auditory-evoked potentials. *Audiology, 26,* 363–368.

Don, M., Allen, A. R., & Starr, A. (1977). Effect of click rate on the latency of auditory brain stem responses in humans. *Annals of Otology, Rhinology and Laryngology, 86,* 186–195.

Don, M., & Eggermont, J. J. (1978). Analysis of the click-evoked brainstem potentials in man using high-pass noise masking. *Journal of the Acoustical Society of America, 63,* 1084–1092.

Don, M., Ponton, C. W., Eggermont, J. J., & Masuda, A. (1993). Gender differences in cochlear response time: An explanation for gender amplitude differences in the unmasked auditory brain-stem response. *Journal of the Acoustical Society of America, 94,* 2135–2148.

Don, M., Ponton, C. W., Eggermont, J. J., & Masuda, A. (1994). Auditory brainstem response (ABR) peak amplitude variability reflects individual differences in cochlear response times. *Journal of the Acoustical Society of America, 96,* 3476–3491.

Don, M., Vermiglio, A. J., Ponton, C. W., Eggermont, J. J., & Masuda, A. (1996). Variable effects of click polarity on auditory brainstem response latencies: Analyses of narrowband ABRs suggest possible explanations. *Journal of the Acoustical Society of America, 100,* 458–472.

Durieux-Smith, A., Edwards, C. G., Picton, T. W., & McMurray, B. (1985). Auditory brainstem responses to clicks in neonates. *Journal of Otolaryngology, 14*(Suppl. 14), 12–18.

Durrant, J. D., Sabo, D. L., & Hyre, R. J. (1990). Gender, head size, and ABRs examined in large clinical sample. *Ear and Hearing, 11,* 10–14.

Edwards, C. G., Durieux-Smith, A., & Picton, T. W. (1985). Neonatal auditory brain stem responses from ipsilateral and contralateral recording montages. *Ear and Hearing, 6,* 175–178.

Eggermont, J. J., & Don, M. (1980). Analysis of the click-evoked brainstem potentials in humans using high-pass noise masking. II. Effect of click intensity. *Journal of the Acoustical Society of America, 68,* 1671–1675.

Elberling, C., & Don, M. (1987). Threshold characteristics of the human auditory brain stem response. *Journal of the Acoustical Society of America, 81,* 115–121.

Fujikawa, S. M., & Weber, B .A. (1977). Effects of increased stimulus rate on brainstem electric response (BER) audiometry as a function of age. *Journal of the American Audiological Society, 3,* 147–150.

Galambos, R., Wilson, M. J., & Silva, P. D. (1994). Identifying hearing loss in the intensive care nursery: A 20-year summary. *Journal of the American Academy of Audiology, 5,* 151–162.

Galbraith, G. C., Olfman, D. M., & Huffman, T. M. (2003). Selective attention affects human brain stem frequency-following response. *NeuroReport, 14,* 735–738.

Gorga, M. P., Kaminski, J. R., Beauchaine, K. A., & Jesteadt, W. (1988). Auditory brainstem responses to tone bursts in normally hearing subjects. *Journal of Speech and Hearing Research, 31,* 87–97.

Hafner, H., Pratt, H., Joachims, Z., Feinsod, M., & Blazer, S. (1991). Development of auditory brainstem evoked potentials in newborn infants: A three-channel Lissajous' trajectory study. *Hearing Research, 51,* 33–47.

Hall, J. W. III. (2006). *New handbook for auditory evoked responses.* Boston, MA: Allyn & Bacon (Pearson Education).

Hecox, K., & Galambos, R. (1974). Brain stem auditory evoked responses in human infants and adults. *Archives of Otolaryngology, 99,* 30–33.

Hirschhorn, T. N., & Michie, P. T. (1990). Brainstem auditory evoked potentials (BAEPS) and selective attention revisited. *Psychophysiology, 27,* 495–512.

Ikeda, K., Sekiguchi, T., & Hayashi, A. (2008). Attention-related modulation of auditory brainstem responses during contralateral noise exposure. *NeuroReport, 19,* 1593–1599.

Ino, T., & Mizoi, K. (1980). Vector analysis of auditory brain stem responses (BSR) in human beings. *Archives of Otorhinolaryngology, 226,* 55–62.

Jewett, D. L. (1987). The 3-channel Lissajous' trajectory of the auditory brain-stem response. IX. Theoretical aspects. *Electroencephalography and Clinical Neurophysiology, 68,* 386–408.

Jewett, D. L., & Williston, J. S. (1971). Auditory-evoked far fields averaged from the scalp of humans. *Brain, 94,* 681–696.

Jiang, Z. D., Brosi, D. M., & Wilkinson, A. R. (1999). Brainstem auditory evoked response recorded using maximum length sequences in term neonates. *Biology of the Neonate, 76,* 193–199.

Jiang, Z. D., & Wilkinson, A. R. (2008). Normal brainstem responses in moderately preterm infants. *Acta Paediatrica, 97,* 1366–1369.

Jiang, Z. D., Zhang, L., Wu, Y. Y., & Liu, X. Y. (1993). Brain stem auditory evoked responses from birth to adulthood: Development of wave amplitude. *Hearing Research, 68,* 35–41.

Jiang, Z. D., Zheng, M. S., Sun, D. K., & Xiang, L. Y. (1991). Brain stem auditory evoked responses from birth to adulthood: Normative data of latency and interval. *Hearing Research, 54,* 67–74.

Kaga, K., & Tanaka, Y. (1980). Auditory brainstem response and behavioral audiometry. *Archives of Otolaryngology, 106,* 564–566.

Kiang, N. Y-S., Watanabe, T., Thomas, E. C., & Clark, L. F. (1965). *Discharge patterns of single fibers in the cat's auditory nerve.* Cambridge, MA: MIT Press.

Kjaer, M. (1979). Differences of latencies and amplitudes of brain stem evoked potentials in subgroups of a normal material. *Acta Neurologica Scandinavica, 59,* 72–79.

Lasky, R. E. (1984). A developmental study on the effect of stimulus rate on the auditory evoked brain-stem response. *Electroencephalography and Clinical Neurophysiology, 59,* 411–419.

Leung, S. M., Slaven, A., Thornton, A. R., & Brickley, G. J. (1998). The use of high stimulus rate auditory brainstem responses in the estimation of hearing threshold. *Hearing Research, 123,* 201–205.

Mackowiak, P., Wasserman, S. S, & Levine, M. M. (1992). A critical appraisal of 98.6°F, the upper limit of the normal body temperature, and other legacies of Carl Reinhold August Wunderlich. *Journal of the American Medical Association, 268,* 1578–1580.

Marshall, N. K., & Donchin, E. (1981). Circadian variation in the latency of brainstem responses and its relation to body temperature. *Science, 212,* 356–358.

McClelland, R. J., & McCrea, R. S. (1979). Intersubject variability of the auditory-evoked brain stem potentials. *Audiology, 18,* 462–471.

McPherson, D. L, Hirasugi, Y., & Starr, A. (1985). Auditory brain stem potentials recorded at different scalp locations in neonates and adults. *Annals of Otology, Rhinology and Laryngology, 94,* 236–243.

Mochizuki, Y., Go, T., Ohkubo, H., & Motomura, T. (1983). Development of human brainstem auditory evoked potentials and gender differences from infants to young adults. *Progress in Neurobiology, 20,* 273–285.

Moore, J. K., Ponton, C. W., Eggermont, J. J., Wu, B. J., & Huang, J. Q. (1996). Perinatal maturation of the auditory brain stem response: Changes in path length and conduction velocity. *Ear and Hearing, 17,* 411–418.

Nuwer, M. R. (1986). *Evoked potential monitoring in the operating room.* New York, NY: Raven Press.

O'Donovan, C. A., Beagley, H. A., & Shaw, M. (1980). Latency of brainstem response in children. *British Journal of Audiology, 14,* 23–29.

Ottaviani, F., Maurizi, M., D'Alatri, L., & Almadori, G. (1990). Auditory brainstem responses in the aged. *Acta Otolaryngologica Supplement, 476,* 110–112.

Parker, D. J., & Thornton, A. R. (1978a). The validity of the derived cochlear nerve and brainstem evoked responses of the human auditory system. *Scandinavian Journal of Audiology, 7,* 45–52.

Parker, D. J., & Thornton, A. R. (1978b). Frequency specific components of the cochlear nerve and brainstem evoked responses of the human auditory system. *Scandinavian Journal of Audiology, 7,* 53–60.

Picton, T. W. (1990). Auditory evoked potentials. In D. D. Daly & T. A. Pedley (Eds.), *Current practice of clinical electroencephalography* (2nd ed., pp. 625–678). New York, NY: Raven Press.

Picton, T. W., & Hillyard, S. A. (1974). Human auditory evoked potentials. II. Effects of attention. *Electroencephalography and Clinical Neurophysiology, 36,* 191–200.

Picton, T. W., Hillyard, S. A., Galambos, R., & Schiff, M. (1971). Human auditory attention: A central or peripheral process? *Science, 173,* 351–353.

Picton, T. W., Hillyard, S. A., Krausz, H. I., & Galambos, R. (1974). Human auditory evoked potentials. I. Evaluation of components. *Electroencephalography and Clinical Neurophysiology, 36,* 179–190.

Picton, T., Hunt, M., Mowrey, R., Rodriguez, R., & Maru, J. (1988). Evaluation of brainstem auditory evoked potentials using dynamic time warping. *Electroencephalography and Clinical Neurophysiology, 71,* 212–225.

Picton, T. W., Ouellette, J., Hamel, G., & Durieux-Smith, A. (1979). Brainstem evoked potentials to tonepips in notched noise. *Journal of Otolaryngology, 8,* 289–314.

Picton, T. W., Stapells, D. R., & Campbell, K. B. (1981). Auditory evoked potentials from the human cochlea and brainstem. *Journal of Otolaryngology, 10*(Suppl. 9), 1–41.

Picton, T. W., & Taylor, M. J. (2007). Electrophysiological evaluation of human brain development. *Developmental Neuropsychology, 31,* 251–280.

Picton, T. W., Taylor, M. J., & Durieux-Smith, A. (2005). Brainstem auditory evoked poten-

tials in pediatrics. In M. J. Aminoff (Ed.), *Electrodiagnosis in clinical neurology* (5th ed., pp. 525–552). Philadelphia, PA: Elsevier Churchill Livingstone.

Ponton, C. W., Moore, J. K., & Eggermont, J. J. (1996). Auditory brain stem response generation by parallel pathways: Differential maturation of axonal conduction time and synaptic transmission. *Ear and Hearing, 17,* 402–410.

Poth, E. A., Boettcher, F. A., Mills, J. H., & Dubno, J. R. (2001). Auditory brainstem responses in younger and older adults for broadband noises separated by a silent gap. *Hearing Research, 161,* 81–86.

Pratt, H., Har'el, Z., & Golos, E. (1984). Geometrical analysis of human three-channel Lissajous' trajectory of auditory brain-stem evoked potentials. *Electroencephalography and Clinical Neurophysiology, 58,* 83–88.

Rowe, M. J., 3rd. (1978). Normal variability of the brain-stem auditory evoked response in young and old adult subjects. *Electroencephalography and Clinical Neurophysiology, 44,* 459–470.

Schulman-Galambos, C., & Galambos, R. (1975). Brainstem auditory evoked responses in premature infants. *Journal of Speech and Hearing Research, 18,* 456–465.

Schwartz, D. M., Morris, M. D., Spydell, J. D., Ten Brink, C., Grim, M. A., & Schwartz, J. A. (1990). Influence of click polarity on the brain-stem auditory evoked response (BAER) revisited. *Electroencephalography and Clinical Neurophysiology, 77,* 445–457.

Sininger, Y. S., & Don, M. (1989). Effects of click rate and electrode orientation on threshold of the auditory brainstem response. *Journal of Speech and Hearing Research, 32,* 880–886.

Sininger, Y. S., Gardi, J. N., Morris, J. H., Martin, W. H., & Jewett, D. L. (1987). The 3-channel Lissajous' trajectory of the auditory brainstem response. VII. Planar segments in humans *Electroencephalography and Clinical Neurophysiology 68,* 368–379.

Stapells, D. R. (2000). Threshold estimation by the tone-evoked auditory brainstem response: A literature meta-analysis. *Journal of Speech-Language Pathology and Audiology*, *24*, 74–83.

Stapells, D. R. (2010). Frequency-specific threshold assessment in young infants using the transient ABR and the brainstem ASSR. In R. C. Seewald & A. M. Tharpe (Eds.), *Comprehensive handbook of pediatric audiology*. San Diego, CA: Plural Publishing.

Stapells, D., Picton, T., & Durieux-Smith, A. (1993). Electrophysiologic measures of frequency-specific auditory function. In J. T. Jacobson (Ed.), *Principles and applications of auditory evoked potentials* (pp. 251–283). New York, NY: Allyn & Bacon.

Starr, A., & Achor, J. (1975). Auditory brain stem responses in neurological disease. *Archives of Neurology, 32*, 761–768.

Starr, A., Amlie, R. N., Martin, W. H., & Sanders, S. (1977). Development of auditory function in newborn infants revealed by auditory brainstem potentials. *Pediatrics, 60*, 831–839.

Starr, A., & Squires, K. (1982). Distribution of auditory brainstem potentials over the scalp and nasopharynx in humans. *Annals of the New York Academy of Sciences, 388*, 427–442.

Stillman, R. D., Crow, G., & Moushegian, G. (1978). Components of the frequency-following potential in man. *Electroencephalography and Clinical Neurophysiology, 44*, 438–446.

Stockard, J. J., Sharbrough, F. W., & Tinker, J. A. (1978). Effects of hypothermia on the human brainstem auditory response. *Annals of Neurology, 3*, 368–370.

Stockard, J. J., Stockard, J. E, & Sharbrough, F. W. (1978). Nonpathologic factors influencing brainstem auditory-evoked potentials. *American Journal of EEG Technology, 18*, 177–193.

Suzuki, T., & Horiuchi, K. (1981). Rise time of pure-tone stimuli in brain stem response audiometry. *Audiology, 20*, 101–112.

Terkildsen, K., & Osterhammel, P. (1981). The influence of reference electrode position on recordings of the auditory brainstem responses. *Ear and Hearing, 2*, 9–14.

Thivierge, J., & Côté, R. (1990). Brain-stem auditory evoked response: Normative values in children. *Electroencephalography and Clinical Neurophysiology, 77*, 309–313.

Woldorff, M., Hansen, J. C., & Hillyard, S. A. (1987). Evidence for effects of selective attention in the mid-latency range of the human auditory event-related potential. *Electroencephalography and Clinical Neurophysiology Supplement, 40*, 146–154.

Yamada, O., Yagi, T., Yamane, H., & Suzuki, J. (1975). Clinical evaluation of the auditory evoked brain- stem response. *Auris Nasus Larynx, 2*, 97–105.

Yamada, O., Yamane, H., & Kodera, K. (1977). Simultaneous recordings of the brain stem response and the frequency-following response to low-frequency tone. *Electroencephalography and Clinical Neurophysiology, 43*, 362–370.

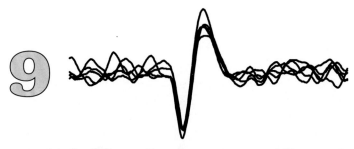

Middle-Latency Responses: The Brain and the Brawn

After all, from the little I know of you, after all the money expended on your education you are entitled to recoup yourself and command your price. You have every bit as much right to live by your pen in pursuit of your philosophy as the peasant has. What? You both belong to Ireland, the brain and the brawn. Each is equally important.

James Joyce, *Ulysses* (Bloom to Dedalus, Eumaeus episode), 1922

The middle-latency responses (MLRs) are the scalp-recorded auditory evoked potentials (EPs) that occur between 10 and 50 ms after a stimulus. Because this is the time when the auditory cortex is first activated, the initial report of these responses suggested that they might represent cortical activity (Geisler, Frishkopf, & Rosenblith, 1958). However, it soon became apparent that reflex responses to sound also could occur in scalp muscles at these latencies. Therefore, it was difficult to distinguish between neurogenic and myogenic responses, to determine what was brain and what was brawn. A particularly striking piece of evidence was that a subject under muscle relaxation with curare showed no clear responses (Bickford, Jacobson, & Cody, 1964). However, later studies (Harker,

Hosick, Voots, & Mendel, 1977; Kileny, Dobson, & Gelfand, 1983) demonstrated that definite MLRs could be recorded in subjects after muscle paralysis induced by succinylcholine or pancuronium. The recordings of Bickford et al. (1964) were designed to record large muscle responses and probably did not average sufficiently to recognize the much smaller cortical MLRs.

The first waves to be recognized in the auditory MLR were a sequence of negative and positive waves called Na, Pa, Nb, and Pb. The last of these waves is essentially the same as the P1 wave of the late auditory evoked potential (LAEP) or vertex potential and often goes by the name of P50 from its peak latency in milliseconds. We consider this particular wave in this chapter, although it can be categorized with either the MLRs or LAEPs. Small early waves, recognized after the initial alphabetical nomenclature, were given the names No and Po. These waves are difficult to distinguish from postauricular muscle (PAM) reflexes when using a mastoid reference and from distorted versions of the ABR when using low-pass filters below 200 Hz.

From the beginning, the interpretation of the MLR has been bedeviled by the possibility that they represent muscle reflexes rather than brain responses. However, the early bitter controversies now have given way to a more reasonable assessment of their source and usefulness. In a relaxed or sleeping subject, scalp-recorded events in the 10- to 50-ms latency range are cerebral in origin, provided we do not use a reference near the PAM in the midmastoid region. The PAM reflex may be a nuisance when we are specifically evaluating brain function, for example, when assessing the transition between wakefulness and anesthesia (Bell, Smith, Allen, & Lutman, 2004; Picton, John, Purcell, & Plourde, 2003). Recordings using a reference electrode on the lateral neck or inion generally eliminate the artifact. This is illustrated in the left half of Figure 9–1. Other reference locations are not immune to muscle artifact. However, the muscle reflexes recorded from the sternomastoid or at the inion are evoked only by high-intensity sounds and only when there is active muscle contraction.

When we are recording the MLRs to assess hearing, the PAM artifact is more of a help than a hindrance. The PAM reflex is mediated through the cochlea. Because of its large size, the reflex may provide a more rapid means to assess hearing than the MLR of cerebral origin. The confusion between muscle reflex and brain response would be detrimental when evaluating central hearing, but would be of no consequence when simply checking for a peripheral hearing loss.

In recent years, the muscle reflexes have assumed a significance of their own. The PAM reflex has become a useful adjunct to other means of objective audiometry and the sternomastoid muscle reflex an important test of vestibular function. This chapter initially reviews the MLRs of cerebral origin and then describes the sound-evoked reflexes that we can record from muscles of the head and neck.

CEREBRAL MLR

Intracranial Sources

We considered the sources for the scalp-recorded MLR in Chapter 4. The MLR recorded with electroencephalography (EEG) is sometimes difficult to model in terms of sources. Magnetoencephalography (MEG) is relatively free of contamination by muscle activity and has greater precision in terms of localizing sources on the superior surface of the temporal lobe. MEG studies of the MLR have shown that the Na and Pa waves of the response likely represent the activation near the primary auditory cortex on Heschl's gyrus (Borgmann, Ross, Draganova, & Pantev, 2001; Pantev et al., 1995; Pelizzone et al., 1987). The Pa wave, the most clearly recognizable component of the MLR, is generated anterior the N1 wave of the slow auditory EP and the two components have oppositely directed tonotopic maps, the Pa generators responding to higher frequencies being more laterally located (Pantev et al., 1995). However, the electrical Pa response shows no clear change in scalp topography with tonal frequency (Woods, Alain, Covarubias, & Zaidel, 1995). This

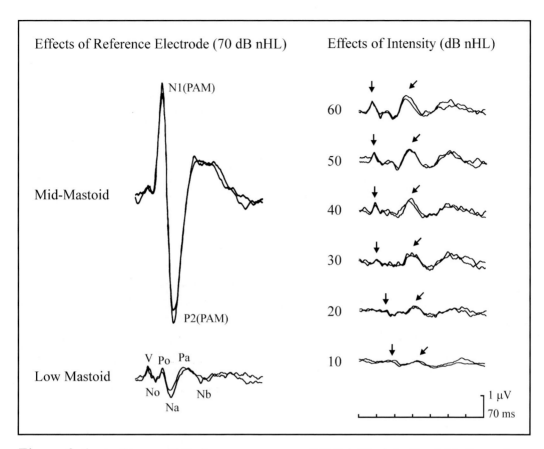

Figure 9–1. *Auditory middle-latency responses (MLRs). The left side of this figure shows the MLR evoked by an 8 ms 2-kHz tone of 70 dB nHL presented to the right ear at a rate of 11/s. Responses were simultaneously recorded between the vertex and midmastoid region and between the vertex and low-mastoid region. Each tracing represents the average of 2000 responses recorded using a bandpass of 25 to 3000 Hz. A large PAM reflex is recorded from the midmastoid region. This consists of a mastoid-negative wave peaking at 14 ms, followed by a positive wave at 20 ms, and a later broad negativity at around 35 ms. Although the initial wave is negative, it shows as an upward deflection on this recording because it originates at the reference electrode. The PAM reflex is much less evident in the recording made using the low mastoid reference. However, the Po wave is quite possibly equivalent to the initial N1 component of the muscle reflex, and the Na is still obscured by the P2 component of the muscle reflex. On the right of the figure is represented a full intensity series using a low mastoid reference. Both wave V of the ABR* (vertical arrow) *and wave Pa* (diagonal arrow) *are recognizable down to 10 dB nHL.*

suggests that that several generators may be involved in the electrical response, thereby obscuring any scalp evidence of tonotopicity. Little is known about the No and Po components of the response. Because they do not show up clearly on

MEG recordings, they may represent activity in the thalamus or thalamocortical radiations. If the filter settings of the recording amplifier are too narrow to accurately reproduce the auditory brainstem response (ABR), the No-Po complex may represent filter-distorted versions of wave V and V' of the ABR.

As discussed in Chapter 4, radial and tangentially oriented scalp-recorded waveforms can cause complex overlapping waveforms during the latency range of the MLR. The response typically is recorded from the vertex using a mastoid or neck reference. At the vertex, we record Na and Pa with latencies of 18 and 28 ms that derive from the vertically oriented dipoles located on the supratemporal plane. If we record from the lateral temporal region using a distant reference, we can obtain evidence of laterally oriented dipole activity—perhaps on the lateral aspect of the superior temporal gyrus or in fissures of the supratemporal plane. EEG source analyses show a laterally (or radially) oriented negative-positive complex with latencies of 27 and 39 ms (e.g., Scherg & von Cramon, 1990). Only the latter wave clearly shows in the scalp-recordings as a distinct temporal positive wave at a latency near 41 ms, the TP41 wave (Cacace & McFarland, 2009; Cacace, Satya-Murti, & Wolpaw, 1990). Scalp-recorded waves generated by radially oriented sources are not measurable with the MEG.

Recording Parameters

The MLR typically is recorded from the vertex using a reference on the mastoid or neck. Recordings using the mastoid contralateral to stimulation reflect preferentially the response of the contralateral cortex (which is larger than the response of the ipsilateral cortex). An ipsilateral reference makes the response symmetric in the central regions. Although reasonable when using the MLR for audiometric purposes, such simple montages do not completely distinguish between the contributions from

the two hemispheres, and the recordings may be within normal limits in patients with lesions affecting one temporal lobe but not the other. If one hemisphere is not responding, the response of the other hemisphere will still be recordable over both sides of the scalp. More extensive measurements of the scalp distribution of the MLR components are essential if we wish to compare the responses of each hemisphere. Early recordings used a set of electrodes in a coronal chain passing from one mastoid through the vertex to the other mastoid. These recordings could demonstrate asymmetries resulting from unilateral lesions (Kileny, Paccioretti, & Wilson, 1987; Kraus, Özdamar, Hier, & Stein, 1982). More extensive studies of the MLR scalp-distribution indicate multiple generators contributing to the waveform (Cacace et al., 1990; Leavitt, Molhom, Ritter, Shpaner, & Foxe, 2007). Source analysis (Leavitt et al., 2007; Scherg & von Cramon, 1990) would be necessary to dissect out these different components (see Figure 4–13). However, this has not yet been validated sufficiently for clinical use. Clearly, further studies are needed.

It is often difficult to be sure that an MLR recording represents a real response rather than background EEG/EMG. When using a very narrow bandwidth such as 20 to 200 Hz, the filtered background activity usually will have two negative-positive deflections in a sweep of 50 ms and we will be tempted to identify these waves as an MLR. Some estimate of the background noise level—either by replications or by more formal statistical assessment—is therefore essential for any recording of the MLR. The MLR has been recorded with many different filter bandpasses. The best advice is to record with a wide bandpass (1–1000 Hz) and then use digital filters with a narrower bandpass

(10–500) to examine the averaged response. Using a wide bandpass during the recording will allow us to evaluate the background EEG and assess the sleep stage. This is important because, as we discuss later, the MLR varies with the sleep stage.

The response typically is recorded using a stimulus rate near 10 Hz. As the line noise from power sources has a frequency (50 or 60 Hz) that is within the range of the frequencies in the MLR, we must attenuate the effects of line noise in the recordings. We do not wish to interpret time-locked line-noise as evidence that a subject is hearing. If necessary, a notch filter may be used, although this can attenuate the response as well as the noise. As discussed in Chapter 2, a stimulus onset asynchrony (SOA) that is equal to an odd-integer multiple of the reciprocal of the line-frequency should ensure clean recordings. Thus, if the line noise is 60 Hz, an SOA of 108.33 ms (stimulus rate of 9.23 Hz) or 91.67 (10.9 Hz) would be preferable to 100 ms.

The MLR is quite resilient to increasing stimulus rates and the Pa wave can be recognized at mean rates of up to 80 Hz using techniques such as maximum length sequences (Bell, Smith, Allen, & Lutman, 2006; Picton, Champagne, & Kellett, 1992) or other deconvolution techniques (Delgado & Özdamar, 2008). Figure 9–2 illustrates the MLRs (and ABRs) recorded using maximum length sequences.

The main components of the vertex-recorded MLR evoked by a moderately loud click are Na at about 16 ms, Pa at 25 ms, Nb at 36 ms, and Pb at 50 ms (Picton, Hillyard, Krausz, & Galambos, 1974). Adjacent negative and positive waves are therefore separated by intervals between 9 and 14 ms. When using regular rates, we should not use rates near 29 Hz (SOA 34 ms) as at these rates the positive waves of one response may overlap the negative waves of the next and attenuate the response. For example, when the SOA is 34 ms, wave Pb of one response will occur at a latency relative to the subsequent stimulus (16 ms) that is similar to the latency of the Na evoked by that stimulus. The opposite effect occurs at rates near 44 Hz (SOA of 23 ms), when Pb to one stimulus occurs near the latency of Pa to the subsequent stimulus. This results in an enhancement of the waves to form the auditory steady-state response (ASSR). These rate effects are discussed more extensively in Chapter 10.

Stimulus-Response Relationships

As seen in Figures 9–1 and 9–2, the MLR can be recognized down to intensities close to behavioral threshold. Figure 9–3 shows the amplitude and latency findings from several studies. The click response generally is larger than the response to tones. The latency increases with decreasing intensity and with decreasing frequency. Several durations of tones have been studied. In terms of audiometry, we should probably evoke MLRs with the 2-1-2 tone that has become widely used in ABR studies. Indeed, we probably should record the ABR and the MLR together by using a filter bandpass that is wide enough for both (e.g., 10–2000 Hz). Typical stimulus rates are between 10 and 20/s if normal averaging is used. Faster rates are possible with maximum length sequences and related procedures.

The MLR to a binaural stimulus is very similar in waveform to that evoked by a monaural stimulus, and the binaural response is only slightly larger than either monaural response. The MLR binaural

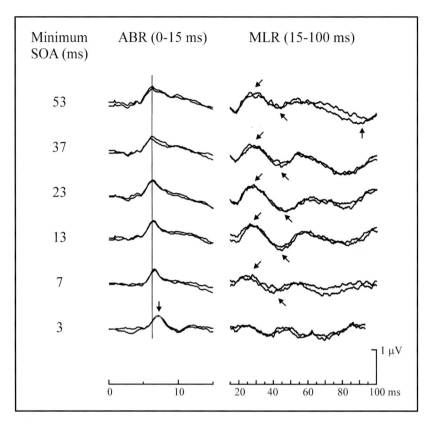

Figure 9–2. *ABR and auditory MLR recorded using maximum length sequences. This figure shows the auditory evoked potentials to a 70 dB nHL rarefaction click. The recordings were obtained using a maximum length sequence of 31, with minimum stimulus onset asynchrony (SOA) between 3 and 53 ms. The average SOAs over the sequence is slightly less than twice the minimum SOA. The analysis was carried out using a 100-ms sweep, except at the minimum SOA of 3 ms when the maximum possible sweep was 93 ms. The first 15 ms of the response is shown on the left and the period from 15 to 100 ms is shown on the right using a narrower time scale. There were no changes in the ABR except for the latency of wave V. This was longer at an SOA of 3 ms than at other SOAs (downgoing vertical arrow). The vertical line occurs at 6.25 ms. The Pa wave in the middle-latency response (downgoing diagonal arrow) is larger at SOAs between 13 and 53 ms than at the intervals 3 or 7 ms. The Nb wave (upgoing diagonal arrow) is larger at intervals 13–37 ms than at shorter or longer intervals. At the longest interval, a late Nc wave (upgoing arrow) is recognizable. This is probably equivalent to the N1 of the late auditory evoked potential. Data derived from Picton et al., 1992.*

interaction components thus become essentially an inverted representation of the monaural response (Junius, Riedel, & Kollmeier, 2007; McPherson & Starr, 1993; Picton & Ross, 2010). This is quite different from the ABR (see Figure 5-11) where the binaural response is almost twice the size of the monaural. Exactly why MLRs

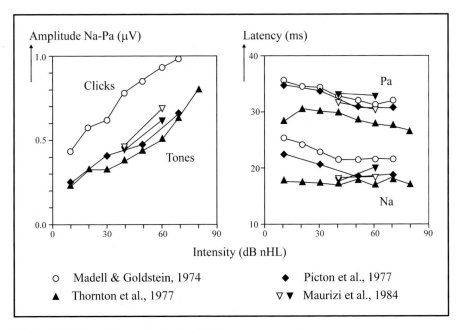

Figure 9–3. Stimulus-response relations of the MLR. The left graph shows the amplitude of Na-Pa as a function of stimulus intensity. Data from several laboratories have been combined in this figure to illustrate that clicks (open symbols) elicit larger MLRs than tones (filled symbols). The right graph shows the latency of Na and Pa components as a function of stimulus intensity. The latencies are not significantly different between clicks and tones.

to binaural stimuli are similar to those to monaural stimuli is not known. As discussed in Chapter 5, the information coming to the auditory cortex from the brainstem probably is already tagged by its spatial location. As the information moves from the brainstem to the cortex, it becomes coded in terms of spatial location rather in terms of ear. Auditory objects from one or the other side or from straight ahead are then treated equally.

In a reverberant environment, an auditory source produces echoes from sounds reflecting off different surfaces. Although the ears receive these reflected sounds in addition to the initial binaural activation, the perceived location of the sound is dominated by the initial input. Liebenthal and Pratt (1999) presented bin-

aural clicks and followed these by an echo (from a different location). By subtracting the response to the click alone from the response to the click and echo, they could record the response to the echo. The ABR to the echo was essentially normal but the Pa wave of the MLR was reduced, suggesting that echo suppression occurs before the level of the auditory cortex where Pa is generated.

MLRs at Different Ages

The MLR can be recorded in infants. However, it has a longer latency than in adults and is much more susceptible to the rate of stimulation, being best recognized at stimulus rates of 1/s and generally invisible at rates greater than 4/s (Jerger, Chmiel, Glaze, & Frost, 1987). Many of the early studies reporting the detection of MLRs in infants likely were measuring the ABR distorted by the filter settings.

At the other end of the range of human ages, the MLR also undergoes dramatic changes. In adults over 60 years of age, the MLR waves are much larger than in young adults, often by a factor of 2 or 3 (Amenedo & Diaz, 1998; Woods & Clayworth, 1986). We do not know the cause for this unexpected increase in responsiveness when everything else is declining with age. One possibility is that the inhibitory connections (mediated by gamma-aminobutyric acid) within the auditory system decline with age.

Attention and Arousal

Early studies of the effects of attention on the MLR reported no clear changes in the response to attended or ignored stimuli (e.g., Picton & Hillyard, 1974). However, when the attentional task was made more demanding, the response to attended stimuli showed an increased positivity over the latencies from 20 to 50 ms, enhancing both waves Pa and Pb (Woldorff & Hillyard, 1991; Woldorff et al., 1993). This may represent a facilitation of the processes that normally underlie Pa and Pb or the addition of some other cerebral process. Whatever its basic physiology, it indicates a selective gating of information at the level of the auditory cortex.

With sleep, the MLR remains clearly recognizable. However, during sleep the amplitudes are smaller and the latencies longer, particularly in the deeper stages of sleep (Jones & Baxter, 1988; Millan, Özdamar, & Bohorquez, 2006; Osterhammel, Shallop, & Terkildsen, 1985). The Nb

and Pb components often become unrecognizable in stage 3 or 4 sleep (stages characterized by EEG delta activity), leaving only a small broad Pa wave. Because of these effects, McGee, Kraus Killion, Rosenberg, and King (1993) recommended that we should monitor the stages of sleep when recording the MLR and evaluate responses only when the level of EEG delta activity is low.

Anesthesia

The MLR is significantly changed during anesthesia (Plourde, 2006; Thornton & Newton, 1989; Thornton & Sharpe, 1998). Therefore, recording the MLR during anesthesia may provide us with information about depth of anesthesia. Before we consider this possibility, we should review some aspects of anesthesia and how it is might be monitored.

General anesthesia is a multidimensional state. Its goals are to make the patient unconscious, to ensure that the patient does not experience pain, to prevent any memory of the surgery, and to stop the muscles from contracting in response to surgical stimulation. Modern anesthesia generally involves administering several medications rather than just one. When muscle relaxants are used, it is impossible to know whether a patient has become aware during an operation as the patient cannot move the muscles to communicate. To prevent inadvertent intraoperative awareness, some objective measure of the effectiveness of anesthesia is needed. Occasionally, anesthetists have used an isolated forearm to allow a patient to communicate. Blood carrying the muscle relaxant is prevented from reaching the forearm and this allows the muscles in the forearm to be activated if the patient becomes aware and wishes to communicate (Thornton et al., 1989). Although this does provide a direct measure of patient responsiveness, the technique is too cumbersome for routine use.

Three simpler methods of measuring anesthetic depth can be used. The first is to measure the levels of the anesthetic in the body—the end-tidal concentration of an inhaled anesthetic (presently available for many agents) or the plasma concentration of an intravenous agent (available after the fact but not immediately). Unfortunately, the relationship between these concentrations and the depth of anesthesia varies among individuals and can change when a particular anesthetic is used in combination with another. What is needed is some measure of the effect of the anesthetic agent or agents on brain function (Bruhn, Myles, Sneyd, & Struss, 2006). Various measurements of the EEG, depending mainly on the amount of slow activity in the EEG, have been widely used. However, the EEG changes differently with different anesthetic agents and EEG measurements may not accurately portray the anesthetic (as opposed to other) effects of the agents (see recent critical report of Avidan et al., 2008).

EPs provide a reasonable alternative to the EEG for monitoring the depth of anesthesia. The advantages of EP studies are that they are specifically related to cortical responsiveness to external stimulation rather than to general cortical activity, and that they are similarly affected by different anesthetic agents. Auditory EPs usually are studied; auditory stimuli are simpler to set up and maintain through the operation than visual or somatosensory stimuli. The usual stimulus for the auditory MLR is a binaural 70 dB nHL (normal hearing level) click presented at a rate near 6/s and the response is recorded from vertex

(or forehead) to mastoid, using a relatively narrow bandpass (e.g., 25–400 Hz) and averaged over 1000 trials (about 3 minutes) using a sweep of 100 ms (Kochs et al., 1999). If we do not wish to have the MLR contaminated by a PAM reflex, an inion or neck reference may be used instead of the mastoid (Bell et al., 2004). The patient's hearing must be checked prior to the operation. Clearly, the technique will not work in a patient with a significant hearing loss (Bell et al., 2006).

Anesthesia is associated with a decreasing amplitude and an increasing latency of the auditory MLR (Gajraj, Doi, Mantzaridis, & Kenny, 1998; Thornton & Newton, 1989; Thornton et al., 1989; Tooley, Stapleton, Greenslade, & Prys-Roberts, 2004). The later waves (Nb and Pb) are affected more than the earlier waves. Because of these increases in latency, the MLR waveform under anesthesia therefore tends to contain two positive waves rather than three over the period of 100 ms. This is illustrated in Figure 9–4. The third positive wave in the unanesthetized recording is likely the notch between N1a and N1b viewed through the typical high-pass filter used for recording the MLR (25 Hz in Thornton et al., 1989). The latency of peak Nb is most clearly related to the awareness: when it exceeds 45 ms, the patient is no longer responsive in the isolated forearm (Thornton et al., 1989). This effect appears to relate to the anesthetic effect of the anesthetics and is independent of the specific plasma concentrations of intravenous anesthetic agents when they are used in combination (Brunner, Nel, Fernandes, & Newton, 2002). However, if the MLR is recorded using maximum length sequences, component latencies do not clearly change with increasing depth of anesthesia and amplitude may be the more important measure (Bell et al., 2006).

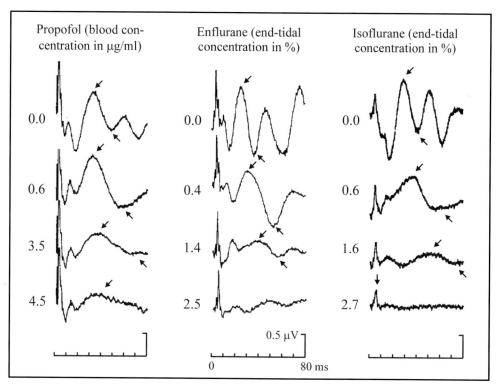

Figure 9–4. **Auditory MLR during anesthesia.** *These recordings show the changes in the MLR with three different anesthetics: the intravenous propofol and the gases isoflurane and enthrone. The propofol and isoflurane were given together with 70% nitrous oxide in oxygen. The MLRs were evoked by a 70 dB nHL click presented at 6/s. The responses were recorded been the vertex and inion, filtered with a bandpass of 25 to 400 Hz and averaged for 512 to 1024 sweeps. As the anesthesia deepens the Pa (downgoing diagonal arrow) and Nb (upgoing diagonal arrow) waves decrease in amplitude and increase in latency. This changes the waveform from 10–100 ms from one containing two positive-negative complexes peaks (Pa-Nb and Pb-Nc) to one with only one. At the deepest levels, the MLR waves are no longer clearly recognizable and only the ABR (vertical arrow) remains. These waveforms are adapted from Thornton and Newton (1989).*

One difficulty with using the MLR to assess depth of anesthesia is that it is not clear what to measure—what peak or what set of latency and amplitudes best discriminates between consciousness and unconsciousness? Computer algorithms can help to distinguish MLR waveforms characteristic of wakefulness and anesthesia without specifically measuring the component peaks and troughs (Kochs, Stockmanns, Thornton, Nahm, & Kalk-mann, 2001). These techniques need further investigation. The 40-Hz response, the steady-state version of the MLR, may be easier to measure and monitor during anesthesia. We consider this in Chapter 10.

We can now return to our initial comments on anesthesia. Because general anesthesia is a multidimensional state (involving changes in consciousness, awareness of pain, memory, and muscle responses), depth of anesthesia cannot be measured on a simple linear scale. We are not sure which aspect of anesthesia is related to the observed changes in the MLR. These changes likely are related to the changes in consciousness but it is difficult to disentangle this from the other effects of anesthesia. Anesthetic changes in the MLR do not predict reflex movement to painful stimulation in a patient who is not paralyzed (Kochs et al., 1999). The effect of the anesthetic agent on these reflexes requires a higher concentration of the anesthetic agent than the changes in the MLR (and one presumes conscious awareness). Monitoring all aspects of anesthesia probably will require measurements as multidimensional as the state.

P50 WAVE OF THE MLR

The P50 wave is a positive wave in the auditory evoked response that occurs between the latencies of the MLR and the LAEPs. It also goes by the name of Pb when considered in the MLR recordings and P1 when considered in the late EPs. Its source in the brain is not known although various regions have been conjectured. Notwithstanding its uncertain origin, it has been tentatively associated with several different neuropsychiatric disorders.

The P50 the wave has been studied extensively in relation to "sensory gating." The concept of sensory gating is that the brain responds less to a repeating stimulus than to one that has not occurred for a while. Such gating might prevent the brain from responding to irrelevant input. Sensory gating is most frequently studied by recording responses to paired stimuli, with the interval between the stimuli being about 500 ms and the interval between

the pairs about 10 seconds (Adler, Pachtman, Franks, Pecevich, & Waldo, 1982; Freedman, Adler, Waldo, Pachtman, & Franks, 1983). In this approach the P50 wave to the second stimulus (S2) in the pair will be smaller than to the first (S1). The amount of "suppression" at S2 can be measured as the difference between the two amplitudes relative to the amplitude of the first: (S1–S2)/S1. This is usually expressed as a percentage with normal values around 75% (Waldo & Freedman, 1983). However, some researchers express the result as a simple S2/S1 ratio (e.g., Boutros, Belger, Campbell, D'Souza, & Krystal, 1999). Because of the long interpair interval, the EPs are averaged over small numbers of trials and are noisy. Dipole modeling can help to reduce the noise (Cardenas, Gerson, & Fein, 1993).

The P50 has been studied extensively in patients with schizophrenia, who show reduced sensory gating, decreased suppression of the response to the second stimulus (Freedman et al., 1987). This abnormality also may occur in unaffected relatives of schizophrenic patients (Clementz, Geyer, & Braff, 1998; Siegel, Waldo, Mizner, Adler, & Freedman, 1984), and is decreased by neuroleptic medication (Freedman et al., 1983). These findings suggest that the P50 effect may indicate some genetic abnormality of the transmitter systems involved in inhibition, with this abnormality predisposing a subject to schizophrenia. Genetic linkage studies have related P50 suppression to a gene sites controlling cholinergic transmitters (Freedman et al., 1997).

Although the sensory gating phenomenon reliably differentiates between groups of schizophrenic patients and groups of normal subjects, the variability of the measurement is such that it cannot be used to assess individual subjects (e.g., Brockhaus-Dumke et al., 2008; Clementz et al., 1998; Patterson et al., 2008). Most studies average approximately 100 responses. Averaging over a greater number of trials might make the measurements more reliable—although the gating effects may decrease with stimulus repetition. Using the larger N1 wave rather than the P50 as the measurement of sensory gating might be more efficient (e.g., Brockhaus-Dumke et al., 2008).

The interpretation of these results is difficult because we are not sure of the intracerebral origin of the P50 wave. The auditory regions of the cortex—in or near Heschl's gyri—are active during the wave but the response of this area does not share the same relationship to the SOA as the scalp-recorded P50 wave (Onitsuka, Ninomiya, Sato, Yamamoto, & Tashiro, 2000). In intracranial recordings, Korzyukov et al. (2007) found that, although the auditory cortices on the superior surface of the temporal lobe contribute to the P50, the neuronal activity contributing to its amplitude reduction during sensory gating is localized to the frontal lobe. The scalp topographies found by Leavitt et al. (2007) indicate multiple components underlying the P50, some generated in the temporal lobe, and others in deeper brain regions.

The P50 effects in schizophrenia also are difficult to relate to the cognitive abnormalities in the disorder (see review by Potter, Summerfelt, Gold, & Buchanan, 2006). How does reduced sensory gating lead to the clinical symptoms of the disorder? Another problem is why does this neurophysiologic finding also occur in other neuropsychiatric disorders, such as Alzheimer's disease (Cancelli et al., 2006), post-traumatic stress disorders (Ghisolfi et al., 2004), and bipolar affective disorders (Lijffijt et al., 2009). Although these disorders all may affect the inhibitory systems involved in sensory gating, each must additionally affect other cerebral processes to give the different clinical presentations. This makes the sensory gating effect very nonspecific.

Another difficulty in the interpretation of sensory gating is the amplitude of the P50 evoked by stimuli repeated at regular rates. Given the concept of decreased sensory gating, we might assume that the response to a regularly repeating stimulus would be larger in schizophrenic subjects. However, Leavitt et al. (2007) found that the P50 amplitude evoked by a repeating tone (SOA of 750 ms) was smaller in schizophrenic patients than in normal subjects. This, in turn, suggests that the observed sensory gating effect may be as much due to a smaller P50 response to S1 rather than a larger (or unsuppressed) response to S2. Such differences occur but usually have not been found to be significant because of intersubject variability (e.g., Brockhaus-Dumke et al., 2008). A recent meta-analysis has indicated that the P50 amplitude to S1 is smaller in schizophrenic subjects (Figure 3 of Patterson et al., 2008).

We have mentioned only some of the many papers on the P50 in schizophrenic patients (a more extensive review is provided by Patterson et al., 2008). The only thing that is clearly apparent in this literature is that schizophrenic subjects differ from normal controls in the responsiveness of the P50 at short SOAs. However, this is too variable a finding to provide any diagnostic information in normal subjects. Exactly what the results indicate in terms of pathophysiology is not known. Further research is needed—recordings should be more detailed in terms of topography and signal-to-noise, and the P50 should be examined together with the later waves of the response such as N1.

A decreased amplitude of the P50 in response to a simple repeating auditory stimulus was reported initially in patients with Alzheimer's disease (Buchwald, Erwin, Rea, van Lancker, & Cummings, 1989). However, this finding was not always replicated (e.g., Phillips, Connolly, Mate-Kole, & Gray, 1997). Golob, Johnson, and Starr (2002) found that the P50 was increased (more than in normal aging) in patients presenting with mild cognitive impairment. This was particularly true of those who later became demented. Patients with Alzheimer's disease no longer showed the increased P50 (Golob, Irimijiri, & Starr, 2007). These variable results may be related to compensatory mechanisms brought to bear when basic perceptual processing starts to fail either with aging or with dementia. Attentional mechanisms may enhance sensory processing (and increase the P50) in aging and in early dementia. When these compensatory mechanisms fail, the P50 decreases and the symptoms of dementia become apparent.

ELECTROMYOGRAPHY (EMG)

To understand some of the different responses that can be evoked in the muscles of the head and neck by sounds, we first review some simple principles of muscle physiology. A muscle is composed of multiple muscle fibers, multinucleated cells a few hundredths to a few tenths of a millimeter across and from several millimeters to several centimeters in length. Within each cell are contractile proteins (myosin and actin) that decrease the length of the fiber when activated. Activation begins at the neuromuscular junction (composed of the termination of the nerve fiber and a specialized region of the muscle membrane called the "endplate"), typically located near the middle of the elongated cell. When the muscle is small or medium in size, this generally is near the belly of the muscle. For longer muscles such as the quadriceps, the endplates may be spread out over the entire length of the muscle. The endplate is depolarized by the neurotransmitter acetylcholine released at the neuromuscular junction by the neuronal action potential. This depolarization causes the muscle fiber membrane to generate its own action potential. The muscle fiber action potential, which is similar to that generated in a nerve fiber although longer lasting (about 2 ms rather than 1 ms), is then transmitted along the muscle fiber in both directions away from the endplate. Because the conduction velocity is of the order of 5 m/s, the muscle fiber action potential will take about 2 ms to travel a centimeter. The membrane of the muscle fiber has deep invaginations called transverse tubules that allow the membrane depolarization to reach the interior of the cell, where it causes the contraction of the actin and myosin filaments within the fiber.

A single motor neuron branches to innervate between 10 and 1000 motor fibers, which together form the "motor unit." Each fiber will be activated when the nerve action potential arrives at the neuromuscular junctions, with the relative timing depending on the lengths of the terminal nerve branches going to the different endplates. If recorded in the extracellular fluid in the vicinity of the endplates, the muscle action potential is a negative-positive complex. If the electrodes are at some distance along the fiber from the end plate, the pattern is a positive-negative-positive complex. The summed activity of all the fibers activated by one neuron is the motor unit action potential. Because of different lengths of the terminal branches of the nerve, there is a latency jitter of several milliseconds in the activation of the different fibers. The motor unit action potential therefore lasts longer than the single fiber discharge, typically 5 to 15 ms, depending on the muscle and the number of fibers in a motor unit. If recorded near the end plate, the motor unit action potential generally will be negative-positive, although there are often smaller deflections on the basic waveform. Away from the end plate, the motor unit action potential usually will be positive-negative or triphasic. The electrical activity of human motor units can be recorded by needle electrodes within the muscle or surface electrodes on the skin overlying the muscle. Surface recordings generally are obtained with the active electrode over the belly of the muscle (where the end plates are usually located and where the muscle action potentials begin). The reference electrode usually is placed near where the tendon of the muscle inserts. Because of the way the extracellular potentials are generated, the waveform at this reference electrode usually is a small inverted version of the waveform recorded over the end plate region. The electrical activity of muscle fibers and motor units is illustrated in Figure 9–5.

The amplitude of a recorded muscle response is quite variable. A major determinant is the distance between the recording electrode and the activated muscle fibers. For the motor unit potential, the amplitude also will vary with the number of muscle fibers in the motor unit. For the muscle potential, the amplitude will vary with the number of motor units activated; this is determined by the number of nerve fibers synchronously activating the muscle. Needle recordings give a typical fiber discharge recorded of around 100 µV and a typical motor unit potential about 0.5 mV. A typical surface-recorded muscle potential around between 0.1 and 20 mV (depending on the size of the muscle).

Sustained muscle contraction is brought about by the repetitive firing of the neurons that innervate the muscle. The strength of the contraction can be increased by increasing either the number of active neurons or the rate at which they fire. The EMG recorded from a needle or a surface electrode will represent the sum of all the motor unit potentials—a random noise with most frequencies between 10 and 100 Hz. If led to an audio speaker, this will give a roaring sound. (One way of providing feedback to a patient contracting a muscle is to connect the EMG to a speaker and ask the patient to "make it roar like a lion"). We can estimate the general level of EMG activity by taking the root-mean-square (rms) value of the recording.

A brief sudden movement, such as might occur in a reflex response, is caused by a multiple neurons firing at about the same time. If the active recording electrode is over the region of the muscle where most endplates are located, the potential will show a negative-positive waveform. Some reflexes, such as that recorded in the sternomastoid muscle after an intense sound, are inhibitory rather than excitatory (Colebatch & Rothwell, 2004). These reflexes occur only when the muscle is contracting. A brief inhibition in a sustained contraction will give a positive-negative wave. The mechanism for this has been examined by Wit and Kingma (2006). During the sustained contraction, the motor unit potentials overlap and, as they occur at different times, they tend to cancel each other out—the negative part of one motor unit action potential occurring at the same time as the positive part of another.

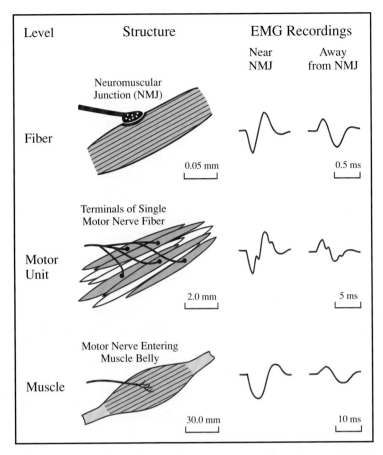

Level	Structure	EMG Recordings	
		Near NMJ	Away from NMJ

Fiber — Neuromuscular Junction (NMJ), 0.05 mm, 0.5 ms

Motor Unit — Terminals of Single Motor Nerve Fiber, 2.0 mm, 5 ms

Muscle — Motor Nerve Entering Muscle Belly, 30.0 mm, 10 ms

Figure 9–5. Basic principles of electromyography (EMG). The top section of this figure shows the muscle fiber, a multinucleated cell containing actin and myosin and serving as the basic contractile unit of the muscle. The diagram shows only the central part of an elongated cell. This is activated by the release of acetylcholine at the neuromuscular junction (NMJ). Once the endplate (the muscle side of the junction) is sufficiently depolarized, an action potential is generated. When recorded by a needle in the extracellular fluid around the muscle fiber, this action potential (also called a "fibrillation") shows as a negative-positive complex. At any distance away from the endplate, the potential is positive-negative. The middle section of the figure shows the motor unit. This is a set of fibers (anywhere from 10 to 100) activated by the terminal branches of a single motor nerve fiber. The fibers composing a motor unit usually are within one region of the muscle, but often are inter-digitated with fibers from other motor units. In this diagram, the motor unit fibers are shaded gray. For simplicity, the diagram exaggerates the width of the fibers. Recorded by a needle electrode, the motor unit potential is the sum of all the electric fields generated by the fibers contained in the motor unit. This gives a waveform that has a dominant negative-positive shape near the NMJs. However, deflections may be superimposed on the basic waveform because the action potentials of individual fiber within the unit are not synchronous and may be spread out over several milliseconds. The lower section of the figure shows the whole muscle. Recordings typically are taken from surface electrodes placed on the skin over the muscle. When all the neurons in the nerve entering the muscle are activated, the sum of all the activated motor unit potentials, gives the muscle potential. This lasts longer than the typical motor unit potential because the motor units are not activated synchronously, and is smoother in its waveform since the smaller deflections are smeared out by the jitter. The EMG recordings in this figure are shown with positivity of the recording electrode relative to a distant reference causing an upward deflection. This is opposite to the normal EMG convention.

When the activation stops, the last motor unit potentials to occur before the inhibition will not overlap with any other and the positive part of their waveforms will not be canceled. Similarly, the negative initial part of the motor unit action potentials that begin after the inhibition will also not be canceled. The different reflex mechanisms are illustrated in Figure 9–6.

Many different muscles in the head and neck respond to sound. The locations of these muscles are shown in Figure 9–7. The responses may be excitatory (the muscle twitches) or inhibitory (the muscle briefly relaxes). The responses may be mediated through the cochlea or through the saccule. We next consider the responses of the postauricular muscle and the sternomastoid muscle in detail.

POSTAURICULAR MUSCLE (PAM)

The postauricular muscle (PAM) is a tiny vestigial muscle located behind the mid portion of the pinna, and innervated by the facial nerve. It arises from the mastoid process and attaches to the middle of the posterior pinna, acting to bring the pinna backward. The electrical responses of the PAM have been extensively (although intermittently) evaluated since they were initially reported by Kiang, Crist, French, and Edwards (1963).

The initial studies were undertaken to determine the nature of the early scalp-recorded auditory responses in human subjects reported by Geisler et al. (1958). Bickford, Jacobson, and Cody (1964) showed that much that could be recorded from the scalp at these early latencies was caused by reflex responses in the muscles of the scalp and neck. These "microreflexes" could

be altered by changing muscle tension and eliminated by muscle relaxants. Two main responses were identified: the PAM response, mediated through the cochlea and recordable down to moderate or low intensities, and the inion response, mediated through the vestibular system and recognized only at high intensities (Cody & Bickford, 1969, Ruhm, Walker, & Flanigin, 1967). We return to the inion response in the next section.

Because the PAM reflex can be recorded down to low intensities of sound, it could be used for objective audiometry. Yoshie and Okudaira (1969) found that the threshold for recognizing the response was between 0 and 20 dB above behavioral thresholds and these findings were replicated by Thornton (1975) and Gibson (1978). However, just as the muscle response can contaminate the recording of brain responses, it also is possible that the brain response can contaminate the recording of the muscle responses, particularly at low intensities and with montages that recorded between mastoid and frontal regions (Buffin, Connell, & Stamp, 1977; Thornton 1975). At low intensities, it often is not clear whether we are recording the PAM reflex or the cortical MLR. This does not matter from the point of view of threshold estimation, but is a concern if we wish to know what we are recording, for example, if we are investigating facial nerve function.

The PAM response did not, however, become widely used for objective audiometry. The main problem was its variability. Early reports found that it was not recognizable in one or both ears in about a third of their subjects (Cody & Bickford, 1969; Robinson & Rudge, 1977). Picton, Hillyard, Krausz, and Galambos (1974) reported the response to be sometimes present and sometimes absent in the same subject.

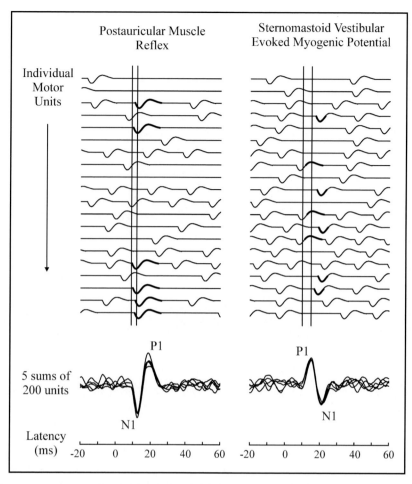

Figure 9–6. Excitatory and inhibitory muscle reflexes. *This figure shows how two types of muscle reflexes—excitatory and inhibitory—can be modeled as the sum of motor unit action potentials in the muscle. On the left is shown what might happen during the postauricular muscle reflex. The muscle is active; motor units occur without stimulation. When the sound occurs (at time 0), a motor unit is synchronized to the sound at a latency between 9 and 12 ms after the sound (the two vertical lines). The motor unit is not activated if it has fired recently (and therefore refractory) or if by chance it is inhibited by other processes. Nevertheless, several motor units (thicker lines) are activated during this time interval. The sum total of the activity is shown below (with five different versions superimposed). The response is a negative-positive sequence. The right half of the figure shows what happens during the vestibular evoked myogenic potential in the sternomastoid muscle. For this response, the motor units are firing more rapidly. Their timing relative to each other is random and the positive and negative parts of the motor unit action potentials tend to cancel each other out in the sum. In the latency between 10 and 15 ms after the sound (vertical lines), there is an inhibition, which prevents the initiation of any motor unit action potential. Because of this, there is a tendency for there to be uncanceled positive waves (thick line) at a latency near 14 ms (from the units that occurred just before the inhibition) and uncanceled negative waves near 21 ms (from the units that occur just after the cessation of the inhibition). This model is derived from the model of Wit and Kingma (2006), although it uses a different waveform for the motor unit action potential. In reality, each motor unit action potential would vary in amplitude and waveform from the general motor unit action potential that we have used in this model, but this would not significantly alter the results.*

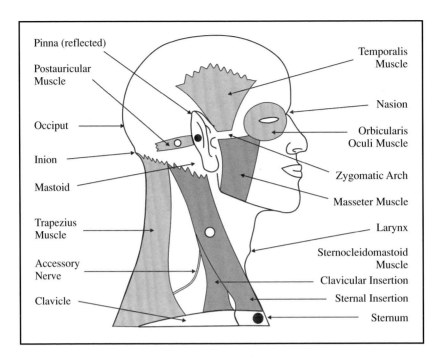

Figure 9–7. Muscles of the head and neck. This diagrammatic lateral view shows the locations of the muscles that can be used to study sound-evoked muscle reflexes. The top layer of muscles in the anterior neck and lateral face has been removed to show the deeper muscles underneath, the dark shaded sternocleidomastoid and the masseter muscles. The location of the active electrode for studying the postauricular muscle is shown by the small white circle. The reference electrode (black circle) can be placed on the posterior surface of the pinna (reflected to show the locations of both the muscle and the electrodes). The active electrode for studying the responses of the sternocleidomastoid muscle is located over the belly of the muscle and the reference on the sternum. The accessory nerve (cranial nerve XI) innervates the sternocleidomastoid and trapezius muscles. For simplicity, the diagram does not show the facial nerve (cranial nerve VII), which innervates the postauricular and oribicularis oculi muscles, or the trigeminal nerve (cranial nerve V), which innervates the masseter and temporalis muscles.

Some of the variability could be explained by the difficulty in locating the active electrode exactly over the belly of the small muscle. However, a much greater proportion of the variability turned out to be related to the direction of gaze.

Patuzzi and O'Beirne (1999a) showed that much of this variability could be attrib-uted to the fact that the PAM response is enhanced by looking toward the side of the stimulus and decreased by looking straight ahead or to the opposite side. This is shown clearly in Figure 9–8. If the response is recorded with the gaze directed toward the stimulus, the response can be recognized in almost all subjects. They did

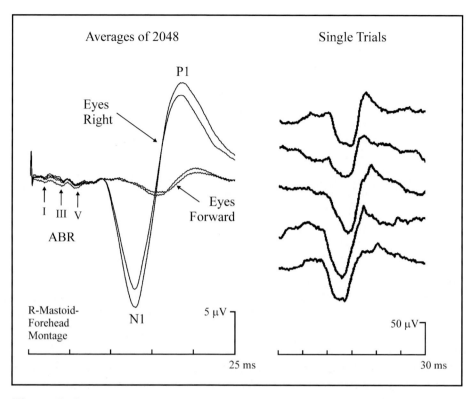

Figure 9–8. *Postauricular muscle (PAM) responses.* *On the left are shown average responses to a 50 dB SL click presented at a rate of 8/s to the right ear in two different conditions: with the eyes looking straight ahead and with the eyes looking to the right. The responses were recorded between the right mastoid and the forehead. When the eyes were looking to the right, a large PAM reflex occurs in the tracing with prominent N1 and P2 waves. With the eyes straight ahead, the reflex is much smaller (and likely distorted with the cerebral MLR). The responses were averaged over 2048 trials in order to show the small waves of the ABR occurring in the first 10 ms of the recording. The waveforms are upside down from those in Figure 9–1. In this particular figure, we are considering the PAM reflex, and the active electrode is on the mastoid, whereas in Figure 9–1 the mastoid electrode serves as the reference. On the right are shown selected single trial responses to the stimulus. The response, which occurs with variable amplitude and latency, is clearly different from the background activity. These waveforms are from O'Beirne and Patuzzi (1999).*

note one subject who did not have a clearly recognizable response even with lateral gaze. In this subject, they were able to record a small response when the subject pushed the head forward. It is difficult in this situation to eliminate some distant record- ing of the sternomastoid response (consid- ered in the next section). Using the lateral gaze manipulations, McCaslin, Jacobson, and Harry (2007) found that the PAM response to a 95 dB nHL click was absent on one or both sides in 15% of subjects.

Recording Parameters

Both Yoshie and Okudaira (1969) and O'Bierne and Patuzzi (1999) mapped the distribution of the response over the mastoid and adjacent regions. The largest and clearest response is recorded from an active electrode placed over the muscle and a reference electrode on the posterior aspect of the ipsilateral pinna. The muscle body is located on the midmastoid about 1.5 cm behind the posterior attachment of the pinna at the level of the external acoustic meatus. The closeness of the recording electrodes decreases the background noise in the recording and makes it very unlikely that other potentials (from the brain or other muscles) might contaminate the response.

The response contains energy between 20 and 300 Hz with the maximum occurring near 50 Hz (O'Bierne & Patuzzi, 1999). Frequency bandpasses narrower than 20 to 300 Hz and line-noise filters can distort the response waveform. For example, Purdy, Agung, Hartley, Patuzzi, and O'Beirne (2005) recorded a triphasic positive-negative-positive waveform when using a high-pass cutoff of 70 Hz. In some subjects, the response can be seen in single trials (see Figure 9–8), but generally we need to average between 20 and 500 recordings to recognize the response. Patuzzi and O'Beirne (1999b) also used a trial-to-trial correlation method to detect the response. This may be helpful when the eye-gaze is variable, for example in a rambunctious infant.

Stimuli can be clicks or brief tones. Clicks generally give much larger responses than tones. PAM responses to increasing-frequency chirps are larger than to clicks, particularly when using transducers with a transfer function that extends further into the high frequencies (Agung, Purdy, Patuzzi, O'Beirne, & Newall, 2005). Yoshie and Okudaira (1969) found that the response decreases with increasing stimulus rates, particularly at rates greater than 12.5/s. The response can nevertheless still be recorded at rates as fast as 81/s (see Figure 8–14). The optimum rate is likely close to 10/s.

Stimulus-Response Parameters

Table 9–1 presents the latencies and amplitudes of the response from several studies. The response is bilateral with very little difference in amplitude between the ipsilateral and contralateral response, the contralateral response being only 0.5 ms later (O'Bierne & Patuzzi, 1999). The response to a binaural click is essentially the sum of the responses to the monaural clicks (O'Bierne & Patuzzi, 1999).

The mean differences between behavioral thresholds and the PAM response detection thresholds were reported as 18 dB at 1 kHz, 26 dB at 2 kHz, and 30 dB at 4 kHz (O'Bierne & Patuzzi, 1999). The response to clicks can be recorded closer to behavioral threshold. With eyes turned to the side of the stimulus, Purdy et al. (2005) found an average difference of 5 dB (SD 12) between the behavioral pure tone average and the threshold (in dB nHL) for detecting the PAM response to clicks in adult subjects with a mild to moderate hearing losses who had a recognizable response (though 3 of the 20 subjects had no response).

The response grows in amplitude and decreases in latency with increasing intensity (O'Bierne & Patuzzi, 1999). The latency change is approximately 2 ms from 100 to 10 dB nHL. For clicks, the amplitude increases rapidly above threshold and then tapers off, whereas for tones the

Table 9–1. Normal Latencies and Amplitudes of Human PAM Reflex*

Study	Stimulus	N1 Latency (ms)	P1 Latency (ms)	N1-P1 Amplitude (μV)
Picton et al., 1974	Monaural 90 dB SL click 10/s	11.8 ± 0.8	16.4 ± 0.7	variable
O'Bierne and Patuzzi, 1999	Monaural 50 dB SL click 8/s	13.8 ± 0.3		72
Purdy et al., 2005	Monaural 80 dB nHL click 17/s	13.9 ± 1.1	18.1 ± 1.4	19.5
McCaslin and Jacobson, 2007	Monaural 95 dB nHL click 8/s	11.7 ± 1.2	16.9 ± 1.9	29.7

*Values presented as means and standard deviations (where available). Findings for ipsilateral stimulation. Latencies measured at peak. Latencies of Purdy et al., were likely delayed a little by use of a high low-pass filter. Amplitudes vary with the lateral gaze. All but the Picton et al. findings are with lateral gaze toward the stimulated ear (and responding muscle).

response grows slowly at low intensities and then very rapidly at intensities above 40 dB SL, likely because of the spread of excitation to regions of the cochlea other than those specific to the nominal frequency of the brief tone.

Subject Factors

A major determinant of the PAM response is the direction of gaze. Patuzzi and O'Beirne (1999a) showed clearly that directing the gaze to one side greatly increased the amplitude of the response on that side to binaural clicks. It is not clear what this effect represents, perhaps it is a vestigial reflex from animals who when looking to one side might move their pinnae out of the visual field and toward possible sounds sources. Whatever its cause, it provides us with a method for facilitating the recognition of a response during objective audiometry (Purdy et al., 2005).

The neuronal pathway underlying the reflex is probably trisynaptic (Hackley,

Woldorff, & Hillyard, 1987). Auditory nerve fibers synapse in the cochlear nucleus, which then sends axons bilaterally to the paralemniscal zones. These send connections to the medial division of the nucleus of the facial nerve. The facial nerve sends a branch to the muscle as it exits from the facial canal behind and inferior to the pinna. The top section of Figure 9–9 provides a diagrammatic view of the reflex.

Patuzzi and O'Beirne (1999a) proposed that lateral eye gaze facilitates the final motor neuron of the reflex, causing a basic subthreshold depolarization that makes it easier for acoustic input to elicit the reflex. In theory, lateral gaze also could facilitate the sensory limb of the reflex, with the subject paying attention to information coming from the side that is being looked at and facilitating the processing of this information. Because the reflex is bilateral, the test would be to record the response contralaterally to the stimulus. Generally, lateral gaze facilitates the response of the muscle toward which the gaze is directed (and not the response to

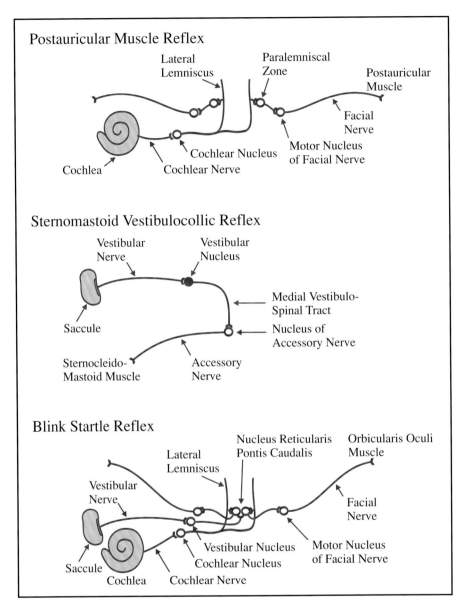

Figure 9–9. *Sound-evoked muscle reflexes. This figure illustrates the reflex pathways activated during three commonly recorded reflexes. The postauricular muscle reflex diagram derives from Hackley et al. (1987), the vestibulocollic reflex diagram from Kushiro et al. (1999) and Uchino et al. (1997), and the startle reflex from Davis et al. (1982). The black vestibular neuron in the vestibulocollic reflex pathway is inhibitory. The vestibulocollic reflex is ipsilateral whereas the postauricular and startle reflex are bilateral.*

the stimulus to which the gaze is directed). However, the sidedness of the gaze enhancement may vary from person to person (Patuzzi, personal communication). Most people have a dominant rise in ipsilateral EMG tone and therefore PAM response in the ear ipsilateral to the gaze direction. However, some subjects show a simultaneous smaller rise in tone in the muscle contralateral to the gaze direction.

As well as changing with the direction of gaze, the PAM response can be enhanced by having the subject activate the muscle voluntarily or by generally tensing the neck muscles. These maneuvers likely enhance the responsiveness of the facial neurons to reflex input so that a larger response is generated. The response clearly is excitatory rather than inhibitory as it can be seen on individual trials (see Figure 9–8). This is quite different from the inhibitory vestibular reflex that we will consider in the next section. For the vestibular evoked myogenic reflex, larger amounts of ongoing activity in the muscle mean that there is more to inhibit.

The PAM response is not affected by paying attention to the eliciting stimulus (Hackley et al., 1987). The response also is not affected by foreperiod manipulations of expectant attention (Sollers & Hackley, 1997). The PAM response is significantly decreased during sleep. However, the response can be recorded during stage I, perhaps in relation to the roving eye movements that occur in that stage of sleep (Picton et al., 2003), and occasionally in other stages (Streletz, Katz, Hohenberger, & Cracco, 1977).

The response can be recorded in young infants although the latency is delayed by several milliseconds compared to normal adults (Agung et al., 2005; O'Beirne & Patuzzi, 1999). The latencies reach adult values by 1 year of age and the response is reasonably easy to record in young children (Buffin et al., 1977; O'Beirne & Patuzzi, 1999). The response can be recorded in elderly subjects (Purdy et al., 2005), but more research is needed to evaluate the effects of aging.

Clinical Uses

The PAM response can be used as an adjunct test of hearing in patients who cannot be tested asleep. Sleep is necessary if we want to record reliable thresholds using the ABR or the ASSR at 80 to 100 Hz. The PAM response is very large compared to the ABR (see Figures 9–1 and 9–8) and often can be seen after averaging only a few recordings. When the PAM response is recognizable, it usually can be recorded at levels close to behavioral threshold after averaging for only a minute or two, provided the response is enhanced by lateral gaze (Purdy et al., 2005). The problem is that the response may not always be recognizable even with gaze facilitation. Therefore, a PAM response testing procedure might be to check if the response is present at a screening level such as 35 dB nHL. If so, we can be reasonably sure that there is no more than a mild hearing loss. If not, further testing will be required. In the young child who does not want to go to sleep and therefore cannot be reliably tested with the ABR or 80-Hz ASSR, PAM response testing could provide important information. However, it will be necessary to compare the effectiveness of the PAM response to recording the slow auditory EPs or the 40-Hz responses in these children.

Neurologically, the response may not be that helpful. The variability of the response makes it difficult to use as a measure of brainstem function. The ipsilateral and contralateral stapedius muscle reflexes are more reliable and more extensively studied (Gelfand, 2009). Because the PAM is the first muscle innervated by the facial nerve after it exits the facial canal, it may be helpful in localizing the pathology of a facial nerve palsy, or in demonstrating return of function in the nerve.

VESTIBULAR-EVOKED MYOGENIC POTENTIAL (VEMP)

Bickford et al. (1964, also Cody & Bickford, 1969) described a large early response that could be recorded from the inion (using a reference electrode on the nose) in response to loud sounds. The inion is the first bony bump you come to when you run your finger up the back of the upper neck, where the extensor neck muscles attach to the skull. It is located just below the larger occipital protuberance of the skull. The inion response contained a large negative peak at 14 ms and a positive peak at 24 ms. Often, this was followed by another more variable negative-positive complex. Most strikingly, the response was present only when the neck muscles were under sustained contraction, typically caused by pulling on a weight attached to a headband. The response was evoked only by very loud sounds (in the 100 dB SPL range). Townsend and Cody (1971) found that the response could be recorded in deaf subjects with preserved vestibular function and therefore proposed that it was mediated through the vestibular system, most likely through otolith receptors in the saccule.

Colebatch, Halmagyi, and Skuse (1994) studied what appeared to be a similar reflex with the active electrode located on the belly of the sternomastoid muscle and the reference electrode on the sternum. The reflex evoked by clicks of 85 or more dB nHL consisted of a positive-negative complex with peaks at 13 and 23 ms. This early response was larger in the muscle ipsilateral to the stimulus. Later (and more variable) responses were recorded bilaterally. The response increased linearly with increasing amplitude of the surface recorded EMG (by pushing the forehead against a bar), and was reduced or absent in patients with reduced vestibular function. They called the response the "vestibulocollic" reflex, but "vestibular evoked myogenic potential" or VEMP (Robertson & Ireland, 1995) has become the most widely used name for the response. These responses can be recorded (with greater amplitude but similar latency) in the trapezius muscle as well as the sternomastoid muscle (Ferber-Viart, Duclaux, Colleaux, & Dubreuil, 1997) when activity in both muscles was maintained by pressing the chin down toward the chest.

The inion response is essentially the same as the VEMP except that is recorded near the insertion rather than the body of the neck muscles muscle. Thus, it is smaller (several tens of microvolts as compared to 50–200 μV) and has an inverted waveform (negative-positive rather than positive-negative). The inion response likely is a combination of responses from the sternomastoid and the trapezius.

Nature of the VEMP

The amplitude of the sternomastoid VEMP varies with the amount of contraction in the muscle (Colebatch et al., 1994; Lim, Clouston, Sheean, & Yiannikas, 1995). Colebatch and Rothwell (2004) used intramuscular needle electrodes to examine the single motor unit action potentials in the muscle and found a brief period of inhibition during which no action potentials occurred. This had been noted earlier in the early reflex response of the jaw muscles by Meier-Ewert, Gleitsmann, and Reiter (1974). This inhibition occurred at the time of the initial positive wave of the reflex. The most likely reason for this is that the positive waves of the last action potentials before the inhibitory period and the negative waves of the first motor units after it are uncanceled in the average recording (Wit & Kingma, 2006). This is illustrated in Figure 9–6.

Colebatch et al. (1994) described the reflex as occurring only in the sternomastoid muscle ipsilateral to the stimulated ear. Some subsequent studies reported that the reflex was bilateral (e.g., Ferber-Viart et al., 1997; Robertson & Ireland, 1995). The reason for the discrepancy likely was related to the recording montages, the sternal reference picking up activity from both sternomastoid muscles (Li, Houlden, & Tomlinson, 1999). If recorded relative to a distant reference (such as an electrode made by linking the two wrists), an electrode located on the sternum can pick up an inverted version of the sternomastoid response. As briefly reviewed in the earlier section on the EMG, the insertion region of a muscle often shows an electrical response—mainly generated by muscle action potentials reaching the ends of the muscle fibers several milliseconds after they were initiated. This response typically is inverted from that recorded over the belly of the muscle. Thus, if we use a reference near the sternal insertion of the muscles, depending on the type of contraction (which could determine the relative activities of the sternal and clavicular sections of the muscle), we could record what looks like a reflex in a "contralateral" recording. Because the belly of the contralateral muscle is actually silent, the recording subtracts the inverted response of the ipsilateral muscle recorded at the sternum (which serves as a reference for both recordings) from zero to give an apparent contralateral response. The picture likely is further complicated by a small excitatory (rather than inhibitory) contralateral response.

Animal studies of the reflex show a simple disynaptic pathway (Kushiro, Zakir, Ogawa, & Sato, 1999; Uchino et al., 1997). Afferent neurons from the saccule with their cell bodies in Scarpa's ganglion synapse in the vestibular nucleus, where they activate neurons that descend through the obex region of the medulla (the central region where the fourth ventricle narrows to become the central canal of the spinal cord) to inhibit the motor neurons of the spinal accessory nerve (cranial nerve XI), which goes to the sternomastoid muscle. These motor neurons are located in the lateral part of the gray matter of the spinal cord near the junction between the spinal cord and medulla oblongata. The spinal accessory nerve also supplies the upper part of the trapezius muscle. The reflex pathway is illustrated in the central part of Figure 9–9.

The function of this very early inhibitory reflex is not known. The acoustic stimulus is not natural for the otolith receptors in the saccule, which together with those in the vestibule are set up to detect linear acceleration. Movements of the head will cause complicated discharge patterns in neurons activated (or inhibited) by the otolith receptors. Some of these movements will activate reflexes to maintain the orientation of the head and body following sudden movements. Why the VEMP reflex is inhibitory and why ipsilateral is not easy to figure out.

Recording Parameters

The reflex is recorded with an active electrode over the belly of the sternomastoid muscle, halfway between its two insertions (skull and sternum). Some investigators suggest that a larger potential can be recorded by placing the electrode a little higher than the middle of the muscle (Sheykholeslami, Murofushi, & Kaga, 2001). The sternomastoid muscle attaches superiorly to the mastoid and the nuchal line of the skull that goes from the mastoid to the inion, and inferiorly to the upper sternum and the medial part of the clavicle. Because of the attachment to the clavicle, the muscle is also called the sternocleidomastoid. Both sternomastoid muscles can be easily recognized by having the subject push the head forward against resistance. The muscle can be activated on only one side by having the subject push the chin up toward the opposite side. The reference electrode usually is located on the sternum or the ipsilateral clavicle. Large electrodes (with diameters of 1.5 cm or more) generally are used. The large surface area reduces the interelectrode impedance and thus reduces extraneous noise in the recording. It also allows a more even integration of the different motor unit action potentials that contribute to the response. We can use simple disk electrodes held in place by adhesive tape or self-attaching disposable electrodes.

The response can be recorded using a bandpass of 10 to 500 Hz. Many investigators use a higher low-pass cutoff (e.g., 2000 Hz). This is not necessary but it will not increase the noise levels very much since there is little spontaneous activity above 500 Hz. The response will need to be averaged, typically for 50 to 500 trials. The recording sweep needs to be at least 50 ms, and many investigators use 100 ms.

Stimulus Parameters

VEMPs can be evoked by either clicks or brief tones. The clicks are the same 100 µs clicks used for the ABR. The polarity of the click is either rarefaction or alternating. The response occurs only at high intensities; the threshold for eliciting a response (provided there is some reasonable ongoing contraction of the muscle) is between 85 and 90 dB nHL in young adults (Akin, Murnane, & Proffit, 2003; Lim et al., 1995; Welgampola & Colebatch, 2005). The

threshold is increased by about 10 dB in subjects older than 50 years (Welgampola & Colebatch, 2001b). When using the response as a clinical test of vestibular function, one typically uses a set level, such as 95 dB nHL.

The VEMP evoked by brief tones are very similar to those evoked by clicks although the latency is slightly longer. The responses are largest for tones with frequencies near 500 Hz (Akin et al., 2003; Murofushi, Matzusaki, & Wu, 1999; Todd, Cody, & Banks, 2000; Welgampola & Colebatch, 2001a), which is similar to what has been found for auditory-responsive nerve fibers in the inferior vestibular nerve of cats (McCue & Guinan, 1997). Figure 9–10 compares some of these data. This frequency specificity is quite different from the PAM reflex, which has similar amplitudes from 500 to 8000 Hz, with the responses at 1000 and 2000 Hz being slightly larger than at the other frequencies (O'Beirne & Patuzzi, 1999). Brief tones with various rise-times and durations have been used to evoke the VEMP. The optimal stimulus is likely that proposed by Welgampola and Colebatch (2001a): a tone with 7-ms duration and with rise- and fall-times of 2.5 ms each. The average VEMP thresholds for such stimuli are around 115 dB peSPL.

The high thresholds for evoking reflex responses to sound through the vestibular system may be one of the reasons that rock and roll music is played at such high levels. Acoustically evoked sensations of self-motion may contribute to the experience of loud music. This idea may account for the desire of rock fans for the music to reach more than 95 dBA SPL and to be accentuated in the lower frequencies (Todd & Cody, 2000).

Although the VEMP can be recorded at short SOAs (Welgampola & Colebatch, 2001a), it is customary to present the stimuli at rates near 5/s, particularly when

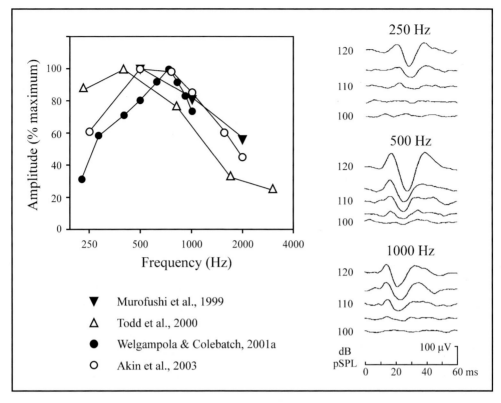

Figure 9–10. *Frequency sensitivity of vestibulocollic reflex. On the left section of the figure are shown data from several studies investigating the effect of tonal frequency on the VEMP amplitude. The maximum amplitude (between 100 and 200 ÌV) occurs at frequencies between 400 and 700 Hz. The right section of the figure shows waveforms from a single subject from Akin et al., 2003. The responses were recorded in 5 dB steps from 120 to 100 dB pSPL. The tones were Blackman gated tones with rise and fall times of 2 cycles each and no plateau. The responses are larger and the thresholds lower at 500 Hz than at the other two frequencies illustrated.*

using stimuli at the higher levels. The stimuli are loud and we should be concerned about possible hair cell damage at rates greater than 10/s. Welgampola and Colebatch (2005) state that the presence of tinnitus is a relative contraindication to click and tone burst VEMP testing. In these subjects, the response may be evoked by bone-conducted stimuli, or galvanic stimulation of the mastoid (Watson & Colebatch, 1998) or skull taps (Welgampola & Colebatch, 2005).

Stimuli presented through bone-conduction evoke reliable VEMPs (Sheyk-holeslami, Kermany, & Kaga, 2001; Sheyk-holeslami, Murofushi, Kermany, & Kaga, 2000). Intriguingly, these stimuli appear to be more effective than air-conducted stimuli, as they evoke responses at lower levels in terms of hearing threshold; the VEMP threshold for bone-conducted stimuli is often near 50 dB nHL (Welgampola & Colebatch, 2005). The response is largest at frequencies near 200 Hz for bone-conducted tones (Sheykholeslami, Kermany, & Kaga, 2001). At frequencies of 200 or 100 Hz, the waveforms suggest that the system responds to both the first and second waves in the tone. The bone-conduction stimulus elicits a bilateral response rather than just an ipsilateral response because the stimulus activates both saccules.

Subject Parameters

The most important subject parameter affecting the VEMP is the level of background EMG activity in the sternomastoid muscle during response recording (Colebatch et al., 1994). The reflex response is linearly related to both the intensity of the sound and the rms level of the EMG level. Li et al. (1995) provide an elegant way of graphing these data as a plane in three-dimensional space. Figure 9–11 replots their data. Because of this relationship, it is essential to ensure that the EMG levels are the same in both muscles when comparing the response between the two sides. Welgampola and Colebatch (2005) have proposed using a "corrected" amplitude —a ratio of the peak-to-peak amplitude of the VEMP divided by the rms value of the

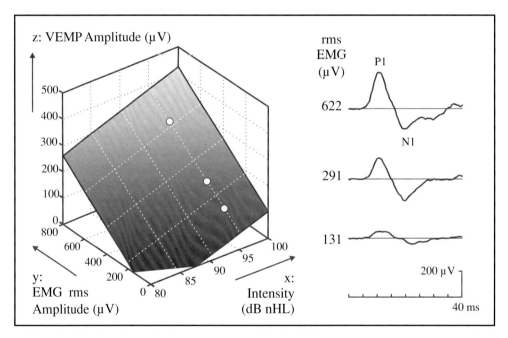

Figure 9–11. Relationship of VEMP to stimulus intensity and background EMG level. The left side of the figure shows the average relationship between the variables according to the equation z = 8.156x + 0.403y − 715 where z is the P1-N1 peak-peak VEMP amplitude, x is the click intensity in dB nHL, and y is the prestimulus EMG root-mean-square (rms) amplitude. The amplitude of the VEMP is shown by the plane that follows this relationship; the shading is such that greater amplitudes are shown by a lighter gray. The dashed lines on the plane show the intensities and the EMG levels. The threshold for recognizing a response occurs on the lower edge of the plane (where the response reaches zero). The graph has been replotted using the published values in Lim et al (1995) On the right are shown responses to a 95 dB nHL click recorded with three different levels of prestimulus EMG. The locations of these responses on the three-dimensional graph are shown by the circles. The VEMP waveforms have been replotted from Lim et al (1995).

tonic background EMG. The usual values are between 0.5 and 3.0 (actual amplitudes 25 to 297 µV).

Every laboratory will use its own technique for having the subject maintain a constant level of background EMG activity. Probably the most common technique is to have the subject lay on the back and raise the head off the bed to an angle of about 30°. The instructions for this are simple and the maneuver activates both sternomastoids equally. This also allows the response to be recorded simultaneously in each muscle to bilateral stimulation, which gives two parallel ipsilateral responses (Huang, Cheng, & Su, 2006; Jacobson & McCaslin, 2007). Other techniques are to have a sitting subject press their forehead against a pressure transducer or their chin down against a chin rest. Maximum muscle exertion would occur when a reclining subject held the head up off the bed and simultaneously turned the head to the other side against a pressure transducer.

The VEMP can be recorded at all ages. In neonates, the response is smaller than in adults and more variable but still easily recorded (Sheykholeslami, Kaga, Megerian, & Arnold, 2005). In elderly subjects, the response has a longer latency, a smaller amplitude, and an increased threshold (Welgampola & Colebatch, 2001a; Zapala & Brey, 2004).

Response Measurements

The main measurements for the response are the amplitudes and latencies of the two peaks P1 and N1. There are later waves in the response but these may be related more to cochlear processing than to vestibular processing and are usually ignored. Table 9–2 provides data from several studies.

Because the most important measurement is the comparison between the sides, Welgampola and Colebatch (2005) propose an "asymmetry ratio"—the absolute difference in amplitude between the two sides divided by the sum of the amplitudes for the two sides and expressed as a percentage. We should remember that this asymmetry is between two ipsilateral reflex recordings (and not between the responses recorded on the two sides for one reflex). In normal subjects, this asymmetry is generally less than 40% provided of course that the amount of ongoing background activity in the two muscles is similar (Welgampola & Colebatch, 2001b). One way to compensate for the differences in background EMG activity is to determine the asymmetry ratio on the basis of the "corrected" amplitudes, the peak-to-peak response amplitudes as a ratio of the mean rectified rms EMG preceding the response (Welgampola & Colebatch, 2001b).

Clinical Applications

The main clinical application of the response is to demonstrate decreased vestibular function in disorders such as Ménière's disease, vestibular neuritis, and acoustic neuroma. By testing otolith function, the VEMP is complementary to caloric testing, which examines the semicircular canals. Zapala and Brey (2004) have reported that, in detecting unilateral vestibular abnormalities, the test has a specificity of 93% and a sensitivity of 52%. These results are similar to those obtained with caloric testing. However, because the two techniques evaluate different vestibular functions, the results are better when both techniques are used together to give a specificity of 89% and a sensitivity of 81%.

Table 9–2. Normal Latencies and Amplitudes of Human Sternomastoid VEMP*

Study	Stimulus	P1 Latency (ms)	N1 Latency (ms)	P1-N1 Amplitude (μV)
Colebatch et al., 1994	Monaural 95 dB nHL click 3/s	13.3 ± 1.5	22.6 ± 2.4	85
Robertson and Ireland, 1995	Monaural 100 dB nHL click 3/s	14.6 ± 2.0	21.3 ± 1.6	10 ± 6
Li et al., 1999	Monaural 95 dB nHL click 9.75/s	11.7 ± 0.7	20.2 ± 1.9	123 ± 51
Welgampola and Colebatch, 2001a	Monaural 123 dB peSPL 500-Hz 7-ms tones 5/s	12.3 ± 1.4	21.4 ± 1.7	91
Zappala and Brey, 2004	Monaural 90 dB nHL 250 Hz 8-ms tones 5.1/s	16.9 ± 1.4	25.2 ± 1.6	181 ± 120
McCaslin and Jacobson, 2007	Monaural 95 dB nHL click 8/s	12.2 ± 2.8	18.6 ± 2.4	103 ± 71

*Values presented as means and standard deviations (where available). Latencies measured at the peak. Amplitudes vary with the amount of ongoing EMG activity in the muscle (see Figure 9–11). Robertson and Ireland did not have their subjects actively contract the muscle.

Although the most common abnormality of the vestibular system results in decreased responsiveness, one disorder results in hypersensitivity. When the temporal bone over the superior semicircular canal is eroded, the resultant superior canal dehiscence creates a "third window," making the labyrinth hypersensitive to sounds. The patients experience vertigo and oscillopsia in response to loud sounds (Tullio phenomenon). These patients have large VEMPs on the side of the lesion with VEMP thresholds that are significantly lower than normal (Colebatch et al., 1998; Struebel, Cremer, Carey, Weg, & Minor, 2001). The final diagnosis requires high-resolution CT scans to demonstrate the dehiscence.

Other uses of the test are reviewed in Welgampola and Colebatch (2005) and discussed further in Chapter 14 of this book. The VEMP is a simple and inexpensive clinical test that does not involve significant patient discomfort and provides important clinical information in patients with vestibular and neurologic disorders.

OTHER ACOUSTIC REFLEXES

We have already mentioned the jaw reflex in our discussion of the mechanisms for the VEMP. This is a transient inhibition in the muscles of the jaw (the masseter and the temporalis) following a loud sound (Deriu et al., 1997; Meier-Ewert et al., 1974). The early part of this reflex, composed of a positive wave at 11 ms and a negative wave at 23 ms, is vestibular in origin.

The startle reflex is a set of motor responses that occur following sudden intense and unexpected stimuli, typically auditory. The reflex consists of a patterned set of bilateral muscle contractions that occur rapidly following the sound, but at latencies significantly longer than we have been considering for the PAM response or the VEMP. In human subjects, the eyes close, the neck muscles tense, the arms flex, the back arches dorsally, the abdominal muscles tense, and the legs flex. Yeomans, Li, Scott, and Franklin (2002) suggest that this is a protective reflex to a sudden blow to the head or the body. The response receives its auditory input from the nuclei of the lateral lemniscus, is organized in the caudal pontine reticular formation, and sends its output to the body through the reticulospinal tract (Davis, Gendelman, Tischler, & Gendelman, 1982). This is illustrated in the bottom section of Figure 9–9. The late components of the VEMP likely represent bilateral startle responses in the neck muscles. The startle reflex is increased in patients with several myoclonic and epileptic syndromes (Wilkins, Hallett, & Wess, 1986). The most reliable part of the startle response is the acoustic blink (Blumenthal et al., 2005). This bilateral response in the orbicularis oculi muscles begins at around 40 ms. The startle blink reflex usually is elicited by brief broadband noise stimuli of high intensity. Table 9–3 compares the startle reflex to the PAM reflex and the VEMP.

Welgampola, Migliaccio, Myrie, Minor, and Carey (2009) have shown that early responses recorded near the eyes to loud low-frequency sounds likely represent activity in the extra-ocular muscles as part of the vestibulo-ocular reflex, perhaps mediated through the superior semicircular canal. This is part of the same reflex as is evaluated using caloric testing.

CONCLUSIONS

The MLR has proven itself useful in many ways. The MLR is a reasonable way to assess hearing thresholds in an awake or lightly sleeping subject. When used for objective audiometry, it should be recorded using a high-pass filter setting that allows the ABR to be measured concomitantly. In this context, we should consider the PAM reflex as a helpful adjunct because it also assesses the function of the cochlea (and can do this more rapidly because of its large size). The cerebral MLR may become helpful in evaluating the function of the

Table 9–3. Sound-Evoked Muscle Reflexes

	PAM Reflex	*Sternomastoid VEMP*	*Startle Blink*
Receptor	cochlea	saccule	cochlea and saccule
Threshold	20 dB nHL	85 dB nHL	70 dB nHL
Main Variable	direction of gaze	contraction of muscle	state of arousal
Laterality	bilateral	unilateral	bilateral
Mechanism	excitatory	inhibitory	excitatory
Onset Latency	9 ms	10 ms	40 ms

auditory cortex but much more work is needed to determine the optimal recording techniques (topography and source analysis) and to delineate the limits of normal for this response at different ages. The MLR provides information about the depth of anesthesia, by evaluating cortical responsiveness. In this use, the PAM reflex is a nuisance and MLR recordings should be obtained using an inion reference. Although helpful in evaluating awareness, the MLR may not indicate the level of unconscious muscle responsiveness. Anesthesia is a multidimensional state and no single measurement will suffice its full assessment. The VEMP has become an important clinical test of the function of the otolith receptors in the saccule. It is now a necessary complement to caloric testing of the semicircular canals in the evaluation of vestibular function. As cerebral response and muscle reflex— as brain and brawn together—the MLR therefore is a full citizen of the EP world.

ABBREVIATIONS

ABR	Auditory brainstem response
ASSR	Auditory steady-state response
EEG	Electroencephalography
EMG	Electromyography
EP	Evoked potential
LAEP	Late auditory evoked potential
MEG	Magnetoencephalography
MLR	Middle-latency response
nHL	Normal hearing level
NMJ	Neuromuscular junction

PAM	Postauricular muscle
rms	Root-mean-square
SOA	Stimulus onset asynchrony
VEMP	Vestibular evoked myogenic potential

REFERENCES

Adler, L. E., Pachtman, E., Franks, R. D., Pecevich, M., Waldo, M. C., & Freedman, R. (1982). Neurophysiological evidence for a defect in neuronal mechanisms involved in sensory gating in schizophrenia. *Biological Psychiatry, 17*, 639–654.

Agung, K., Purdy, S. C., Patuzzim, R. B., O'Beirne, G. A., & Newall, P. (2005). Rising-frequency chirps and earphones with an extended high-frequency response enhance the post-auricular muscle response. *International Journal of Audiology. 44*, 631–636.

Akin, F. W., Murnane, O. D., & Proffitt, T. M. (2004). The effects of click and tone-burst stimulus parameters on the vestibular evoked myogenic potential (VEMP). *Journal of the American Academy of Audiology, 14*, 500–509.

Amenedo, E., & Díaz, F. (1998). Effects of aging on middle-latency auditory evoked potentials: A cross-sectional study. *Biological Psychiatry, 43*, 210–219.

Avidan, M. S., Zhang, L., Burnside, B. A., Finkel, K. J., Searleman, A. C., Selvidge, J. A., . . . Evers, A. S. (2008). Anesthesia awareness and the bispectral index. *New England Journal of Medicine, 358*, 1097–1108.

Bell, S. L., Smith, D. C., Allen, R., & Lutman, M. E. (2004). Recording the middle latency response of the auditory evoked potential as a measure of depth of anaesthesia: A technical note. *British Journal of Anaesthesia, 92*, 442–445.

Bell, S. L., Smith, D. C., Allen, R., & Lutman, M. E. (2006). The auditory middle latency response, evoked using maximum length sequences and chirps, as an indicator of adequacy of anesthesia. *Anesthesia and Analgesia, 102*, 495–498.

Bickford, R. G., Jacobson, J. L., & Cody, D. T. (1964). Nature of average evoked potentials to sound and other stimuli in man. *Annals of the New York Academy of Sciences, 112*, 204–223.

Blumenthal, T. D., Cuthbert, B. N., Filion, D. L., Hackley, S., Lipp, O. V., & van Boxtel, A. (2005). Guidelines for human startle eyeblink electromyographic studies. *Psychophysiology, 42*, 1–15.

Borgmann, C., Ross, B., Draganova, R., & Pantev, C. (2001). Human auditory middle latency responses: Influence of stimulus type and intensity. *Hearing Research, 158*, 57–64.

Boutros, N. N., Belger, A., Campbell, D., D'Souza, C., & Krystal, J. (1999). Comparison of four components of sensory gating in schizophrenia and normal subjects: A preliminary report. *Psychiatry Research, 88*, 119–130.

Brockhaus-Dumke, A., Schultze-Lutter, F., Mueller, R., Tendolkar, I., Bechdolf, A., Pukrop, R., . . . Ruhrmann, S. (2008). Sensory gating in schizophrenia: P50 and N100 gating in antipsychotic-free subjects at risk, first-episode, and chronic patients. *Biological Psychiatry, 64*, 376–384.

Bruhn, J., Myles, P. S., Sneyd, R., & Struys, M. M. (2006). Depth of anaesthesia monitoring: What's available, what's validated and what's next? *British Journal of Anaesthesia, 97*, 85–94.

Brunner, M. D., Nel, M. R., Fernandes, R., Thornton, C., & Newton, D. E. (2002). Auditory evoked response during propofol anaesthesia after pre-induction with midazolam. *British Journal of Anaesthesia, 89*, 325–327.

Buchwald, J. S., Erwin, R. J., Read, S., Van Lancker, D., & Cummings, J. L. (1989). Mid-latency auditory evoked responses: differential abnormality of P1 in Alzheimer's disease. *Electroencephalography and Clinical Neurophysiology, 74*, 378–384.

Buffin, J. T., Connell, J. A., & Stamp, J. M. (1977). The post-auricular muscle response in children. *Journal of Laryngology and Otology*, 91, 1047–1062.

Cacace, A. T., & McFarland, D.J. (2009). Middle latency auditory evoked potentials. In J. Katz (Ed.), *Handbook of clinical audiology* (6th ed., pp. 373–394). Baltimore, MD: Lippincott Williams & Wilkins.

Cacace, A. T, Satya-Murti, S., & Wolpaw, J. R. (1990). Human middle-latency auditory evoked potentials: Vertex and temporal components. *Electroencephalography and Clinical Neurophysiology, 77*, 6–18.

Cancelli, I., Cadore, I. P., Merlino, G., Valentinis, L., Moratti, U., Bergonzi, P., . . . Valente, M. (2006). Sensory gating deficit assessed by P50/Pb middle latency event related potential in Alzheimer's disease. *Journal of Clinical Neurophysiology, 23*, 421–425.

Cardenas, V. A., Gerson, J., & Fein, G. (1993). The reliability of P50 suppression as measured by the conditioning/testing ratio is vastly improved by dipole modeling. *Biological Psychiatry, 33*, 335–344.

Clementz, B. A., Geyer, M. A., & Braff, D. L. (1998). Poor P50 suppression among schizophrenia patients and their first-degree biological relatives. *American Journal of Psychiatry, 155*, 1691–1694.

Cody, D. T. R., & Bickford, R. G. (1969). Averaged evoked myogenic responses in normal man. *Laryngoscope, 79*, 400–416.

Colebatch, J. G., Day, B. L., Bronstein, A. M., Davies, R. A., Gresty, M. A., Luxon, L. M., & Rothwell, J. C. (1998). Vestibular hypersensitivity to clicks is characteristic of the Tullio phenomenon. *Journal of Neurology, Neurosurgery and Psychiatry, 65*, 670–678.

Colebatch, J. G., Halmagyi, G. M., & Skuse, N. F. (1994). Myogenic potentials generated by a click evoked vestibulocollic reflex. *Journal of Neurology, Neurosurgery and Psychiatry, 57*, 190–197.

Colebatch, J. G., & Rothwell, J. C. (2004). Motor unit excitability changes mediating vestibulocollic reflexes in the sternocleidomastoid muscle. *Clinical Neurophysiology, 115*, 2567–2573.

Davis, M., Gendelman, D. S., Tischler, M. D., & Gendelman, P. M. (1982). A primary acoustic startle circuit: Lesion and stimulation studies. *Journal of Neuroscience, 2,* 791–805.

Delgado, R. E, & Özdamar, O. (2004). Deconvolution of evoked responses obtained at high stimulus rates. *Journal of the Acoustical Society of America, 115,* 1242–1251.

Deriu, F., Ortu, E., Capobianco, S., Giaconi, E., Melis, F., Aiello, E., . . . Tolu, E. (2007). Origin of sound-evoked EMG responses in human masseter muscles. *Journal of Physiology, 580,* 195–209.

Ferber-Viart, C., Duclaux, R., Colleaux, B., & Dubreuil, C. (1997). Myogenic vestibular-evoked potentials in normal subjects: A comparison between responses obtained from sternomastoid and trapezius muscles. *Acta Otolaryngologica, 117,* 472–481

Freedman, R., Adler, L. E., Waldo, M. C., Pachtman, E., & Franks, R. D. (1983). Neurophysiological evidence for a defect in inhibitory pathways in schizophrenia: Comparison of medicated and drug-free patients. *Biological Psychiatry, 18,* 537–551.

Freedman, R., Coon, H., Myles-Worsley, M., Orr-Urtreger, A., Olincy, A., Davis, A., . . . Byerley, W. (1997). Linkage of a neurophysiological deficit in schizophrenia to a chromosome 15 locus. *Proceedings of the National Academy of Sciences, USA, 94,* 587–592.

Gajraj, R. J., Doi, M., Mantzardis, H., & Kenny, G. N. C. (1998). Analysis of the EEG bispectrum, auditory evoked potentials and the EEG power spectrum during repeated transitions from consciousness to unconsciousness. *British Journal of Anaesthesia, 80,* 46–52.

Geisler, C. D., Frishkopf, L. S., & Rosenblith, W. A. (1958). Extracranial responses to acoustic clicks in man. *Science, 128,* 1210–1211.

Gelfand, S. A. (2009). The acoustic reflex. In J. Katz (Ed.), *Handbook of clinical audiology* (6th ed., pp. 189–221). Baltimore, MD: Lippincott Williams & Wilkins.

Ghisolfi, E. S., Margis, R., Becker, J., Zanardo, A. P., Strimitzer, I. M., & Lara, D. R. (2004). Impaired P50 sensory gating in post-traumatic stress disorder secondary to urban violence. *International Journal of Psychophysiology, 51,* 209–214.

Gibson, W. P. R. (1978). The myogenic (sonomotor) responses. In W. P. R. Gibson, *Essentials of clinical electric response audiometry* (pp. 133–156). New York, NY: Churchill-Livingston.

Golob, E. J., Irimajiri, R., & Starr, A. (2007). Auditory cortical activity in amnestic mild cognitive impairment: Relationship to subtype and conversion to dementia. *Brain, 130,* 740–752.

Golob, E. J., Johnson, J. K., & Starr, A. (2002). Auditory event-related potentials during target detection are abnormal in mild cognitive impairment. *Clinical Neurophysiology, 113,* 151–161.

Hackley, S. A., Woldorff, M., & Hillyard, S. A. (1987). Combined use of microreflexes and event-related brain potentials as measures of auditory selective attention. *Psychophysiology, 24,* 632–647.

Harker, L. A., Hosick, E., Voots, R. J. & Mendel, M. I. (1977). Influence of succinylcholine on middle component auditory evoked potentials. *Archives of Otolaryngology, 103,* 133–137.

Huang, T.-W., Cheng, P.-W., & Su, H.-C. (2006). The influence of unilateral versus bilateral clicks on the vestibular-evoked myogenic potentials. *Otology and Neurotology, 27,* 193–196.

Jacobson, G. P., & McCaslin, D. L. (2007) The vestibular evoked myogenic potential and other sonomotor evoked potentials. In R. F. Burkard, M. Don, & J. J. Eggermont (Eds), *Auditory evoked potentials: Basic principles and clinical applications* (pp. 572–598). Baltimore, MD: Lippincott Williams & Wilkins.

Jerger, J., Chmiel, R., Glaze, D., & Frost, J. D., Jr. (1987). Rate and filter dependence of the middle-latency response in infants. *Audiology, 26,* 269–283.

Jones, L.A., & Baxter, R. J. (1988). Changes in the auditory middle latency responses during all-night sleep recording. *British Journal of Audiology, 22,* 279–285.

Junius, D., Riedel, H., & Kollmeier, B. (2007). The influence of externalization and spatial cues on the generation of auditory brainstem responses and middle latency responses. *Hearing Research, 225,* 91–104.

Kiang, N. Y., Crist, A. H., French, M. A., & Edwards, A. G., (1963). Postauricular electrical response to acoustic stimuli in humans. *Massachusetts Institute of Technology Quarterly Progress Report, 68*, 218–225.

Kileny, P., Dobson, D., & Gelfand, E. T. (1983). Middle-latency auditory evoked responses during open-heart surgery with hypothermia. *Electroencephalography and Clinical Neurophysiology, 55*, 268–276.

Kileny, P., Paccioretti, D., & Wilson, A. F. (1987). Effects of cortical lesions on middle-latency auditory evoked responses (MLR). *Electroencephalography and Clinical Neurophysiology, 66*, 108–120.

Kochs, E., Kalkman, C. J., Thornton, C., Newton, D., Bischoff, P., Kuppe, H., . . . Stockmanns, G. (1999). Middle latency auditory evoked responses and electroencephalographic derived variables do not predict movement to noxious stimulation during 1 minimum alveolar anesthetic concentration isoflurane/nitrous oxide anesthesia. *Anesthesia and Analgesia, 88*, 1412–1417.

Kochs, E., Stockmanns, G., Thornton, C., Nahm, W., & Kalkman, C. J. (2001). Wavelet analysis of middle latency auditory evoked responses: Calculation of an index for detection of awareness during propofol administration. *Anesthesiology, 95*, 1141–1150.

Korzyukov, O., Pflieger, M. E., Wagner, M., Bowyer, S. M., Rosburg, T., Sundaresan, K., . . . Boutros, N. N. (2007). Generators of the intracranial P50 response in auditory sensory gating. *NeuroImage, 35*, 814–826.

Kraus, N., Özdamar, Ö., Hier, D., & Stein, L. (1982) Auditory middle latency responses (MLRs) in patients with cortical lesions. *Electroencephalography and Clinical Neurophysiology, 54*, 275–287.

Kushiro, K., Zakir, M., Ogawa, Y., & Sato, H. (1999). Saccular and utricular inputs to sternocleidomastoid motoneurons of decerebrate cats. *Experimental Brain Research, 126*, 410–416.

Leavitt, V. M., Molholm, S., Ritte, W., Shpaner, M., & Foxe, J. J. (2007). Auditory processing in schizophrenia during the middle latency period (10–50 ms): High-density electrical mapping and source analysis reveal subcortical antecedents to early cortical deficits. *Journal of Psychiatry and Neuroscience, 32*, 339–353.

Li, M. W., Houlden, D., & Tomlinson, R. D. (1999). Click evoked EMG responses in sternocleidomastoid muscles: Characteristics in normal subjects. *Journal of Vestibular Research, 9*, 327–334.

Liebenthal, E., & Pratt, H. (1999). Human auditory cortex electrophysiological correlates of the precedence effect: Binaural echo lateralization suppression. *Journal of the Acoustical Society of America, 106*, 291–303.

Lijffijt, M., Moeller, F. G., Boutros, N. N., Steinberg, J. L., Meier, S. L. Lane, S. D., & Swann, A. C. (2009). Diminished P50, N100 and P200 auditory sensory gating in bipolar I disorder. *Psychiatry Research, 167*, 191–201.

Lim, C. L., Clouston, P., Sheean, G., & Yiannikas, C. (1995). The influence of voluntary EMG and click intensity on the vestibular click evoked myogenic potential. *Muscle and Nerve, 18*, 1210–1213.

Madell, J. R., & Goldstein, R. (1972). Relation between loudness and the amplitude of the early components of the averaged electroencephalic response. *Journal of Speech and Hearing Research, 15*, 134–141.

Maurizi, M., Ottaviani, F., Paludetti, G., Rosignoli, M., Almadori, G., & Tassoni, A. (1984). Middle-latency auditory components in response to clicks and low- and middle-frequency tone pips (0.5–1 kHz). *Audiology, 23*, 569–580.

McCaslin, D. L. Jacobson, G. P., & Harry,T. (2008). The recordability of two sonomotor responses in young normal subjects *Journal of the American Academy of Audiology, 19*, 542–547

McCue, M. P., & Guinan, J. J., Jr. (1997). Sound-evoked activity in primary afferent neurons of a mammalian vestibular system. *American Journal of Otology, 18*, 355–360.

McGee, T., Kraus, N., Killion, M., Rosenberg, R., & King, C. (1993). Improving the reliability of the auditory middle latency response by monitoring EEG delta activity. *Ear and Hearing, 14*, 76–84.

McPherson, D. L. & Starr, A. (1993). Binaural interaction in auditory evoked potentials: Brainstem, middle- and long-latency components. *Hearing Research, 66,* 91–98.

Meier-Ewert, K., Gleitsmann, K., & Reiter, F. (1974). Acoustic jaw reflex in man: Its relationship to other brainstem and microreflexes. *Electroencephalography and Clinical Neurophysiology, 36,* 629–637.

Millan, J., Ozdamar, O., & Bohórquez, J. (2006). Acquisition and analysis of high rate deconvolved auditory evoked potentials during sleep. *Conference Proceedings of IEEE Engineering in Medicine and Biology Society, 1,* 4987–4990.

Murofushi, T., Matsuzaki, M., & Wu, C. H. (1999). Short tone burst-evoked myogenic potentials on the sternocleidomastoid muscle: Are these potentials also of vestibular origin? *Archives of Otolaryngology-Head and Neck Surgery, 125,* 660–664.

O'Beirne, G. A., & Patuzzi, R. B. (1999). Basic properties of the sound-evoked post-auricular muscle response (PAMR). *Hearing Research, 138,* 115–132.

Onitsuka, T., Ninomiya, H., Sato, E., Yamamoto, T., & Tashiro, N. (2000). The effect of interstimulus intervals and between-block rests on the auditory evoked potential and magnetic field: Is the auditory P50 in humans an overlapping potential? *Clinical Neurophysiology, 111,* 237–245.

Osterhammel, P. A., Shallop, J. K., & Terkildsen, K. (1985). The effect of sleep on the auditory brainstem response (ABR) and the middle latency response (MLR). *Scandinavian Audiology, 14,* 47–50.

Pantev, C., Bertrand, O., Eulitz, C., Verkindt, C., Hampson, S., Schuierer, G., & Elbert, T. (1995). Specific tonotopic organizations of different areas of the human auditory cortex revealed by simultaneous magnetic and electric recordings. *Electroencephalography and Clinical Neurophysiology, 94,* 26–40.

Patterson, J. V., Hetrick ,W. P., Boutros, N. N., Jin, Y., Sandman, C., Stern, H., . . . Bunney, W. E., Jr. (2008). P50 sensory gating ratios in schizophrenics and controls: A review and data analysis. *Psychiatry Research, 158,* 226–247.

Patuzzi, R. B., & O'Beirne, G. A. (1999a). Effects of eye rotation on the sound-evoked post-auricular muscle response (PAMR). *Hearing Research, 138,* 133–146.

Patuzzi, R. B., & O'Beirne, G. A. (1999b). A correlation method for detecting the sound-evoked post-auricular muscle response (PAMR). *Hearing Research, 138,* 147–162.

Pelizzone, M., Hari, R., Mäkelä, J. P., Huttunen, J., Ahlfors, S., & Hämäläinen, M. (1987). Cortical origin of middle-latency auditory evoked responses in man. *Neuroscience Letters, 82,* 303–307.

Phillips, N. A., Connolly, J. F., Mate-Kole, C. C., & Gray, J. (1997). Individual differences in auditory middle latency responses in elderly adults and patients with Alzheimer's disease. *International Journal of Psychophysiology, 27,* 125–136.

Picton, T. W., Champagne, S. C., & Kellett, A. J. C. (1992) Auditory evoked potentials recorded using maximum length sequences. *Electroencephalography and Clinical Neurophysiology, 84,* 90–100.

Picton, T. W., & Hillyard, S. A. (1974). Human auditory evoked potentials. II Effects of attention. *Electroencephalography and Clinical Neurophysiology, 36,* 191–200.

Picton, T. W., Hillyard, S. A., Krausz, H. I., & Galambos, R. (1974). Human auditory evoked potentials I: Evaluation of components. *Electroencephalography and Clinical Neurophysiology, 36,* 179–190.

Picton, T. W., John M. S., Purcell, D. W., & Plourde, G. (2003). Human auditory steady-state responses: effects of recording technique and state of arousal. *Anesthesia and Analgesia, 97,* 1396–1402.

Picton, T. W., & Ross, B. (2010). Physiological measurements of human binaural processing. In J. Buchholz, T. Dau, T. Poulsen, & J. Dalsgaard-Christensen (Eds.). *Binaural processing and spatial hearing. 2nd International Symposium on Auditory and Audiological Research (ISAAR 2009),* Copenhagen, Denmark: Centertryk A/S.

Picton, T. W., Woods, D. L., Baribeau-Braun, J., & Healey, T. M. G. (1977). Evoked potential audiometry. *Journal of Otolaryngology, 6,* 90–119.

Plourde, G. B. (2006). Auditory evoked potentials. *Best Practice and Research in Clinical Anaesthesiology, 20,* 129–139.

Potter, D., Summerfelt, A., Gold, J., & Buchanan, R.W. (2006). Review of clinical correlates of P50 sensory gating abnormalities in patients with schizophrenia. *Schizophrenia Bulletin, 32,* 692–700.

Purdy, S. C., Agung, K. B., Hartley, D., Patuzzi, R. B., & O'Beirne, G. A. (2005). The post-auricular muscle response: An objective electrophysiological method for evaluating hearing sensitivity. *International Journal of Audiology, 44,* 625–630.

Robertson, D. D., & Ireland, D. J. (1995). Vestibular evoked myogenic potentials. *Journal of Otolaryngology, 24,* 3–8.

Robinson, K., & Rudge, P. (1977). Abnormalities of the auditory evoked potentials in patients with multiple sclerosis. *Brain, 100,* 19–40.

Ruhm, H., Walker, E. Jr., & Flanigin, H. (1967). Acoustically-evoked potentials in man: Mediation of early components. *Laryngoscope, 77,* 806–822.

Scherg, M., & von Cramon, D. (1990). Dipole source potentials of the auditory cortex in normal subjects and in patients with temporal lobe lesions. In F. Grandori, M. Hoke & G.L. Romani (Eds.), *Auditory evoked magnetic fields and electric potentials. Advances in Audiology* (Vol. 6, pp. 165–193). Basel, Switzerland: Karger.

Sheykholeslami, K., Kaga, K., Megerian, C. A., & Arnold, J. E. (2005). Vestibular-evoked myogenic potentials in infancy and early childhood. *Laryngoscope, 115,* 1440–1444.

Sheykholeslami, K., Kermany, M., & Kaga, K. (2001). Frequency sensitivity range of the saccule to bone-conducted stimuli measured by vestibular evoked myogenic potentials. *Hearing Research, 160,* 58–62.

Sheykholeslami, K., Murofushi, T., & Kaga, K. (2001). The effect of sternocleidomastoid electrode location on vestibular evoked myogenic potential. *Auris Nasus Larynx, 28,* 41–43.

Sheykholeslami, K., Murofushi, T., Kermany, M. H., & Kaga, K. (2000). Bone-conducted evoked myogenic potentials from the sternocleidomastoid muscle. *Acta Otolaryngologica, 120,* 731–734.

Siegel, C., Waldo, M.. Mizner, G., Adler, L. E.; & Freedman, R. (1984). Deficits in sensory gating in schizophrenic patients and their relatives. *Archives of General Psychiatry, 41,* 607–612.

Sollers, J. J., & Hackley, S. A. (1997). Effects of foreperiod duration on reflexive and voluntary responses to intense noise bursts. *Psychophysiology, 34,* 518–526.

Streletz, L. J., Katz, L., Hohenberger, M., & Cracco, R. Q. (1977). Scalp recorded auditory evoked potentials and sonomotor responses: An evaluation of components and recording techniques. *Electroencephalography and Clinical Neurophysiology, 43,* 192–206.

Streubel, S. O., Cremer, P. D., Carey, J. P., Weg, N., & Minor, L. B. (2001). Vestibular evoked myogenic potentials in the diagnosis of superior canal dehiscence syndrome. *Acta Otolaryngologica Supplement, 545,* 41–49.

Thornton, A. R. D. (1975). The use of post-auricular muscle responses. *Journal of Laryngology and Otology, 89,* 997–1010.

Thornton, A. R., Mendel, M. I., & Anderson, C. V. (1977). Effects of stimulus frequency and intensity on the middle components of the averaged auditory encephalic response. *Journal of Speech and Hearing Research, 20,* 81–94.

Thornton, C., Barrowcliffe, M. P., Konieczko, K. M., Ventham, P., Dore, C., & Newton, D. E. F. (1989). The auditory evoked response as an indicator of awareness. *British Journal of Anaesthesia, 63,* 113–115.

Thornton, C., & Newton, D. E. F. (1989). The auditory evoked response: A measure of depth of anaesthesia. *Balliere's Clinical Anaesthesiology, 3,* 559–585.

Thornton, C., & Sharpe, R. M. (1998) Evoked responses in anaesthesia. *British Journal of Anaesthesia, 81,* 771–781.

Todd N. P., & Cody, F. W. (2000). Vestibular responses to loud dance music: A physiological basis of the "rock and roll threshold"? *Journal of the Acoustical Society of America, 107*, 496–500.

Todd, N. P, Cody, F. W., & Banks, J. R. (2000). A saccular origin of frequency tuning in myogenic vestibular evoked potentials? Implications for human responses to loud sounds. *Hearing Research, 152*, 173–175.

Tooley, M. A., Stapleton, C. L., Greenslade, G. L., & Prys-Roberts, C. (2004). Mid-latency auditory evoked response during propofol and alfentanil anaesthesia. *British Journal of Anaesthesia, 92*, 25–32.

Townsend, G. L., & Cody, D. T. R. (1971). The averaged inion response evoked by acoustic stimulation: its relation to the saccule. *Annals of Otology, Rhinology and Laryngology, 80*, 121–131.

Uchino, Y., Sato, H., Sasaki, M., Imagawa, M., Ikegami, H., Isu, N., & Graf, W. (1997). Saculocollic reflex arcs in cats. *Journal of Neurophysiology, 77*, 3003–3012.

Waldo, M., & Freedman, R. (1986). Gating of auditory evoked responses in normal college students. *Psychiatry Research, 19*, 233–239.

Watson, S. R., & Colebatch, J. G. (1998). Vestibulocollic reflexes evoked by short duration galvanic stimulation in man. *Journal of Physiology, 513*, 587–597.

Welgampola, M. S., & Colebatch, J. G. (2001a) Characteristics of tone burst-evoked myogenic potentials in the sternocleidomastoid muscles. *Otology and Neuro-Otology, 22*, 796–802.

Welgampola, M. S., & Colebatch, J. G. (2001b) Vestibulocollic reflexes: normal values and the effect of age. *Clinical Neurophysiology, 112*, 1971–1979.

Welgampola, M. S., & Colebatch, J. G. (2005). Characteristics and clinical applications of vestibular-evoked myogenic potentials. *Neurology, 64*, 1682–1688.

Welgampola, M. S., Migliaccio, A. A., Myrie, O. A., Minor, L. B., & Carey, J. P. (2009). The human sound-evoked vestibulo-ocular reflex and its electromyographic correlate. *Clinical Neurophysiology, 120*, 158–166.

Wilkins, D. E., Hallett, M., & Wess, M. M. (1986). Audiogenic startle reflex of man and its relationship to startle syndromes. A review. *Brain, 109*, 561–573.

Wit, H. P., & Kingma, C. M. (2006). A simple model for the generation of the vestibular evoked myogenic potential (VEMP). *Clinical Neurophysiology, 117*, 1354–1358.

Woldorff, M. G., Gallen, C. C., Hampson, S. A., Hillyard, S. A., Pantev, C., Sobel, D., & Bloom, F. E. (1993). Modulation of early sensory processing in human auditory cortex during auditory selective attention. *Proceedings of the National Academy of Sciences, USA, 90*, 8722–8726.

Woldorff, M. G., & Hillyard, S. A. (1991). Modulation of early auditory processing during selective listening to rapidly presented tones. *Electroencephalography and Clinical Neurophysiology, 79*, 170–191.

Woods, D. L., Alain, C., Covarrubias, D., & Zaidel, O. (1995). Middle latency auditory evoked potentials to tones of different frequency. *Hearing Research, 85*, 69–75.

Woods, D. L., & Clayworth, C. C. (1986): Age-related changes in human middle latency auditory evoked potentials. *Electroencephalography and Clinical Neurophysiology, 65*, 297–303.

Yeomans, J. S., Li, L., Scott, B. W., & Frankland, P. W. (2002). Tactile, acoustic and vestibular systems sum to elicit the startle reflex. *Neuroscience and Biobehavioral Reviews, 26*, 1–11.

Yoshie, N., & Okudaira, T., (1969). Myogenic evoked potential responses to clicks in man. *Acta Otolaryngologica Supplement, 252*, 89–103.

Zapala, D. A., & Brey, R. H. (2004). Clinical experience with the vestibular evoked myogenic potential. *Journal of the American Academy of Audiology, 15*, 198–215.

10

Auditory Steady-State and Following Responses: Dancing to the Rhythms

Hay quien baila al son que le tocan, quien baila al suyo solamento, y quien no baila de ninguna manera.

(There are those who dance to the rhythm played to them, those who only dance to their own rhythm, and those who do not dance at all.)

José Bergamin, *El Cohete y la Estrella* (The Rocket and the Star), 1923

The brain is full of rhythms. Some dance to the music of external stimuli, others generate themselves, and others disappear when a stimulus occurs. This chapter deals with those that follow the frequencies of external sounds. Because they are both initiated by and composed of rhythms, these following responses usually are evaluated in the frequency domain rather than the time domain (see Chapter 3). Many different following responses can be recorded from the human scalp in response to many different types of stimuli. Auditory steady-state responses (ASSRs) are one type of following response. ASSRs occur when the amplitude and frequency content of the stimulus remains constant over time and the response becomes stable in terms of its amplitude and phase relationship to that stimulus. The basic requirements for steady-state responses are a periodically presented stimulus and a part of the brain capable of following this periodicity and generating fields that can be recorded from the scalp. When the stimulus changes over time, the brain may still follow the sound but the response (like the stimulus) is not constant. We then use the more general term "following response." In order to evaluate responses to stimuli that change their amplitude and frequency characteristics over time, we can use techniques like the Fourier analyzer (discussed in Chapter 3) or correlation procedures. As well as the ASSRs, this chapter also considers following responses evoked by a sound that changes the frequency of its amplitude modulation (AM) over time and responses that follow the amplitude of the speech envelope. The frequency-following response (FFR) elicited by the actual frequency of a tone (rather than its modulation) was discussed briefly in Chapter 8.

Following responses usually are divided into those that follow the spectral frequency of a sound and those that follow its envelope frequency. The cochlear microphonic (CM) of the electrocochleogram (Chapter 7) is the quintessential FFR. Like the signal transduced by a microphone, the CM follows the acoustic waveform of the stimulus. The human brainstem also generates an FFR. This has a similar waveform to the CM but a significantly longer latency as it is generated by neurons in the brainstem rather than by hair cells in the cochlea. In the literature, the term FFR generally is used to denote this brainstem response as distinct from the CM.

Often, the CM and the brainstem FFR are recorded together and we must disentangle them by evaluating their latency and scalp topography. Both responses also can be contaminated by stimulus artifact from the earphone. The artifact can be distinguished by using an acoustic delay line, typically a tube connecting the transducer to the ear. This delays the physiologic responses as the sound takes time to travel though the tube after the artifact has been generated before the physiologic response is initiated. It also decreases the amplitude of the artifact as the transducer is moved away from the head. The brainstem FFR is best distinguished from the

CM by using a brief tone (allowing us to measure the longer onset latency of the brainstem response) and a two-channel recording montage: between the vertex and the contralateral mastoid and between the vertex and ipsilateral mastoid (Picton, Woods, Baribeau-Braun, & Healey, 1977). The CM is larger in the ipsilateral recordings whereas the FFR is approximately equal in the two channels. Another elegant way to distinguish the brainstem FFR from the CM uses forward masking to eliminate the FFR and leave the CM (which is unaffected by the masking). Subtracting the masked response from the unmasked response gives the FFR without CM contamination (Chimento & Schreiner, 1990).

When a sound changes its amplitude over time, the brain can follow its amplitude envelope as well as its spectral frequency. These responses can follow modulations of the amplitude that are either periodic or variable All responses can be called "envelope following response" or "amplitude-modulation following responses." These responses are "ASSRs" when the modulation is periodic and the response stable. In order to evoke ASSRs the modulation also can be set up to pass (or "window") a brief stimulus in a periodic manner or the modulation envelope can be a simple sinusoidal modulation of the amplitude or frequency of a tone. Because the acoustic spectrum of such a modulated stimulus does not contain energy at the modulation frequency (provided there is no distortion), the transduction process will not generate artifact at the frequency of the modulation. Energy at the modulation frequency only occurs when the signal passes through the transduction process of the cochlea—with compression in the initial conversion of acoustic to electric signals and then complete rectification at the synapse between hair cell and afferent nerve fibers. These processes are illustrated in Figure 10–1.

However, a sinusoidally modulated tones still can generate artifact at the carrier frequency and its sidebands. There-fore, we must be careful not to let these alias themselves back into the spectrum near the modulation frequency (see Figure 2–6). This problem is discussed at greater length by Picton and John (2004) and Small and Stapells (2004). Provided

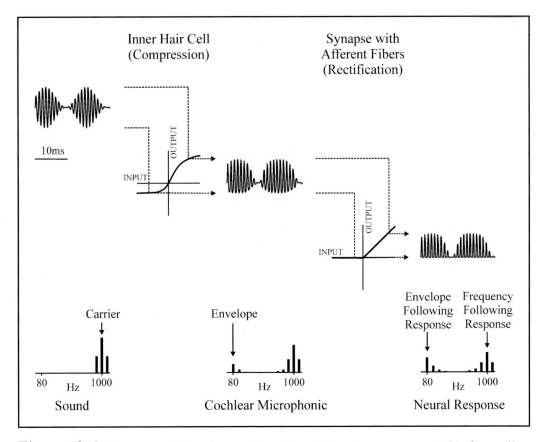

Figure 10–1. Frequency-following and envelope-following responses. This figure illustrates what happens to an amplitude-modulated tone (carrier frequency of 1000 Hz and modulation frequency of 80 Hz) as it is converted into neuronal signals through the cochlea. The input-output curve of the inner hair cell is close to linear near the origin but is compressed as the sound gets more intense. The compression is asymmetric, being greater for a condensation than rarefaction movement. The synapse between the hair cell and the afferent fiber causes a rectification of the signal. At the bottom of the figure, the signal is shown in the frequency domain. The energy in the sound is located at the carrier frequency and at the two side-bands (separated from the carrier by the modulation frequency). The energy carried by the neurons into the brain contains energy both at the carrier frequency (plus the side-bands) and at the modulation or envelope frequency (plus harmonics). Responses to the carrier frequency are called frequency-following responses and responses to the modulation frequency are called envelope-following responses. This figure is revised from Lins et al. (1995).

we prevent the aliasing by using steep low-pass filters and/or choose appropriate analog-to-digital conversion rates so that any aliased artifact is not mistaken for a physiological response, we can be confident that the recorded ASSR is physiologic and not artifactual.

FREQUENCY-FOLLOWING RESPONSE (FFR)

The brainstem FFR typically has been recorded in response to a brief tone. With a sustained tone, we run into the problem of electromagnetic artifacts. When activating a speaker, a pure tone generates electromagnetic fields that can induce currents in the recording circuits. For a brief tone, these artifacts should be over before the brainstem FFR occurs, but when the tone is continuous, the response and the artifact will occur simultaneously. As discussed, an acoustic delay line can help to further separate the artifact and response.

An elegant way to separate the FFR evoked by a brief tone and wave V of the auditory brainstem response (ABR) evoked by the onset of the tone is to record responses to tones of opposite polarity. Adding the responses together gives the transient wave V and middle latency response (MLR), whereas subtracting one response from the other gives the FFR (Yamada, Yamane, & Kodera, 1977). Figure 10–2 illustrates this technique and also presents the basic relations between the FFR and the intensity and frequency of the tone. Krishnan (2007) provides a recent review of the literature on the brainstem FFR.

The FFR decreases in amplitude with increasing frequency and becomes difficult to recognize at frequencies above 1500 Hz

(Moushegian, Rupert, & Stillman, 1973). The response probably is mediated through the phase-locking of neural discharges. Single auditory neurons cannot fire at rates more than several hundred per second but a population of neurons (each neuron phase-locking every several cycles) can mediate the FFR up to about 1500 Hz (see Figure 1–10).

When more than one tone is presented to the ear, distortion products can be generated because of the nonlinearities in the cochlear transduction process. These form the basis for recording the distortion product OAEs. In addition to generating acoustic energy recorded in the OAEs, these distortion products also activate the afferent nerves and can be recorded in the FFR (Pandya & Krishnan, 2004; Rickman, Chertoff, & Hecox, 1991). Indeed, the envelope following response to two beating tones is essentially a simple (second-order) distortion-product response. In the OAEs, the 2f1-f2 third-order (cubic) distortion product is most prominent, whereas in the ASSR, the f2-f1 second-order (quadratic) distortion product is the largest (Purcell, John, & Picton, 2003).

The FFR recorded from the human scalp is composed of several components (Stillman, Crow, & Moushegian, 1978). If the recording is taken between vertex and ipsilateral mastoid or earlobe, the CM can contribute to the response. There are likely several brainstem sources for the FFR. The main generator is in the ascending fibers of the lateral lemniscus, but pontine nuclei also may contribute to the scalp fields, particularly when recorded using a horizontal montage (mastoid to mastoid).

The amplitude of the FFR decreases linearly with decreasing intensity, reaching threshold at about 30 to 40 dB nHL (normal hearing level) when using brief

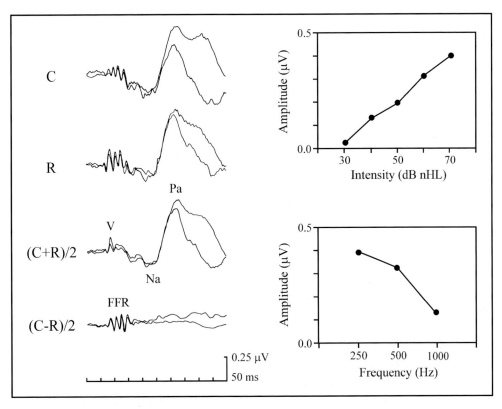

Figure 10–2. *Brainstem frequency-following response (FFR). The left section of the figures shows the responses recorded to 500-Hz tones of 7.5 ms duration (2.5 ms each for rise, fall, and plateau). The tones were presented at a rate of 10/s and an intensity of 50 dB nHL. Responses were obtained for tones with opposite polarities: condensation (C) and rarefaction (R). Each of the two different responses at each polarity was averaged over 2048 trials. Averaging the two responses together gives the transient EP with clearly recognizable waves V, Na, and Pa. Taking the difference between the two recordings (and dividing by 2) gives the FFR without any transient EP. The graphs on the right show the effects of stimulus intensity (at 500 Hz) and tonal frequency (at 60 dB nHL) on the amplitude of the FFR (measured peak-to-peak during plateau). Data are from Picton et al. (1977).*

500-Hz tonebursts (Picton et al., 1977). Studies with high-pass masking noise indicate that the responses to low-frequency tones at low to moderate intensities are mediated by the apical regions of the cochlea (Yamada, Kodera, Hink, & Suzuki, 1979). Therefore, the FFR may be used to evaluate low-frequency hearing (Stillman, Moushegian, & Rupert, 1976). However, in this context, it has been largely super-seded by either the tone-ABR or the ASSR to AM tones, both of which provide more precise threshold-estimations.

Early studies did not demonstrate any clear effects of attention on the FFR (Hillyard & Picton, 1979). One recent study showed no effect of attention on the amplitude of the FFR but some minimal effects on its latency (Hoorman, Falkenstein, & Hohnsbein, 2000). Another study showed an enhancement of the FFR with attention (Galbraith, Olfman, & Huffman, 2003), although this effect was measured in terms of signal-to-noise ratio (SNR) and it is not clear if the noise was constant across the different experimental conditions. The most convincing evidence for an effect of attention on the FFR comes from a study in which subjects listened to dichotic vowels, with the vowels in one ear spoken by a female voice and those in the other ear by a male voice (Galbraith, Bhutra, Choate, Kitahara, & Mullen, 1998). The FFR to the fundamental of the voice was enhanced by attention to that voice.

Indeed, the major present interest in the FFR concerns the response to speech sounds. Following the fundamental of voiced sounds is important for their perception. Whispered speech (which has no definite fundamental) is difficult to understand even when presented at the same intensity as normal speech. In Chapter 5, we considered the brainstem response to the onset of a "da" syllable (Johnson, Nicol, & Kraus, 2005). This contains an FFR to the vocal pitch when the vowel begins (see Figure 5–15). We will return to the FFR evoked by speech sounds at the end of this chapter.

FOLLOWING RESPONSES AT DIFFERENT STIMULUS RATES

When following responses are recorded from the vertex using a neck or mastoid reference, the responses are larger for particular stimulus rates compared to others. This effect of rate is crucial to understanding these responses. As well as indicating which stimulus rates might be most appropriate in different situations, the rate function suggests how to differentiate responses deriving from different intracerebral generators.

The responses at stimulus rates near 40 Hz are larger than at other frequencies. On either side of this peak in responsiveness are null regions—near 27 Hz and near 68 Hz—where the response is often so small as to be unrecognizable. These findings are illustrated in Figure 10–3 which shows the amplitude and phase of ASSRs to AM white noise presented at modulation rates from 10 to 100 Hz. Rather than recording separate responses at multiple separate rates, the modulation frequency was swept from low to high and back again and the responses analyzed using a Fourier analyzer (Purcell, John, Schneider, & Picton, 2004). This technique is explained more fully in Chapter 3 (particularly in relation to Figure 3–11).

Perception of Different Modulation Rates

The amplitude-rate functions shown in the upper left of Figure 10–3 do not easily relate to what we perceive. Measuring the threshold at which the modulation of a broadband noise can be detected at different modulation frequencies gives a relatively simple "temporal modulation transfer function" (Bacon & Viemeister, 1985; Viemeister, 1979). As stimulus rate is increased, we perceive AM in a stable manner until a cutoff frequency near 50 Hz, above which our perceptual acuity decreases at a rate of 4 dB per octave (see left section of Figure 10–4). The transfer function for a modulated pure tone can be more complex because the modulation may be perceived spectrally. The sidebands that make up the modulation become separately perceptible when they exceed the filter bandwidth for the carrier frequency.

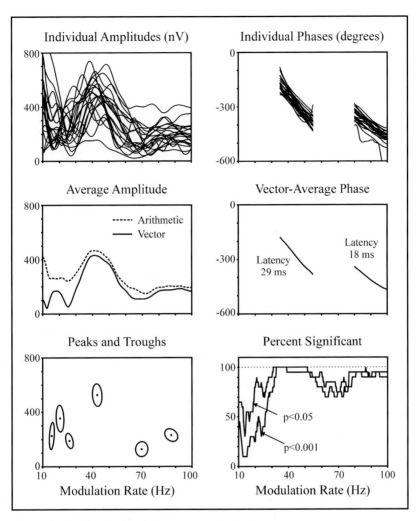

Figure 10–3. *Effect of stimulus rate on envelope-following responses. The stimulus was a 60-dB SPL white noise that was amplitude modulated to a depth of 100%. The modulation frequency was swept between 10 and 100 Hz (and back again), and the amplitude and phase of the response calculated for each modulation frequency using a Fourier analyzer (see Figure 3–11). The top left diagram shows the amplitudes of 20 individual subjects between the ages of 20 and 39 years. Below that are shown the average results combined over all the subjects using either arithmetic or vector-averaging. The amplitudes of the two types of averages are close together when the phases of the responses for the individual subjects are similar. If the phases are different, the vector average is small because of cancellation between the individual waveforms in the vector-averaging process. At the bottom left are shown the average measurements for the different peaks and troughs in the rate function. The ellipses represent the p <0.05 confidence limits for the mean values. The top right diagram shows the individual phase plots over the regions where the phases were consistent from one subject to the next. Below that are shown the vector averaged phases and the apparent latencies that can be calculated from the slope of these phases versus rate. The lower right diagram shows the percentage of responses judged significantly greater than the residual background noise at two different criteria. The recordings were taken over a period of 90 minutes in order to get good responses at all modulation frequencies. However, because the subjects were awake, the signal-to-noise ratio at the 80-Hz region was less than optimal and not all subjects showed significant responses (unlike at the 40-Hz region where all responses were significant). These previously unpublished results were obtained using programs from Purcell et al. (2004) with the assistance of Nic Petrescu and Patricia van Roon.*

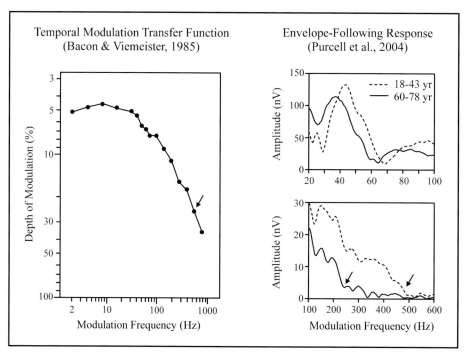

Figure 10–4. Effects of modulation rate. The left side of the figure shows the temporal modulation transfer function of Bacon and Viemeister (1985). The function plots the threshold for recognizing modulated white noise (as different from unmodulated noise). At low modulation frequencies subjects can detect modulation at a depth of about 5%. At frequencies higher than about 40 Hz, the subjects become progressively less sensitive, the threshold increasing to about 35% at 800 Hz. The arrow points to the 500 Hz frequency at which a 25% modulation is just detectable. The right side of the figures shows the amplitude of the envelope following response recorded during a sweep of modulation frequencies from 20 to 600 Hz (Purcell et al., 2004). Responses were recorded in groups of young and elderly subjects. The depth of modulation was maintained constant at 25%. Because the recorded response is much larger at the lower modulation frequencies, the findings are plotted using a more sensitive amplitude scale for the higher frequencies. The response becomes indistinguishable from the background EEG noise at about 500 Hz for the young subjects and near 250 Hz for the elderly subjects (arrows). The response is plotted using linear scales for both the amplitude and the modulation frequency, unlike the temporal modulation transfer function which uses logarithmic scales.

Sometimes this can be seen as an increased sensitivity in the 40- to 50-Hz region for a 1000 Hz carrier (see Figure 1 of Viemeister, 1979), but this is not likely related to the 40-Hz accentuation in the ASSR, which is as clear for modulated noise as it is for tones.

Our suprathreshold perceptions ("What does it sound like?" rather than "Can it be heard?") change significantly with increasing rate. At rates below 15 Hz, we hear "beats" or "fluctuations," whereas at rates from 15 to 150 Hz (centering near 50 Hz), we perceive "flutter" or "roughness." The latter sensation may be related to the bandpass response functions of neurons in the inferior colliculus (Fastl & Zwicker, 2007). A sensitive listener may resolve the stimuli even more finely into separate sounds (<3 Hz), fluctuations (3–10 Hz), flutter (10–50 Hz), and residual pitch (>50 Hz), with all sounds above 10 Hz sounding rough.

Intracerebral Sources at Different Envelope Frequencies

As well as not relating to perceptual studies, the ASSR rate function does easily fit with physiologic studies of how neurons respond to different modulation frequencies (Joris, Schreiner, & Rees, 2004). Neurons lower in the auditory nervous system respond temporally—they follow the envelope of the stimulus, whereas neurons at higher stations respond to particular stimulus rates by increasing their rate of discharge (rather than by synchronizing their firing to the envelope). In this manner, time-codes in a population of neurons are transferred to rate-codes in a set of neurons that each respond specifically to a particular modulation rate. The higher we travel in the auditory system, the lower the range of modulations to which neurons respond in a synchronous manner. Cortical neurons cease synchronizing to the envelope at rates above 50 to 100 Hz, even though our brainstem neurons can follow (and we can perceive) modulations out to 1000 Hz or more.

One difficulty in mapping the ASSRs to either the neuronal or the perceptual findings is that several different intracerebral generators contribute to the scalp-recording. Most important are the auditory brainstem, particularly in the region of the

inferior colliculus and thalamus, and the auditory cortex. These different generators will have different latencies and different response patterns. The overlapping responses may add to each other at some rates and cancel each other out at other rates (Purcell et al., 2004). This is illustrated in Figure 10–5. If the cortex responds at a delay of 29 ms and with a low-pass function cutting off above 50 Hz, and the brainstem responds at a latency of 8 ms to all frequencies within the range tested (10–100 Hz), the actual amplitude-rate function of the envelope following response can be modeled reasonably well.

Apparent latencies for the ASSRs can be calculated from the relations between the phase of the response and the frequency of modulation (see Chapter 3). In Figure 10–2 (middle section) the latencies are estimated as 29 ms for the 40-Hz response and 19 ms for the 80-Hz response. Apparent latencies vary from study to study. Part of this variability may be due to the problem of estimating the latency of a response when it is generated by multiple generators, each with its own latency. The apparent latency measured in the region of 40 Hz is typically near 30 ms, with the carriers of lower frequency having longer latencies. Different studies have reported values between 20 and 41 ms (reviewed by Picton, John, Dimitrijevic, & Purcell, 2003). At frequencies above 150 Hz, the latencies have been consistently around 8 to 10 ms (range 7–18 as reviewed by Picton et al., 2003). This is the latency region that might be expected for a brainstem response to tones. The apparent latency in the region of the 80-Hz response is the most variable—between 9 and 31 ms (Picton et al., 2003). This may be because the response in this frequency region is generated by several brain sources in brainstem, thalamus, and cortex. Another

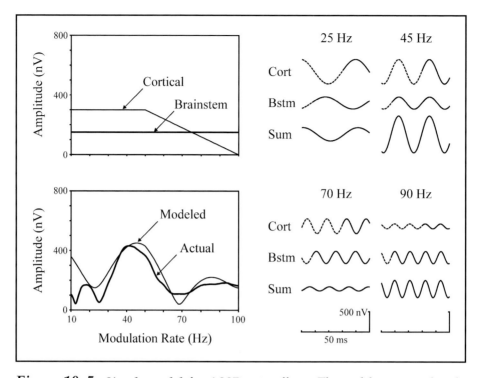

***Figure 10–5.** Simple model for ASSR rate effects. The model proposes that the response recorded from the scalp represents the overlapping fields from simultaneously active brainstem and cortical sources. As shown in the upper left diagram, the brainstem source (thick line) is equally active at all modulation rates, whereas the larger cortical response (thin line) is most active at slow rates and decreases its amplitude at rates above 50 Hz. This model is similar to that proposed by Purcell et al. (2004). The waveforms in the right half of the figure show the responses when the latencies are 8 ms for the brainstem generator (Bstm) and 29 ms for the cortical generator (Cort). The latencies are illustrated diagrammatically by the dotted line response. The responses are of opposite polarity at 25 and 70 Hz and tend to cancel each other when summed together. At 45 and 90 Hz, the responses are in phase and sum to give a large response. The results at all frequencies, as plotted in the modeled waveform (thin line) in the lower right diagram, are close to the actual data (thick line). The amplitudes plotted in the graphs are measured baseline to peak.*

possibility is that muscle reflexes may contribute to the response. We have already seen that the postauricular muscle can follow at rates of 80 Hz (see Figure 8–15).

A simple two-component (brainstem-cortex) model, such as illustrated in Figure 10–5, does not explain the response pattern in the lower frequency range (e.g., the tendency to a null near 27 Hz). Another

response, perhaps in secondary auditory cortex, might be responding with a longer latency and only at the lower frequencies. This slow response might overlap with the primary cortical response and cancel responses in the 27-Hz null region. It also is possible that the cortex, by reason of its connectivity, may respond best or "resonate" at frequencies near 40 Hz, and that this resonant response might not occur at frequencies above 50 or below 30 Hz. These possibilities lead to complicated models that are difficult to fit; the more components to the model the more difficult it is to disentangle one component from another.

A different way to explain the response null near 27 Hz follows from the fact that the cortical MLR contains most of its energy near 40 Hz. The 40-Hz ASSR may result largely from the superposition of repeated responses as initially suggested by Galambos, Makeig, and Talmachoff (1981) (see Figure 1–14). If this is the case, overlapping MLRs evoked at a stimulus onset asynchrony (SOA) equal to an odd number of half cycles of 40 Hz (12.5 ms), should cancel themselves out because each successive response will be of opposite polarity to the preceding one. This would occur at 80 Hz (SOA of 12.5 ms), 27 Hz (SOA of 27.5 ms), and 16 Hz (SOA of 62.5 ms). This logic works for the 27 Hz null, but it does not explain the 68 Hz null, and incorrectly identifies nulls at 80 and 16 Hz.

If we could distinguish the fields generated by the different intracerebral sources, we could perhaps allocate the ASSRs recorded using multichannel scalp-recordings to the different sources, and find out which sources predominate at which rate. However, the two main sources, high brainstem and primary auditory cortex, generate similar fields at the scalp. Both sources have vertically oriented equivalent dipoles. Nevertheless, source analysis suggests that the 40-Hz responses are generated mainly in the auditory cortex and that the 90-Hz responses are generated mainly in the brainstem (Herdman et. al., 2002). On MEG examination, the 40-Hz sources are larger in the right hemisphere than in the left (Ross, Herdman, & Pantev,

2005a). This asymmetry may have some relation to the asymmetry noted in fMRI studies between left and right hemispheres (Zatorre & Belin, 2001), but the relationship is not clear. An initial speculation would be to relate the 40-Hz response more to temporal than to spectral processing, but temporal processing appears more left-sided on the fMRI studies. Hemodynamic studies of the of the brain during the perception of 40-Hz modulated sounds indicate activation in the primary auditory cortices, but also in regions outside the temporal lobe—right middle frontal gyrus and the anterior cingulate (Reyes et al., 2004).

ASSRs at Slow Rates

The data that we have been considering so far have concerned the following responses at rates near 40 Hz and 80 Hz. Significant following responses also can occur at rates below 30 Hz. Because of the higher levels of background noise in the electroencephalogram (EEG) at these frequencies, particularly the large alpha rhythms that occur at 10 Hz, these slow responses can take longer to record than those at higher stimulus rates. Nevertheless, several authors have identified reliable responses in the low-frequency regions, usually near 5 Hz, 10 Hz, and 20 Hz (Alaerts, Luts, Hofmann, & Wouters, 2009; Picton, Skinner, Champagne, Kellett, & Maiste, 1987; Rees, Green, & Kay, 1986; Wong & Stapells, 2004). The amplitudes and the frequencies at which the responses reach maximum vary with the type of stimulus. Responses to modulations of a speech-weighted broadband noise (Alaerts et al., 2009) showed a higher SNR than the responses to amplitude or frequency-modulated tones (Picton et al., 1987). Furthermore, the responses often are larger when recorded at the second harmonic of the stimulus rate. This type of response is effectively reacting to the modulation changing in either direction. Second harmonic responses are particularly prominent in response to frequency-modulation (Maiste & Picton, 1989) and changes in interaural correlation or interaural latency differences (Dajani & Picton, 2006). For these stimuli, the response is best recorded at 8 Hz in response to a 4-Hz modulation. The choice of 4 rather than 5 Hz leads to the second harmonic response being less obscured by the EEG alpha rhythm, which is generally larger at 10 than 8 Hz. Maintaining an eyes-open alert state, which attenuates the alpha activity in the EEG, also is important in ensuring a good SNR for these responses.

Apparent latencies for the slow ASSRs have given latencies that vary between 30 and 200 ms. The difficulty in measuring apparent latencies when there are multiple underlying generators may explain the variability of these latencies. In their original description of the ASSRs at different rates, Rickards and Clark (1984) suggested that the apparent latencies calculated from phase-rate plots were related to the peak latencies of the transient EPs generated in the same regions as the ASSRs. Thus, we could relate the 80-Hz responses to the ABR, the 40-Hz responses to the MLR, and the slow ASSRs to the late auditory evoked potentials (LAEPs).

A full model for the rate function, extending coverage down into lower frequencies than the model presented in Figure 10–4, would then include another source with a frequency bandpass cutting off above about 10 Hz and a latency between 100 and 200 ms. However, this source is likely multiple, involving different areas of cortex activated at many different latencies. Herdman et al. (2002) found that both tangential and radial sources occurred in both temporal lobes during the ASSRs to 12-Hz stimuli. The rate function in the low frequencies therefore would be much less consistent from subject to subject than the initial activation of cortex that shows as the 40-Hz peak and the brainstem that shows in the frequencies above 70 Hz.

Despite the intersubject variability, slow ASSRs do tap into cerebral functions that are close to perception. Alaerts et al. (2009) found that a combination of measurements of the signal-to-noise ratio of the ASSRs at rates 4, 10, and 20 Hz correlated well ($r = 0.82$) with the phoneme identification score when both the psychophysical and physiologic tests were done in different levels of noise. Wong and Stapells (2004) found that the slow ASSRs were related to the perceptual effects of the binaural masking level difference whereas the 40-Hz and 80-Hz responses were not.

Overview of the Rate Effects

We started our evaluation of the following responses with some clear facts (the pattern of the response to different stimulus rates) and some difficult interpretations (where in the brain responses are generated at each of the stimulus rates). Life is not simple but it can be considered so if we are cautious. Therefore, in the following discussions, we refer often to three main categories of response. Two of these are named for the rate near which they are best recorded: the 40-Hz and 80-Hz ASSRs. Although named the 40-Hz response and the 80 Hz response, the actual recordings may be obtained at nearby rates such as 37 or 83 Hz. The third category of following response is the slow ASSR, which can be recorded using envelope rates of less than 25 Hz. We begin our discussions with the subject factors that affect the following responses differently at different modulation rates.

SUBJECT FACTORS

Effects of age

In infants, where the auditory cortex is not mature, there is no accentuation of the amplitude near 40 Hz—the responses are similar in amplitude to those at faster stimulus rates. Because the background noise levels in the recording decrease with increasing frequency, the responses at higher rates have better SNRs. Rickards et al. (1994) found the responses much more detectable from 70 to 100 Hz than at 40 Hz in sleeping infants. Levi, Folsom, and Dobie (1993, 1995) examined the ASSRs in adults and infants. The responses were more detectable near 40 Hz for awake adults and near 80 Hz for sleeping infants. In sleeping adults, the responses also were more detectable near 80 Hz. Later findings suggested that the ASSRs to low-level stimuli in sleeping adults were still better at 40 Hz than at 80 Hz (Dobie & Wilson, 1998).

Pethe, Mühler, Siewert, and von Specht (2004) examined the development of the ASSR in children from age 2 months to 14 years. They recorded responses to a 1-kHz tone modulated at frequencies of either 40 or 80 Hz and presented at intensities between 50 and 10 dB nHL. Infants below the age of 2 years were tested asleep but all other recordings were in wakefulness. All responses increased in amplitude with increasing age but the rate of change was greater for the 40-Hz response. Below 1 year of age, the 40-Hz response was about the same amplitude as the 80-Hz response but by age 14 years the 40-Hz response was considerably larger; at 50 dB nHL, the amplitudes were about 150 nV for the 40-Hz response and 80 nV for the 80-Hz response. Because the residual background EEG was higher for the 40-Hz response, the SNR for the younger children was better for the 80-Hz response, and it was not until the age of 13 years that the SNR became better for recording the 40-Hz responses.

As well as changing in infancy and childhood, the amplitude-rate function of the following response changes with increasing age in adolescents and adults. The frequency at which the 40-Hz response is maximal changes with age. Purcell et al. (2004) found that this peak occurred at a significantly lower frequency (37 Hz compared to 41 Hz) in elderly subjects (age 60–78 years) than in young adults (age 18–43 years) when evaluating responses to white noise amplitude-modulated at a depth of 25% and swept over a range of frequencies. Poulsen, Picton, and Paus (2007), using 100% AM noise, found an increase in the peak frequency with increasing age from 19 to 45 years, and Poulsen Picton and Paus (2009) found that the peak occurred earlier in young adolescents (age 10–12 years) than in the previously studied adult group. The right side of Figure 10–6 combines the data from these two studies with some unpublished data obtained by Nic Petrescu and Patricia van Roon in 60 adults from 20 to 80 years. The combined data show that the frequency at which the 40-Hz response peaks increases with increasing age up to about 45 years and then decreases with further increase in age.

In addition, the combined data provide information about age-related changes in the amplitude and latency of the 40-Hz response. The apparent latency measured

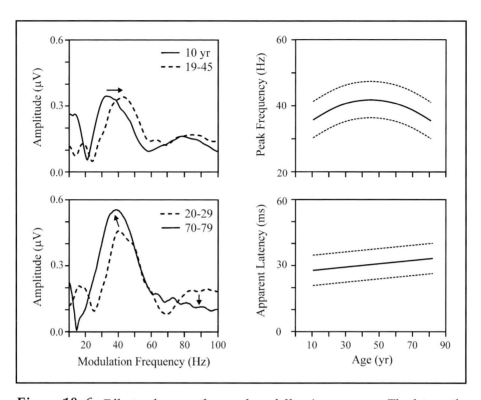

Figure 10–6. *Effects of age on the envelope following response. The data on the left were obtained using the sweep technique for white noise amplitude-modulated at a depth of 100%. The upper set of data from Poulsen et al (2009) compares the results in children age 10 years with a set of adults ages 19–45 years. The main effect (horizontal arrow) is an increase in the frequency at which the 40-Hz peak occurs. The lower set of data, obtained with Petrescu and van Roon (unpublished), compares the responses in subjects in their 20s to subjects in their 70s. With increasing age, the 40-Hz peak increases in amplitude and decreases in frequency and the 80-Hz response decreases in amplitude (arrows). The Poulsen et al. data were recorded using a slightly lower intensity (55 instead of 60 dB SPL) than the data of Petrescu and van Roon. The right half of the figure shows regression analyses that combined the data from Poulsen et al. with the data from Petrescu and van Roon. The 40-Hz peak frequency shows a quadratic regression with the maximum peak occurring near 45 years. The apparent latency of the 40-Hz response increases linearly with increasing age at a rate of 0.08 ms per year. The dotted lines represent ±1 standard error of the regression estimate.*

around the peak of the function shows a small but regular increase (0.08 ms/ year) with increasing age. The amplitude at the peak of the function also shows a small linear increase (2 nV/year) with increasing age. (To evaluate the latter relation we compensated the data from the two Poul-sen et al. papers to account for the slightly lower stimulus intensity compared to the new data.) Previous studies of the 40-Hz response have found a similar small increase in amplitude with increasing age, although this sometimes did not reach significance (Boettcher, Madhotra, Poth,

& Mills, 2002; Boettcher, Poth, Mills, & Dubno, 2001; Picton et al., 2003). These changes are very small when compared with the intersubject variability at each age. The age-related effects for the following response may be related to the age-related increases in the amplitude and latency of the Pa wave of the MLR (Woods & Clayworth, 1986). Rojas et al. (2006) found an increase in the amplitude of the 40-Hz ASSR recorded using magnetoencephalography (MEG) from age 5 to 52 with most of the change occurring between 5 and 20 years. These findings are compatible with the EEG recordings of Pethe et al. (2004) that were discussed earlier in this section. In both studies, the response were all obtained at 40 Hz and thus did not consider the effect of the response being larger at lower modulation-frequencies in the younger subjects.

The 80-Hz responses also change amplitude and latency with age. Data for the newborn and infants have not yet been recorded using many stimulus rates. Response latencies therefore are estimated directly from phase without using apparent latencies. The responses of the newborn infant are about half the size of the adult response (reviewed in Chapter 13). The response is larger in older infants, but exactly when in infancy or childhood the 80-Hz ASSR reaches adult amplitudes is not known. The latencies of the responses in the newborn infant are difficult to determine as the number of cycles of stimulation between stimulus and response is not known (Alaerts, Luts, Van Dun, Desloovere, & Wouters, 2010; John, Brown, Muir, & Picton, 2004; Lins et al., 1996). A recent study by Alaerts et al. (2010) proposed that the response is about 10 ms later in infants than in adults and that the latency decreases significantly over the first few weeks of age. When the latency reaches

adult values is unknown. By the age of 10 years, the 80-Hz response has roughly the same amplitude and latency as in adults age 20 to 40 years (see Figure 10–6, upper left).

In adulthood, the amplitude of the 80-Hz response generally decreases with increasing age (Picton, Dimitrijevic, Perez-Abalo, & van Roon, 2005). This shows up in the right side of the amplitude-rate functions (see Figure 10–6, lower left). This effect may be related in part to the cochlear hearing loss that occurs with increasing age and in part to changes in the central auditory system that interfere with its ability to follow rapidly changing sounds.

Purcell et al. (2004) found that elderly subjects showed smaller following responses at modulation rates over 100 Hz than young adults. Furthermore, the responses ceased to be significantly different from the background EEG and electromyographic (EMG) noise at modulation frequencies above 165 Hz (compared to 260 Hz in young subjects). These physiologic results were roughly similar to the changes in threshold for modulation detection in the elderly (e.g., He, Mills, Ahlstrom, & Dubno, 2008). Leigh-Paffenroth and Fowler (2006) found that elderly subjects were less able to phase-lock ASSRs to modulated sounds than younger subjects. Grose, Mamo, and Hall (2009) found reduced ASSR amplitudes in older listeners compared to young listeners for a modulation rate of 128 Hz but not for a modulation rate of 32 Hz. These results indicated a reduced ability to follow at rapid rates in elderly subjects but the findings did not clearly relate to psychophysical evaluations of speech perception in modulated noise, where the elderly showed deficits at 32 Hz modulation.

The ability to follow sounds as they change is necessary to the perception of speech. However, as we will see, following speech occurs at many different acoustical levels from the vocal pitch to the speech envelope, and at many different physiologic levels from brainstem to cortex. Each type of following likely changes differently with both development and aging.

Gender

The combined adult and adolescent data set we have been examining showed no significant effects of gender on the following responses at either 40 Hz or 80 Hz. Occasionally, we have noted that the 80-Hz responses tend to be a little larger and a little earlier in female compared to male subjects (John & Picton 2000a; Picton et al., 2009), but these small differences do not always replicate. However, they are similar to the findings with the transient ABR reviewed in Chapter 8.

Effects of Arousal

Sleep significantly reduces the amplitude of the 40-Hz response. The amplitude of this response in slow-wave sleep is about one half its amplitude in wakefulness (Linden, Campbell, Hamel, & Picton, 1985; Picton, John, Purcell, & Plourde, 2003). Cohen, Rickards, and Clark (1991) investigated the effect of sleep on the ASSRs recorded at different stimulus rates and found a striking decrease in the amplitude of the response at rates near 40 Hz. They also found a decrease in the response at rates near 80Hz, but this was a much smaller change. Part of the decrease in the 80-Hz response during sleep may have been due to the concomitant reduction in the background noise from the residual

EEG and EMG noise in the recordings. This is clear in the left side of Figure 10–7 where the background noise (measured in the frequency bins between the stimulus frequencies) during sleep is less than half its waking amplitude. The amplitudes measured for the responses combine both the actual response amplitudes and the amplitude of the background noise. The right side of Figure 10–7 shows graphs from Cohen et al. (1991) and from Purcell et al. (2004). The latter data had lower levels of background noise and showed no significant effect of sleep on the responses at rates near 80 Hz.

The simple model of the ASSR with brainstem and cortical responses occurring at different latencies (see Figure 10–5) can explain the effects of sleep or anesthesia on the responses, most particularly the decrease in the 40 Hz peak (Cohen et al., 1991; Linden et al., 1985; Purcell et al., 2004). This would be caused by sleep reducing the cortical (or thalamo-cortical) response more than the brainstem response. This would change the apparent latency of the response near 40 Hz toward the latency of the brainstem response. Lins and Picton (1995) found that this occurred; the apparent latency for the 40-Hz responses to a 1000-Hz tone changed from 34 ms awake to 27 ms asleep, but the difference was small and the latency for the 40-Hz response was still later than for the ASSRs at 80 Hz. Similar results were obtained by Purcell et al. (2004) for amplitude modulated broadband noise and by Linden et al. (1985) for 500-Hz tones, but these differences were variable and not statistically significant. These results need to be replicated. The nature of the 40-Hz response recorded during sleep—how much is cortical and how much brainstem—still needs to be determined.

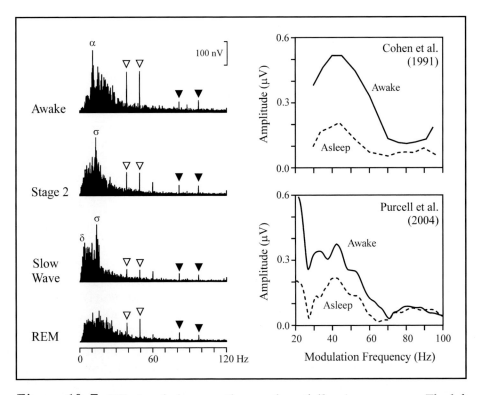

Figure 10–7. *Effects of sleep on the envelope-following response. The left section of this figure shows responses to a 1000-Hz tone of 60 dB SPL that was simultaneously modulated at 39, 49, 81, and 93 Hz. Responses then could be measured at each of the modulation rates. During sleep, the responses at 39 and 49 Hz were significantly reduced in amplitude. The responses at 81 and 93 Hz were slightly smaller during sleep but this was likely just caused by the lower level of background noise during the sleep recordings. This can be estimated in the recording at the frequencies adjacent to the actual responses. The lower frequencies of the spectra show evidence of the alpha rhythm (α) during wakefulness and spindle or sigma activity (σ) and delta activity (δ) during the sleep stages. These data are from Lins and Picton (1995). The right half of the figures shows graphs from two papers showing the effects of sleep at different modulation rates. The data from Cohen et al. (1991) are for a 1-kHz binaural tone presented at 30 dB HL with combined amplitude and frequency modulation. The data from Purcell et al. (2004) are for white noise at 60 dB SPL amplitude-modulated at 25% depth. Estimated noise levels were lower in the Purcell et al. recordings and these show no effect of sleep on the response amplitudes near 80 Hz. Both studies showed that sleep significantly reduced the response amplitude near 40 Hz.*

Anesthesia

The 40-Hz responses are dramatically attenuated by most anesthetics (Meuret, Backman, Bonhomme, Plourde, & Fiset, 2000; Plourde & Picton, 1990; Plourde, Villemure, Fiset, Bonhomme, & Backman, 1998). Therefore, the 40-Hz responses might be useful when monitoring an anesthetized patient for inappropriate intraoperative awareness (Tonner & Scholz, 2006). We considered the physiology of anesthesia and the effects of anesthesia on the MLR in the preceding chapter. The mechanisms underlying the change in the 40-Hz ASSR with anesthesia probably are related to those that affect the MLR, provided the effects of stimulus rate are considered (McNeer, Bohórquez, & Özdamar, 2009). The 40-Hz response likely is generated by an interaction between cortical and subcortical sources, and anesthesia disrupts this interaction (Plourde et al., 2008).

The main advantage of the 40-Hz ASSR over the transient MLR as a monitor for consciousness is the simplicity of the measurement (Plourde, 2006). We do not have to pick peaks or measure latencies; the amplitude of the response is either measurable or not. The decision about whether a response is present or absent can be made within a brief recording period. The response to a repeating tone of 75 to 95 dB pSPL is recognizable in most awake adult subjects within 16 seconds and in all subjects within a minute and a half (Picton et al., 2003). Appropriate care has to be taken, in particular, employing vector averaging and using a neck reference that does not record the postauricular muscle reflex. The effects of different anesthetic agents on the 40-Hz response are generally similar; the response goes away when consciousness goes away. However, although most anesthetics decrease the 40-Hz ASSR, the agent ketamine actually increases the amplitude of the response. This suggests that ketamine causes unconsciousness by a different mechanism than other anesthetics (Plourde, Baribeau, & Bonhomme, 1997).

The 80-Hz ASSR has not been studied extensively during anesthesia. Luts, Des-loovere, and Wouters (2006) were able to record reasonable 80-Hz ASSR thresholds in young infants tested under anesthesia with ketamine, midazolam, and clonidine. A reasonable assumption might be that the 80-Hz ASSRs share the transient ABR's resilience to sedative and anesthetic agents. If this hypothesis is indeed validated, one way to ensure the integrity of the recording system when monitoring the cerebral effects of anesthetics would be to record responses to sounds simultaneously modulated at independent rates near 40 and 80 Hz (e.g., 41 and 87 Hz). The decrease in the 40-Hz response would monitor the anesthetic effect while the preservation of the 80-Hz response would ensure that this change was not caused by some problem with the stimulus or recording system. The left side of Figure 10–7 illustrates this procedure for monitoring natural sleep (Lins & Picton, 1995).

Effects of Attention

Early studies showed that the 40-Hz response was sensitive to the general level of alertness. In a drowsy subject, "minute rhythms" occurred as the ASSR increased and decreased in amplitude over periods close to a minute (Galambos & Makeig, 1988). When a subject attended to foreground stimuli, the 40-Hz response to a background train of auditory stimuli changed in amplitude or phase, perhaps in association with a general orienting response (Makeig & Galambos, 1989; Rohrbaugh, Varner, Paige, Eckardt, & Ellingson, 1990). The initial studies of the effects of specific attention to the intensity or frequency of recurring auditory stimuli, however, did not show any significant change in the 40-Hz response (Linden, Picton, Hamel, & Campbell, 1987).

If attention is paid to the temporal structure of the modulated sound in order to detect occasional changes in the modulation frequency, then there are definite changes in the 40-Hz ASSR (Ross, Picton, Herdman, & Pantev, 2004; Saupe, Widmann, Bendixen, Müller, & Schröger, 2009; Skosnick, Krishnan, & O'Donnell, 2007). The response is enhanced by attention and this effect is greater in the right auditory cortex than in the left.

As yet studies have not evaluated the effect of attention on the 80-Hz ASSR. A reasonable hypothesis would be that this is unaffected by attention, like the transient ABR.

CARRIER FREQUENCY

We now consider the effects of different stimulus parameters on the following responses. At the beginning of this chapter, we considered the effects of modulation frequency. In this section, we review the effects of carrier frequency. There are significant differences between the two most commonly studied ASSRs—the 40-Hz and 80-Hz responses.

40-Hz Responses

One of the most striking things about the 40-Hz-response is that it is much larger in amplitude for lower carrier frequencies (Galambos et al., 1981; Picton et al., 1987). Figure 10–8 compares data from different studies. The amplitude at 500 Hz is typically about twice the amplitude at 2 kHz. Why is not known. One possible explanation revolves around the idea that the scalp-recorded 40-Hz response is the sum of brainstem and cortical responses. The 500-Hz ABR contains more energy at

40 Hz and has a longer latency than the response to higher frequencies. These characteristics allow the ABR to sum with the cortical response to give a larger recording when carrier-frequencies are low. However, these effects do not explain why the response recorded magnetically, which contains little in the way of brainstem activity, also is much larger for lower carrier frequencies (Ross, Borgmann, Draganova, Roberts, & Pantev, 2000). Another explanation might be that at high intensity a low-frequency tone activates the basilar membrane from base to apex, whereas a high-frequency tone activates the basilar membrane only near the stapes. Such an explanation would require a smaller frequency-effect at lower intensities when the cochlear activation patterns are more circumscribed, but this does not seem to be the case. Rodriguez, Picton, Linden, Hamel, and Laframboise (1986) found that the amplitudes of the 40-Hz responses were linearly related to intensity for both 500-Hz (17 nV/dB) and 2000-Hz tones (14 nV/dB). These relationships did not change at low intensities, and the difference between the frequencies persisted when notched noise was used to limit any spread of activation in the cochlea. Furthermore, if the breadth of activation on the basilar membrane is the cause, the 80-Hz response generated in the brainstem should show a similar effect. However, these responses tend to be larger for midfrequency (1 and 2 kHz) carriers. We are left with a clear finding with no obvious explanation—the increase in amplitude of the 40-Hz ASSR with decreasing carrier frequency.

80-Hz Responses

When evoked by singly presented stimuli, the 80-Hz responses are roughly equal in

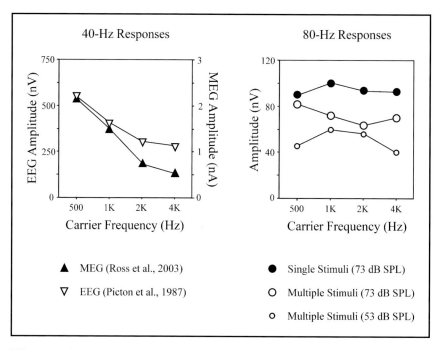

Figure 10–8. *Effects of carrier frequency. On the left are shown the effects of carrier frequency on the 40-Hz response recorded using either MEG (Ross et al., 2003) or EEG (Picton et al., 1987). The stimuli for the MEG recordings were 100% amplitude modulated and presented at 70 dB SL. The stimuli for the EEG recordings were 50% modulated and presented at 77 dB SPL. On the right are shown the effects of carrier frequency on the 80-Hz responses. These data are combined across several conditions reported in Picton et al. (2009). All stimuli were 100% amplitude modulated. In the single-stimulus condition and low-intensity multiple stimulus conditions, the responses were about the same amplitude across carrier frequencies (with a tendency to be larger at the midfrequencies). When multiple stimuli were presented simultaneously at high intensity, the responses were larger at 500 and 4000 Hz.*

amplitude across the different frequencies (Lins et al., 1995; Lins & Picton, 1995). At low or moderate intensities, there is a tendency for the responses to be larger at 1 and 2 kHz than at lower or higher frequencies. Most subsequent measurements have been obtained using multiple simultaneous stimuli where interactions occur between the response to the different stimuli (Picton, van Roon, & John, 2009). Therefore, we now review the effects of these interactions.

INTERACTIONS BETWEEN STIMULI WITH DIFFERENT CARRIER FREQUENCIES

Masking and Tuning Curves

The simplest interaction between stimuli of different carrier-frequencies involves two simultaneous stimuli. Various processes can occur between stimuli of different frequencies. We already have considered the distortion products from different carrier frequencies, responses that occur at frequencies representing some combination of the f1 and f2. Here, we are concerned with interactions between the two stimuli that are manifest in the response at each frequency (at f1 or f2) rather than at a combination frequency (such as f1-f2 or 2f1-f2). The effects at f1 or f2 can be measured by recording the ASSR to the modulation of one or both these frequencies. When two tones occur together, we can observe masking, suppression, and facilitation.

First, we will briefly review the idea of the tuning curve originally considered in earlier chapters (see Figure 5–5 and Figure 7–8). A probe tone is presented at an intensity near threshold. Then, a masking tone or narrowband noise is presented and its intensity is raised until the probe tone becomes inaudible. A tuning curve is then constructed by changing the masking frequency and plotting the intensity of the masker needed to prevent the probe from being heard (Stelmachowicz & Jesteadt, 1984). The left side of Figure 10–9 illustrates this procedure. Tuning curves have been obtained using 80-Hz ASSRs. The probe was an amplitude-modulated tone presented at 10 dB above the physiologic threshold, and the intensity of a narrowband masker necessary to make the response no longer recognizable was determined for different frequencies of masker (Markessis et al., 2009). Decisions about the presence or absence of the response were made after only 90 seconds. Although this allowed the authors to construct tuning curves within a reasonable period of time, some low-level responses could have been missed because of SNR problems. However, using the same SNR criterion for the masked and unmasked response should result in tuning curves that were correctly shaped. The ASSR tun-

ing curves obtained by Markessis et al. (2009) were indeed similar to the psychophysical curves. There was a "detuning" effect; the tip of the tuning curve was shifted to a higher frequency than that of the probe. This is likely due to suppression (Moore, 1978). Such detuning does not occur when a forward masking paradigm is used as suppression occurs only when the probe and masker are presented simultaneously. Unfortunately, forward masking paradigms are not easily compatible with recording ASSRs.

Another approach to investigating the interactions between masker and probe is to present the masker and probe at the same or similar intensity and to measure the effect of the masker on the amplitude of the probe response. This technique of determining a masking function is illustrated in the left half of Figure 10–10. This evaluates the interactions between stimuli more rapidly than the tuning curve because only one recording is needed for each pairing of masker and probe. We do not need multiple recordings to determine the lowest intensity of the masker needed to completely attenuate the probe response. The masking function is similar to the tuning curve but the theoretical relationships between these techniques need to be worked out. John, Lins, Boucher, and Picton (1998) showed that the masking function for the 80-Hz response was complex and a little unexpected—the masking was greater when the masker frequency was higher than that of the 80-Hz probe rather than lower. In addition, low-frequency maskers showed some tendency to enhance the response amplitude. The greater masking by higher frequency maskers was also seen for the 40-Hz response examined using MEG (Ross, Draganova, Picton, & Pantev, 2003), although this study did not find the low-frequency enhancement.

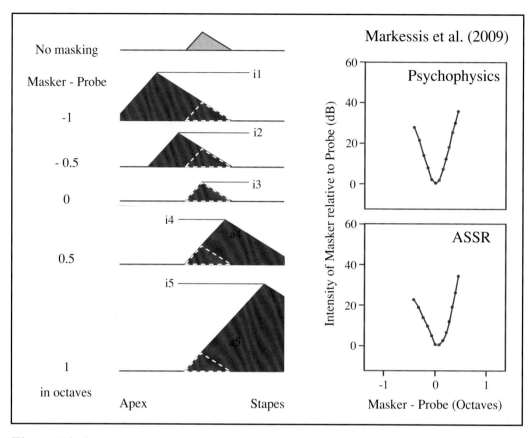

Figure 10–9. *Tuning curves. The left section of the figure shows how tuning curves are constructed. The activation patterns of both the masker (black) and the probe (gray) are shown on the basilar membrane. The basilar membrane is diagrammed going from the stapes on the right to the apex on the left. This differs from the usual convention but it allows us to place the high frequencies on the right as they are usually plotted for the tuning curve. To construct the tuning curve, the intensity of the masker is increased until the subject no longer perceives the probe (dashed line) or there is no recognizable ASSR. We then plot the intensity of the masker (i1, i2, i3, etc.) against the masker frequency. Because of the asymmetry of the activation pattern, the tuning curve generally has a steeper slope when the masker is higher than the probe than vice versa. The right side of the figure shows data from Markessis et al. (2009). The psychophysical and ASSR tuning curves are shown for a 2-kHz probe.*

Sweep techniques allow us to measure the masking functions quite elegantly. The amplitude of the response to a constant 80-Hz AM tone is monitored while the frequency of the masking noise is swept from high to low and back again (Wilding, McKay, Baker, Picton, & Kluk, submitted). The right side of Figure 10–10 shows some results from the sweep paradigm together with those obtained using stimuli at discrete frequencies. Further developments of this paradigm might make it possible to evaluate masking functions at several different frequencies simultaneously. For example, two continuous AM tones can be presented at 500 and 2000 Hz (each modulated at a different frequency) while two narrowband

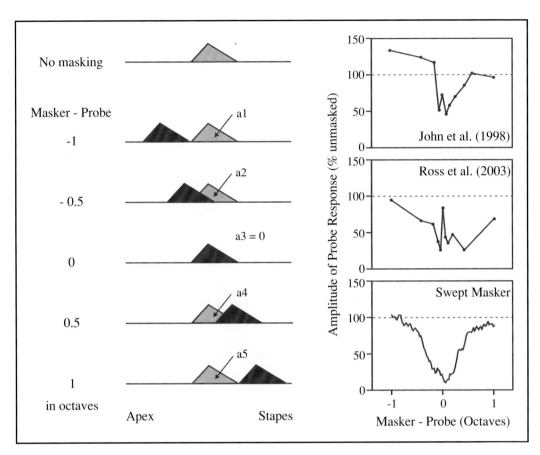

Figure 10–10. *Masking functions. The left section of this figure shows the activation patterns on the basilar membrane when a masking stimulus (black) is presented together with the probe stimulus (gray). The masking effect is then evaluated by plotting the amplitude (a1, a2, a3, etc.), usually expressed relative to the amplitude when the probe is presented alone, against the frequency of the masker. The right section of the figures shows masking functions obtained in three different studies. The study of John et al. (1998) used tone-on-tone masking and recorded electrical 80-Hz responses to a 1-kHz tone. The study of Ross et al. (2003) used tone-on-tone masking and recorded the magnetic 40-Hz response to a 1-kHz tone. When pure tones are used as maskers, a glitch occurs when the probe and masker have the same frequency; the probe effectively becomes louder and has less modulation. Therefore, this point could be discounted in the graphs. The graph in the lower right shows some pilot data obtained by sweeping a narrowband noise through the octave below and above the probe tone. More extensive data are presented by Wilding et al. (2010). The electrical response to the probe was evoked by the 80-Hz modulation of a 2-kHz tone occurring continuously together with the tone. Because the masker was a narrowband noise, no glitch occurs when the masker and tone are the same frequency. The tip of the masking function occurs at a frequency slightly above the frequency of the probe.*

noises are simultaneously swept from 250 to 1000 Hz and from 1000 to 2000 Hz.

The high-pass masking technique used to derive narrowband responses (see Chapter 5, in particular Figure 5–7) also can be used to assess the width of the activation pattern on the basilar membrane that leads to the ASSR. Herdman, Picton, and Stapells (2002) examined the 80-Hz ASSRs in the presence of noise that was high-pass filtered at different frequencies. The masking noise would prevent ASSRs from being initiated in the regions of the basilar membrane activated by the noise. As the high-pass cutoff was decreased and entered the region of the basilar membrane being activated by the ASSR, the amplitude of the ASSR would begin to decrease. The high-pass cutoff was decreased further until the noise completely masked the response. The difference between the two cutoffs then gives the region of the basilar membrane being activated by the ASSR. This width is determined both by the width of the tuning curves of the neurons responding to the modulated tone and the activation pattern of the stimulus (related to its acoustic spectrum and to the traveling wave). For the 80-Hz response to a 60 dB SPL tone, the width was between one half and one octave.

Multiple Simultaneous Stimuli

Having considered the interactions between two stimuli, we now can consider the interactions among several stimuli. Lins and Picton (1995) showed that 80-Hz responses could be recorded to four stimuli presented simultaneously in each ear with little change in amplitude from when the responses were recorded to just a single stimulus. We considered these results in Chapter 6 (see Figure 6–13). Figure 10–11 illustrates similar findings with some more recent data. The procedure of recording multiple different responses simultaneously is the basis for the clinical instrument that goes by the acronym MASTER (*M*ultiple *A*uditory *Ste*ady-*S*tate *R*esponses; John et al., 1998; John & Picton,

2000b). The lack of effect of other stimuli has limits. As pointed out by John et al. (1998), the 80-Hz responses get smaller when the carrier frequencies are separated by a half octave or less and when the intensity is greater than 60 dB SPL. Even outside these limits, multiple stimulation sometimes reduces response amplitude of the 80-Hz responses although usually by only a small amount (e.g., Purcell et al., 2003). The 40-Hz responses show much greater interactions than 80-Hz responses (John et al., 1998).

John, Purcell, Dimitrijevic, and Picton (2002) point out some of the advantages and caveats associated with using multiple simultaneous stimuli. As discussed in Chapter 6, responses are more efficiently recorded using multiple stimuli provided the amplitudes do not decrease by a factor of more than $\sqrt{K}$ where K is the number of simultaneous stimuli. If there is no change in the amplitude with multiple stimuli, responses to eight stimuli can be recognized in the same time it takes to recognize one. However, thresholds usually cannot be estimated eight times faster. We have to continue the multiple-stimulus recording until the smallest response is recognized. Furthermore, when testing patients, thresholds occur at different levels. We may need to record for a prolonged period at one intensity to be sure that there is indeed no response at one particular frequency, even though responses at other frequencies have already been clearly recognized. Thus, when eight stimuli are presented simultaneously (four to each ear) the time advantage of the multiple-stimulus technique is between two and three times rather than eight times. John et al. (2002) suggested that more efficient programs—programs that allow the intensity for each stimulus to be changed "on the fly"—would significantly improve

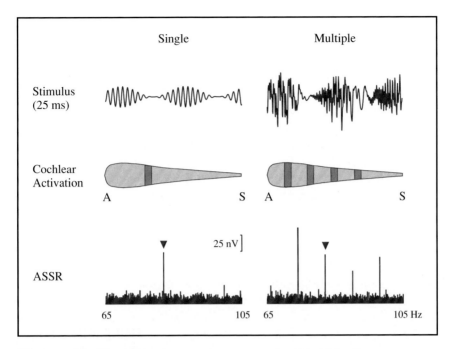

Figure 10–11. ***Multiple simultaneous stimuli.*** *This figure compares ASSRs to a single stimulus (left) with ASSRs to multiple simultaneous stimuli (right). The single stimulus was a 1-kHz tone amplitude modulated at 82 Hz and presented at an intensity of 60 dB SPL. In the multiple-stimulus condition, this stimulus was presented simultaneously with tones of 0.5, 2, and 4 kHz, modulated at 74, 90, and 98 Hz, respectively. The upper part of the figure shows the acoustic waveform. The middle section shows the presumed activation of the basilar membrane (darker gray regions). The membrane is shown with the apex (A) on the left and the stapes (S) on the right; although the opposite of the usual plot, this allows us to keep the stimuli and responses in order. The lower part of the figure shows the ASSRs. The amplitude of the response to the 1-kHz tone (arrowhead) is not significantly different between the two recording conditions. Only part of the response spectrum (from 65 to 105 Hz) is shown.*

the time-advantage of using multiple stimuli. Some of these ideas have recently been implemented (Van Dun et al., 2008).

Interactions Between Modulation Rate and Carrier Frequency

When using multiple stimuli, there has been a tendency to use lower modulation frequencies with lower carrier frequencies. Early studies of newborns suggested that that the optimum modulation frequency for recording the 80-Hz ASSR varied with the carrier frequency: 72 Hz for 500 Hz, 85 Hz for 1500 Hz, and 97 Hz for 4000 Hz (Rickards et al., 1994). Later studies in adults showed no clear interaction between modulation rate and carrier frequency, though intersubject variability may have obscured subtle effects (John & Picton,

2000a). Purcell and John (in press) looked at the effect of modulation frequency on the ASSRs to 500- and 2000-Hz tones using a sweep technique. The 500-Hz response was generally larger between 80 and 90 Hz than at lower or higher frequencies, but the most striking finding was the inter-subject variability in the frequency at which the response was largest. The 2-kHz response appeared to reach its maximum between 90 and 100 Hz, although higher modulation frequencies were not studied. Knowing which modulation frequencies would give optimal recordings for each carrier frequency in each subject would greatly speed threshold testing. However, it is not yet clear how this information can be quickly obtained.

TIMING

The ASSR for a 40-Hz modulation develops over a period of about 200 ms and then continues as a stable response (Ross, Picton, & Pantev, 2002). The initial development of the ASSR can be obscured by the transient gamma-band response (GBR), a brief burst of activity with frequencies near 40 Hz that it evoked by the onset of a stimulus. The ASSR can be distinguished from the GBR by using stimuli with modulations that begin with opposite phase. The GBR occurs in response to the onset of modulation regardless of its phase. Calculating the difference between the responses removes the GBR, but doubles the size of the ASSR; subtracting an inverted response is the same as adding a response of similar polarity. Once developed, the ASSR returns to baseline more quickly (over about 50 ms) when the modulation ceases. If a 40-Hz ASSR is disrupted, for example, with a concomitant short burst of noise, it takes about 200 ms for the response

to develop again (Ross, Herdman, & Pantev, 2005b). The 200-ms period that the 40-Hz takes to develop (or reinstate itself) may reflect some basic property of cortical processing, perhaps related to the binding of properties into objects, and may be the basis for the integration time observed in the psychophysics for perceptual processes such as loudness estimation.

These original results were obtained with MEG recordings. Figure 10–12 shows some electrical recordings that replicate the 200-ms development time for the 40-Hz response and demonstrate a shorter integration period of about 100 ms for the 80-Hz response.

INTENSITY

As the intensity of the stimulus increases the amplitude of the ASSR increases and the latency decreases. When brief tones of 500 Hz are presented at rates of 40 Hz, the amplitude (baseline-to-peak) of the response increases linearly with increasing intensity up to 90 dB HL with slopes between 5 and 20 nV/dB, and the latency decreases with a slope of approximately 100 to 200 μs/dB (Galambos et al, 1981; Rodriguez et al., 1986; Stapells, Linden, Suffield, Hamel, & Picton, 1984). The amplitude slopes are smaller for tones of higher frequency (Rodriguez et al, 1986). Similar changes occur when the stimulus is the AM of a continuous tone rather than separate tones, although the changes with intensity in both amplitude (3–9 nV/dB) and latency (80–100 μs/dB) are less (Parker & O'Dwyer, 1998; Picton et al, 1987).

At modulation rates near 80 to 100 Hz, the ASSR is smaller and the amplitude change with intensity correspondingly less, approximately 1 to 2 nV/dB for intensities below 60 dB SPL (Lins Picton, Picton,

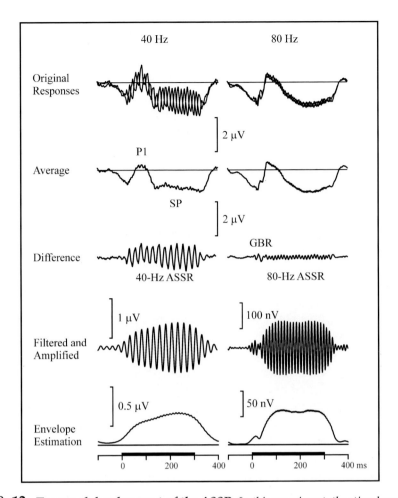

Figure 10–12. *Temporal development of the ASSR.* *In this experiment, the stimulus was a continuous 1-kHz tone presented at 65 dB SPL. Every 500 ms there was a 300-ms period of amplitude-modulation at either 40 or 80 Hz. The modulation alternated in its onset phase and the responses recorded from vertex to posterior neck were averaged separately on the basis of the onset phase. The upper tracings represent the superimposed responses averaged across 10 subjects, with the 80-Hz responses being averaged over four times as many trials as the 40-Hz responses (because the ASSR is much smaller in amplitude). Averaging the responses together (second set of tracings) gives the cerebral response to the modulation. This shows a negative sustained potential (SP) through the duration of the modulation and a P1 wave following the onset of the modulation. Because of the regularity of stimulus timing the SP anticipates the actual onset of the stimulus; it therefore may represent an expectancy wave as well as a sensory response. Because the stimuli were coming twice a second, there is no recognizable N1 wave. The difference between the two original tracings (actually the difference divided by 2) shows the ASSR with most of the onset response removed. However, in the 80-Hz response, there appears to be a small onset gamma-band-response (GBR) that is not completely removed by the subtraction—it is likely triggered by modulation in one direction more than in another and therefore is not completely canceled. The top three sets of data are all at the same amplitude scale. The tracings in the fourth line have been band-pass filtered (35–45 Hz or 70–90 Hz) and amplified with the 80 Hz amplified more than the 40-Hz response. These waveforms show the rise and fall of the ASSR over the period of the modulation. The lowest set of tracings estimates the envelope of this filtered response. This estimate of the envelope was obtained by rectifications and low-pass filtering. The 40-Hz ASSR develops over about 250 ms and ceases within about 80 ms after the end of the modulation. The 80-Hz ASSR develops over about 100 ms (there is a glitch in the first 50 ms that is likely the result of the uncanceled GBR). The 80-Hz ASSR falls back to baseline within 50 ms after the end of the modulation.*

Champagne, &, 1995). The latency change of 60 to 80 μs/dB is similar across carrier frequencies (John & Picton, 2000). At intensities higher than 60 dB, the response shows a greater amplitude increase with increasing intensity and the harmonics in the response become more prominent (Lins et al, 1995).

Ménard, Gallégo, Berger-Vachon, Collet, and Thai-Van (2008) related the amplitude intensity functions for the 80-Hz responses to psychophysical estimates of loudness. They used an unbiased estimate of amplitude, obtained by subtracting noise power away from the measured response power before the amplitude is calculated (discussed in Chapter 6). Like Lins et al. (1995), they found that the slope of the amplitude-intensity function increased when the intensity increased beyond 60 dB HL. Most importantly, they found a high correlation with loudness estimates ($r = 0.9$). Similar results, with correlation coefficients between 0.8 and 0.9, were obtained by Zenker-Castro, Barajas de Prat, and Zabala (2008). These results suggest that ASSR amplitudes might be useful as an objective measure of loudness when fitting hearing aids (see discussion in Zenker-Castro & Barajas de Prat, 2008). Picton et al. (2005) found that the slope of the amplitude-intensity function of the ASSR was higher in subjects with sensorineural hearing loss than in those with normal hearing. This likely represents "physiologic recruitment," although the authors did not relate the amplitudes to psychophysical estimates of loudness. Zenker Castro and Barajas de Plat (2008) have proposed ways to calculate the compression factor of a hearing aid to compensate for loudness recruitment. These techniques need to be evaluated further.

The relationship of the ASSR to stimulus intensity can be directly measured by sweeping the stimulus through a range of intensities (Picton, van Roon, & John, 2007). Four separate carrier frequencies can then be examined simultaneously in each ear. The slope of the amplitude-intensity function was greater at 500 Hz (1.4 nV/dB) than at 1kHz (0.9 nV/dB) or 2 kHz (0.8 nV/dB) with the slope at 4 kHz (1.3 nV/dB) being intermediate. At intensities of greater than 60 dB SPL the amplitude-intensity function flattened off for the midfrequencies, indicating significant interactions between stimuli when multiple stimuli occurred simultaneously. These effects are illustrated in Figure 10–13.

Interactions between amplitude-modulated stimuli can involve processes other than simple masking or suppression. Picton et al. (2009) found complex effects of modulation frequency when stimuli were presented dichotically. The response at the higher modulation frequency was larger than that at the lower modulation frequency but only for carriers of 500 or 1000 Hz and modulation frequencies less than 90 Hz.

THRESHOLD

40-Hz Responses

One of the main clinical applications for the ASSRs has been the objective evaluation of hearing thresholds (Picton, 2007). When the 40-Hz response was initially reported (Galambos et al., 1981), one of the hopes was that it might provide a better way to estimate thresholds at low frequencies than was possible with the tone-ABR. As can be seen in Table 10–1, the response estimates thresholds in waking adults with a mean physiologic-behavioral difference of about 10 dB and a standard deviation of about 10 dB. Unfortunately,

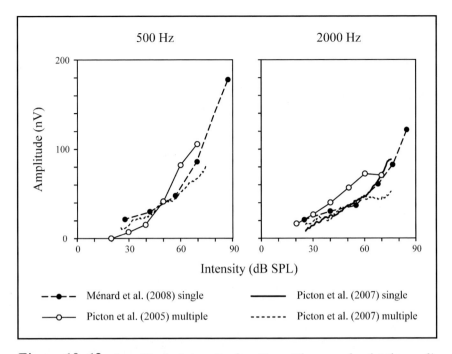

Figure 10–13. Amplitude-intensity functions. These graphs plot the amplitude of the 80-Hz ASSR relative to stimulus intensity in normal subjects. The data from Ménard et al. (2008) have been changed from HL to SPL. The data from Picton et al. (2007) were obtained using a sweep of intensities rather than a set of discrete intensities.

the 40-Hz response was attenuated by sleep (Linden et al., 1985) and was difficult to record in infants (Stapells, Galambos, Costello, & Makeig, 1988). Because assessment of infant hearing was the major application for objective audiometry, the response soon fell out of favor. However, it remains an important way to assess hearing in adult patients (or adolescents) when behavioral thresholds are inconsistent or unreliable. In this context, either the 40-Hz response or the LAEPs (see Chapter 11) may provide objective estimates of threshold, one paper preferring the former (Van Maanen & Stapells, 2005), one the latter (Tomlin, Rance, Graydon & Tsialios, 2006), and another finding the results about the same (Yeung & Wong, 2007).

Various factors explain the variability of the data in Table 10–1. The early studies used brief tones instead of modulated tones and these give physiologic thresholds that are closer to the behavioral thresholds. However, these behavioral thresholds are for brief tones and because of temporal integration it is not always clear how nHL for brief tones relates to HL for longer tones. The more recent studies use modulated tones, but differ in terms of the amount of time allowed in assessing whether a response is present or not. Studies that use the Audera equipment (Ozdek et al., 2010; Tomlin et al., 2006) are limited to a recording period of less than 2 minutes, and this usually is not enough to recognize responses at low intensities. If 40-Hz responses are recorded for periods

Table 10–1. 40-Hz responses: Physiologic-Behavioral Threshold Differences (in dB), Means, and SD. (Studies using Adults or Older Children)

Group	Study	Frequency (Hz)			
		500	1000	2000	4000
Normal	Sammeth and Barry, 1985	9 ± 7	10 ± 10	9 ± 5	16 ± 7
	Aoyagi et al., 1993	11 ± 10	11 ± 11	13 ± 10	18 ± 12
	Tomlin et al. , 2006	17 ± 10			42 ± 14
	Tlumak et al, 2007*	10 ± 10	10 ± 9	11 ± 8	13 ± 10
	Ozdek et al., 2010	15 ± 12	10 ± 7	14 ± 8	15 ± 9
Hearing-Impaired	Kankkunen and Rosenhall, 1985**	8 ± 11	5 ± 9	4 ± 7	3 ± 8
	Aoyagi et al., 1993	8 ± 7	9 ± 6	13 ± 8	12 ± 6
	Van Maanen and Stapells, 2005	14 ± 7	11 ± 6	12 ± 14	0 ± 9
	Tomlin et al., 2006	11 ± 9			23 ± 8
	Tlumak et al., 2007*	5 ± 10	11 ± 11	12 ± 13	9 ± 13
	Ozdek et al., 2010	8 ± 6	9 ± 6	9 ± 7	14 ± 10

*Tlumak, Rubenstein, and Durrant (2007) is a meta-analysis of many published papers.
**Kankkunen and Rosenhall (1985) results are for groups containing both normal and hearing-impaired subjects.

of 15 minutes at each intensity, the response can be recognized down to within ±10 dB of behavioral thresholds (Stapells, Makeig, & Galambos, 1987). When recording one response at a time, this would take too long for clinical use. Some compromise between time and accuracy is necessary. We discussed this issue in Chapter 6, and will return to it when we examine the more extensive set of threshold data for the 80-Hz response. Van Maanen and Stapells (2005) recorded 40-Hz responses to four different frequencies simultaneously. The 40-Hz responses show more interaction between frequencies than the 80-Hz responses (John et al., 1998) and the responses are smaller when four stimuli are presented simultaneously than when each is presented singly. The increased efficiency from recording four responses simultaneously therefore is balanced by the decrease in amplitude. At 40 Hz, using multiple simultaneous stimuli has about the same level of efficiency as using separate recordings with single stimuli.

80-Hz Responses

Since the 80-Hz responses are little affected by sleep (Cohen et al., 1991) and can be readily recorded in infants (Rickards et al., 1994), they have been studied much more extensively as a means for objective audiometry. Table 10–2 provides data from some of the many published studies. This particular table is limited to the results in older children and adults. The results with infants are considered more fully in Chapter 13. The choice of studies in the

Table 10–2. 80-Hz Responses: Physiologic-Behavioral Threshold Differences (in dB), Means, and SD. Studies Using Multiple Simultaneous Stimulation in Adults or Older Children

Group	Study	Frequency (Hz)			
		500	*1000*	*2000*	*4000*
Normal	Lins et al., 1996	14±11	12±11	11±8	13±11
	Herdman and Stapells, 2001	14±10	8±7	8±9	15±9
	Dimitrijevic et al., 2002	17±10	4±11	4±8	11±7
	Luts and Wouters, 2004 (5 min)	15±9	10±11	12±7	18±9
	Luts and Wouters, 2004 (15 min)	12±7	7±7	9±7	13±7
	Picton et al., 2005 (2 min)	35±16	16±8	19±9	23±15
	Picton et al., 2005 (12 min)	21±8	7±8	10±6	13±7
	Tlumak et al., 2007*	17±12	13±12	11±10	15±10
	Elberling et al., 2007	11±7	10±7	6±5	13±4
	D'haenens et al., 2009	19±10	15±8	10±8	13±8
	Ishida et al., in press (bone conduction)	14±11	12±13	11±11	8±7
Hearing-Impaired	Lins et al., 1996	9±9	13±12	11±10	12±13
	Dimitrijevic et al., 2002	13±11	5±8	5±9	8±11
	Herdman and Stapells, 2003	14±13	8±9	10±10	3±10
	Van Maanen and Stapells, 2005	17±11	15±7	19±9	4±10
	Picton et al., 2005 (12 min)	11±18	−4±9	3±11	5±12
	Vander Werff and Brown, 2005	15±8	9±6	8±6	6±5
	Tlumak et al., 2007*	14±13	10±13	9±12	8±13
	Lin, Ho, and Wu, 2009	17±14	15±9	14±8	11±8
	D'haenens et al., 2009 (mild)	14±11	13±8	14±7	13±6
	D'haenens et al., 2009 (moderate)	14±7	10±10	9±6	11±9
	Ishida et al., in press (bone conduction)	17±13	11±11	9±10	5±8

*Tlumak et al. (2007) is a meta-analysis of many published papers.

table has been limited to those using multiple simultaneous stimuli and those that can adjust the amount of time for a recording. Therefore, the listing does not include any results with Audera equipment, which limits its recording time to less than 2 minutes. The justification for this is that the physiologic-behavioral differences will be elevated in subjects with behavioral thresholds near normal. Other sources that provide a more extensive review of these and other threshold-data are Vander Werff, Johnson, and Brown (2008) and Cone-Wesson and Dimitrijevic (2009).

Accurate threshold estimation depends on being able to distinguish small responses from the residual background electrical noise (from EEG and muscle activity). As the background EEG reduces with increased recording time (see Chapters 3 and 6), the longer we record, the smaller the ASSR we can recognize. Figure 10–14 shows data recorded from the same subject after two different recording periods: 1.6 and 9.8 min-

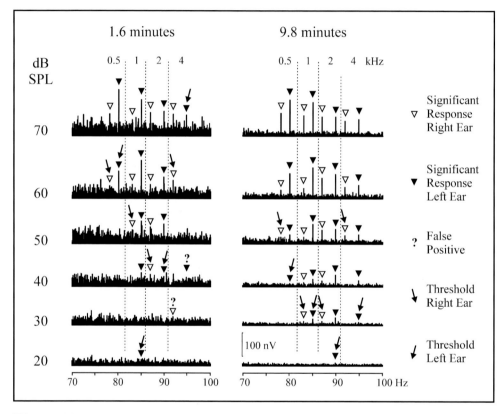

Figure 10–14. Threshold estimations. *This figure illustrates how thresholds are determined after different analysis times. In this paradigm, four stimuli (0.5, 1, 2, and 4 kHz carriers) were simultaneously presented in each ear. The modulation rates were set up so that the higher-frequency carrier and the left ear had the higher modulation frequency. With a longer analysis time, the background noise is reduced to a lower level and responses of smaller amplitude become recognizable. The ASSR threshold was determined as the lowest intensity at which a significant (p <0.05) response was recognized, provided the response was present at all higher intensities, with the proviso that the response might have been missed at one intensity. The qualifications were to ensure against the system detecting a false positive response (as shown by the ? examples in the figure) or occasionally missing a response that was there. The longer analysis time gives thresholds that are closer to the behavioral threshold (between 10 and 20 dB SPL), and much less variable (range 20 to 50 dB rather than 20 to 70 dB SPL). Data from Picton et al. (2005).*

utes (Picton et al., 2005). After 1.6 minutes, the noise level remains high and responses are recognized on average between 30 and 40 dB above behavioral thresholds (between 10 and 20 dB SPL). After 9.8 minutes, the responses can be recognized at lower intensities and there is less variability in the differences between physiologic and behavioral thresholds.

If we record for less than 2 minutes, we often will not be able to recognize ASSR responses of less than 40 nV. As demonstrated in Figure 10–15, this occurs about 36 dB above behavioral thresholds

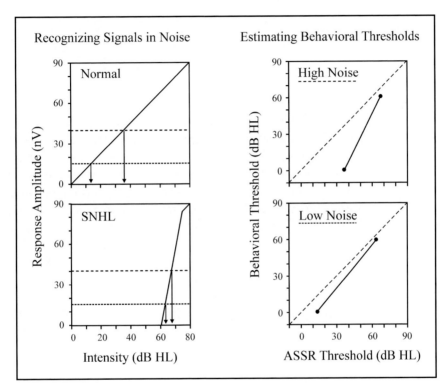

Figure 10–15. Effects of residual noise on threshold estimation. *This figure illustrates how well thresholds are estimated at different levels of background noise. On the left are shown representative ASSR amplitude-intensity functions for subjects with normal-hearing and subjects with sensorineural hearing loss (SNHL). Two levels of noise are shown: the high noise (dashed line) being the confidence limits for recognizing a signal after 1.6 minutes and the low noise (dotted line) after 9.8 minutes (cf. Figure 10–14). For the normal subject, the threshold for recognizing the ASSR occurs at 36 dB above behavioral threshold for high noise and 13 dB above behavioral threshold for low noise. In the SNHL subject, the ASSR amplitude increases rapidly from zero to normal amplitudes over the first 10 dB above threshold—physiologic recruitment. The difference between ASSR and behavioral threshold-estimations at high and low noise levels is small: 8 and 3 dB, respectively. The right side of the figure shows the relations between ASSR and behavioral thresholds at the two different noise levels (i.e., after analyzing data for 1.6 or 9.8 minutes).*

in a subject with normal hearing but about 13 dB above behavioral thresholds in a subject with a sensorineural hearing loss. If the hearing-impaired patient has recruitment, the amplitude of the response (like the perceived loudness) grows more rapidly with increasing intensity above threshold than in a normal subject. Several of the studies listed in Table 10–2 that compare normal and hearing-impaired subjects have found that the threshold differences are smaller and less variable in hearing-impaired subjects.

As illustrated in the lower section of Figure 10–15, we can plot the estimated behavioral thresholds (on the *y*-axis) relative to physiologic thresholds (*x*-axis) and calculate a regression line. If we use short recording periods, the regression line is farther away from the diagonal at low intensities than at high. This makes the slope greater than 1, usually between 1.2 and 1.4. The intercept on the *y*–axis is an estimate of the difference between the physiologic and behavioral thresholds at 0 dB. If we use recording periods that decrease the background noise enough so that we can detect responses of 15 nV, the regression line runs almost parallel to the diagonal of the graph with a slope near 1. Unfortunately, the literature is complicated because regression lines have been plotted with reversed axes (e.g., Rance, Rickards, Cohen, De Vidi, & Clark, 1995). It probably is better to put the predicted value—the behavioral thresholds—on the *y*-axis. Figure 10–16 plots data from two studies, Dimitrijevic et al. (2002) and Rance and Rickards (2002). These issues concerning the relations between estimated behavioral thresholds and the residual noise level are covered at greater length in Picton, John, Dimitrijevic, and Purcell (2003) and Picton et al. (2005). Several studies have compared the physiologic

and behavioral thresholds using different recording times; the data of Luts and Wouters (2004) and Picton et al. (2005) are included in Table 10–2. Luts and Wouters (2005) directly compared the Audera and Master instruments and found that, though both perform well for hearing-impaired subjects, thresholds obtained with the Audera in normal subjects are both elevated and variable.

Regression statistics can be used to calculate an expected difference between physiologic and behavioral thresholds at each intensity. This then can be used to compensate for the increased difference at lower intensities when the recording time is short (Rance & Rickards, 2002; Rance et al., 1995). Usually, we subtract the mean physiologic-behavioral difference when we estimate thresholds (discussed in Chapter 6). When using the regression approach, what is subtracted varies with the physiologic threshold. A sample regression is illustrated in the right side of Figure 10–16. For example, 35 dB is subtracted when the physiologic threshold is 40 dB HL and 5 dB when the physiologic threshold is 80 dB. However, the variance of the threshold estimates is also increased when the residual noise levels are high. This variance increases the error of the estimated behavioral threshold, often making them "discordant" with behavioral thresholds, particularly when the thresholds are at low or moderate levels (Hatzopoulos et al., 2010). If we measure thresholds using sufficient analysis time to allow us to recognized ASSRs at low amplitude, the regression line of the behavioral thresholds versus physiologic thresholds usually has a slope near 1, as in the left side of Figure 10–16. If we were to use the regression approach in this situation, we would subtract the same amount regardless of the physiologic threshold.

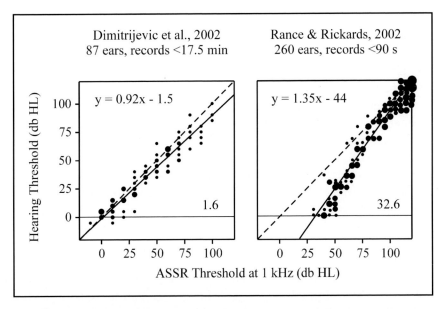

Figure 10–16. *Estimating hearing thresholds from ASSR thresholds. These two graphs show regression analyses relating the behavioral thresholds (y-axis) to the ASSR thresholds at 1 kHz (x-axis). If the hearing thresholds could be perfectly predicted from the ASSR thresholds, the data would line up along the diagonal (*dashed line*). The data tend to be located to the right of the diagonal indicating that the hearing thresholds are lower than ASSR thresholds. Dimitrijevic et al. (2002) determined thresholds using recording periods that extended out to 17.5 minutes at the lowest intensities to be sure that a small response was present or absent. Rance and Rickards (2002) did not extend their recordings beyond 90 s and therefore could not recognize small responses. The slope of the regression (*continuous line*) is close to 1 in the Dimitrijevic regression and significantly higher than 1 in the Rance regression. The number at the lower right in each graph gives the intercept of the regression line with the x-axis; this is the mean ASSR threshold when the hearing threshold is 0 dB HL.*

When estimating behavioral thresholds from ASSR thresholds we should bear in mind a general principle presented in Chapter 6—we cannot conquer time. If we want to obtain accurate estimates of behavioral thresholds, we need to spend the time necessary to reduce the background EEG and EMG noise sufficiently to recognize small ASSRs. This is particularly true when we are considering thresholds that are only mildly or moderately elevated and/or when the hearing loss we are investigating is not characterized by recruitment. The SNR for the expected amplitude of the response is what determines whether we can reliably decide that the response is present or not.

Time still can be saved without sacrificing the SNR. Using multiple simultaneous stimuli can decrease the amount of time required as this does not significantly alter the amplitudes of the 80-Hz response or the background noise when the responses are near threshold. Multiple responses then can be evaluated in the same time that it takes for one. Protocols that monitor the recording and move to another intensity as soon as a response is reliably declared present or absent need to be made available in clinical instruments (John and Purcell, 2008; Luts, Van Dun, Alaerts, & Wouters, 2008). The future of ASSR audiometry will depend on programs that track thresholds efficiently, making automatic decisions about the presence or absence of responses and using intelligent protocols to bracket thresholds. John et al. (2002) have shown that 80-Hz ASSRs are not affected by simultaneously presenting stimuli of different frequencies with intensities differing by up to 20 dB. The limits of this multiple-intensity approach need to be further evaluated in terms of how great an intensity-difference can be tolerated and whether this varies with the type of hearing loss.

Choice of Stimuli for ASSR Audiometry

A plethora of different stimuli have been used to evoke ASSRs. The acoustic parameters of these stimuli were reviewed in Chapter 5. Originally, ASSRs were evoked by periodically presented brief tones. Responses to simple AM are more frequency-specific in acoustic terms but are smaller than the responses to brief tones. Various techniques have been proposed to enhance the amplitude of the ASSR (and therefore increase the speed of the recording) without losing too much in the way of frequency-specificity. The original paper of Cohen et al. (1991) suggested a combination of AM and FM (frequency modulation). The difficulty with this is that the amplitude enhancement will depend on the relative phases of the two modulations (John, Dimitrijevic, van Roon, & Picton, 2001), and this may change among subjects. John,

Dimitrijevic, and Picton, (2002) proposed using an exponential envelope that causes a larger response at lower carrier frequencies. A similar stimulus was proposed by Stürzebecher, Cebulla, and Pschirrer, 2001. A combination of exponential envelope AM and FM has also been used (D'haenens et al., 2007). Most recently, bandpass chirps designed to compensate for cochlear delay times have been proposed (Elberling, Cebulla, &. Stürzebecher, 2007). Which stimulus is optimum is unclear. Comparative studies have assessed response amplitude rather than threshold accuracy or have compared protocols in which both the stimuli and the analysis protocols differ (e.g., Vander Werff, 2009). My intuition is that the effects of different stimuli are small and that either exponential amplitude-modulation (AM^2) or bandpass chirps might be best.

Evaluation of Suprathreshold Hearing

The ASSRs are well suited to the evaluation of suprathreshold hearing. AM and FM tones can be amplified through hearing aids without the significant distortion that occurs with transient stimuli (Picton et al., 1998). Because the threshold for recording a modulation following response is similar to the threshold for detecting the modulation (Picton et al., 1987), ASSRs might become useful as an objective means for demonstrating a subject's ability to discriminate between stimuli differing in intensity or frequency. Dimitrijevic, John, and Picton (2004) found significant relationships between word recognition and the number of ASSRs detected using stimuli that were independently modulated in frequency and amplitude (Dimitrijevic, John, van Roon, & Picton, 2001). Alaerts et al (2009) found even better correlations using ASSRs at slower modulation rates.

The objective evaluation of suprathreshold hearing needs to be developed further. Fitting hearing aids and programming implants in infants require some estimate of what the infants are actually hearing and whether it is sufficient for them to make the discriminations necessary for speech perception. It is possible that speech stimuli may be used in this context—we dream of talking through the hearing aid or implant and seeing in the recorded brain responses whether the speech has been reliably transmitted to the brain. To this end, we briefly look at some research on speech-following responses.

SPEECH-FOLLOWING RESPONSES

Speech is produced by manipulating multiple rhythms (see Figure 5–13). Vowel sounds and voiced consonants are based on the rhythmic opening and closing of the vocal folds—between 50 and 250 Hz during normal speech, although a wider range occurs during singing. Many phonemes are defined by accentuated bands of frequencies, "formants," that move momentarily to indicate stop consonants or remain briefly stable during vowels. The most important formants occur between 200 and 5000 Hz. Other phonemes are distinguished by the relative timing of different sound components. Voice onset time differentiates between "pa" and "ba" in European languages and between "ba" and "mba" in some African languages. The ongoing amplitude of the speech sound— the "speech envelope"—changes over time according to its own rhythms, usually in the range of 1 to 20 Hz. Sometimes, these are the relaxed rhythms of everyday

speech but at other times they can become the more definite rhythms of oratorical cadence and poetic meter. The perception of speech depends on the brain's ability to follow all these different rhythms.

Speech FFRs

The response to the normal voicing rhythm is most easily studied using synthesized speech where the rhythm is held constant. Responses then can be recorded and the voicing response measured by means of a frequency transform. Krishnan (2002) showed that the response to a synthesized vowel contains a series of harmonics of the voicing frequency or fundamental, with the harmonics accentuated near the first formant and much less prominent for the second formant. The brainstem response represents the acoustic waveform as seen through a low-pass filter with a cutoff beginning near 1000 Hz.

Normal speech does not have a constant voicing frequency. In European languages, the speech fundamental varies both randomly and in response to various intonation patterns such as the rising pitch at the end of a question. In tonal languages, vowels are categorized on the basis of the pitch track during the vowel. Measuring the brainstem response to such changes in intonation cannot be performed using frequency transforms, which assume that a signal is constant for the duration of the analysis. However, they can be measured using techniques such as the short-term autocorrelation algorithm (Krishnan, Xu, Gandour, & Cariani, 2004), the Fourier analyzer (Aiken & Picton, 2006, 2008a), or other short-term frequency techniques (Dajani, Purcell, Wong, Kunov, & Picton, 2005). High-pass masking studies show that the response at the fundamental or voicing frequency is a combination of two processes: an FFR that follows the spectral energy in the signal at the voicing frequency and an envelope-following response that follows the modulation-frequency of the higher frequency harmonics. Aiken and Picton (2008a) called these components the spectral FFR and the envelope FFR. Figure 10–17 shows the response to a natural vowel recorded using a frequency transform and a Fourier analyzer.

The accuracy of pitch tracking in the human brainstem varies with the subject's language experience. Subjects who used tonal languages showed a much greater ability to synchronize their brainstem response to the changing pitch of a sound

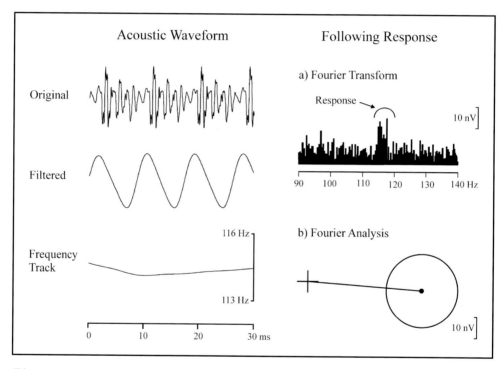

Figure 10–17. Response to a natural vowel. *The tracing in the upper left shows the acoustic waveform of the vowel "a" spoken in a normal voice. If we filter the waveform to show the fundamental frequency we can construct the frequency-track of the speaker's vocal pitch. Over a sustained vowel (lasting 1.5 seconds) this pitch varies over a range from 113 to 118 Hz. If we average the brain response to the vowel and then submit it to a Fourier transform (upper right), we find that the response to the vocal pitch is spread out over multiple different frequency bins (spanning from 113 to 118 Hz). In this particular recording, the response is recognizable over this region in the spectrum, but the SNR is low and in recordings from other subjects we are unable to see a definite response. If we analyze the following response using a Fourier analyzer, which allows the reference-frequency to vary through the duration of the analysis, we find a large response with a high SNR. The response is plotted using a polar plot with the circle representing the* $p < 0.05$ *confidence limits of the mean response. This polar plot uses the same amplitude-scale as the Fourier transform; the analyzed response is about three times larger than in the transformed data. Data from Aiken and Picton (2006).*

(Krishnan, Xu, Gandour, & Cariani, 2005) and this occurred even for pitch patterns that were not native to their particular language (Krishnan, Gandour, & Bidelman, 2010). The brainstem's ability to follow pitch is plastic and depends on experience. Musical experience also may enhance the ability of the brainstem to track pitch (Wong, Skoe, Russo, Dees, & Kraus, 2007).

Response to the Speech Envelope

The speech envelope is the changing amplitude of the energy in continuous speech as it sequences through the different phonemes and syllables of the spoken words. Following this envelope is crucially important to speech perception. The overlapping frequencies that make up the incoming acoustic signal must be parsed and categorized and ultimately put back together as a comprehensible message. Clearly, the spectral content of the signal is essential to identifying the different phonemes, but the amplitude-envelope is equally important. A set of four frequency limited bands of noise, modulated by the temporal envelopes for four matching frequency bands of the incoming signal, can provide enough speech information to support near-perfect identification of vowels, consonants, and sentences (Shannon, Zeng, Kamath, Wygonski, & Ekelid, 1995). This finding explains why speech can be recognized through a cochlear implant, where the incoming spectrum is divided up across a small number of electrodes rather than thousands of different neurons. Even without any spectral information at all (with white noise modulated with the overall speech envelope) sentence recognition is above chance. Envelope fre-

quencies between 4 and 16 Hz contribute most to the intelligibility of speech. Recording the brain's response to the speech envelope, which changes from moment to moment over a relatively wide range, is not possible using either a frequency transform or a Fourier analyzer.

Aiken and Picton (2008a) used correlation techniques to look at the response of the human auditory cortex to the speech envelope of sentences. The envelope of the spoken sentence was abstracted from the speech signal by rectification and low-pass filtering. This was then correlated with the EEG signals coming from the auditory cortices using various delays. The highest correlation occurred at a latency of about 190 ms; the auditory cortex following the speech envelope after this delay. Figure 10–18 shows some of the findings. This latency suggests that the LAEPs likely are involved in following speech. The morphology of the transient LAEP then might represent the impulse function of the cortex, which is convolved with the incoming sensory signal to give the cortical response. Lalor and Foxe (2010) used a different mathematical approach to obtain a similar impulse response that they call "auditory evoked spread spectrum analysis." Abrams, Nicol, Zecker, and Kraus (2008) found that the cortical response that followed the speech envelope was greater in the right hemisphere than the left. Ahissar et al (2001) found that the ability of the auditory cortex to follow the envelopes of speech that had been temporally compressed was correlated with the ability of the subject to perceive the speech signals. These results are promising. We need more studies assessing how the human cortex follows the speech envelope.

We have begun to see how the speech envelope is converted to electrical rhythms

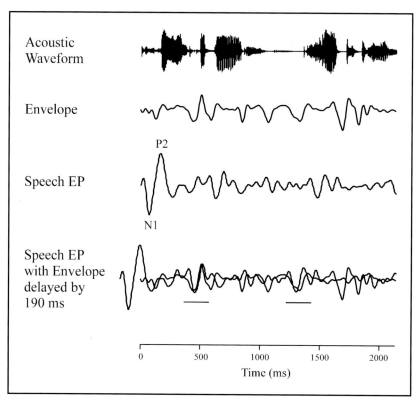

Figure 10–18. Response to speech envelope. *The top tracing shows the acoustic waveform of the beginning of the sentence, "To find the body, they had to drain . . ." The envelope of this waveform was obtained by rectification, log transformation, and then filtering. The evoked potential recorded from the brain shows a large N1-P2 response to the onset of the sentence, followed by a sequence of waves. As shown at the bottom, this sequence of waves show positive correlations with the speech envelope when the brain response is shifted to the left by 190 ms (i.e., when the brain response occurs 190 ms after what is happening in the stimulus). Lines show regions of high correlation. Data from Aiken and Picton (2008b).*

in the brain. The envelope is more complex than a single waveform; there are likely multiple envelopes, each for a particular spectral region. Furthermore, the processing of the envelope must be more complex than simply representing it in electrical form. Interactions must occur between the envelope and the regions of the brain that process phonemes, syllables, words, and sentences. These processes all occur in this brave new world of cerebral speech processing.

CONCLUDING COMMENTS

We have reviewed many different following responses that can be recorded as the human brain processes sounds. These responses most commonly are evoked by periodic stimuli and studied as ASSRs. These responses have become a useful tool for the objective evaluation of hearing threshold. They also provide a possible means to assess suprathreshold hearing. This would be useful in fitting hearing aids and programming implants, and might become useful in evaluating patients with auditory processing disorders.

In addition, our studies have raised some general questions about the brain. What is the nature of these following responses? Our understanding of how the brain perceives the world has been largely based on the idea of "labeled lines." In this formulation, the physical parameters of a sensory stimulus are coded by the rates of firing in neurons that are specific to each of these parameters. The frequency spectrum of a sound is thus coded in terms of the activation of neurons connected to different regions of the basilar membrane. However, sensory attributes might also be coded in the timing of the neuronal discharges. This has always been part of our understanding of hearing— that pitch might be coded in the synchronous discharges of groups of neurons. This concept leads to the idea that synchronization may play a role in other aspects of perception (Uhlhaas et al., 2009). Features may be linked together to form objects using synchronous oscillations and perceptual information may be carried by EEG rhythms.

In the epigraph for this chapter, Bergamin described people who dance to the rhythms played to them, people who dance to their own rhythms and people who do not dance at all. His categorization also may apply to the neurons of our brain.

ABBREVIATIONS

ABR	Auditory brainstem response
AM	Amplitude modulation
ASSR	Auditory steady-state response
CM	Cochlear microphonic
EEG	Electroencephalogram
EMG	Electromyogram
FFR	Frequency-following response
FM	Frequency modulation
GBR	Gamma band response
LAEP	Late auditory evoked potential
MASTER	Multiple Auditory Steady-State Responses
MEG	Magnetoencephalography
MLR	Middle latency response
nHL	Normal hearing level
SNHL	Sensorineural hearing loss
SNR	Signal-to-noise ratio
SOA	Stimulus onset asynchrony

REFERENCES

Abrams, D., Nicol, T., Zecker, S., & Kraus, N. (2008). Right-hemisphere auditory cortex is dominant for coding syllable patterns in speech. *Journal of Neuroscience, 28*, 3958–3965.

Ahissar, E., Nagarajan, S., Ahissar, M., Protopapas, A., Mahncke, H., & Merzenich, M. M. (2001). Speech comprehension is correlated with temporal response patterns recorded from auditory cortex. *Proceedings of the National Academy of Sciences, USA, 98*, 13367–13372.

Aiken, S. J., & Picton, T. W. (2006). Envelope following responses to natural vowels. *Audiology and Neurotology, 11*, 213–232.

Aiken, S. J., & Picton, T. W. (2008a). Envelope and spectral frequency following responses to vowel sounds. *Hearing Research, 245*, 35–47.

Aiken, S. J., & Picton, T. W. (2008b). Human cortical responses to the speech envelope. *Ear and Hearing, 15*, 139–157.

Alaerts, J., Luts, H., Hofmann, M., & Wouters, J. (2009). Cortical auditory steady-state responses to low modulation rates. *International Journal of Audiology, 48*, 582–593.

Alaerts, J., Luts, H., Van Dun, B., Desloovere, C., & Wouters, J. (2010) Latencies of auditory steady-state responses recorded in early infancy. *Audiology and Neurotology, 15*, 116–127.

Aoyagi, M., Kiren, T., Kim, Y., Suzuki, Y., Fuse, T., & Koike, Y. (1993). Frequency specificity of amplitude-modulation-following response detected by phase spectral analysis. *Audiology, 32*, 293–301.

Bacon, S. P., & Viemeister, N. F. (1985). Temporal modulation transfer functions in normal-hearing and hearing-impaired listeners. *Audiology, 24*, 117–134.

Boettcher, F. A., Madhotra, D., Poth, E. A., & Mills, J. H. (2002). The frequency-modulation following response in young and aged human subjects. *Hearing Research, 165*, 10–18.

Boettcher, F. A., Poth, E. A., Mills, J. H., & Dubno, J. R. (2001). The amplitude-modulation following response in young and aged human subjects. *Hearing Research, 153*, 32–42.

Chimento, T. C., & Schreiner, C. E. (1990). Selectively eliminating cochlear microphonic contamination from the frequency-following response. *Electroencephalography and Clinical Neurophysiology, 75*, 88–96.

Cohen, L. T., Rickards, F. W., & Clark, G. M. (1991). A comparison of steady-state evoked potentials to modulated tones in awake and sleeping humans. *Journal of the Acoustical Society of America, 90*, 2467–2479.

Cone-Wesson, B., & Dimitrijevic, A. (2009). The auditory steady-state response. In J. Katz (Ed.), *Handbook of clinical audiology* (6th ed., pp. 322–350). Baltimore, MD: Lippincott Williams & Wilkins.

Dajani, H. R., & Picton, T. W. (2006). Human auditory steady-state responses to changes in interaural correlation. *Hearing Research, 219*, 85–100.

Dajani, H., Purcell, D., Wong, W., Kunov, H., & Picton T., (2005). Recording human evoked potentials that follow the pitch contour of a natural vowel. *IEEE Transactions in Biomedical Engineering, 52*, 1614–1618.

D'haenens, W., Dhooge, I., De Vel, E., Maes, L., Bockstael, A., & Vinck, B. M. (2007). Auditory steady-state responses to MM and exponential envelope AM^2/FM stimuli in normal-hearing adults. *International Journal of Audiology, 46*, 399–406.

D'haenens, W., Dhooge, I., Maes, L., Bockstael, A., Kepler, H., Philips, B., . . . Vinck B. M. (2009). The clinical value of the multiple-frequency 80-Hz auditory steady-state response in adults with normal hearing and hearing loss. *Archives of Otolaryngology-Head and Neck Surgery, 135*, 496–506.

Dimitrijevic, A., John, M. S., & Picton, T. W. (2004). Auditory steady-state responses and word recognition scores in normal-hearing and hearing-impaired adults. *Ear and Hearing, 25*, 68–84.

Dimitrijevic, A., John, M. S., Van Roon, P., & Picton, T. W. (2001). Human auditory steady-state responses to tones independently modulated in both frequency and amplitude. *Ear and Hearing, 22*, 100–111.

Dimitrijevic, A., John, M. S., Van Roon, P., Purcell, D. W., Adamonis, J., Ostroff, J., . . . Picton, T. W. (2002). Estimating the audiogram using multiple auditory steady-state responses. *Journal of the American Academy of Audiology, 13*, 205–224.

Dobie, R. A., & Wilson, M. J. (1998). Low-level steady-state auditory evoked potentials: effects of rate and sedation on detectability. *Journal of the Acoustical Society of America, 104*, 3482–3488.

Elberling, C., Cebulla, M., & Stürzebecher, E. (2007). Simultaneous multiple stimulation of the auditory steady-state response (ASSR). In T. Dau, J. M. Buchholz, J. M. Harte, & T. U. Christiansen (Eds.), *Auditory signal processing in hearing-impaired listeners (ISAAR 2007)* (pp. 201–209). Copenhagen, Denmark: Centertryk (GN ReSound Audiological Library).

Fastl, H., & Zwicker, E. (2007). *Psychoacoustics: Facts and models.* Berlin, Germany: Springer.

Galambos, R., & Makeig, S. (1988). Dynamic changes in steady-state potentials. In E. Basar (Ed.), *Dynamics of sensory and cognitive processing by the brain* (pp. 178–199). Berlin, Germany: Springer.

Galambos, R., Makeig, S., & Talmachoff, P. J. (1981). A 40-Hz auditory potential recorded from the human scalp. *Proceedings of the National Academy of Sciences, USA, 78,* 2643–2647.

Galbraith, G. C., Bhuta, S. M., Choate, A. K., Kitahara, J. M., & Mullen, T. A., Jr. (1998). Brain stem frequency-following response to dichotic vowels during attention. *Neuro-Report, 9,* 1889–1893.

Galbraith, G. C., Olfman, D. M, & Huffman, T. M. (2003). Selective attention affects human brain stem frequency-following response. *NeuroReport, 14,* 735–738.

Grose, J. H., Mamo, S. K., & Hall, J. W., 3rd. (2009). Age effects in temporal envelope processing: Speech unmasking and auditory steady state responses. *Ear and Hearing, 30,* 568–575

Hatzopoulos ,S., Prosser, S., Ciorba, A., Giarbini, N., Kochanek, K., Sliwa, L., . . . Martini, A. (2010). Threshold estimation in adult normal- and impaired-hearing subjects using auditory steady-state responses. *Medical Science Monitor, 16,* CR21–CR27.

He, N-J., Mills, J. H., Ahlstrom, J. B., & Dubno, J. R. (2008). Age-related differences in the temporal modulation transfer function with pure-tone carriers. *Journal of the Acoustical Society of America, 124,* 3841–3849.

Herdman, A. T., Lins, O., van Roon, P., Stapells, D. R., Scherg, M., & Picton, T. W. (2002). Intracerebral sources of human auditory steady-state responses. *Brain Topography, 15,* 69–86.

Herdman, A. T., Picton, T. W., & Stapells, D.R. (2002) Place specificity of multiple auditory steady-state responses. *Journal of the Acoustical Society of America, 112,* 1569–1582.

Herdman, A. T., & Stapells, D. R. (2001). Thresholds determined using the monotic and dichotic multiple steady-state response technique in normal-hearing subjects. *Scandinavian Audiology, 30,* 41–49.

Herdman, A. T., & Stapells, D. R. (2003) Auditory steady state response thresholds of adults with sensorineural hearing impairment. *International Journal of Audiology, 42,* 237–248.

Hillyard, S. A., & Picton, T. W. (1979). Event-related brain potentials and selective information processing in man. In J. E. Desmedt (Ed.), *Cognitive components in cerebral event-related potentials and selective attention. Progress in clinical neurophysiology* (Vol. 6., pp. 1–52). Basel, Switzerland: Karger.

Hoormann, J., Falkenstein, M., & Hohnsbein, J. (2000). Early attention effects in human auditory-evoked potentials. *Psychophysiology, 37,* 29–42.

Ishida, I. M., Cuthbert, B. P., & Stapells, D. R. (in press). Multiple-ASSR thresholds to bone-conduction stimuli in adults with normal and elevated thresholds. *Ear and Hearing.*

John, M. S., Brown, D. K., Muir, P. J., & Picton, T. W. (2004). Recording auditory steady-state responses in young infants. *Ear and Hearing, 25,* 539–553.

John, M. S., Dimitrijevic, A., & Picton, T. W. (2002). Auditory steady-state responses to exponential modulation envelopes. *Ear and Hearing, 23,* 106–117.

John, M. S., Dimitrijevic, A., van Roon, P., & Picton, T. W. (2001). Multiple auditory steady-state responses to AM and FM stimuli. *Audiology and Neuro-Otology, 6,* 12–27.

John, M. S., Lins, O. G., Boucher, B. L., & Picton, T. W. (1998). Multiple auditory steady-state responses (MASTER): Stimulus and recording parameters. *Audiology, 37,* 59–82.

John, M. S., & Picton, T. W. (2000a). Human auditory steady-state responses to amplitude-modulated tones: phase and latency measurements. *Hearing Research, 141,* 57–79.

John, M. S., & Picton, T. W. (2000b). MASTER: A Windows program for recording multiple auditory steady-state responses. *Computer Methods and Programs in Biomedicine, 61,* 125–150.

John, M. S., & Purcell, D.W. (2008). Introduction to technical principles of auditory steady-state response testing. In G. Rance (Ed.), *Auditory steady-state response: Generation, recording, and clinical applications* (pp. 11–53). San Diego, CA: Plural Publishing.

John, M. S., Purcell, D. W., Dimitrijevic, A., & Picton, T. W. (2002). Advantages and caveats when recording steady-state responses to multiple simultaneous stimuli. *Journal of the American Academy of Audiology, 13,* 246–259.

Johnson, K. L., Nicol, T. G., & Kraus, N. (2005). Brain stem response to speech: A biological marker of auditory processing. *Ear and Hearing, 26,* 424–434.

Joris, P. X., Schreiner, C. E., & Rees, A. (2004). Neural processing of amplitude-modulated sounds. *Physiological Reviews, 84,* 541–577.

Kankkunen, A., & Rosenhall, U. (1985). Comparison between thresholds obtained with pure-tone audiometry and the 40-Hz middle latency response. *Scandinavian Audiology, 14,* 99–104.

Krishnan, A. (2002). Human frequency-following responses: Representation of steady-state synthetic vowels. *Hearing Research, 166,* 192–201.

Krishnan, A. (2007). Frequency-following response. In R. F. Burkard, M. Don, & J. J. Eggermont (Eds.), *Auditory evoked potentials: Basic principles and clinical applications* (pp. 313–333). Baltimore, MD: Lippincott Williams & Wilkins.

Krishnan, A., Gandour, J. T., & Bidelman, G. M. (2010). The effects of tone language experience on pitch processing in the brainstem. *Journal of Neurolinguistics, 23,* 81–95.

Krishnan, A., Xu, Y., Gandour, J. T., & Cariani, P. A. (2004). Human frequency-following response: Representation of pitch contours in Chinese tones. *Hearing Research, 189,* 1–12.

Krishnan, A., Xu, Y., Gandour, J. T., & Cariani, P. A. (2005). Encoding of pitch in the human brainstem is sensitive to language experience. *Cognitive Brain Research, 25,* 161–168.

Lalor, E. C., & Foxe, J. J. (2010). Neural responses to uninterrupted natural speech can be extracted with precise temporal resolution. *European Journal of Neuroscience, 31,* 189–193.

Leigh-Paffenroth, E. D., & Fowler, C. G. (2006). Amplitude-modulated auditory steady state responses in younger and older listeners. *Journal of the American Academy of Audiology, 17,* 582–597.

Levi, E. C., Folsom, R. C., & Dobie, R. A. (1993). Amplitude-modulation following response (AMFR): effects of modulation rate, carrier frequency, age, and state. *Hearing Research, 68,* 42–52.

Levi, E. C., Folsom, R. C., & Dobie, R. A. (1995). Coherence analysis of envelope-following responses (EFRs) and frequency-following responses (FFRs) in infants and adults. *Hearing Research, 89,* 21–27.

Lin, Y. H., Ho, H. C., & Wu, H. P. (2009). Comparison of auditory steady-state responses and auditory brainstem responses in audiometric assessment of adults with sensorineural hearing loss. *Auris Nasus Larynx, 36,* 140–145.

Linden, R. D., Campbell, K. B., Hamel, G., & Picton, T. W. (1985). Human auditory steady state evoked potentials during sleep. *Ear and Hearing, 6,* 167–174.

Linden, R. D., Picton, T. W., Hamel, G., & Campbell, K. B. (1987). Human auditory steady state evoked potentials during selective attention. *Electroencephalography and Clinical Neurophysiology, 66,* 145–159.

Lins, O. G., Picton, P. E., Picton, T. W., Champagne, S. C., & Durieux-Smith, A. (1995). Auditory steady-state responses to tones amplitude-modulated at 80–110 Hz. *Journal of the Acoustical Society of America, 97,* 3051–3063.

Lins, O. G., & Picton, T. W. (1995). Auditory steady-state responses to multiple simultaneous stimuli. *Electroencephalography and Clinical Neurophysiology, 96,* 420–432.

Lins, O. G., Picton, T. W., Boucher, B. L., Durieux-Smith, A., Champagne, S. C., Moran, L. M., . . . Savio, G. (1996). Frequency-specific audiometry using steady-state responses. *Ear and Hearing, 17,* 81–96.

Luts, H., Desloovere, C., & Wouters, J. (2006). Clinical application of dichotic multiple-stimulus auditory steady-state responses in high-risk newborns and young children. *Audiology and Neurotology, 11,* 24–37.

Luts, H., Van Dun, B., Alaerts, J., & Wouters, J. (2008). The influence of the detection paradigm in recording auditory steady-state responses. *Ear and Hearing, 29,* 638–650.

Luts, H., & Wouters, J. (2004). Hearing assessment by recording multiple auditory steady-state responses: The influence of test duration. *International Journal of Audiology, 43*, 471–478.

Luts, H., & Wouters, J. (2005). Comparison of MASTER and AUDERA for measurement of auditory steady-state responses. *International Journal of Audiology, 44*, 244–253.

Maiste, A., & Picton, T. (1989). Human auditory evoked potentials to frequency-modulated tones. *Ear and Hearing, 10*, 153–160.

Makeig, S., & Galambos, R. (1989). The CERP: Event-related perturbations in steady-state responses. In E. Basar & T. H. Bullock (Eds.), *Brain dynamics: Progress and perspectives* (pp. 373–400). Berlin, Germany: Springer.

Markessis, E., Poncelet, L., Colin, C., Coppens, A., Hoonhorst, I., Kadhim, H., & Deltenre, P. (2009). Frequency tuning curves derived from auditory steady state evoked potentials: A proof-of-concept study. *Ear and Hearing, 30*, 43–53.

McNeer, R. R., Bohórquez, J., & Özdamar, O. (2009). Influence of auditory stimulation rates on evoked potentials during general anesthesia: relation between the transient auditory middle-latency response and the 40-Hz auditory steady state response. *Anesthesiology, 110*, 1026–1035.

Ménard, M., Gallégo, S., Berger-Vachon, C., Collet, L., & Thai-Van, H. (2008). Relationship between loudness growth function and auditory steady-state response in normal-hearing subjects. *Hearing Research, 235*, 105–113.

Meuret, P., Backman, S. B., Bonhomme, V., Plourde, G., & Fiset, P. (2000). Physostigmine reverses propofol-induced unconsciousness and attenuation of the auditory steady state response and bispectral index in human volunteers. *Anesthesiology, 93*, 708–717.

Moore, B. C. (1978). Psychophysical tuning curves measured in simultaneous and forward masking. *Journal of the Acoustical Society of America, 63*, 524–532.

Moushegian, G., Rupert, A. L., & Stillman, R. D. (1973). Scalp-recorded early responses in man to frequencies in the speech range.

Electroencephalography and Clinical Neurophysiology, 35, 665–667.

Ozdek, A., Karacay, M., Saylam, G., Tatar, E., Aygener, N., & Korkmaz, M. H. (2010). Comparison of pure tone audiometry and auditory steady-state responses in subjects with normal hearing and hearing loss. *European Archives of Oto-Rhino-Laryngology, 267*, 43–49.

Pandya, P. K., & Krishnan, A. (2004). Human frequency-following response correlates of the distortion product at 2f1-f2. *Journal of the American Academy of Audiology, 15*, 184–197.

Parker, D., & O'Dwyer, D. (1998). The 40 Hz modulation-following response: Prediction of low-frequency uncomfortable loudness levels in normally hearing adults. *Audiology, 37*, 372–381.

Pethe, J., Mühler, R., Siewert, K., & von Specht H. (2004). Near-threshold recordings of amplitude modulation following responses (AMFR) in children of different ages. *International Journal of Audiology, 43*, 339–345.

Picton, T. W. (2007). Audiometry using auditory steady-state responses In R. F. Burkard, M. Don, & J. J. Eggermont (Eds.), *Auditory evoked potentials: Basic principles and clinical applications* (pp. 441–462). Baltimore, MD: Lippincott Williams & Wilkins.

Picton, T. W., Dimitrijevic, A., Perez-Abalo, M. C., & van Roon, P. (2005). Estimating audiometric thresholds using auditory steady-state responses. *Journal of the American Academy of Audiology, 16*, 143–156.

Picton, T. W, Durieux-Smith, A., Champagne, S. C., Whittingham, J., Moran, L. M., Giguère, C., & Beauregard, Y. (1998). Objective evaluation of aided thresholds using auditory steady-state responses. *Journal of the American Academy of Audiology, 9*, 315–331.

Picton, T. W., & John, M. S. (2004). Electromagnetic artifacts when recording auditory steady-state responses. *Journal of the American Academy of Audiology, 15*, 541–554.

Picton, T. W., John, M. S., Dimitrijevic, A., & Purcell, D. W. (2003). Human auditory steady-state responses. *International Journal of Audiology, 42*, 177–219.

Picton, T. W., John, M. S., Purcell, D. W., & Plourde, G. (2003). Human auditory steady-state responses: the effects of recording technique and state of arousal. *Anesthesia & Analgesia, 97*, 1396–1402.

Picton, T. W., Skinner, C. R., Champagne, S. C., Kellett, A. J., & Maiste, A. C. (1987). Potentials evoked by the sinusoidal modulation of the amplitude or frequency of a tone. *Journal of the Acoustical Society of America, 82*, 165–178.

Picton, T. W., van Roon, P., & John, M. S. (2007). Human auditory steady-state responses during sweeps of intensity. *Ear and Hearing, 28*, 542–557.

Picton, T. W., van Roon, P., & John, M. S. (2009). Multiple auditory steady-state responses (80–101 Hz): Effects of ear, gender, handedness, intensity and modulation rate. *Ear and Hearing, 30*, 100–109.

Picton, T. W., Woods, D. L., Baribeau-Braun, J., & Healey, T. M. G. (1977). Evoked potential audiometry. *Journal of Otolaryngology, 6*, 90–119.

Plourde, G. (2006). Auditory evoked potentials. *Best Practice and Research Clinical Anaesthesiology, 20*, 129–139.

Plourde, G., Baribeau, J., & Bonhomme, V. (1997). Ketamine increases the amplitude of the 40-Hz auditory steady-state response in humans. *British Journal of Anaesthesia, 78*, 524–529.

Plourde, G., Garcia-Asensi, A., Backman, S., Deschamps, A., Chartrand, D., Fiset, P., & Picton, T. (2008). Attenuation of the 40-Hz auditory steady-state response by propofol involves the cortical and subcortical generators. *Anesthesiology, 108*, 233–242.

Plourde, G., & Picton, T. W. (1990). Human auditory steady-state response during general anesthesia. *Anesthesia & Analgesia, 71*, 460–468.

Plourde, G., Villemure, C., Fiset, P., Bonhomme, V., & Backman, S. B. (1998). Effect of isoflurane on the auditory steady-state response and on consciousness in human volunteers. *Anesthesiology, 89*, 844–851.

Poulsen, C., Picton, T. W., & Paus, T. (2007). Age-related changes in transient and oscil-latory responses to auditory stimulation in healthy adults 19 to 45 years old. *Cerebral Cortex, 17*, 1454–1467.

Poulsen, C., Picton, T. W., & Paus, T. (2009). Age-related changes in transient and oscillatory brain responses to auditory stimulation during early adolescence. *Developmental Science, 12*, 220–235.

Purcell, D. W., & John, M. S. (in press). Evaluating the modulation transfer function of auditory steady state responses in the 65- to 120-Hz range. *Ear and Hearing, 31.*

Purcell, D. W., John, M. S., & Picton, T. W. (2003). Concurrent measurement of distortion product otoacoustic emissions and auditory steady state evoked potentials. *Hearing Research, 176*, 128–141.

Purcell, D. W., John, S. M., Schneider, B. A., & Picton, T. W. (2004). Human temporal auditory acuity as assessed by envelope following responses. *Journal of the Acoustical Society of America, 116*, 3581–3593.

Rance, G., & Rickards, F. (2002). Prediction of hearing threshold in infants using auditory steady-state evoked potentials. *Journal of the American Academy of Audiology, 13*, 236–245.

Rance, G., Rickards, F. W., Cohen, L. T., De Vidi, S., & Clark, G. M. (1995) The automated prediction of hearing thresholds in sleeping subjects using auditory steady state evoked potentials. *Ear and Hearing, 16*, 499–507.

Rees, A., Green, G. G., & Kay, R. H. (1986). Steady-state evoked responses to sinusoid-ally amplitude-modulated sounds recorded in man. *Hearing Research, 23*, 123–133.

Reyes, S. A., Salvi, R. J., Burkard, R. F., Coad, M. L., Wack, D. S., Galantowicz, P. J., & Lockwood, A. H. (2004) PET imaging of the 40 Hz auditory steady state response. *Hearing Research, 194*, 73–80.

Rickards, F. W., & Clark, G. M. (1984). Steady-state evoked potentials to amplitude-modulated tones. In R. H. Nodar & C. Barber (Eds.), *Evoked potentials II* (pp. 163–168). Boston, MA: Butterworth.

Rickards, F. W., Tan, L. E., Cohen, L. T., Wilson, O. J., Drew, J. H., & Clark, G. M. (1994) Auditory steady-state evoked potential in newborns. *British Journal of Audiology, 28,* 327–337.

Rickman, M. D., Chertoff, M. E., & Hecox, K. E. (1991). Electrophysiological evidence of nonlinear distortion products to two-tone stimuli. *Journal of the Acoustic Society of America, 89,* 2818–2826.

Rodriguez, R., Picton, T., Linden, D., Hamel, G., & Laframboise, G. (1986). Human auditory steady state responses: Effects of intensity and frequency. *Ear and Hearing, 7,* 300–313.

Rohrbaugh, J. W., Varner, J. L., Paige, S. R., Eckardt, M. J., & Ellingson, R. J. (1990). Auditory and visual event-related perturbations in the 40 Hz auditory steady-state response. *Electroencephalography and Clinical Neurophysiology, 76,* 148–164.

Rojas, D. C., Maharajh, K., Teale, P. D., Kleman, M. R., Benkers, T. L., Carlson, J. P., & Reite, M. L. (2006). Development of the 40 Hz steady state auditory evoked magnetic field from ages 5 to 52. *Clinical Neurophysiology, 117,* 110–117.

Ross, B., Borgmann, C., Draganova, R., Roberts, L. E., & Pantev, C. (2000). A high-precision magnetoencephalographic study of human auditory steady-state responses to amplitude-modulated tones. *Journal of the Acoustic Society of America, 108,* 679–691.

Ross, B., Draganova, R., Picton, T. W., & Pantev, C. (2003). Frequency specificity of 40-Hz auditory steady-state responses. *Hearing Research, 186,* 57–68.

Ross, B., Herdman, A. T., & Pantev, C. (2005a). Right hemispheric laterality of human 40 Hz auditory steady-state responses. *Cerebral Cortex, 15,* 2029–2039.

Ross, B., Herdman, A. T., & Pantev, C. (2005b). Stimulus induced desynchronization of human auditory 40-Hz steady-state responses. *Journal of Neurophysiology, 94,* 4082–4093.

Ross, B., Picton, T. W., Herdman, A. T., & Pantev, C. (2004). The effect of attention on the auditory steady-state response. *Neurology and Clinical Neurophysiology, 2004, 22,* 1–4.

Ross, B., Picton, T. W., & Pantev, C. (2002). Temporal integration in the human auditory cortex as represented by the develop-ment of the steady-state magnetic field. *Hearing Research, 165,* 68–84.

Sammeth, C. A., & Barry, S. J. (1985) The 40-Hz event-related potential as a measure of auditory sensitivity in normals. *Scandinavian Audiology, 14,* 51–55.

Saupe, K., Widmann, A., Bendixen, A., Müller, M. M., & Schröger E. (2009). Effects of inter-modal attention on the auditory steady-state response and the event-related potential. *Psychophysiology, 46,* 321–327.

Shannon, R. V., Zeng, F. G., Kamath, V., Wygonski, J., & Ekelid, M. (1995). Speech recognition with primarily temporal cues. *Science, 270,* 303–304.

Skosnik, P. D., Krishnan, G. P., & O'Donnell, B. F. (2007). The effect of selective attention on the gammaband auditory steady-state response. *Neuroscience Letters, 420,* 223–228.

Small, S. A., & Stapells, D. R. (2004). Artifactual responses when recording auditory steady-state responses. *Ear and Hearing, 25,* 611–623.

Stapells, D. R., Galambos, R., Costello, J. A., & Makeig, S. (1988). Inconsistency of auditory middle latency and steady-state responses in infants. *Electroencephalography and Clinical Neurophysiology, 71,* 289–295.

Stapells, D. R., Linden, D., Suffield, J. B., Hamel, G., & Picton, T. W. (1984). Human auditory steady-state potentials. *Ear and Hearing, 5,* 105–113.

Stapells, D. R., Makeig, S., & Galambos, R. (1987). Auditory steady-state responses: Threshold prediction using phase coherence. *Electroencephalography and Clinical Neurophysiology, 67,* 260–270.

Stelmachowicz, P. G., & Jesteadt, W. (1984). Psychophysical tuning curves in normal-hearing listeners: test reliability and probe level effects. *Journal of Speech and Hearing Research, 27,* 396–402.

Stillman, R. D., Crow, G., & Moushegian, G. (1978). Components of the frequency-following potential in man. *Electroencephalography and Clinical Neurophysiology, 44,* 438–446.

Stillman, R. D., Moushegian, G., & Rupert, A. L. (1976). Early tone-evoked responses in normal and hearing-impaired subjects. *Audiology. 15*, 10–22.

Stürzebecher, E., Cebulla, M., & Pschirrer, U. (2001). Efficient stimuli for recording of the amplitude modulation following response. *Audiology, 40*, 63–68.

Tlumak, A. I., Rubinstein, E., & Durrant, J. D. (2007). Meta-analysis of variables that affect accuracy of threshold estimation via measurement of the auditory steady-state response (ASSR). *International Journal of Audiology, 46*, 692–710.

Tomlin, D., Rance, G., Graydon, K., & Tsialios, I. (2006). A comparison of 40 Hz auditory steady-state response (ASSR) and cortical auditory evoked potential (CAEP) thresholds in awake adult subjects. *International Journal of Audiology, 45*, 580–588.

Tonner, P. H., & Scholz, J. (2006). The sinking brain: How to measure consciousness in anaesthesia. *Best Practice and Research Clinical Anaesthesiology, 20*, 1–9.

Uhlhaas, P. J., Pipa, G., Lima, B., Melloni, L., Neuenschwander, S., Nikolić, D., & Singer, W. (2009). Neural synchrony in cortical networks: history, concept and current status. *Frontiers in Integrative Neuroscience, 3, Article 17*, 1–19.

Vander Werff, K. R. (2009). Accuracy and time efficiency of two ASSR analysis methods using clinical test protocols. *Journal of the American Academy of Audiology, 20*, 433–452.

Vander Werff, K. R., & Brown, C. J. (2005). Effect of audiometric configuration on threshold and suprathreshold auditory steady-state responses. *Ear and Hearing, 26*, 310–326.

Vander Werff, K. R., Johnson, T. J., & Brown, C. J. (2008). Behavioural threshold estimation for auditory steady-state response. In G. Rance (Ed.), *Auditory steady-state response: Generation, recording, and clinical applications* (pp. 125–147). San Diego, CA: Plural Publishing.

Van Dun, B., Verstraeten, S., Alaerts, J., Luts, H., Moonen, M., & Wouters, J. (2008). A flexible research platform for multi-channel auditory steady-state response measurements. *Journal of Neuroscience Methods, 169*, 239–248.

Van Maanen, A., & Stapells, D. R. (2005). Comparison of multiple auditory steady-state responses (80 vs. 40 Hz) and slow cortical potentials for threshold estimation in hearing-impaired adults. *International Journal of Audiology, 44*, 613–624.

Viemeister. N. F. (1979). Temporal modulation transfer functions based upon modulation thresholds. *Journal of the Acoustical Society of. America, 66*, 1364–1380.

Wilding, T., McKay, C. Baker, R., Picton, T., & Kluk, K. (2010). Using the auditory steady-state response to record electrophysiological tuning curves: A possible fast objective method for diagnosing dead regions. *Ear and Hearing*, Manuscript submitted for publication.

Wong, P. C., Skoe, E., Russo, N. M., Dees, T., & Kraus, N. (2007). Musical experience shapes human brainstem encoding of linguistic pitch patterns. *Nature Neuroscience, 10*, 420–422.

Wong, W. Y. S., & Stapells, D. R. (2004). Brainstem and cortical mechanisms underlying the binaural masking level difference in humans: An auditory steady-state response study. *Ear and Hearing, 25*, 57–67.

Woods, D. L., & Clayworth, C. C. (1986). Age-related changes in human middle latency auditory evoked potentials. *Electroencephalography and Clinical Neurophysiology, 65*, 297–303.

Yamada, O., Kodera, K., Hink, R. F., & Suzuki, J. I. (1979). Cochlear distribution of frequency-following response initiation. A high-pass masking noise study. *Audiology, 18*, 381–387.

Yamada, O., Yamane, H., & Kodera, K. (1977). Simultaneous recordings of the brain stem response and the frequency-following response to low-frequency tone. *Electroencephalography and Clinical Neurophysiology, 43*, 362–370.

Yeung, K. N. K., & Wong, L. L. N. (2007). Prediction of hearing thresholds: Comparison of cortical evoked response audiometry and auditory steady state response audiometry techniques. *International Journal of Audiology, 46*, 17–25.

Zatorre, R. J., & Belin, P (2001). Spectral and temporal processing in human auditory cortex. *Cerebral Cortex, 11*, 946–953.

Zenker-Castro, F., & Barajas de Prat, J. (2008). The role of auditory steady-state responses in fitting hearing aids. In G. Rance (Ed.), *Auditory steady-state response: Generation,* *recording, and clinical applications* (pp. 241–258). San Diego, CA: Plural Publishing.

Zenker-Castro, F., Barajas de Prat, J., & Zabala, E. L. (2008). Loudness and auditory steady-state responses in normal-hearing subjects. *International Journal of Audiology, 47,* 269–275.

11

Late Auditory Evoked Potentials: Changing the Things Which Are

> Observe constantly that all things take place by change, and accustom thyself to consider that the nature of the Universe loves nothing so much as to change the things which are and to make new things like them. For everything that exists is in a manner the seed of that which will be.
>
> Marcus Aurelius Antoninus, *Meditations* IV-46, 167 CE
> (translated by George Long, 1891)

As reviewed in Chapter 1, the late auditory evoked potentials (LAEPs) were the first human evoked potentials (EPs) to be recorded from the scalp and the first to be used for objective audiometry. These achievements were based on the fact that LAEPs are significantly larger than earlier potentials. The greater amplitude of the LAEPs is caused by their generation in regions of the brain that are close to the recording electrodes on the scalp. LAEPs derive from activation of dipole fields in multiple areas of cortex, most prominently the auditory regions on the superior surface of the temporal lobe. They are the most delayed and the most prominent of the transient auditory responses, the culmination of the brain's response to change.

The LAEPs have more names than other auditory EPs. Initially, they were called "vertex responses" or "vertex potentials" because they were recorded with largest amplitude from electrodes placed on the top of the head. Because their waveforms were similar in the different sensory modalities, vertex responses were considered nonspecific responses to any change in the environment, the reticular formation theoretically causing widespread activation of the cortex so that a new event could be properly registered and understood. However, it soon became apparent that responses in different modalities actually showed distinctly different scalp topographies, and that the auditory responses were generated mainly in the auditory regions of cortex. These potentials therefore could represent highly specific processing of the auditory stimulus. Another name was "cortical auditory evoked potentials," but this does not differentiate them from the middle latency responses (MLRs), which also are generated in the cortex. Various terms using the word "change," for example, "acoustic change complex" (Martin & Boothroyd, 2000), have been used to indicate that the responses can be evoked by any change in a stimulus and not just by its onset. However, this is true for all transient EPS and not just those occurring at the later latencies. The most commonly used names relate to latency—"slow" or "late" auditory EPs, or "auditory late responses." For our purposes, we call them the "late auditory evoked potentials" (LAEPs), with the proviso that they are still very much alive.

Despite the fact that we have studied them for longer than the earlier potentials, we understand little about the mechanisms of their generation or their role in human perception. One problem is that multiple different areas of cortex contribute to what we record from the scalp during the LAEPs, and the overlapping fields from these different generators are extremely difficult to disentangle. Another reason for our lack of understanding is that these potentials are affected as much by the psychological expectancy of the perceiver as by the physical nature of the acoustic event. This led to their description as "mesogenous," at the interface between the earlier exogenous responses (determined by the stimulus) and the later endogenous responses (determined by its meaning) (Hillyard, Picton, & Regan, 1978).

For the purposes of this chapter, the LAEPs include waveforms between 50 and 250 ms after a stimulus: the N1-P2-N2 waves of the transient auditory EP, the auditory sustained potential (SP), which begins at about 120 ms, and the mismatch negativity (MMN). The P1 wave was considered with the auditory MLRs in Chapter 9. The vertex N1 wave typically peaks at 100 ms, but there are several N1 deflections with peak latencies between 70 and 150 ms, each recorded maximally at different scalp locations. The P2 wave usually occurs at a peak latency of 180 ms but it may be earlier (and smaller in amplitude) if the stimulus lasts longer than 50 ms and an SP occurs. The N2 wave at around 250 ms occurs as a small wave in the normal waking response but becomes greatly enhanced in sleep. Many different processes, which are considered in Chapter 12, can overlap during the waking N2 wave. One of these is the MMN, an additional negative wave in the response to a deviant stimulus occurring in a train of standard stimuli. It can be manifest as an enhancement of the later part of the N1 wave, as a separate N2 wave or as an attenuation of the P2 wave.

As we saw in Chapters 1 and 2, EP waveforms can be considered in terms of a set of overlapping components. Based on their contribution to experimental variance or their origin within the brain, various analyses of the scalp-recorded LAEPs can distinguish different components of these waveforms. Näätänen and Picton (1987) considered a component as the contribution to the recorded waveform of a particular generator process. This process would occur in a specific location within the brain and be determined by the specific pattern of input to that region. In terms of the LAEPs the input could be both the sensory information being transmitted to the cortex and the attentional influences that determine what should be processed further. The main LAEP components identified in the Näätänen-Picton review were the vertical and tangential N1-P2 dipoles originating in the temporal lobes, a frontal N1 wave, the MMN, and two components of the processing negativity (originating in the temporal and frontal lobes).

This chapter considers the aspects of the LAEPs that are mainly under exogenous control: the N1, P2, SP wave, and the MMN. Chapter 12 considers the components that are more endogenous in nature: the processing negativity, Nd, N2, and P300, and the effects of attention and task-relevance on these potentials. In this chapter, we describe the relationship of LAEPs to the physical parameters of the sound (intensity, duration, frequency), and then consider the temporal aspects of the responses. The way in which different stimuli occur in time will lead us to issues of probability and predictability, and the differentiation between standard and deviant stimuli. Neither this chapter nor the next should be considered in isolation. Within these two chapters, we move from the physical world to the psychological perception of that world. This progress is not a simple transition, but a continual interaction between stimulus and meaning, between bottom-up and top-down processes. Key to this processing is the registration of change. Therefore, before we review the precise ways in which LAEPs react to change, we briefly consider some general concepts of change. We will return to this at the end of the chapter, but we need some basic ideas before we begin—a brief shower before entering the pool of data.

AUDITORY CHANGE

The LAEPs occur whenever there is a change in the acoustic world. LAEPs typically are evoked by a brief stimulus such as a click or short tone. When the stimulus lasts longer than several hundred milliseconds, LAEPs occur at both the onset and the offset (Clynes, 1969; Hillyard & Picton, 1978; Onishi & Davis, 1968; Pantev, Eulitz, Hampson, Ross, & Roberts, 1996). Figure 11–1 shows the onset and offset responses recorded with different stimulus durations. The onset response decreases in amplitude when the interval from the preceding offset response becomes less than 5 seconds. The onset response is about twice the size of the offset response at equal on-off duty cycles.

LAEPs also are recorded when a continuing stimulus changes in some way, for example, when the amplitude or frequency of an ongoing tone changes (Clynes, 1969; Kohn Lifshitz & Litchfield, 1978, 1980). The left section of Figure 11–2 compares the response to a frequency change to the responses to the onset or offset of a tone. The responses to a change in frequency are very similar in morphology to the onset/offset responses even though the stimulus is always on. In particular, they follow the same temporal rules: a larger response is evoked by the change when it follows a longer period of constancy. For frequency modulation, the responses are equal for changes of either direction, but for amplitude modulation the responses are smaller for amplitude decreases. The initial experiments of Clynes (1969) found no response to a change in the rate at which an ongoing change was occurring, for example, when a tone that was increasing in intensity began to increase more rapidly. They suggested that the LAEPs were evoked only by a change from rest to motion. However,

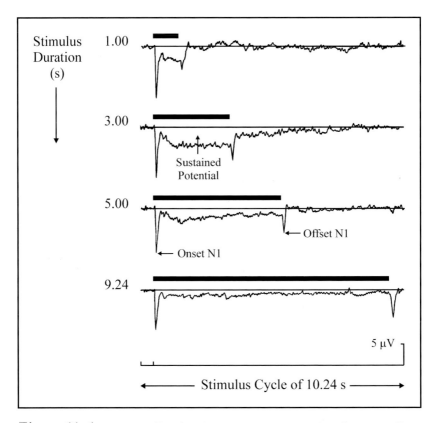

Figure 11–1. Onset, offset, and sustained potentials. These recordings represent the responses evoked by 1-kHz tones of 80 dB HL with different durations. The tones were presented at a rate of one tone every 10.24 seconds (stimulus cycle). Responses were recorded from the vertex using a balanced frontal to mastoid reference adjusted to cancel out the effects of eye-blinks. The filter bandpass was 0-20 Hz. Each tracing represents the average of 128 individual responses. With increasing tone duration, the onset response and the sustained potential get smaller and the offset response gets larger. Waveforms adapted from Hillyard and Picton (1978).

Kohn, Lifshitz, and Litchfield (1978, 1980) showed small LAEPs when an ongoing ramp in frequency or amplitude changed its rate, even when it did not change its direction. The reaction time for behaviorally detecting these changes was very variable. The authors therefore proposed that the brain actually generated responses to the changes, but that the average responses were often small or invisible because of the trial-to-trial latency-jitter.

These results are important as they suggest that LAEPs occur whenever there is a perceptible change in the auditory world.

LAEPs also can be elicited by more complicated changes than simple shifts in the intensity or frequency of an ongoing tone. As considered in Chapter 5, changes in the interaural timing of a binaural stimulus are perceived as a change in the location of the sound These changes evoke LAEPs that are similar to those occurring

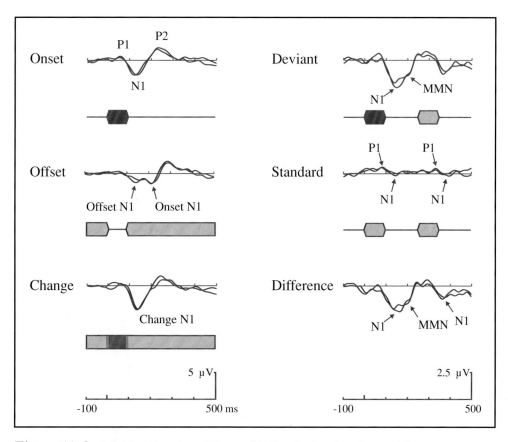

Figure 11–2. **LAEPs related to different kinds of stimulus change.** *The responses were recorded at the midfrontal electrode relative to an average reference. All tones were 60 dB SPL. The waveforms on the left show responses to a brief tone, to a brief gap in a continuous tone, and to a brief change in frequency. In separate blocks, the frequencies changed from 1000 to 1200 Hz or vice versa (and the waveforms were averaged across blocks). All stimuli occurred at a rate of 1/s. For the recordings on the right, tones were presented at a rate 4/s and occasionally (p = 0.1) one of the stimuli changed frequency from 1000 to 1200 Hz (or vice versa). The responses to the deviant contained both an N1 response and a later MMN wave. The responses to the standard stimuli are very small because of the rapid stimulus rate but distinct P1 and N1 waves are recognizable. These are enhanced when the standard follows a deviant. The difference-waveform obtained by subtracting the standard from the deviant recordings shows that the stimulus change evokes a broad negative wave that contains two components. The first represents a change in the N1 response whereas the second represents the additional MMN. The smaller version of this response occurring after the second stimulus probably represents a change in the N1 and some mismatch processing of the standard stimulus following a deviant.*

at the onset of the sound except for the fact that they have a longer latency, the vertex N1 wave peaking at about 135 ms rather than 100 ms (McEvoy, Picton, Cham-

pagne, Kellett, & Kelly, 1990). Figure 5–12 illustrates these responses. Jones and Perez (2002) have recorded LAEPs, which they called "C-processes" (or change processes), to changes in musical notes. Similar responses followed changes in either pitch (from A to A-flat played on a clarinet) or timbre (from clarinet to oboe both playing A). Because the response to the pitch change occurred even when the fundamental was removed, they proposed that the response is mainly elicited by changes in the spectral profile. Martin and Boothroyd (2000) recorded LAEPS, which they called the "acoustic change complex," in response to a change from one synthetic vowel to another, which also is essentially a change in spectral profile.

Another type of change is between two separate stimuli. Näätänen and Picton (1987) differentiated between change-1 or "level change" (from an immediately preceding stimulus parameter) and change-2 or "stimulus change" (from a previously presented stimulus). When a deviant stimulus occurs in a train or standard stimuli, the deviant stimulus elicits an MMN in addition to the onset response. This is illustrated in the right section of Figure 11–2. One simple way to demonstrate the MMN is to subtract the response to the standard from the response to the deviant. When the difference between the stimuli is large, this can show two different negative waves: one at the latency of the N1 to the standard and another later wave. The first wave may be ascribed to the specificity of the refractory period of N1. As shown later in this chapter, the LAEPs have a prolonged refractory period and are very small when one stimulus follows another at intervals of several hundred milliseconds (e.g., the response to the repeating standard stimuli in the middle recordings on the right half of Figure 11–2). If the stimulus changes in some way, some of the activated neurons will differ from those activated by the preceding stimuli and therefore will not be refractory.

Instead, they will respond as though they had not been stimulated before, like "fresh afferents." The second component of the difference waveform, which differs from the N1 both in its longer latency and more frontal scalp topography, may represent a process that automatically compares the present stimulus to the preceding stimuli. However, exactly how this works is not yet known, and we will return to this discussion later in the chapter.

The stimulus onset asynchrony (SOA) between the repeating standard stimuli has different effects on the onset response and the MMN. Although the onset-response is much smaller when the SOA decreases below one second, the MMN to the deviant stimulus may actually get larger, provided the interval between the deviants remains constant (Näätänen, Paavilainen, Alho, Reinikainen, & Sams, 1987a). For the recordings on the right side of Figure 11–2, the stimuli were occurring with an SOA of 250 ms; the responses to the standards are barely recognizable but the response to the deviant is large. If we look at the difference between the responses to the standard and deviant stimulus, we can see two peaks. The first likely represents the increased size of the N1 in the deviant response, caused by the activation of neurons that have not been made refractory by the repeating standard stimuli, and the second is what might be considered a true MMN.

These two processes can be distinguished using various experimental manipulations. When the difference between the standard and deviant stimuli is large, the MMN rides on the N1. As the difference between the deviant and the standard stimuli is made smaller, the earlier of the two peaks in the difference waveform becomes smaller and the latency of the later peak increases. These effects can be seen in Figure 11–3 (Scherg, Vajsar, & Pic-

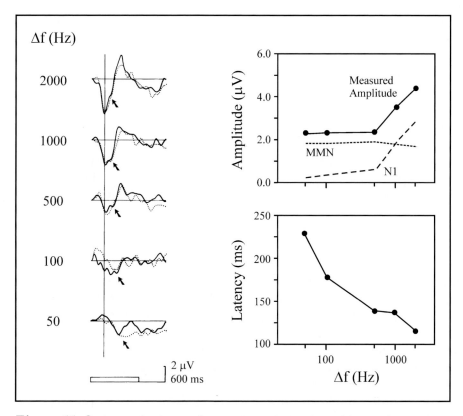

Figure 11–3. *N1 and mismatch negativity (MMN). In this experiment tones, lasting 400 ms were presented with an SOA of 0.9 s at an intensity of 75 dB SPL. In each recording block, two tones were presented, one of 1000 Hz and another of 1050, 1100, 1500, 2000, or 3000 Hz. One of the tones (the deviant) occurred improbably (p = 0.2). In counterbalanced design, this could be either the 1000-Hz tone or the other. On the left half of this figure are shown the responses to the deviant tones, which could occur either irregularly (dotted line) or regularly once every five tones (continuous line). The responses were recorded from the midfrontal scalp using a sternovertebral reference. The vertical line indicates the latency of the N1 wave. The arrow indicates the MMN, which rides on an N1 when the frequency difference (Δf) between the standard and deviant tones is large. When the difference is small, very little N1 occurs and the latency of the MMN peak is increased. On the right are graphed the amplitudes and latencies of the MMN peak. This amplitude measurement can be considered a combination of a constant MMN component (dotted line) and an N1 (dashed line) that adds to the MMN when the frequency difference is large. Unpublished data from Scherg et al. (1989).*

ton, 1989). At large differences, the measurement taken at the peak latency of the MMN will contain as much N1 as MMN. As the difference gets small, the N1 becomes small and the MMN increases in latency; then what is measured is predominantly MMN.

Another way to disentangle the MMN from the N1 effect is by using a control condition with multiple stimuli all differing from each other (Jacobsen, Schröger, Horenkamp, & Winkler, 2003). In the control condition, the responses will show the N1 effect but no MMN as the MMN only occurs when the deviant is improbable—a stimulus cannot be a deviant if it is not unusual. Thus, responses from the control condition (recorded with 10 different standards each occurring 10% of the time) can be subtracted from the deviant response (recorded with a paradigm with 10% deviants and 90% standards) to give a true MMN. We will return to this paradigm later.

As in Figure 11–2, the MMN often is recorded when stimuli are presented very rapidly. As the interval between the stimuli decreases, the subject will perceive a continuous sound that fluctuates in amplitude rather than a series of discrete stimuli. Ultimately, the subject will not be able to distinguish the fluctuations in amplitude and the perception will be truly continuous. In this case, the deviant stimulus will be like a change in an ongoing tone. If this is so, should there not be a MMN to the change in a continuous tone in addition to the N1 change response? Lavikainen, Huotilainen, Ilmoniemi, Simola, and Näätänen (1995) found that the N1m to a frequency change in an ongoing tone recorded with magnetoencephalography (MEG) could be analyzed into two overlapping responses: a response peaking near 100 ms that was similar to the onset N1 response in its source-location and a response peaking about 30 ms later that was generated more anteriorly. They proposed that the two responses were triggered by the onset of the new frequency and the deviance of this frequency from the preceding frequency. However, exactly what differentiates these two responses is not clear, and we will return to them later when we discuss the cerebral processes that occur during the LAEPs.

PHYSICAL PARAMETERS OF THE SOUND

Onset Parameters

The latency and the amplitude of the LAEPs vary with stimulus rise-time—how rapidly the stimulus changes. The latency of the N1 peak increases as the rise-time increases from several to several hundred milliseconds, the increase being only a small proportion (about 10%) of the change in rise-time (Onishi & Davis, 1968). At lower intensities, the increase was greater than at higher. The amplitude of the response is relatively constant provided the rise-time is between several milliseconds and about 50 ms. At longer rise times, the response is smaller (Onishi & Davis, 1968; Skinner & Jones, 1968). This effect is likely because of the latency jitter of the response; exactly when the system recognizes that a stimulus is occurring will vary from trial to trial. At very short rise-times, the response to a tonal stimulus will be larger because of spectral splatter; the rapid onset causes a click-like spectrum (Prasher, 1980). This effect does not occur when using noise stimuli with very rapid rise-times as their spectrum is already broad.

The amplitude of the N1-P2 complex also varies with the duration of the stimulus (Alain, Woods, & Covarrubias, 1997; Milner, 1969; Onishi & Davis, 1968). Duration can be described in several ways—the total duration from beginning to end, the duration between the beginning of the onset and the beginning of the offset, or the plateau duration between the end of the onset and the beginning of the offset. If the rise-time is fast (3 to 5 ms), the response gets larger as the duration of the plateau increases up to 70 ms although the growth of amplitude decreases at longer durations. For longer rise-times, the N1-P2 complex likely is responding to the duration of both the rise time and the plateau. As a rough rule of thumb, we can suggest that the response integrates the stimulus with a time constant of about 50 ms. This is more rapid than perceptual integration. As stimulus duration gets longer than 50 ms, the perceived loudness of a sound continues to increase but the onset N1-P2 complex does not change. Suprathreshold loudness increases and the threshold of detection decreases by about 12 dB as the stimulus duration increases from several milliseconds to several hundred milliseconds. However, the perceptual processing underlying loudness integration likely involves multiple looks rather than constant accumulation (Viemesister & Wakefield, 1991). The LAEPs might be related more to the looks than to the final perception.

Näätänen and Winkler (1999) discuss the time course over which auditory sensory information is integrated into a stimulus representation. The N1 wave of the LAEP occurs before the different features of an auditory object have been joined together, and might represent the process of arraying the features for later integration into a full representation. The MMN, as reviewed later in this chapter, can be used to assess this integration process.

The effects of rise-time and duration on the N1-P2 have several implications. First, the optimal stimulus for recording N1-P2 waves of the LAEP would have a rise- (and fall-) time of between 10 and 20 ms and a plateau duration of 30 ms or more. A common stimulus is a tone with rise and fall times of 10 ms and a plateau of 30 ms. Second, when evaluating thresholds we should be aware of differences between short tones and longer tones. For example, when we use a tone with a 200-ms plateau-duration, we should expect

the LAEP threshold to be higher than the perceptual threshold, since the LAEP is evoked by only the initial 30 to 50 ms of the tone whereas perception is based on the whole tone. The third implication of these findings is that the human auditory system has a system that integrates stimulus energy over periods of around 50 ms. We need to find out more about how this system works and how it relates to the longer time for perceptual integration.

Stimulus Intensity

The early studies of the LAEPs were concerned mainly with how they were affected by intensity of the stimulus, and how close to auditory threshold they were recognizable. The left section of Figure 11–4 shows some early recordings from the author's scalp. The N1-P2 waves of the LAEP decrease in amplitude and increase in latency as the intensity of the stimulus decreases, but still remain recognizable at 10 dB above threshold. The graphs on the right section of the figure show some mean data from a later study (Picton, Woods, Baribeau-Braun, & Healey, 1977).

The rate of change for the amplitude-intensity function of the LAEP tends to decrease with increasing intensity. The data plotted in Figure 11–4 are representative of the findings in many other papers (early studies are reviewed in Picton et al., 1977; more recently Ross, Lütkenhöner, Pantev, & Hoke, 1999). The function therefore does not fit well with any power function for loudness, which would show an increasing rate of change with increasing intensity. Some aspects of the LAEP amplitude do relate reasonably well to loudness. For example, the amplitude of the LAEP does increase rapidly when the intensity of stimuli

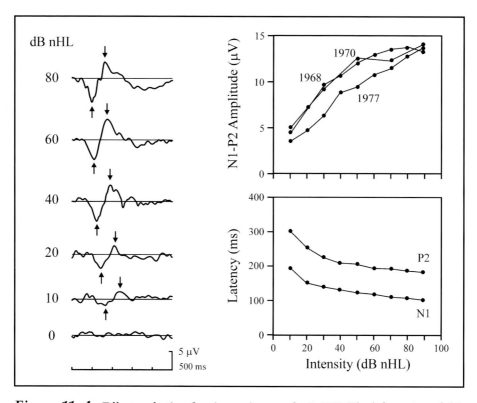

Figure 11–4. ***Effects of stimulus intensity on the LAEP.*** *The left section of this figure shows the responses to a 32 ms 1000-Hz tone presented at various intensities with an SOA of 2.5 s. These LAEPs were recorded from the vertex of the author in 1968 using a mastoid reference. On the right are some mean data from several studies to illustrate the effects of stimulus intensity on the amplitude and latency of the response. In the amplitude graph, three sets of mean data are presented: one from 1968 (the same unpublished study as the recordings on the left), one from Picton et al. (1970), and one from Picton et al. (1977). The average standard deviations are about 2 μV for the amplitudes, about 5 ms for the N1 latency and 10 ms for the P2 latency. The standard deviations of the latencies become larger near threshold. All data were obtained using 1000-Hz tones presented with an SOA of 2.5 s. The data in the latency graph are from the 1977 study (in which the rise time of the tone was 10 ms).*

presented in noise is increased above threshold when just like the perceived loudness of these stimuli (Davis, Bowers, & Hirsh, 1968). However, other aspects do not fit at all, in particular the SOA, which dramatically alters the N1-P2 waves but has no effect on loudness for intervals of greater than several hundred milliseconds. Some early studies found a relation between the shape of the amplitude-intensity function, particularly whether the response amplitude increased or decreased at higher intensity, and personality characteristics related to sensation-seeking ("augmenting-reducing"). However, such relations are quite variable and of doubtful meaning (Prescott, Connolly, & Gruzelier, 1984).

Signals in Noise

Although the LAEPs clearly are related to the intensity of the sound, the background acoustic noise in which the sounds occur also plays a role in determining their amplitude. Billings, Tremblay, Souza, and Binns (2007) found that the LAEPs to 1000-Hz tones presented in free field were not significantly altered when the tones were amplified 20 dB by a hearing aid. One possible reason is that the hearing aid amplified the background acoustic noise as well as the stimulus. The signal-to-noise ratio (SNR) did not change between aided and unaided conditions. The LAEP amplitude may have depended more on the SNR than the absolute intensity of the sound. A follow-up study (Billings, Tremblay, Stecker, & Tolin, 2009) compared the responses to 60 and 75 db SPL 1000-Hz tones in various levels of background noise and found a significant effect of background noise without any effect of absolute intensity. The lack of any effect of intensity was perhaps due to the saturation of the amplitude of the response at these intensities (Picton, Goodman, & Bryce, 1970) (see Figure 11–4). At lower intensities, we might expect effects of both SNR and intensity. Nevertheless, using the LAEPs to assess the effects of hearing-aids will require attention to both the acoustic noise and the amount of amplification.

Although acoustic noise, when presented at levels near the intensity of the stimulus, reduces the LAEP (Davis et al., 1968), low levels of noise may actually enhance the LAEPs (Alain, Quan, McDonald, & van Roon, 2009). Exactly how this effect is mediated remains to be determined. Stochastic resonance, the improvement in a system's performance when noise is added, often occurs in nonlinear systems (Moss, Ward, & Sannita, 2004; Zeng, Fu, & Morse, 2000). Typically, adding noise makes a previously subthreshold signal detectable. The noise allows the signal to be measured, and once the signal has been measured, the noise can be attenuated by scaling or averaging.

Audiometric Evaluation With LAEPs

After the advent of averaging, the LAEPs were investigated extensively as a way to estimate behavioral thresholds in subjects who could not respond on behavioral testing or whose thresholds were unreliable (reviewed by Hyde, 1993). As shown in Table 11–1, the early studies found that the LAEPs could be recognized very close to threshold. Many of the studies used 10-dB steps and then estimated the threshold 5 dB lower than the level of the last clearly recognizable response. However, even considering this extrapolation (a few dB on average), the results were more accurate than we would now expect. This may have been partly related to the subjects, who were probably very cooperative, stayed very still during the recording, and attended closely to the tones, and partly related to the examiners, who probably were aware of the behavioral audiogram and may have prolonged the testing at a particular level when they knew that a response should have been present.

The LAEPs should be recognizable on average at about 10 dB above threshold. Closer to threshold, they probably vary in latency from trial to trial and this could make them difficult to recognize in average recordings. This 10 dB physiologic-behavioral difference is similar to the most recent findings listed in Table 11–1.

Table 11–1. Estimation of Behavioral Thresholds Using LAEPs

Study	Ears Tested	Dur (ms)	SOA (s)	Swps	Physiologic-Behavioral Difference (dB) 500	1000	2000	4000	PTA
Davis et al. (1967)	46 HI children	40	1	64					0±7
Beagley and Kellogg (1969)	40 NH 36 HI	25	1.25	60	4±4 3±6	2±5 1±6	6±5 4±7		4±3 3±5
Coles and Mason (1984)	129 HI	200	1.5	64	0±10	−1±6	−1±11	−2±7	
Prasher et al. (1993)	27 Ménière's	200	1	?		2±8		−1±8	
van Maanen and Stapells (2005)	23 adults	60	1.1	50	20±6	20±9	22±12		
Lightfoot and Kennedy (2006)	24 adults	80	1.4	10		11±6		10±10	10±5
Tomlin et al. (2006)	36 NH 30 HI	100	1.4	60	10±6 9±7			12±4 14±14	
Yeung and Wong (2007)	19 NH 44 HI	200	0.8	64	6±9	8±7	8±8	−2±15	

Differences are expressed as means ± standard deviations. NH is normal hearing: HI is hearing impaired. Dur is the duration of the tones. SOA is stimulus onset asynchrony. Swps is the number of sweeps (or trials) in the average response when near threshold (fewer could be recorded at higher intensities). PTA is the pure-tone average threshold for frequencies 500, 1000, and 2000 Hz (1000, 3000, and 8000 Hz for Lightfoot and Kennedy). In the Lightfoot and Kennedy study, the tones were at 1000 and 3000 Hz. The stimuli in this study varied in ear and frequency within the same run, this sequence giving a large responses (and allowing a small number of sweeps in the average).

Ross, Lütkenhöner, Pantev, and Hoke (1999) reviewed almost 2000 threshold estimations with the LAEP, and estimated a true electrophysiologic threshold (at which supra-threshold EP measurements could be extrapolated to zero amplitude) that was 7.5 dB below the detection level at which a significant EP waveform was recorded. They used a powerful phase coherence approach to detecting significant waveforms (see Figure 6–5). Therefore, we should consider 7.5 dB above behavioral threshold to be the minimum level at which the EP should be recognized. Other techniques based on the visual or computer evaluation of replicate waveforms (see Chapter 6) may lead to higher recognition thresholds, as they are not as powerful as the phase-coherence approach.

One factor that we need to consider when comparing LAEP and pure-tone thresholds is the integration time of the LAEP, which is significantly shorter than the perceptual integration time. Using HL thresholds (based on tones lasting a half second or more) may not be appropriate for the LAEP, which is evoked by only the first 50 ms or so of the tone. This may in part explain the higher thresholds found by van Maanen and Stapells (2005), where the intensity calibration for the brief tones evoking the LAEPs was the same as for the longer tones used in pure-tone audiometry.

A final consideration in the use of the LAEPs to evaluate hearing threshold is the state of the subject (to which we shall return in a later section of this chapter). In drowsy or sleeping subjects, the threshold for recognizing the LAEP is considerably higher than that found in an alert subject. Mendel et al. (1975) found LAEP thresholds 25 to 30 dB above behavioral thresholds in subjects who were sleeping or drowsily preparing to fall asleep.

The LAEPs are widely used in the evaluation of hearing loss in adults or older children when the behavioral thresholds are unreliable and a functional hearing loss suspected (e.g., Coles & Mason, 1984; Hone, Norman, Keogh, & Kelly, 2003; Hyde, Alberti, Matsumoto, & Li, 1986). The decision to use the LAEPs or the 40-Hz auditory steady-state response (ASSR) in this context depends on the laboratory and its experience (Tomlin, Rance, Graydon, & Tsialios, 2006; van Maanen & Stapells, 2005). Whatever technique is used, the examiner should be careful to make accurate threshold measurements in addition to simply demonstrating the presence of physiologic responses below the behavioral threshold. The most common cause for exaggerated thresholds on behavioral testing is an underlying hearing loss of less severity than that being claimed.

The stimulus and recording parameters for recording the N1-P2 waves for audiometric purposes are reasonably well established. Tones with rise times of 10 or 20 ms and durations of at least 50 ms should be presented with an SOA of between 1 and 2 seconds. The response should be recorded from the vertex to the mastoid using a filter bandpass of 1 to 15 Hz and averaging should be performed over between 10 and 100 responses (depending on whether the response is recognized). A second recording channel should monitor ocular artifacts and reject from the averaging any trial contaminated by blinks or eye-movements. Stapells (2009) has summarized similar parameters. Tones of longer duration are helpful because of the additional SP. As discussed later in this chapter, refractory effects allow multistimulus paradigms, such as those used by Ross et al. (1999) and by Lightfoot and Kennedy (2006), to speed the recognition of responses at different stimulus frequencies.

In addition to evaluating thresholds, the LAEPS may be useful in indicating how well sounds are processed. The LAEPs indicate that the sounds have reached the cortex. They show that the sounds have been processed further than what would be indicated by the auditory brainstem response. The presence of normal LAEPs therefore is helpful when evaluating the ability of a young child with a hearing impairment to hear sounds when provided with a hearing aid (Golding et al., 2007).

Stimulus Frequency and Spectral Patterns

The LAEPs evoked by brief tones decrease in size with increasing frequency of the tone (Antinoro, Skinner, & Jones, 1969; other papers reviewed by Reneau & Hnatiow, 1975). This change of amplitude with increasing frequency was more evident for stimuli with frequencies higher than 1000 Hz and for stimuli of higher intensities. The latency of the LAEP N1 wave decreased with increasing frequency (Jacobson, Lombardi, Gibbens, Ahmad, & Newman, 1992; Woods, Alain, Covarrubias, & Zaidel, 1993), with the main latency change (about 15 ms) between 250 and 1000 Hz and much less change for higher frequencies. MEG studies have indicated a similar latency decrease for N1m from 100 to 1000 Hz, but then found an increasing latency for tones of higher frequency (Roberts & Poeppel, 1995). The effects of frequency on amplitude (especially the interaction with intensity) may be related to the extent of the basilar membrane (and hence the number of afferent neurons)

activated by the sound. The latency effects are greater than what might be expected from the cochlear delay. Low-frequency sounds take more time to process and this time increases as the analysis proceeds up the auditory pathway (Woods, Alain, Covarrubias, & Zaidel, 1993).

Tones of different frequency activate different regions of the auditory cortex, with low-frequency tones generally activating more lateral and anterior areas of the superior surface of the temporal lobe. This tonotopic organization of the cortex is evident in the source analyses of the LAEP from MEG (e.g., Pantev et al., 1988, 1995) and activation patterns from functional magnetic resonance imaging (MRI) (e.g., Woods et al., 2009). However, this particular tonotopic organization is not always found in MEG studies and may vary with the hemisphere and with the ear of stimulation (Gabriel et al., 2004). In electrical studies, source dipoles cannot be easily distinguished in terms of location. Nevertheless, the scalp topography often is quite different for tones of different frequency; responses to high-frequency tones have a more anterior scalp distribution than those to low frequency tones (Alain et al., 1997; Verkindt, Bertrand, Perrin, Echallier, & Pernier, 1995). This topographic difference shows up on dipole source analysis as a difference in orientation rather than source location. A possible explanation is that the different frequencies activate separate regions on a curved surface (such as a gyrus or the curved superior surface of the temporal lobe). Regions not sufficiently far apart to distinguish in terms of location would then still have distinct orientations. A similar explanation has been used for the orientation of the MEG dipoles of both the N1 and the MMN (Tiitinen et al., 1993).

What these tonotopic findings mean is not easy to determine. Given the gyral variability of the auditory cortex, it is unclear that any curvature would be consistent from one subject to the next. The LAEP probably is generated simultaneously in widespread regions of the superior surface of the temporal lobe. Each region may have a tonotopic distribution of sources that is oriented along different directions. What we record from the scalp as magnetic or electric fields is likely the sum of activity in many different regions. If we track the location of a source dipole through the duration of the N1m, we find that it moves (typically from medial to lateral) as the latency increases, with the "tracks" for tones of different frequencies having different beginnings and endings (Ozaki et al., 2003; Zouridakis, Simos, & Papanicolaou, 1998). This suggests a "progressive excitation" of different regions of the superior surface of the temporal lobe during the sensory analysis of the stimulus (Zouridakis et al., 1998).

The perceived pitch of a tone depends as much on the periodicity of the sound as on its spectral content. Tones composed of a series of harmonics of one fundamental are heard with a pitch equal to the fundamental even when the fundamental is absent. The pitch of a sound composed of harmonics of 250 Hz beginning at 1000 Hz (e.g., 1000, 1250, 1500, and 1750 Hz) has a dominant pitch of 250 Hz (the "missing fundamental") even though the energy of its spectrum is above 1000 Hz. In an elegant study, Pantev, Hoke, Lütkenhöner, and Lehnertz (1989) found that the source location for the magnetic N1 evoked by tones depends more on pitch than spectral energy. However, there still are differences between tones whose pitch is determined by a missing fundamental and

pure tones—perceptual processing in the cortex of the superior surface of the temporal lobe is as complex as the sounds (Fujioka et al., 2003).

Many musical sounds are harmonic in nature. The timbre (or quality) of a musical note of a particular pitch and loudness is specific to the instrument generating the sound. This depends in part on the pattern of the harmonics. The flute has most of its energy in the fundamental and sounds "pure," whereas brass instruments have multiple higher harmonics and sound "rich." Musical notes evoke LAEPs with a larger P2 wave than simple pure tones, with this difference being more evident in musicians than in nonmusicians (Shahin, Roberts, Pantev, Trainor, & Ross, 2005). The anterior regions of the temporal lobe, particularly in the right hemisphere, may be the source of these effects (Shahin, Roberts, Pantev, Aziz, & Picton, 2007).

Harmonic sounds also have allowed us to look at the separation of auditory objects. If we present a series of harmonics all at the same intensity, they will sound like a buzzing at the frequency of the fundamental. If we then mistune one of the harmonics, it will become perceptible as an independent sound. The stimulus then indicates two auditory objects: a pure tone and a buzz. The LAEP evoked by such a stimulus will differ from that evoked by a stimulus with all harmonics in tune by having a smaller P2 wave. By calculating a difference waveform, we can isolate a small negative wave associated with the perception of the mistuned harmonic—the "object-related negativity" (Alain, Arnott, & Picton, 2001). This is illustrated in Figure 11–5. Like the N1, this object-related negativity can be enhanced by low levels of background acoustic noise (Alain et al., 2009).

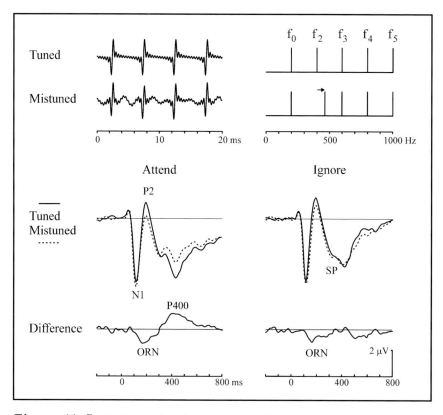

Figure 11–5. Object-related negativity. *The upper section of the figure shows the types of stimuli used to record the object-related negativity. On the left are the time waveforms (limited to 20 ms) and on the right the spectra (limited to 1000 Hz). The "tuned" stimulus contained 12 harmonics of the 200-Hz fundamental, all of equal amplitude. In the "mistuned stimulus the second harmonic is shifted higher by 16% (from 400 to 460 Hz). The lower section of the figure shows the frontocentral LAEPs recorded to the tuned and mistuned stimuli during two experimental conditions: in one the subject was actively attending in order to detect the mistuned stimuli, and in the other the subject was ignoring the stimuli and watching a silent subtitled movie. In both conditions, the mistuned-tuned difference waveforms which shows an object related negativity (or ORN) from 100 to 300 ms. In the attend condition, a P400 also occurs. Data adapted from Alain et al. (2001).*

TEMPORAL ASPECTS

Stimulus Onset Asynchrony (SOA)

Early studies of the LAEPs showed that the response was significantly affected by the interval between stimuli (Davis, Mast, Yoshie, & Zerlin, 1966; Milner, 1969; Nelson & Lassman, 1968). The amplitude of the response increased with increasing intervals between the stimuli, with the rate of increase decreasing as the intervals increased and the amplitudes asymptoting at intervals somewhere between 10 and 20 seconds. If we fit the data from the early studies using an exponential equation of the format illustrated in the bottom right of Figure 11–6 as suggested by Milner (1969), we find time constants between 1 and 5 seconds. Milner found a time constant of 4.3 seconds. Nelson and Lassman (1968) fitted their data using an amplitude versus log(SOA) equation, but this does not easily relate to any physiologic process.

Intensity interacts with SOA in determining the N1-P2 amplitude (Picton et al., 1970), with stimuli of lower intensity showing less of an SOA effect. Response amplitudes tend to saturate at high intensities (60 dB HL or more) when the stimuli

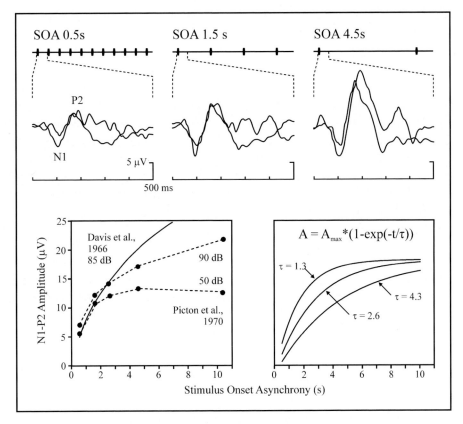

Figure 11–6. Effects of stimulus onset asynchrony (SOA) on the LAEP. The upper section of the figures shows the LAEPs recorded from two different subjects in response to 70-dB 1-kHz 32-ms tones presented at different SOAs. These are unpublished data from studies reported in Picton et al. (1970). The upper line shows the tones over a 5-second period and the LAEPs are recorded over a 500-ms period. The dashed-line data in the graph on the lower left compares the effects of SOA at two different stimulus intensities (from Picton et al., 1970). The graph also plots the original data published by Davis et al., (1966). The lower right graph shows the estimated recovery curves for the SOA effects with different time constants. In the formula, the t value is the SOA and τ is the time constant. The 1.3- and 2.6-second values are from Sams et al. (1993) for the posterior and anterior N1m, respectively. The 4.3-second value is from Milner (1969) for the LAEPS evoked by an 80-dB 1-kHz 350-ms tone.

are presented at more rapid rates (with SOAs of less than 3 s) but the amplitudes continue to increase when the stimuli occur at slower rates. This makes the SOA effect much larger for louder stimuli. Müller-Gass, Marcoux, Jamshidi, and Campbell (2008) found that long SOAs caused only a small increase the amplitude of LAEPs to peri-threshold stimuli and did not alter the estimated physiologic threshold.

MEG studies have provided some interesting ideas concerning the SOA effect on the LAEP. Hari, Kaila, Katila, Tuomisto, and Varpula (1982) found that both the vertex-recorded electrical N1 wave and the N1m response to an 80-dB SPL tone increased in amplitude with increasing SOA. However, the magnetic response saturated at SOAs of less than 4 seconds whereas the vertex response had still not saturated at 16 seconds. Lü, Williamson, and Kaufman (1992) were able to identify two sources for the N1 wave of the LAEP: one on the superior surface of the temporal lobe having a time constant of 1 to 3 seconds and another located more inferiorly, perhaps in the superior temporal gyrus, with a time constant of 3 to 5 seconds. Sams, Hari, Rif, and Knuutila (1993) also identified two magnetic sources, both on the superior surface of the temporal lobe, one anterior (and inferior) to the other. Both increased with increasing SOA, the time constant being 2.6 s for the anterior source and 1.4 s for the posterior source. Both MEG studies clearly indicate that the scalp-recorded N1 is generated by more than one source within the brain and that these different sources are differently affected by SOA. Neither fully explains the SOA data for the electrical responses to high-intensity sounds, which have a longer time constant. These findings would require another source, likely not on the superior surface of the temporal lobe, perhaps in the frontal lobe.

Repetition: Adaptation and Sensitization

SOA effects can be clearly seen when stimuli are presented in pairs or in brief trains. If we present brief trains of stimuli with the train onset asynchrony (TOA) much longer than the SOA of the stimuli in the train, the LAEP to the first stimulus is much larger than to the responses to the succeeding stimuli, which have amplitudes that depend mainly on the SOA (Fruhstorfer, Soveri, & Järvilehto, 1970; Picton, Hillyard, & Galambos, 1976; Ritter, Vaughan, & Costa, 1968). This is illustrated in Figure 11–7. At SOAs of 3 seconds, the response to the second stimulus is larger than that to the following stimuli, but at briefer SOAs, the response does not change much after its initial decrement between the first and second stimulus.

This decrease in amplitude has gone by various names: habituation, adaptation, rate-effect, and refractoriness. None of these terms ideally suit the phenomenon. Habituation usually means a decrease in response with stimulus repetition that can be reinstated by some extra dishabituating stimulus without altering the repeating stimulus. Adaptation usually indicates some fatigue in the receptors or synapses of a sensory system, which requires rest and metabolic recuperation to return the response to normal. However, adaptation also is used in terms of perception or behavior to indicate that an individual has become accustomed to an environment. Rate-effects do not easily contain any idea of specificity. Refractoriness typically is used in the context of action potentials; an axon is unable to respond to stimulation within a brief absolute refractory period after it has discharged and requires greater than normal stimulation to respond during the subsequent relative refractory period. The decrements in the LAEP with

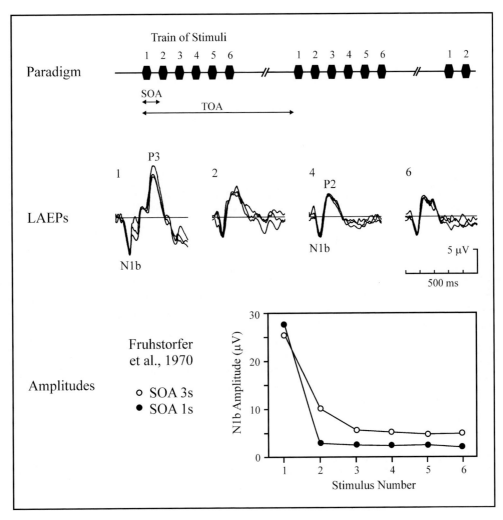

Figure 11–7. *Short-term adaptation of the LAEPs. The top section of this figure shows the stimulus paradigm: trains in which stimuli repeat at a regular SOA are themselves repeated with a train-onset asynchrony (TOA) that is much longer than the SOA. The middle section shows some LAEPs in response to a train of ten 60 dB nHL (normal hearing level) clicks presented with an SOA of 1 s and a TOA of 30 s. The LAEPs are shown for selected positions in the train. These data are adapted from Picton et al. (1976). The bottom section shows a graph of the N1 amplitudes from Fruhstorfer et al. (1970), who used a TOA of 100s and SOAs of 1 and 3 s (data estimated from their Figure 4).*

stimulus repetition are like the refractoriness of the action potential in the sense that the amplitude simply depends on the interval from the preceding response. However, the intervals are much longer than neural refractory periods. Long-term decrements in the LAEP that occur over minutes to hours (rather than the seconds measured in the usual rate-effect studies) might be considered true habituation because these decrements can be dishabituated by manipulations such as having the subject attend to the stimuli (Picton et al., 1976).

Close analysis of the LAEP waveforms at the different positions in the train indicates at least two components of the N1 wave, an early one (at 70–100 ms) with a short refractory period of about 1 second and a later one (after 100 ms) with a much longer refractory period lasting up to 10 seconds (Budd, Barry, Gordon, Rennie, & Michie, 1998). These results probably are related to the two MEG components (posterior and anterior) found in the MEG studies of the N1m that we have already discussed.

Because of refractoriness, the LAEPs to the second stimulus of a pair or to stimuli following the first in a train thus become smaller as the SOA decreases from 10 to 0.5 s. However, at intervals shorter than 0.5 s, there is an enhancement of the response so that the second stimulus of a pair (or later stimuli in a train) evokes a response that is equal to or larger than the first. This was initially recognized in MEG studies (Loveless, Hari, Hamalainen, & Tiihonen, 1989; Loveless, Levanen Jousmaki, Sams, & Hari, 1996) where the response components following N1 are small and do not significantly interfere with measuring the response to the second stimulus. The effect also can be seen in electrical recordings, provided the response to the initial stimulus is subtracted out from the responses to the paired or repeating stimuli (Budd & Michie, 1994; Sable, Low, Maclin, Fabiani, & Gratton, 2004). Wang, Mouraux, Liang, and Iannetti (2008) have found that this enhancement at short SOA also is present for EPs in other sensory modalities.

Several mechanisms have been proposed to explain this enhancement. Loveless and his colleagues (Loveless et al., 1996; McEvoy, Levanen, & Loveless, 1997) suggest that the process reflects temporal integration. Sounds presented close to-

gether are considered together, that is, perceived as a pair or a train rather than discrete stimuli. They found that their results could be best explained using two separate sources for the N1 with the anterior source, occurring some 30 ms later than the posterior source, contributing most to the enhancement effect. Sable et al. (2004) propose that the prolonged refractoriness of the response is mediated by inhibitory processes that take several hundred milliseconds to develop. Stimuli occurring before these processes have developed (during the period when the inhibition remains latent) are not reduced in amplitude whereas later stimuli are. Wang et al. (2008) found that the P2 wave was not enhanced at the short SOA and proposed that an additional negative wave might be evoked by the second stimulus of a pair. This could increase the N1 and decrease the P2 waves. Wang et al. suggested that such a wave might be an MMN to the second stimulus perceived as deviant because the memory representation of the preceding stimulus has not had enough time to form. As discussed later, the MMN and the anterior N1m may be related.

Specificity of the Refractory Period

When a stimulus occurs within the refractory period, the amplitude of the LAEP varies inversely with the similarity between the present and preceding stimuli. This was first demonstrated by Butler (1968) using a paradigm wherein a test stimulus occurred once every 5 s. In the control condition, the test stimuli occurred alone. In experimental conditions, three intervening stimuli of a frequency either the same as or different from that of the test stimuli were presented (once every 1.25 s) between the test stimuli. The amplitude of the LAEP to the test stimulus expressed as a percentage of its amplitude in the control condition varied with the frequency of the intervening stimuli. The basic idea of this paradigm is shown in Figure 11–8. Butler, Spreng, and Keidel (1969) extended these results to consider the ear of stimulation; the LAEP to the test stimulus was larger when the intervening and test stimuli were presented to different ears

Butler proposed that these results indicated a specificity of the SOA-dependent refractoriness of the LAEP. Each stimulus activated a population of neurons, and once activated these neurons would be refractory to stimulation for several seconds. The closer the intervening stimuli

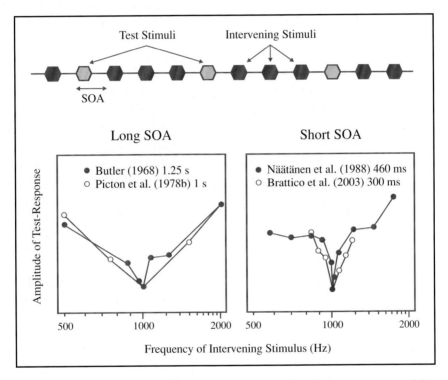

Figure 11–8. Selective adaptation of the LAEPs. The upper section of this figure shows the paradigm for studying selective adaptation; test stimuli are separated by several intervening stimuli. Separate recordings are obtained in separate blocks with test stimuli differing across blocks in terms of some parameter such as tonal frequency. The amplitude of the response to the test stimulus is then plotted as a function of that parameter. The two graphs in the lower section of the figures show the selective adaptation curves from different studies using a 1-kHz tone as the test stimulus. The scales have been arbitrarily adjusted to allow the graphs to be superimposed. The studies with the longer SOA show a broader (less specific) adaptation. curve. The studies of Butler (1968) and Picton et al. (1978b) used three intervening stimuli. The Näätänen et al. (1988) study used one and the Brattico et al. (2003) study used five intervening stimuli. Brattico et al. used a reverse paradigm (see Figure 11–10): the intervening stimulus stayed at 1000 Hz and the test-stimulus changed randomly.

were in frequency (or space) to the test stimuli, the more the neuronal populations that they activated would share common neurons. When the test stimulus differed from the intervening stimuli, it would activate some neurons ("fresh afferents") that had not been activated by the intervening stimuli as well as the refractory neurons activated by both types of stimuli. The response to the test stimulus therefore would be larger than when the intervening stimuli were the same as the test stimulus, and this difference would increase as the difference between the stimuli increased. The effect—the specificity of the refractory period—thus can be attributed to a selective adaptation of neurons responding to the test stimuli that also respond to the intervening stimuli and therefore are in a refractory state when the test stimulus occurs (May & Tiitinen, 2010).

Although we are discussing these processes in terms of refractory periods, similar effects can be obtained using other mechanisms. For example, we can conceive of a network of interacting neurons as instantiating at a certain level of activity the perception of a particular sound. As the sound ceases, the activity in the network will decline but it will not become completely inactive for a while. A new stimulus that shares some of the network components with the preceding stimulus will need to activate only a few other components to make its own network reach a perceptible level. The activation process therefore is smaller than if the new stimulus did not share any components with the preceding stimuli. Such an explanation is discussed further in the legend for Figure 11–9.

In terms of frequency, the effects of selective adaptation plotted against the frequency of the intervening stimuli has some similarities to the tuning curves of individual neurons (see Figure 5–6). However, the relationship is not simple (see modeling and discussion in Näätänen et al., 1988). Tuning curves show how the response of a neuron with a particular characteristic frequency will respond to other frequencies at a higher intensity. Thus, at a set intensity above threshold, a neuron that responds best to the test stimulus may also respond to (and become adapted by) the intervening stimulus. This overlap should increase with increasing intensity. The effects of intensity on the selective adaptation curves has not been fully examined, all reported studies using stimuli near 60 to 70 dB HL.

The results of Butler (1968) with tones of different frequencies have been replicated many times (Brattico, Tervaniemi, & Picton, 2003; Näätänen et al., 1988; Picton, Woods, & Proulx, 1978b). However, as indicated in Figure 11–8, the sharpness of the tuning has varied from study to study. Some of the variance may be related to stimulus intensity; at higher intensities, we might expect greater overlap in the neuronal populations responding to the different tones. The rate of stimulus presentation also may have an effect. The intervening stimuli were presented at an SOA of 460 ms in the Näätänen et al. and 300 ms in the Brattico et al. studies both of which found a very narrow tuning near the frequency of the test stimulus. These stimuli were occurring much more rapidly than in the original Butler studies which used SOAs of 1.25 s. It is not clear how this mediates the more specific adaptation curve. However, at the rapid stimulus rates, we might presume that sensitization may occur. This may make neurons that are affected by sensitization (those generating the anterior N1m) contribute more to the adaptation curves than the others.

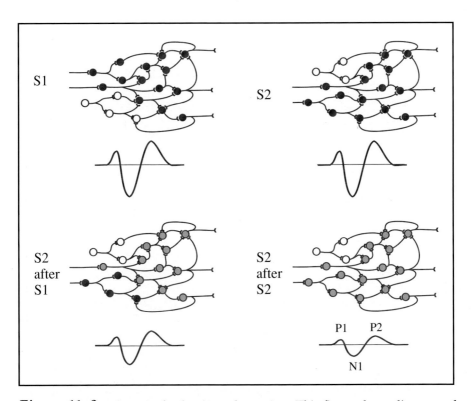

Figure 11–9. Theory of selective adaptation. *This figure shows diagrams of an interactive network of cortical neurons that respond to sounds. This is highly schematic—we have to consider the neurons as being in many different cortical areas and being much more numerous (and much more connected). Below each network is represented the field potential recorded at a distance from the activated network. In the upper left, the network responds to one stimulus (S1) and in the upper right to a different stimulus (S2). Neurons activated by the stimulus are shown in black. If S2 is repeated shortly after S1 (lower left), many of the neurons in the network do not need to be fully activated again because they remain active from the previous stimulation. These are shown in gray. The response therefore is smaller than if S2 occurred without any preceding stimulus (upper right). If S2 is repeated (lower right), all of the neurons are in an adapted state (gray) and the activation potential is lower than if the S2 followed S1.*

Brattico et al. (2003) reversed the original Butler paradigm so that the test stimulus changed and the intervening stimulus stayed the same. If the test stimuli were then randomized within each recording block of recording, multiple interstimulus effects could be evaluated concomitantly, the EPs for the test stimuli being averaged separately on the basis of their frequency. This paradigm (illustrated at the top of Figure 11–10) decreased any variability that might occur between blocks. The results were similar to those recorded using the original paradigm.

If, however, we maintained a constant test stimulus and randomized the frequency of the sets of intervening stimuli, we lost most of the tuning. The response

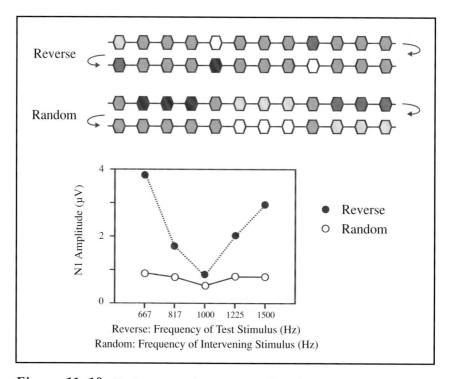

Figure 11–10. Variant paradigms to study selective adaptation. The upper section of this figure shows two paradigms derived from the original Butler paradigm The "Reverse" paradigm keeps the intervening stimulus constant (at 1000 Hz) and changes the test stimulus. In this paradigm, we also randomized the frequencies of the test stimuli within a recording block (frequency is coded as the darkness of the shading). The effects (shown by the filled circles in the lower graph) *were similar to those obtained in the original Butler paradigm. The "Random" paradigm kept the test stimulus constant and just randomized the sets of intervening stimuli. When the SOA was short, there was a cumulative effect on the test stimulus; the intervening stimuli from preceding cycles added their adaptation-effect to that of the set immediately prior to the test stimulus. This resulted in very general adaptation.*

to the test stimulus was small regardless of the frequency of the immediately preceding set of intervening stimuli. These results are illustrated in Figure 11–10 as the "Random" paradigm. The reason was a carryover of refractoriness from one cycle to the next caused by the rapid stimulus presentation (SOAs of 400 ms). For example, some neurons responding to the 1000-Hz test stimulus after a set of 1500-Hz intervening stimuli would be refractory

because their response fields included 1500 Hz. However, because of the short SOA, other neurons that shared different response fields with the intervening stimuli of the preceding cycle (occurring only 2 seconds before) also would remain refractory.

As well as providing theoretical information about how the auditory system works, the Butler paradigm and its variants have several practical advantages. LAEPs are more efficiently recorded if multiple different stimuli are presented concomitantly rather than in separate stimulus blocks. This was discussed in general terms in Chapter 6. In terms of the LAEPs, several techniques are possible. We can alternate the ears to which the stimuli are presented while keeping the within-ear rate the same. The responses will be a little smaller than if there were just presented to one ear alone but this is more than compensated for by the fact that we can record responses at twice the overall rate. We also can present tones of different frequency in each ear by setting up sequences that have an overall rate that is faster than when tones of only one frequency are presented in a block. Both Ross et al. (1999) and Lightfoot and Kennedy (2006) describe multiple-stimulus paradigms that can be used when recording the LAEPs for audiometric purposes.

SEQUENCES OF STANDARD AND DEVIANT STIMULI

The selective adaptation paradigms usually present different auditory stimuli in regular sequences. If we examine the responses evoked by the test stimuli more closely, we often can see an additional component of the LAEP—the MMN—that becomes more distinct when the physical difference between the intervening and test stimuli becomes smaller. We considered this in our initial overview of change detection (see Figure 11–3). The extra peak increases in latency as the difference becomes smaller. Measured using a simple baseline-to-peak difference, the amplitude gets larger as the difference gets larger. However, this change in amplitude is related mainly to the N1 component, which overlaps more with the MMN when the difference is large (and the

MMN latency short). This is suggested by the dotted and dashed lines in the graph in the right section of Figure 11–3.

Typically, the MMN is not studied using the selective adaptation paradigm. Rather, it usually is recorded in response to a deviant stimulus (as opposed to a test stimulus) that occurs randomly (rather than regularly) in a train of standard (as opposed to intervening) stimuli: the "oddball" paradigm. The MMN in these irregular sequences is often followed by a later positive wave—the P3a—that reflects the subject noticing the stimulus changes. We consider this component in Chapter 12. First, we must try to understand the MMN.

Even when the paradigm is irregular, the selective adaptation of the N1 remains problematic for the identification and measurement of the MMN. Any subtraction of standard from deviant will contain an N1 adaptation effect as well as the MMN. This is not a major problem when the deviant is very similar to the standard ,the N1 effect is small and the MMN is delayed beyond any overlap. When the difference between standard and deviant becomes large, controls are needed to account for the N1 adaptation effect. One approach is to subtract the response to the same stimulus as the deviant when it is presented in a paradigm with multiple equiprobable tones (e.g., Jacobsen et al., 2003). This technique is diagramed in Figure 11–11. These recordings reveal a MMN that does decrease in amplitude as the difference between the stimuli decreases. However, this occurs only as the difference approaches discrimination-threshold. For near-threshold deviations, the decreased MMN amplitude therefore may reflect the decreased rate of deviance detection. The concept is that the MMN has a constant amplitude but occurs only

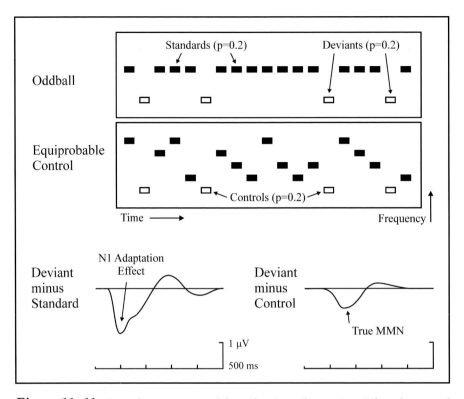

Figure 11–11. *Paradigm to control for selective adaptation.* When the normal oddball paradigm is used to evaluate the MMN, the difference waveform obtained by subtracting the deviant from the standard contains both a MMN and the N1 adaptation effect. One way to control for the effect of adaptation is to use an equiprobable control condition as illustrated in the upper section of the figure. This approach is based on that to Jacobsen and Schröger (2003) but the illustrated paradigm is different in that the average tonal frequency of the noncontrol stimuli in the equiprobable condition is the same as the frequency of the standard in the oddball condition. As diagrammed in the lower section of the figure, subtracting control from deviant should give the true MMN without any overlay from the N1 adaptation effect. However, the MMN might itself be reduced as there may be a very small MMN in the control condition. In that condition, the control stimulus can be considered at the limits of a varying standard (cf. Winkler et al., 1990)

on trials when the deviation is indeed registered by the brain (Horvath et al., 2008).

Mismatch Negativity to Changes in Stimulus Features

The classic MMN is recorded in the response to an occasional change in the frequency of a repeating tone (Sams, Paavilainen, Alho, & Näätänen, 1985). As we have noted, the peak latency of this wave increases as the difference between standard and deviant stimuli decreases (see the lower right graph of Figure 11–3). This latency runs parallel to the reaction time for discriminating between the stimuli (obtained in different experiments from those in which the MMN was measured), which occurs 150 to 200 ms later

(Horvath et al., 2008; Tiitinen, May, Reini-kainen, & Näätänen, 1994). This suggests that the MMN indexes the discrimination process. Although the early research suggested that the MMN amplitude decreased with decreasing frequency difference (Tiitinen et al., 1994), the studies of Horvath et al. (2008) suggest that this change in amplitude is more related to whether the discrimination occurred than to the ease whereby it was made.

The source of the MMN to a frequency deviant is located on the superior surface of the temporal lobe. The scalp topography of the MMN typically is more frontal than that of the N1, and several studies have found the MMN source to be anterior to the N1 source (e.g., Sams, Kaukoranta, Hämäläinen, & Näätänen, 1991; Scherg et al., 1989). Giard, Perrin, Pernier, and Bouchard (1990) proposed that a frontal source (more on the right than the left) occurred during the generation of the MMN in addition to those on the superior temporal surface. Such a radial source might not be visible in MEG recordings.

The MMN can also be evoked by occasional changes in many other physical characteristics (or "features") of the repeating stimulus, such as intensity, duration, spectral pattern, location, and so forth (reviewed in Näätänen, Paavilainen, Rinne, & Alho, 2007; Picton, Alain, Otten, & Ritter., 2000). Of these, the intensity MMN is interesting because it clearly distinguishes the MMN from the usual N1 (Näätänen, Paavilainen, Alho, Reinikainen, & Sams, 1987b). When the deviant stimulus has a lower intensity than the standard, there is a decrement (or little change) in the N1, but a clear MMN still occurs. The duration MMN distinguishes the MMN from the N1 in another way (Näätänen, Paavilainen, & Reinikainen, 1989). The latency of the duration MMN is determined by the offset of the shorter of the two stimuli

(the time at which the duration change first becomes apparent) rather than to the onset of the deviant stimulus. This makes it relatively easy to distinguish the MMN from the N1. Thus, if the standard has a duration of 100 ms and the deviant a duration of 200 ms (or vice versa), the MMN peaks at a latency of about 225 ms from the onset of the deviant stimulus (125 ms after the moment—100 ms—at which the deviant becomes discriminable). If the stimuli are 50 and 100 ms, the MMN peaks at 175 ms (125 ms after 50 ms). For all stimuli (standards or deviants, long or short), the N1 peaks at about 100 ms after the stimulus onset.

A deviance from an ongoing standard may involve the conjunction of two features rather than just a single feature (Takegata, Paavilainen, Näätänen, & Winkler, 1999). A paradigm to elicit a MMN to a "conjunction deviant" would involve presenting two concomitant trains of standard stimuli (each occurring with a probability of 0.45), with the two standards differing in frequency and intensity. A conjunction deviant ($p = 0.1$) would be a stimulus that had the frequency of one standard and the intensity of the other. The deviant can be detected only by evaluating both features together.

The MMN evoked by changing one characteristic of the ongoing stimuli is independent of that evoked by changing a different characteristic (Takegata et al, 1999). Thus, a stimulus that changes from a standard in two ways (a double deviant), for example, in the conjunction of frequency and intensity and in location, elicits a MMN that is equivalent to the sum of the MMNs elicited by either deviant when presented alone. These results indicate that there are parallel and independent systems in the brain that evaluate each of the different features of a stimulus and determine whether it can be predicted from preceding stimuli or not. Further evidence for this independence comes from studies that have found differences in scalp topography between the MMNs evoked by different kinds of deviance (Giard et al., 1995), although these differences are not always significant, particularly when the discriminability of the deviant is controlled (e.g., Deouell & Bentin, 1998).

Because of this independence of the different MMNs, several MMNs can be evaluated concomitantly using one stimulus sequence (Näätänen, Pakarinen, Rinne, & Takegata, 2004). In the paradigm described as "Optimum-1," a standard tone with a defined frequency, intensity, duration, location, and gap occurs as every second stimulus. In between these standards, various deviants occur. These can be of different types (e.g., frequency, intensity, duration, location, or gap) and the response to each deviant will show a MMN when compared to the standard response. Figure 11–12 compares this paradigm to the usual oddball paradigms for recording different MMNs, with the overall probability kept constant for any one type of deviant. The MMNs in the optimum paradigm essentially were the same as those recorded in multiple separate oddball paradigms. Because five times as many deviants were recorded in the same time as one in the single-deviant paradigm, the efficiency of the recording was greatly increased. The other interesting aspect of the paradigm is that a deviant along one dimension is still standard along the other dimensions being examined. Pakarinen, Takegata, Rinne, Huotilainen, and Näätänen (2007) have extended this paradigm so that various levels of deviance can be examined for each type of deviant. They used four dimensions of deviant, with six levels of deviance within

each dimension (for a total of 24 deviants), in order to obtain an objective assessment of discrimination, a "discrimination profile" for the auditory system. This approach can evaluate the discrimination of phonetic as well as acoustic changes (Pakarinen et al., 2009). A further development to increases the efficiency of the recording has been to remove the standard stimulus and to present just the deviant stimuli, with the invariant properties of the deviant stimuli serving as a standard against which the brain detects the sound changes (Pakarinen, Huotilainen, & Näätänen, in press). This requires that the MMN be distinguished from the other LAEP waves by some means such as latency or intracerebral source analysis.

Objective Evaluation of Stimulus Discrimination

Because the presence of a MMN indicates that the deviant stimulus has been discriminated from the standard, the MMN has been used as an objective measurement of auditory perception. Kraus et al. (1996) showed that children with learning problems showed no MMN to a phonemic discrimination between /da/ and /ga/ though there was a MMN to the easier /da/ and /wa/ discrimination. This suggests some basic underlying disorder in the auditory system of these children. The relation between this disorder and the children's learning problems remains to be determined (see Bishop, 2007 for a review of the issues and problems).

The MMN in infants and children is difficult to detect as the background electroencephalogram (EEG) is larger and more variable than in adults. Signal-to-noise issues, severe enough to make the MMN problematic in some adults (Cacace

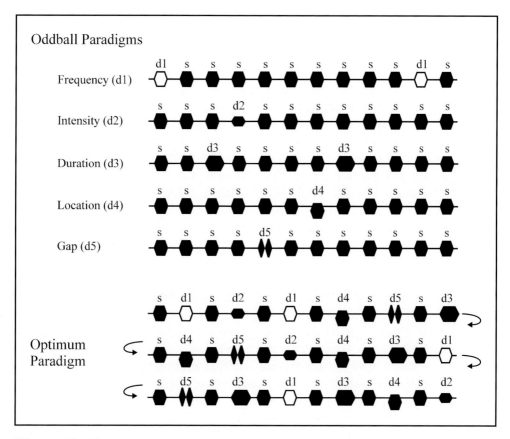

Figure 11–12. Optimum paradigm for recording the MMN. The upper section of the figure illustrates the usual way in which the MMN is recorded using the oddball paradigm. For each type of deviance, a sequence of standard and deviant stimuli is presented, with the deviant stimulus occurring with a probability of 0.1. Different deviant stimuli (d1 frequency, d2 intensity, d3 duration, d4 location, and d5 gap) are examined in separate recording sessions. Näätänen et al. (2004) proposed an optimum paradigm wherein multiple types of deviants were presented concomitantly. This is illustrated in the lower section. One of the five deviants occurred every second stimulus, separated from the previous deviant by a standard stimulus. The overall probability of any particular deviant was the same, but five deviants occurred within the same time as one in the single-deviant paradigms, thus greatly improving the efficiency of the recording.

& McFarland, 2003; Wunderlich & Cone-Wesson, 2001) have not been properly considered in infants and children. Measuring difference waveforms is not a simple process when the recording is noisy. It is particularly problematic when the peak latency (or polarity) of the response is undetermined. We can easily wind up picking peaks in the residual background noise. Only when the changes are constant across replications can we be sure that deviance detection is occurring and that the auditory system is discriminating the sounds. Because of the signal-to-noise issues, the MMN may be able to show discrimination difficulties in a group of subjects compared to normal but may not be able to determine much about any individual subject (see discussion in Picton et al., 2000).

The routine paradigm for recording the MMN as an objective demonstration of auditory discrimination uses an SOA of about 500 ms and a deviant that occurs with a probability of between 0.1 and 0.2. Responses are recorded using a bandpass of 0.1 to 15 Hz and averaged separately for the standard and the deviant. Multiple channel recordings are needed (including at least the Fz and Cz channels and an EOG monitor. The deviant average requires several hundred trials, depending on the size of the MMN. Stapells (2009) provides more extensive advice. The new optimum paradigms that we have discussed (see Figure 11–12) may become the method of choice in the future. These paradigms allow multiple discriminations to be assessed simultaneously and may be able to provide more extensive and more reliable information than the routine MMN paradigms. This approach has been used successfully in children (Lovio et al., 2009).

Mismatch Negativity to Stimulus Patterns and Abstract Features

The MMN can be evoked by a deviance in the pattern of stimulus presentation rather than in the simple features of the stimuli. A simple pattern deviance would be the unpredicted repetition of a stimulus in a sequence that regularly alternated between two stimuli. The repeating stimulus elicits a clear MMN (Alain & Woods, 1997; Nordby, Roth, & Pfefferbaum, 1988). This would be unexpected on the basis of simple stimulus features as the repeating

stimulus is the same as that immediately preceding. The MMN to this pattern deviance differs in its scalp topography from the MMN to a simple frequency deviance, indicating that the systems that evaluate recurring patterns use different neuronal populations (Alain, Achim, & Woods, 1999).

The standard pattern can involve several stimuli. Tervaniemi, Maury, and Näätänen (1994) presented a repeating pattern of 10 tones, the frequency of which descended regularly from one tone to the next. An increase in frequency or a stimulus repetition evoked a MMN, regardless of where in the sequence it occurred. The system responsible for generating the MMN therefore was coding the fact that the pitch was descending from one stimulus to the next. Alain, Cortese, and Picton (1999) found that changes in the frequency or timing of any stimulus within a repeating sequence of tones evoked a MMN. Sample results are shown in Figure 11–13.

The pattern can be abstract rather than specifically related to particular sequences of stimuli. Saarinen, Paavilainen, Schröger, Tervaniemi, and Näätänen (1992) presented pairs of tones in which the frequencies increased, decreased or stayed the same. However, the actual frequencies varied from one standard to the next. A MMN was evoked by a deviant pair that changed frequency (or not) differently from the repeating standard pair. The system thus was abstracting the direction of frequency change from the various standard pairs and applying that abstract rule to determine if a deviant pair had occurred. This ability to form abstract rules from particular instances indicates a "primitive intelligence" in the auditory cortex (Näätänen, Tervaniemi, Sussman, Paavilainen, & Winkler, 2001).

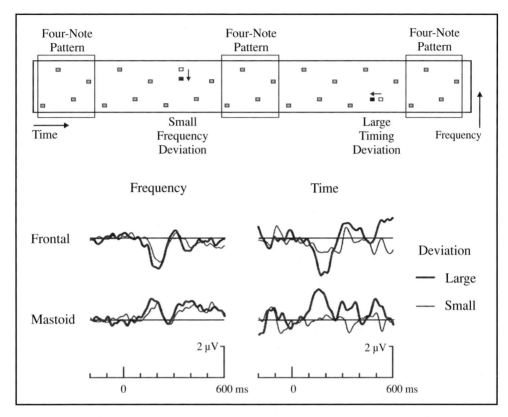

Figure 11–13. ***MMN to change in stimulus-pattern.*** *The upper section of the figure shows the stimulus paradigm. A four-note pattern repeats every 800 ms. With a probability of 0.05, one of the notes deviates from the pattern in either its frequency or its timing. For each type of pattern-deviance, two different levels were used. The difference in frequency from the preceding tone was decreased by 25 or 75%, or the interval from the preceding tone was decreased by 25 or 75% timing. The lower section of the figure shows the grand-mean deviant-standard difference waveforms. A frontal MMN with a peak-latency near 200 ms occurs for both types of deviant. This inverts in polarity at the mastoid. Data from Alain et al. (1999).*

Time and the MMN: Event Integration, Trace Duration, and Refractoriness

The process underlying the MMN integrates the information in an auditory event over a period 150 ms; this has been termed the "temporal window of integration" (Yabe et al., 1998). The paradigm wherein a stimulus is occasionally omitted from a regular train can be used to estimate the time required to integrate an auditory event. If the stimuli occur rapidly such that the integration time includes more than one stimulus, then an occasional omission will be detected as a deviant stimulus and a MMN will occur in response to the omission. At slower rates, the system simply will consider the omission as part of the irregular rate and no MMN will occur. If the subject is actively attending to the stimulus, an N2-P3 complex will occur when the missing stimulus is consciously detected (Picton et al., 1976). However, if the subject is not attending, there is no clear response at these long intervals. A MMN occurs only if the SOA is 150 ms or less.

Studies of the SOA between the repeating stimuli can help determine how long information about the preceding stimulus (or stimulus event) is maintained. As the SOA between the stimuli in a train was increased, the magnetically recorded MMN evoked by a deviant stimulus (occurring with probability of 0.14) became smaller until it was no longer distinguishable from noise when the SOA exceeded 9 s (Sams et al., 1993). This duration is similar to the estimated trace duration for the anterior N1m component (see Figure 11–6), and for sensory memory as tested behaviorally.

Another approach to estimating the timing parameters of the MMN is to present brief trains of stimuli with a short SOA (610 ms) and a longer train onset asynchrony (TOA) of 11 to 15 s (Cowan, Winkler, Teder, & Näätänen, 1993). This paradigm derives from those used to evaluate the short-term habituation or adaptation of the LAEPs that we reviewed earlier in this chapter (see Figure 11–7). However, the focus of the Cowan et al. experiments was to see what happened with deviant stimuli. If the standard stimulus was constant from train to train, a MMN did not occur when the deviant was the first stimulus in a train. The system did not maintain any memory of the previous set of standards, which occurred more than 10 seconds before. However, a deviant occurring at the second stimulus elicited a large MMN. The system therefore can quickly reinstate a previous memory (Ritter, Sussman, Molholm, & Foxe, 2002). However, if the standard stimulus changed

from train to train (the "roving standard paradigm"), the MMN did not occur at the first position and was very small at the second position (Cowan et al., 1993). The authors therefore proposed that it takes two or more repeating standards to establish a trace that can be used to register a deviant.

The initial studies of the time duration of the MMN process were concerned with how long the memory of a repeating standard stimulus lasts. We also might consider the effects of the relative probabilities of the deviant and the standard stimuli. In this discussion, we are considering probability in terms of sequential probability, the number of times a deviant occurs in a sequence of stimuli. If the SOA is maintained constant, the MMN decreases as the deviant becomes more probable and becomes nothing as the deviant and standard become equiprobable (reviewed by Näätänen et al., 2007). This may have something to do with trace strength, the more standard stimuli occurring before a deviant, the stronger the trace and the greater the detected deviance. In addition, as the deviant becomes more probable, it may itself form a trace and a standard stimulus following a deviant can then evoke a small MMN (Sams, Ahlo, & Näätänen, 1984). This would attenuate the MMN as measured in the deviant-standard difference waveform.

We also might consider the effects of temporal probability of a deviant, the number of times it occurs within a period of time, as opposed to the sequential probability. Maintaining the SOA and changing the probability of the deviant will change the intervals between the deviant stimuli. Sabri and Campbell (2001) compared the MMN evoked under various conditions of temporal and sequential probability. The MMN clearly increased as the temporal probability became lower. However, the MMN also varied with the number of intervening stimuli: the fewer there were (the shorter the overall SOA, and higher the sequential probability) the smaller the MMN. These results suggest that the MMN depends on two processes: the strength of the trace (determined by the temporal probability of the standards) and the refractoriness of the deviance detection mechanism (determined by the temporal probability of the deviants). Time has a similar effect on the process that detects the mismatch and the process that lays down a memory of the standard. Both processes seem to have a time course of about 10 seconds; the memory trace lasts that long and the deviance detection mechanism becomes nonrefractory within that time.

Another way to look at the refractory effects is to evaluate the MMN to deviants that occur with a set probability but with a longer or shorter interval from the previous deviant (as determined by the random sequencing of the stimuli). Separately averaging the deviant responses on the basis of the time since the preceding deviant, Picton et al (2000) found that the MMN increased in amplitude as the interdeviant interval increased from 1 to more than 2.5 s. Pincze, Lakatos, Rajkai, Ulbert, and Karmos (2002) studied the effect of interdeviant interval on the MMN recorded in cat cortex and found a relationship between MMN amplitude and the log of the interdeviant interval. The data could have also been fitted with an exponentially asymptoting function with a time constant of several seconds (cf. the Nelson and Lassman data for N1-P2 discussed on p. 351).

A trace duration of about 10 s also can explain some of the results with repeating sequences of sounds. The MMN process can detect a repeating sequence of several stimuli, and only generates a MMN if one of the stimuli in the sequence changes in some way. If this is so, why should the sequences of stimuli used in the selective adaptation paradigm (three or four intervening stimuli followed by one test stimulus) still generate a MMN in the response to the test stimulus as shown in Figure 11–3? In that experiment (Scherg et al., 1989), a MMN occurred whether the test stimuli occurred either regularly once every fifth stimulus or randomly with a probability or 0.2. A random presentation typically is used to elicit a MMN. In a regular paradigm, because the test stimulus is predictable from sequence to sequence, we might think that the deviant test stimulus should not elicit a MMN. However, it does (see dotted-line results in Figure 11–3). The reason lies in the span over which the MMN evaluates sequences. This time period is likely related to the time course of echoic memory, around 8 to 10 s. The regular stimuli in the Scherg et al experiment occurred once every 4.5 s. In order to detect a repeating sequence, the MMN system would have to maintain in memory at least two sequences (lasting at least 9 seconds) and preferably more. Only if it can evaluate two or more sequences can the system recognize that a sequence is repeating itself in a predictable manner. If two sequences lasted 9 seconds, a system that had a time span of 8 seconds could not determine that there was a regularly repeating sequence and would just react to the change in frequency of the tone. If the stimuli are repeated at a more rapid rate, if the SOA is decreased to 100 ms so that the full sequence lasted only 500 ms, no MMN occurs (Sussman, Vaughan, & Ritter, 1998). Several regular sequences then occur during the MMN time span and the change in frequency can be considered part of a repeating sequence and not considered deviant. If the deviant stimulus occurs randomly at the rapid ISI with the same probability as that in the regular presentation (but with no predictable sequence), a clear MMN occurs.

In summary, the MMN is characterized by two time periods. Stimulus information is integrated over between 100 and 200 ms. This integration time is longer than the 50-ms integration time of the N1 wave. We might be tempted to suggest an N1 system that quickly scans for the occurrence of a stimulus, and an MMN system that evaluates whether the stimulus is new or simply repeating. These distinctions may be related to posterior and anterior regions of the auditory cortex. The second MMN time period is about 10 seconds long. This is the duration over which a stimulus trace can last for comparison to incoming stimuli, the time over which a stimulus sequence is scanned for regularity, and the period from a preceding MMN within which the MMN remains partially refractory. This time is of the same order of magnitude as the refractory period of the N1 wave, or at least the components of the N1 that are generated more anteriorly on the superior surface of the temporal lobe. The period is similar to that proposed for auditory sensory memory, and may represent the operating time of the networks of neurons in the auditory cortex.

The Organization of Perception

The sounds diagrammed in Figure 11–14 can be perceived in two ways. Sometimes they can sound like a galloping horse— dum-di-dum, dum-di-dum. At other times, they may sound like two birds: one peeping di-di-di at a slow rate and the other independently peeping dum-dum-dum at

a more rapid rate. These different percepts result from auditory scene analysis (Bregman, 1990), cerebral processes that divide up the sounds we hear and attribute them to different objects in different places. To perceive the galloping horse, we attribute all the sounds to one source and give it a temporal pattern. To perceive the two birds, we attribute each sound to an independent source, streaming sounds of similar frequency together. Streaming is facilitated by increasing the frequency difference (Δf) between the two sounds or by decreasing the SOA. As the frequency difference was increased, the LAEP evoked by the middle tone of the triplet increased in size; this increase involved both N1 and P2 components of the vertex response and the N1c wave of the right temporal response (Snyder, Alain, & Picton, 2006). These effects could be examined by subtracting from the recorded LAEPs a control recording in which all the stimuli had the same frequency. Like the perception of streaming, the difference-waveform became larger as the train of stimuli continued. These results probably are related to the selective adaptation of the sounds; as the tones become less adapted by intervening tones, they become more independently recognizable. Gutschalk et al. (2005), recording the MEG responses to a similar set of stimuli, found that the same set of stimuli sometimes could be perceived as two streams and sometimes as one. If the responses were separately averaged on the basis of how the sounds were being perceived, the response to the different tone was larger when the stimuli were being streamed.

The mechanisms for streaming are not fully understood (see reviews by Micheyl et al., 2007, and Snyder & Alain, 2007). Sounds likely are segregated into different streams based on simple cues like frequency prior to arriving at the cortex.

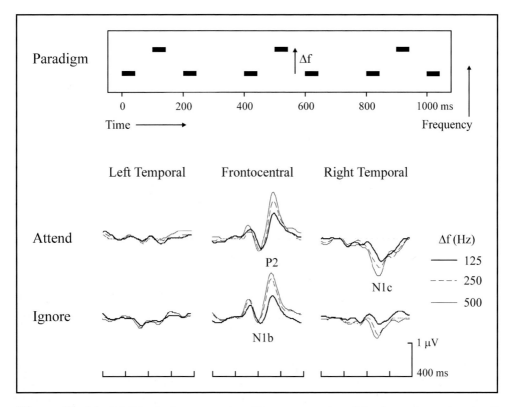

Figure 11–14. *LAEPs during streaming. The upper section of the figure shows the stimuli that could be perceived as a gallop or as two separate streams of sounds (depending on the SOA and the Δf). For this experiment, the low-frequency tone always had a frequency of 500 Hz, the SOA within the triplet was 100 ms, and the interval between the onset of each triplet was 400 ms. When Δf increased, the perception of streaming became more pronounced and the response to the second tone in the triplet became larger. The lower section of the figure shows difference-waveforms calculated by subtracting the response in a control condition with no Δf from the LAEP to the triplet. This clearly shows the enhanced LAEP in the frontocentral and right temporal recordings. Data from Snyder et al. (2006).*

However, cortical mechanisms play a role when streaming is based on more complex features (such as periodicity pitch rather than frequency). Attention plays a large role in setting up and adapting the different streams, perhaps through manipulating thalamocortical interactions.

When stimuli of similar frequency are perceived together in auditory stream, the MMN is determined by the stream in which the deviant occurs rather than the complete set of stimuli presented (Sussman,

2005; Winkler et al., 2003). Experiments using alternating stimuli can provide an example of how this occurs (Yabe et al., 2001). As seen earlier, the infrequent omission of stimulus from a repeating train can evoke a MMN provided that the stimuli are occurring faster than the temporal window for integrating an auditory event (about 150 ms). If two tones alternate regularly with an SOA of 125 ms and the frequencies of the two tones are sufficiently close together so that only one stream of sounds is heard, an omission evokes a MMN. If, however, the frequencies of the two tones are far enough apart so that two streams of sounds are heard, no MMN occurs. Each of the two perceived streams contains stimuli with an SOA of 250 ms, which is beyond the temporal window of integration. Streaming precedes deviance detection.

Sensory information is organized in many other ways in addition to streaming. Pairs of stimuli are perceived as pairs rather than as discrete stimuli (Müller & Schröger, 2007). Stimuli that vary slightly from moment to moment can be perceived as variants of one standard (Winkler et al., 1990). Like streaming, these other automatic processes of auditory scene analysis occur prior to the MMN process. In the variable standard paradigm, the brain makes a fuzzy model of the standard that takes into account its variability. However, the standards near the limits of the variability also may evoke a small MMN.

In addition to automatic sensory processes, the MMN system can have access to long-term memory processes. What we have become most familiar with—what has become a perceptual prototype—is detected more easily as a deviant than sounds we have not experienced before. Huotilainen, Kujala, and Alku (2001) recorded MMNs to infrequent stimuli occurring in trains of phonemes that were either prototypes of native language phonemes or nonprototypes matched in terms of the physical differences between the standard s and deviants. Fewer standards were needed to produce a prominent MMN when using prototype phonemes than nonprototypes. These results indicate faster trace development if the system has access to particular phonemes in long-term memory.

Learning, Experience, and the MMN

Näätänen, Schröger, Karakas, Tervaniemi, and Paavilainen (1993) studied the effect of learning on the MMN in a paradigm that used a standard stimulus that changed frequency seven times within 365 ms and a deviant that was a small change in one of these frequencies. Subjects who were able to detect a slightly deviant pattern in a behavioral discrimination task showed an MMN to this deviant when the stimuli were presented while the subjects read a book. Subjects who initially were not able to discriminate the stimuli did not show any MMN. However, after they learned to discriminate the two stimuli (with repeated practice), an MMN was elicited by the deviant. Interestingly, the MMN to the deviant was larger after a night of sleep, suggesting that sleep consolidates the memory traces for stimuli experienced during wakefulness (Atienza, Cantero, & Stickgold, 2004).

The MMN also can demonstrate how subjects learn to discriminate speech sounds. Tremblay, Kraus, Carrell, and McGee (1997) trained monolingual English-speaking adults to discriminate the prevoiced labial stop sound "mba: from the normally voiced "ba" (a distinction that is not used phonemically in the English language). As the subjects learned the discrimination, the MMN was measured using a paradigm wherein one stimulus was deviant and the other standard. The MMN increased as the subjects became able to make the discrimination.

Discriminating the sounds of language is the most important ability that is learned by our auditory system. As we learn the different prototype phonemes of our mother tongue, we set up traces in the auditory cortex that can be accessed when we discriminate speech sounds. Näätänen et al. (1997) found that a deviant vowel sound that did not fit the prototypes of Finnish vowels did not elicit as large a MMN in Finnish subjects as other deviants that did fit Finnish prototypes, whereas Estonian subjects, for whom the deviant vowel was prototypical, showed a large MMN. Furthermore, this language-related MMN showed much more activity in the left hemisphere than in the right on MEG source analysis. A larger MMN in the left hemisphere for the detection of a deviant stop-consonant was also found by Shtyrov et al. (2000). This asymmetry correlated significantly with the right-ear advantage found on behavioral testing with a dichotic listening test.

P2 WAVE AND LEARNING

As well as the change in the MMN, the P2 of the LAEP increases dramatically as subjects learn to discriminate stimuli that they previously found indistinguishable (recently reviewed by Alain, 2007). This finding initially was reported by Tremblay, Kraus, McGee, Ponton, and Otis (2001) for training in the discrimination of voice-onset times. In English, we normally discriminate between voiced and unvoiced stop consonants, such as "b" and "p." For the "b" phoneme the voicing (vocal fold vibration) occurs as the onset of the sound, whereas for the "p" sound it is delayed by about 30 ms. Languages such as Swahili also use an "mb" phoneme wherein the voicing begins before the lips open. English-speaking subjects cannot normally distinguish "mb" and "b" but most can be trained to make this discrimination. Training increases the P2

wave of the LAEP evoked by these stimuli. This P2 enhancement with perceptual learning was confirmed by Atienza, Cantero, and Dominguez-Martin (2002) who trained subjects to discriminate the seventone patterns of Näätänen et al. (1993), and by Reinke, He Wang, and Alain (2003) who trained subjects to separate superimposed vowels.

It remains unclear how much of the P2 effect is specifically related to training and how much related to a nonspecific effect of exposure to the sounds (Sheehan, McArthur, & Bishop, 2005). Tremblay, Shahin, Picton, and Ross (2009) found effects of perceptual training on a voiceonset time cue on both the trained stimuli and on other auditory stimuli (a simple "a" vowel sound). Using source analysis, they found that the training-specific effects were greater in the left hemisphere, whereas the nonspecific effects were bilateral. The P2 enhancement occurred only in subjects who improved their ability to discriminate the stimuli. In addition, the subjects who improved showed larger N1 waves (before and after training) than the subjects who did not learn the discrimination. Some of these results are illustrated in Figure 11–15. Using MEG, Ross and Tremblay (2009) confirmed that experience alone without specific attention to the sounds can increase the amplitude of the P2. The auditory cortex will alter its responsiveness to sounds on the basis of its experience. Attention during the experience will organize this increased responsiveness to alter the way in which these sounds are categorized and perceived.

The P2 wave of the LAEP is much less understood in terms of its nature and origin than the N1 wave. The P2 is generated mainly on the superior surface of the temporal lobe with a location anterior to

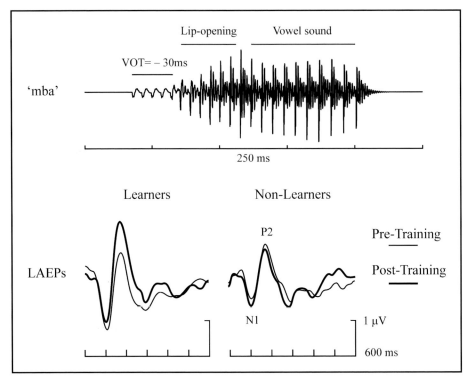

Figure 11–15. Effects of discrimination training on the LAEPs. The upper section of the figure shows an "mba" sound with the voice-onset time (VOT) occurring 30 ms prior to lip opening. Subjects were trained to discriminate between sounds with a VOT of –20 and –10 ms. The lower section shows the effects of training on their LAEPs. Subjects who learned to discriminate the sounds showed a larger N1 before training and a larger P2 after training than subjects who were unable to learn. Data from Tremblay et al. (2009).

that of the N1 generator, which is itself centered on the planum temporale region posterior to the primary auditory cortex (Hari et al., 1987). However, the P2 may have multiple origins (Godey, Schwartz, de Graaf, Chauvel, & Liégeois-Chauvel, 2001). Some of these may be radial and therefore not show up on MEG recordings (Shahin, Roberts, Miller, McDonald, & Alain, 2007). However, the most clearly defining nature of the P2 is that it follows the N1. Therefore, we might be tempted to suggest that the two waves represent two different stages in information processing, perhaps the evaluation of the incoming

information and the transmission of what has been resolved to other cortical areas for further evaluation. This is overly simplistic but it does fit with the learning effects. The output of processing should be greater for the same amount of information input after we have learned how to process the information more effectively.

MUSIC AND MUSICIANS

The subjects who have become most adept at discriminating sounds for their pitch and spectral patterns are musicians. Shahin,

Bosnyak, Trainor, and Roberts (2003) found that the P2 wave and the N1c wave of the LAEP were enhanced in musicians compared to nonmusicians, especially for musical sounds. Source analyses found that the effects were larger in the right temporal lobe. They attributed these findings to a lifetime of training with these sounds. Prior MEG studies had found that musicians had a larger N1m to musical sounds than nonmusicians (Pantev et al., 1998) but these findings are not always significant (Lütkenhöner, Seither-Preisler, & Seither, 2006). Kuriki, Kanda, and Hirata (2006) have used MEG to confirm the P2 enhancement in musicians when stimulated with musical sounds. Musicians also show a larger MMN to music-related deviances than nonmusicians (e.g., Fujioka, Trainor, Ross, Kakigi, & Pantev, 2005; Tervaniemi, Rytkönen, Schröger, Ilmoniemi, & Näätänen, 2001). The early right anterior negativity elicited in musicians by harmonically inappropriate chords differs from the MMN elicited by frequency or pattern deviances by occurring later and having a more anterior and right-sided topography (Koelsch et al., 2001; Koelsch, Schmidt, & Kansok, 2002).

SUSTAINED POTENTIALS

So far we have been considering the LAEPs evoked by the onset of a stimulus. The continuation of a stimulus elicits a sustained potential (SP). This is a negative wave that is recorded maximally over the frontocentral regions of the scalp. This wave is generated mainly on the superior surface of the temporal lobe, with its equivalent dipole occurring anterior to that for the N1 (Scherg et al., 1989). It lasts through the duration of the sound although it decreases in amplitude over time if

sound continues past several seconds (see Figure 11–1). Its beginning is difficult to determine as it occurs during the transient LAEPs evoked by the onset. Picton, Woods, and Proulx (1978a) estimated an onset at about 120 ms. The SP reacts differently from the onset response in response to many stimulus manipulations (Picton, Woods, & Proulx, 1978b). As illustrated in Figure 11–16, the SP is less susceptible to increasing stimulus rates than the onset response, does not saturate at higher intensity, and decreases more regularly with increasing frequency. Furthermore, the SP is less affected by selective adaptation to frequency using the Butler paradigm. This may be because frequency is determined in the first few milliseconds. The SP would be more concerned with processing that lasts longer, for example, the evaluation of stimulus duration.

SUBJECT FACTORS

Sleep

Sleep is a complex state. It generally is classified into periods with rapid-eye-movements (REM) and without (non-REM or NREM). NREM sleep is further categorized into transitional sleep (stages 1 and 2) and slow-wave sleep (stages 3 and 4) on the basis of the amount of delta (0 to 3 Hz) activity in the EEG. Various transients occur during sleep. Spindles (or sigma activity) occur during stages 2, 3, and 4 of NREM sleep. Vertex sharp waves are prominent in stage 2 sleep, and K-complexes (a large delta wave with an associated spindle) occur in stages 2, 3, and 4. The vertex sharp waves and K-complexes can occur spontaneously or they can be evoked by sounds. Indeed, prior to the advent of averaging techniques, determining whether

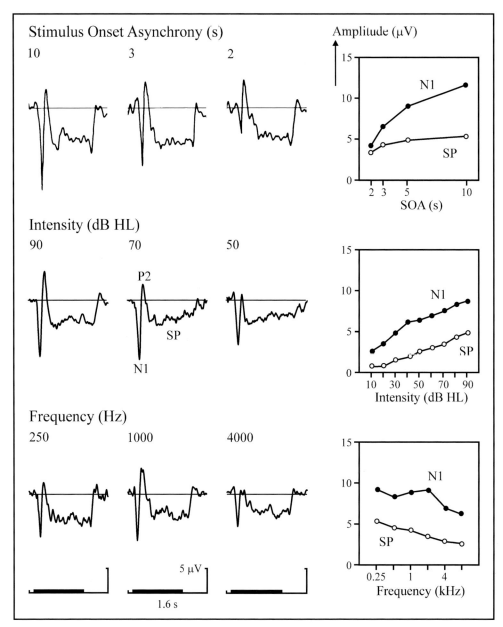

Figure 11–16. *Auditory sustained potentials (SPs).* This figure shows the effects of different experimental manipulations on the SP to a tone lasting 1 s, and on the transient response to the onset of the tone. On the left are shown sample EP waveforms. The waveforms within each of the experimental manipulations come from the same subject but the subjects differ between manipulations. On the right are graphed the average amplitudes for the N1 and the SP for sets of 10 or 12 subjects (the P2 wave was very variable and is not plotted). For the SOA manipulation, the tone had an intensity of 80 dB HL and a frequency of 1 kHz. The N1 decreases with decreasing SOA much more than the SP. For the intensity manipulation, the 1-kHz tone was presented every 3 s. The rate of increase in the N1 amplitude decreases with increasing intensity whereas the SP increases much more regularly. For the frequency manipulation, the 80-dB tone was presented once every 3 s. The amplitude of the N1 remains relatively stable until frequencies of 2 kHz whereas the SP decreases regularly with increasing frequency. Data from Picton et al. (1978b).

these responses could be evoked by sounds during sleep was one way to evaluate a child's hearing (Derbyshire, Fraser, Mc-Dermott, & Bridge, 1956). With averaging, we were able to record more reliable responses while a subject was sleeping. As seen in Chapter 1 (see Figure 1–6), the LAEPs showed waveforms that varied with the different stages of sleep (Osterhammel, Davis, Wier, & Hirsh, 1973; Williams, Tepas, & Morlock, 1962). Figure 11–17 illustrates the LAEP changes that occur with sleep.

Campbell and Colrain (2002) examined the changes in the LAEPs as a subject falls asleep. As the N1 gradually decreases in amplitude to reach baseline, the positive peaks, P1 and P2, increase in amplitude. The change in the positive waves may reflect the dissipation of a long-lasting processing negativity that overlaps with these peaks during the waking state (Campbell, 2000). This may be related to some basic wakeful processing afforded to all stimuli regardless of whether they are the focus of interest. When awake, we are not oblivious of sounds even when we are not paying attention to them. In stage 1 NREM sleep (drowsiness), the background EEG fluctuates between periods of mainly alpha activity and periods of theta activity; the

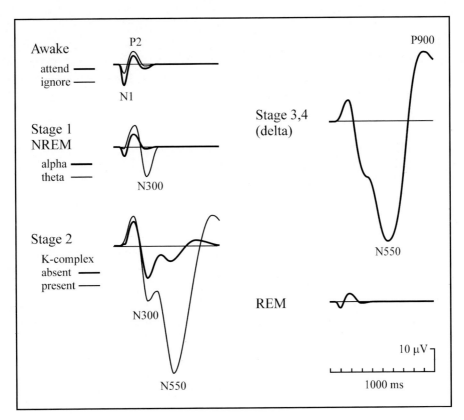

Figure 11–17. LAEPs during sleep. This figure illustrates the typical patterns that the LAEP takes during the various stages of sleep. These patterns are based on Campbell (2000), Colrain et al. (2000), Campbell and Colrain (2002), and Colrain and Campbell (2007).

organized EEG is becoming fragmentary just as consciousness is dissolving. The LAEP is smaller when the background EEG is predominantly theta rather than alpha (Colrain, di Parsia, & Gora, 2000). A large sleep N2 wave or N300 occurs in the NREM stages of sleep, and is particularly prominent during stage 2. This wave and the occurrence of spontaneous spindles herald the loss of normal waking consciousness. The N300 in the LAEP is related to the vertex sharp waves that are seen in the unaveraged EEG, occurring either spontaneously or in response to external stimuli. The spontaneous waves may be triggered by various internal stimuli (such as heartbeats or intestinal contractions) that are not observable other than by the sleeping subject. In slow wave sleep, there also is a late large negative-positive complex with peaks near 550 ms and 900 ms (Bastien, Crowley, & Colrain, 2002; Colrain & Campbell, 2007). These waves may be related to the K-complexes that occur spontaneously, although the relationship has not been fully worked out. Exactly what these sleep-specific waves (N300, N550, and P900) represent in terms of cerebral processing remains unknown. Intracranial recordings show that they are maximally recorded in the superior regions of the frontal lobes (Wennberg, 2010). They could represent a failed attempt to arouse the subject or an inhibitory process to prevents arousal and maintain the sleeping state (or both). The LAEP in REM sleep is similar to that recorded in wakefulness although smaller in amplitude.

In general, the MMN does not occur during NREM sleep (Paavilainen et al., 1987; recent review by Sculthorpe, Ouellet, & Campbell, 2009). Sleep recordings need to be examined over more trials than in wakefulness because of the larger amounts of background EEG activity in sleep. Small deviants evoke no MMN. There may be a difference between the sleep LAEPs evoked by standards and deviants when the differences between the stimuli are large, but this is more likely a difference in the N2 (or N300) related to selective adaptation. This would be akin to the N1 adaptation effect that is differentiated from a true MMN in the waking records. One possible reason for the lack of the MMN might be that sensory memory does not persist as long in sleep as in wakefulness. However, the MMN remains absent in NREM sleep even when the SOA is very short, suggesting inhibition of sensory input occurs before entry into the MMN generating system rather than more rapid memory decay (Sabri & Campbell, 2005). Unlike NREM sleep, MMN responses do occur in REM sleep although they are (like the other LAEPs) smaller than in wakefulness (Atienza, Cantero, & Gomes, 1997; Sabri & Campbell, 2005).

Development

The LAEP changes dramatically during development (reviews by Picton & Taylor, 2007; Wunderlich & Cone-Wesson, 2006). Most EP studies of young infants are performed when the infant is asleep. Only in older infants is it possible to record reliable LAEPs during wakefulness. The studies of sleeping newborn infants show LAEP waveforms that are similar in waveform to those of sleeping adults although the latencies decrease with age (Barnet, 1975). In the normal awake infant, the most prominent wave of the LAEP is a large positive component, which is recorded with maximal amplitude over the fronto-central regions of the scalp. As illustrated in the left section of Figure 11–18, as

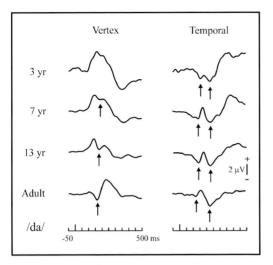

Vertex   Temporal

3 yr

7 yr

13 yr

2 µV

Adult

/da/

-50   500 ms

***Figure 11–18.** Development of the LAEPs in childhood. This figure shows ERPs evoked by the syllable /da/ recorded at different ages from two separate locations, the vertex and the mid-temporal region. The vertex recording shows dramatic changes from a large monophasic positive wave to the adult P1-N1b-P2 waveform. The main process appears to be the growth of the N1b wave (upward arrow) in the middle of the positive wave. The temporal regions show more regular changes with two negative waves (N1a and N1c, upward arrows) shortening in latency with increasing age. These data were originally published in Pang and Taylor (2000) and the actual figure is from Picton and Taylor (2007).*

Guan, 2001; Ponton, Eggermont, Khosla, Kwong, & Don, 2002; Ponton, Eggermont, Kwong, & Don, 2000). The cortical activation in infants and children would then be concentrated in the deeper layers of the cortex (causing a surface positive wave) and would not extend fully into the dendritic trees (to generate a surface negative wave). However, this explanation does not easily fit with the responses recorded from lateral scalp (Tonnquist-Uhlen, Ponton, Eggermont, Kwong, & Don, 2003). These waveforms show two surface negative waves (often called N1a and N1c to differentiate them from the vertex N1b) even in infants. As children become older, these waves develop quite regularly, decreasing in latency but not changing polarity (see right side of Figure 11–18). The child's auditory response generated in the superior surface of the temporal lobe therefore may contain a large positive wave with a peak latency between 100 and 200 ms that obscures a smaller negative component (Picton & Taylor. 2007). The child's LAEP is larger and has a more mature morphology (containing an N1 wave) when evoked by speech sounds than by simple tones (Wunderlich, Cone-Wesson, & Shepherd, 2006). Another factor that plays a role in the development of the LAEP in childhood is the more prolonged refractory period of the N1 component in younger children. The N1 response can be seen even in younger children but only when using longer SOAs (Gilley, Sharma, Dorman, & Martin, 2005).

Unfortunately, the MMN in infants remains controversial (reviewed by Picton & Taylor, 2007). Although the original studies showed a frontal-negative difference wave (Alho, Sainio, Sajaniemi, Reinikainen, & Näätänen, 1990), other studies

age increases, this monophasic response changes slowly into the triphasic P1-N1-P2 waveform of the normal adult.

The vertex N1 wave in the response to simple sounds does not become clear until early adolescence (Bruneau, Roux, Guérin, Barthélémy, & Lelord, 1997; Pang & Taylor, 2000; Poulsen, Picton, & Paus, 2009; Tonnquist-Uhlen, Borg, & Spens, 1995). The development of the N1 wave may relate to the formation of functioning synaptic connections within the upper layers of the auditory cortex (Moore &

have recorded a positive difference wave (e.g., Dehaene-Lambertz & Gliga, 2004). Therefore, we might refer to the waveform as the "mismatch response (MMR)," which is neutral as to its actual polarity. Several possible reasons might explain these discrepant findings. The MMR may mature in a similar way to the N1, with a positive MMR in early infancy (when the synapses on the dendrites are not mature) developing into the negative MMR as the superficial levels of cortex become activated. Trainor et al. (2003) reported that the MMR to a deviant stimulus containing a gap is positive at age 2 months and negative at age 6 months. Different infants may respond differently to the deviant stimulus, perhaps because of different cerebral states. Friederici, Friedrich, and Weber (2002) reported that the infant MMR was more negative in the awake state. Wakefulness in the infant may not be as consistent a state as in older children. Indeed, the infant cortex may only intermittently process incoming information even when the infant is awake. A final reason is that there may be two overlapping waves (Kushnerenko et al., 2002): a negative wave that is later than the MMN of an older child or adult, and a positive wave similar to the adult P3a. The negative wave may index the detection of the deviant and the positive wave may reflect orientation to this stimulus. Depending on the relative timing and sizes of these waves, a negative or positive MMR might result when they are combined.

Aging Effects

The P1, N1, and P2 waves of the LAEP show only small changes in elderly compared to young adults. With increasing age, the N1 and P2 waves increase in latency and decrease slightly in amplitude but the changes are small and often not significant (Goodin, Squires, Henderson, & Starr, 1978; Iraqui, Kutas, Mitchiner, & Hillyard, 1993; Picton, Stuss, Champagne, & Nelson, 1984; Polich, 1997). This robustness of the N1 and P2 waves is in stark contrast to the age-related changes in the later endogenous waves of the LAEP that we consider in the next chapter. Of interest is that the P1 wave is often significantly larger in the elderly (e.g., Alain, McDonald, Ostroff, & Schneider, 2004; Ross, Fujioka, Tremblay, & Picton, 2007). This might be related to the age-related disinhibition in the generation of the Na and Pa waves of the MLR that we discussed in Chapter 9. However, it might also be caused by a small age-related decrease in the overlapping N1 wave.

The MMN generally is smaller in elderly than in young adults (Gaeta, Friedman, Ritter, & Cheng, 1998; Woods, 1992). However, this effect is most clearly seen when the deviance is small (Alain et al., 2004; Gaeta et al., 1998). Therefore, it might relate more to the decreased precision of precortical sensory analysis than to changes in the cortical MMN process itself. Furthermore, the decrease in the MMN is more evident when the interval between stimuli is increased (Pekkonen, Jousmäki, Partane, & Karhu, 1993). This might be caused by a shorter persistence of the auditory memory trace with increasing age. Alain et al. (2004) showed that the elderly can still perceive occasional stimulus deviances (and generate the N2-P3 waves associated with the detection) even if such deviances do not elicit any recognizable MMN when the stimuli are unattended. They attributed these results to top-down compensation for age-related deficits in automatic stimulus evaluation.

MULTIPLE COMPONENT VIEW OF THE LAEPS

Close examination of the N1 peak of the LAEP often reveals several deflections, particularly when recordings are evaluated at multiple electrode sites. McCallum and Curry (1979) differentiated three separate waves—N1a (70 ms) maximal at frontotemporal sites, N1b (100 ms) maximal at the vertex and N1c (140 ms) maximal at the temporal sites. Note that the N1a terminology also has been used for the "anterior" magnetic source dipole (as opposed to the posterior N1p) underlying the magnetic N1 wave; this is not the same as the scalp recorded N1a. Wolpaw and Penry (1975) proposed that the LAEP contained a vertex response consisting of P1-N1-P2 and a temporal or T-complex consisting of a positive wave Ta at around 110 ms and a negative wave Tb around 150 ms. As already discussed in Chapter 4, these findings likely are related to vertically (tangentially) oriented and radially oriented dipole generators located on the superior and lateral surfaces of the temporal lobes (e.g., Scherg et al., 1989).

Näätänen and Picton (1987) suggested that six components could contribute to the scalp-recorded N1 wave. Two of these were generated in the superior and lateral surface of the temporal lobe, causing the vertex N1b and the temporal N1c. A third was generated in the motor or premotor regions of the frontal cortex. These three were considered true N1 components in that they were elicited by an auditory stimulus without regard to its physical or psychological context. Three other components, the MMN and the temporal and frontal components of the processing negativity, could overlap with the N1 but these occurred only in particular contexts. The context could be bottom-up (an organized sequence of stimuli) or top-down (selective attention to the stimuli).

In describing the different experimental studies of the LAEP, we have reviewed several lines of MEG evidence indicating two N1m components generated on the superior surface of the temporal lobes. The magnetic response to a frequency change in an ongoing tone might consist of two separate waves rather than a single N1m. Refractory period studies differentiated an anterior N1m component with a prolonged refractory period from a posterior component with a shorter refractory period. The sensitization at very short SOAs is mainly related to the anterior N1m component and not the posterior component. Other evidence such as the different frequency-specificity curves shown in Figure 11–8 also suggests that two different processes might be active during the N1, one specifically tuned and another broadly tuned.

Jääskeläinen et al. (2004) used a combination of MEG and functional MRI to localize active areas on the superior surface of the temporal lobe. The magnetic measurements provided timing information and the hemodynamic measurements indicated localization. The authors proposed two main sources of N1 activity, an early posterior source (peaking around 85 ms) with very broad tuning and a later anterior source with very specific tuning. The authors suggested that these two responses were likely related to the "what?" and "where?" systems that have been localized to anterior and posterior parts of the auditory cortex (e.g., Rauschecker & Tian, 2000). The longer latency of the anterior component may depend on the longer time required to identify an object than to register its occurrence somewhere in auditory space. Jääskeläinen et al. also suggested that the early N1 component may serve to gate incoming information for further analysis in the object-processing system.

As considered in Chapter 4, the auditory cortex contains many different areas. Each has its own connections to the thalamus and to adjacent regions of the cortex. As activation expands from the primary or core cortex into the belt and parabelt regions, the auditory areas make reciprocal connections to other areas of cortex in temporal, frontal, and parietal regions. Each of the auditory areas on the superior surface of the temporal lobe and on the adjacent regions of the superior temporal gyrus generates a P1-N1-P2-like wave as it is activated. These waveforms provide a very simplified view of the underlying physiology. However, the processing likely involves dendritic activation (largely excitatory and thus causing a surface negativity) and ultimately the discharge of neurons that will conduct information to other regions of cortex (such activity occurring in the cell bodies and axons and causing a surface positivity). How the transfer of information from one region to the next occurs remains unknown. Possibly, rhythmic oscillations between neurons (thalamic and cortical) cause a pulsatile forward transfer of information. For example, as information arrives in cortex it might trigger a thalamocortical circuit that feeds back after a delay. This feedback signal then causes the neurons, which have been integrating the original input patterns in their dendrites, to transfer that analyzed information forward to other regions of cortex.

The sequence for each region of cortex involves three steps: sensory patterns are input, the dendrites integrate the incoming information, and a delayed signal then causes the processed information to be read out for further evaluation. The timing of the steps may depend on the region of cortex (the anatomy of its thala-mocortical and cortico-cortical connections) and on the information it receives (how long before a particular dendritic discrimination is made). Dendritic activation is easily susceptible to top-down control, this being greater the farther away from the primary cortex. Attentional processes mediated in the frontal region can predispose the dendrites of a particular region of the auditory cortex to make particular distinctions. Figure 11–19 provides a simple model of cortical activity as information flows in a pulsatile manner from one region to the next. As well as being pulsatile, the flow of information may activate only certain areas of the auditory cortex, depending on both the physical stimulus and the psychological expectancy. Beyond the core regions, the activation would then be patchwork in its distribution.

The electrical activity generated in the auditory cortex and recorded from the scalp derives from many different P1-N1-P2 generators, each located within a particular region of the auditory cortex. The latency and amplitude of each generator would depend on the anatomy of the region and its connections, the pattern of inputs that it receives, and the top-down goals of the individual. Clearly, the number of generators can equal the number of neurons active. However, because the neurons within one anatomic region should all react similarly to a particular set of physical stimuli and psychological expectancies, basing the number on the number of cortical regions rather than neurons might be reasonable. Each region will have its own time signature in terms of when the activation begins and how long it takes to die away.

We can conceive of two main flows of information in the posterior and anterior regions of the cortex, one related to where something has occurred and the other to

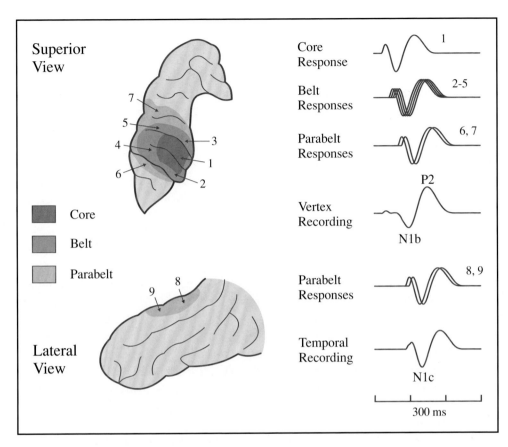

Figure 11–19. *Multicomponent view of the LAEP.* On the left of this figure are shown the superior and lateral surfaces of the left temporal lobe. The location of the main auditory areas on these surfaces are indicated by shading. On the right are shown the hypothetical responses of the different auditory regions to the onset of a sound. The activation begins in the core region of the auditory cortex and then spreads to adjacent regions of the belt and then the parabelt. The activation of the anterior regions occurs later than that of the posterior regions. The responses on the superior surface of the temporal lobe (1, 2, 3, 4, 5, 6, and 7) contribute to the vertex recording, whereas the responses on the superior temporal gyrus (8 and 9) contribute to the temporal recording. These scalp recordings sum the responses of the different contributing regions. This is a highly simplified model of what might be occurring. Each of the regions likely has a particular EP morphology and the response often spreads beyond the parabelt regions farther onto the planum temporale posteriorly, onto the superior temporal gyrus laterally, and toward the temporal pole anteriorly.*

what it is. The posterior flow is faster both in terms of onset and in terms of the duration of activity. As well as being organized into the two main flows, the activation process spreads away from the primary cortex like the ripples from a stone. The farther we move from the core area of the auditory cortex, the later the latency becomes. Thus, the generators on the lateral aspect of the temporal lobe have a later latency (negativity near 140 ms) than the generators on the superior surface (negativity near 100 ms). Zouridakis et al. (1998) have mapped these flows of excitation by tracking equivalent dipole sources through the duration of the N1m. Regions involved in the complex identification of exactly what was heard (musical attributes, speech sounds, etc.) will take a longer time than those regions in simpler analyses such as localization. "What?" is slower than "where?" We integrate information about the frequency and loudness of sounds over one to several hundred milliseconds but we decide on where a sound is coming from within a few tens of milliseconds.

Each and every sound therefore will initiate a specific set of different N1-P2 processes. A change in the frequency of a tone might elicit an early response that detects that the frequency has changed and a later response that determines the spectral and temporal characteristics of the new stimulus. A stimulus with a mistuned harmonic will elicit a response to the onset of the harmonic stimulus and a later response that detects the harmonic that does not fit with the fundamental and therefore considers it as a new object.

What we record from the scalp is the sum of the fields generated in all the auditory regions as they process the sensory information they receive. This summed field will have the general morphology of the P1-N1-P2 potential but will show subtle differences depending on the set of auditory areas contributing to the overall electrical field. It is difficult to disentangle the responses of these different areas of auditory cortex in the scalp recorded electrical fields. Nevertheless, we can recognize the later N1 waves that are generated on the lateral surface of the temporal lobe as the N140 or Tb component. Using MEG source analyses and various experimental manipulations, we can distinguish the early posterior response from the later anterior response, but each of these likely represents responses from several different regions.

In this view, the P1-N1-P2 recorded from the vertex and midfrontal regions is largely determined by a pulsatile patchwork activation of the various regions of auditory cortex on the superior surface of the temporal lobe. Each of these regions may be more or less active depending on the physical characteristics of the sound and the attentional requirements of the individual; each sound in each context activates its own patchwork of auditory cortex.

However, we are left with one nagging problem. As discussed in Chapter 4, lesion studies show that damage to the posterior temporal lobe (that spare the core regions and the anterior belt and parabelt regions of the auditory cortex) can severely attenuate the N1-P2 complex (Knight, Scabini, Woods, & Clayworth, 1988; Woods, Clayworth, Knight, Simpson, & Naeser, 1987). One possibility is that the posterior regions of the auditory cortex gate further processing in the more anterior regions (cf. Jääskeläinen et al., 2004). If the gating mechanism were damaged, the anterior regions might not process information properly.

So far, we have considered only how the auditory cortex contributes the scalp recorded LAEPs. The auditory regions will always project to other regions of the brain. In particular, they will activate different areas of the frontal lobe, such as the premotor, cingulate, and prefrontal cortices. Activation of these areas mainly comes into play when the subject is attending to the stimuli, making cognitive decisions about them and responding to them behaviorally. We deal with these effects more fully in the following chapter. Much of this frontal activity will involve radial sources and will not be clearly picked up in the MEG. Furthermore, the frontal regions of the brain process information with a longer time perspective than the sensory regions; the working memory mediated in the frontal lobes lasts much longer than the echoic memory of the auditory system. Therefore, these frontal activations are the likely reason for the original temporal distinctions that Hari et al. (1982) found between the vertex-recorded LAEPs and the response recorded using MEG.

The Nature of the MMN

The psychophysiologic processes underlying the MMN remain unknown. Two main theories have been proposed to account for the difference between the response to a repeating standard and the response to an occasional deviant. The first involves "memory comparison" (Näätänen, 1992; Näätänen, & Alho, 1995, Näätänen et al., 2007). The invariant features of a repeating stimulus or stimulus-sequence are automatically identified and then maintained in sensory memory for a brief period of time (generally about 10 seconds). The more a stimulus repeats itself, the stronger this memory (or set of memories) becomes. Each incoming stimulus (or sequence of stimuli) is then compared to the memory for the preceding stimuli. A MMN is generated when a discrepancy is noted between present and preceding stimuli, when the system notices that the sensory model maintained in the cortex does not fully account for what has just happened. The MMN process may then signal other regions of the brain to respond to the unpredicted stimuli in some way. One possible response would be to revise the cortical model of the sensory world to take into consideration the deviant occurrence. Because of this, the theory has also been called the "model-adjustment"

theory (Garrido et al., 2009). However, such responses may occur only if those other regions of the brain are disposed to respond. More often than not, we simply notice deviant stimuli and pay them no further attention. To make an adequate model perfect may require more effort than we wish to expend.

The second theory of the MMN is that it is caused by the "selective adaptation" of neurons that respond specifically to different stimuli or to different aspects of these stimuli (May & Tiitinen, 2010). These neurons (or neuronal networks) respond less to stimuli that occur during their refractory period than to stimuli that occur after a longer interval. The partial refractory period lasts for about 10 seconds. When a deviant stimulus occurs, it activates neurons (or neuronal circuits) that were not activated by the preceding stimuli and these give a larger response than if the stimulus were another standard (and all the neurons that it activated were refractory). The deviant response will not be as large if the deviant stimulus simply occurred with no intervening standards as there is always some overlap in the receptive fields between neurons that respond to standards and those that respond to deviants. Nevertheless, some neurons will be nonrefractory, and this will cause a larger response. Because of the concept of nonrefractory neurons, the theory also has gone by the name of "fresh afferents." Clear evidence for selective adaptation is provided through Butler's paradigm in which test stimuli of different frequencies are separated by repeating intervening stimuli. The response to the test stimulus is larger the more different it is from the intervening stimulus (and the fewer shared neurons are activated).

An important addition to this basic idea is that some of the neurons (or networks) that respond to the deviant stimulus will delay their response as the difference between standard and deviant decreases. This effect is related to lateral inhibition between neurons that respond best at different locations on a frequency continuum. For example, a standard of 1000 Hz will delay the response to a deviant of 1050 Hz much more than the response to a deviant tone of 2000 Hz. Thus, refractoriness may be indicated not only by a decrease in amplitude of the response but also by an increase in the latency of the responses to stimuli that have overlapping response fields. May et al. (1999) used neuronal modeling based on physiologic studies of cortical neurons to demonstrate the feasibility of such latency changes. The selective adaptation theory thus proposes that the MMN represents the delayed response of neurons that respond to stimuli similar to but not the same as preceding stimuli. This theory suggests that the N1 and the MMN are similar processes.

The experiments of Jääskeläinen et al. (2004) evaluated the idea of selective adaptation to repeating sounds. One of the arguments for a memory-based MMN process is that it takes more than one standard stimulus to set up a memory trace. Thus, in the roving standard paradigm wherein the trains are separated by a long enough period to attenuate any prior sensory memory (Cowan et al., 1993), no MMN is generated to the first stimulus in the train or to a deviant that occurs in the second position, because the memory cannot yet determine what is invariant about incoming stimuli. Jääskeläinen et al. found a MMN to the second of two tones in a pair when the tones were different, as would be expected by selective adaptation. However, as pointed out by Näätänen, Jacobsen, and Winkler (2005), they should have controlled for differences in the selective

adaptation of standards and deviants in the repeating pairs; selective adaptation occurs but the MMN can still be detected (or not) if it is controlled for.

Different variables have either similar or different effects on the MMN and N1. Some similarities between the MMN and the N1 are striking. For example, both the N1 and the MMN are absent in NREM sleep and present in REM sleep. However, many other variables have distinct effects on the MMN and the N1 wave of the LAEP as recorded from the scalp (e.g., Näätänen et al., 2005, 2007). These might still be accommodated in the selective adaptation theory (May & Tiitiinen, 2010), as briefly considered below.

First, Näätänen et al. (2005) pointed out that the MMN occurs for deviances from abstract patterns involving an upward or downward change in frequency regardless of the frequency of the stimuli. They suggest that such findings could not be explained by selective adaptation because the frequencies were continually changing. However, neurons responding to such abstract features independently of the actual stimulus frequency probably exist in the auditory cortex and these could be selectively adapted. Selective adaptation need not be limited to simple stimulus features.

Second, the MMN occurs in children even when they show no evidence of a vertex N1 wave. This may be related to the duration of the refractory periods as the deviant stimuli are occurring at longer intervals from each other than the standards (May & Tiitinen, 2010). As we have seen, the N1 in children is more prominent when the SOA is longer.

Third, the N1 and the MMN have different scalp topographies and different locations for their source dipoles. The MMN tends to have a source location that is significantly more anterior than the N1 (e.g., Scherg et al., 1989). However, we could still consider the responses similar, the N1 being generated in the posterior regions of the auditory cortices and the MMN in the anterior regions. Rosburg, Hauesin, and Kreitschmann-Andermahr (2004) found that the time-track of the dipoles underlying the MMN was similar to that of the N1 in its posterior to anterior shift but differed significantly in that it did not shift from superior to inferior. This also might be related to flow of information in the more anterior regions of the auditory cortex. These differences do not necessarily indicate completely different processes, if we accept that the scalp distribution of the N1 can itself vary with the SOA and with stimulus features (e.g., musical notes versus pure tones). If we are considering multiple different generators in the auditory cortex, different sets of these generators can contribute to the N1 and to the MMN.

Fourth, old age has different effects on the N1 and the MMN. As discussed, the N1-P2 waves of the LAEP are much less affected by old age than the MMN. This might be due to age-related deterioration in the information reaching cortex; more precise information is required to determine that a stimulus is different from another than just to determine where it has occurred.

Fifth, some pharmacologic manipulations such as the administration of antagonists of the N-methyl-D-aspartic acid (NMDA) receptor can selectively decrease the MMN while not affecting (or even enhancing) the N1 (Javitt, Steinschneider, Schroeder, & Arezzo,1996; Umbricht et al., 2000). Perhaps the more anterior regions of the auditory cortex on the superior surface of the temporal lobes are more susceptible to these neurotransmitter effects.

Despite the extensive arguments for each of the two theories, they are in fact not that dissimilar. The adaptation model stems from physiology and fits more gracefully with the anatomy of the auditory cortex and physiologic mechanisms such as habituation and lateral inhibition. The memory-based model derives from psychology and fits more easily with behavioral data. The pattern of adaptation resulting from prior stimulation is basically the same as a memory. In the study of memory, we usually begin with the habituation of simple reflexes, where the habituating pathway "learns" that a particular stimulus has occurred before. The adaptation theory is simpler than the memory-comparison theory in that it does not require a separate comparison between input and memory; the comparison is carried out as the information is transferred through the variously adapted pathways. It also considers change-1 (from nothing to stimulus) in the same way as change-2 (from one stimulus to another). Both types of change involve the activation of neurons that have not been made refractory by previous stimulation

In the same way that the generation of the N1 activates other regions of the cortex, the generators of the MMN in the auditory cortex project to frontal and parietal regions of the brain (Molholm, Martinez, Ritter, Javitt, & Foxe, 2005). Garrido et al. (2008) have used dynamic causal modeling to demonstrate network interactions between the auditory cortex, superior temporal gyrus, and right inferior frontal gyrus. They have interpreted these findings as evidence that the auditory system is involved in reducing the prediction error between the sensory model based on past experience and the sensory information from the present world (Garrido, Kilner, Stephan, & Friston, 2009).

When reviewing the generation of the N1, we considered two major flows of information in the auditory cortex, the posterior processing related to where and the anterior processing related to what. The MMN can be generated in both systems, although it will occur more commonly in the anterior system. The anterior regions of the auditory cortex are most involved when we decide what a sound might be and how it might relate to those we previously heard.

The Hedgehog and the Fox

An old proverb that goes back at least as far as ancient Greece states that the fox knows many things but the hedgehog knows one big thing. The proverb has many levels of interpretation, one of which one involves two modes of thinking: one that considers the infinite variety of things and the other their inherent unity. We might bear this proverb in mind when we consider the N1 and the MMN. On the one hand, we have differentiated between different negative waves generated in the auditory cortices. The main differentiation has been between the N1 responses to the onset or offset of sounds (change-1) and the MMN response to the deviance of one stimulus from those that precede it (change-2). The N1 wave may be related mainly to the posterior regions of the auditory cortex that rapidly process the occurrence of a new sound source and locate it in space, whereas the MMN may be related to the anterior regions of the cortex that take the necessary time to process the actual identity of the sound source. However, each of these waves can be differentiated further. The MMN responses to a change in the pattern of repeating

sounds or to a change in an abstract feature of the sounds clearly involve different cerebral mechanisms from the simple MMN evoked by a change in the frequency of a sound. Furthermore, we also can record other negative waves, such as the object-related negativity associated with detecting two different objects within one sound or the early right anterior negativity associated with harmonically deviant musical sounds. The hedgehog might consider all these negative waves as representing the same phenomenon — the processing of incoming information in the context of what has happened before. The fox might attribute each of the negative waves to a localized region of the auditory cortex (or a particular network of neurons with the cortex) that processes a particular aspect of our sound environment. Both views are correct.

CONCLUSION

We have wandered around the land of the LAEPs, and spent time with many different potentials. These responses provide us with information about how the auditory cortex processes what is happening in our world. The results we have considered are complex. At present, we have only a beginning understanding of how the cortex processes the sounds we hear. Our knowledge causes us to wonder more. Further research is required.

This chapter looks mainly at how the cortex processes sounds to which we are not attending. The next chapter considers how attention might affect this processing. Incoming information interacts with perceptual expectancy to complete the phenomenon of hearing. Although the material has been divided into two chapters to facilitate reading, the processes are not at all separate. Top-down and bottom-up are simultaneous.

We considered change and how it is registered in the brain. Initially, we considered two types of change: from no stimulus to stimulus or from one stimulus to another. The one was related to the N1 wave of the LAEP and the second to the MMN. However, these processes likely are more similar than they are different. Both relate to neuronal activity in many areas of the auditory cortex, with the actual areas contributing to each determined by the specific stimulus change being processed. Both the N1 and the MMN register changes in the auditory world and initiate the processing that may be required for the brain to adapt to such changes. Prior experience allows changes to be detected and determines how they are handled. As Marcus Aurelius noted in the epigraph, what has occurred before is the seed for everything that will occur after.

ABBREVIATIONS

ASSR	Auditory steady-state response
EEG	Electroencephalography
EP	Evoked potential
LAEP	Late auditory evoked potential
MEG	Magnetoencephalography
MLR	Middle-latency response
MMN	Mismatch negativity
MMR	Mismatch response
MRI	Magnetic resonance imaging

nHL	Normal hearing level
NMDA	N-methyl-D-aspartic acid
SNR	Signal-to-noise ratio
SOA	Stimulus onset asynchrony
TOA	Train onset asynchrony
SP	Sustained potential

REFERENCES

Alain, C. (2007). Breaking the wave: Effects of attention and learning on concurrent sound perception. *Hearing Research, 229*, 225–236.

Alain, C., Achim, A., & Woods, D. L. (1999). Separate memory-related processing for auditory frequency and patterns. *Psychophysiology, 36*, 737–744.

Alain, C., Arnott, S. R. & Picton, T. W. (2001) Bottom-up and top-down influences on auditory scene analysis: Evidence from event-related brain potentials. *Journal of Experimental Psychology. Human Perception and Performance, 27*, 1072–1089.

Alain, C., Cortese, F., & Picton, T. W. (1999). Event-related brain activity associated with auditory pattern processing. *NeuroReport, 10*, 2429–2434.

Alain, C., & Izenberg, A. (2003). Effects of attentional load on auditory scene analysis. *Journal of Cognitive Neuroscience, 15*, 1063–1073.

Alain, C., McDonald, K. L., Ostroff, J. M., & Schneider, B. (2004). Aging: A switch from automatic to controlled processing of sounds. *Psychology and Aging, 19*, 125–133.

Alain, C., Quan, J., McDonald, K., & van Roon, P. (2009). Noise-induced increase in human auditory evoked neuromagnetic fields. *European Journal of Neuroscience, 30*, 132–142.

Alain, C., & Woods, D. L. (1997). Attention modulates auditory pattern memory as indexed by event-related brain potentials. *Psychophysiology, 34*, 534–546.

Alain, C., Woods, D. L., & Covarrubias, D. (1997). Activation of duration-sensitive auditory cortical fields in humans. *Electro-encephalography and Clinical Neurophysiology, 104,* 531–559.

Alho, K., Sainio, K., Sajaniemi, N., Reinikainen, K., & Näätänen, R. (1990). Event-related brain potential of human newborns to pitch change of an acoustic stimulus. *Electroencephalography and Clinical Neurophysiology, 77,* 151–155.

Antinoro, F., Skinner, P. H., & Jones, J. J. (1969). Relation between sound intensity and amplitude of the AER at different stimulus frequencies. *Journal of the Acoustical Society of America, 46,* 1433–1436.

Atienza, M., Cantero, J. L., & Dominguez-Marin, E. (2002). The time course of neural changes underlying auditory perceptual learning. *Learning and Memory, 9,* 138–150.

Atienza, M., Cantero, J. L., & Gómez, C. M. (1997). The mismatch negativity component reveals the sensory memory during REM sleep in humans. *Neuroscience Letters, 237,* 21–22

Atienza, M., Cantero, J. L., & Stickgold, R. (2004). Post-training sleep enhances automaticity in perceptual discrimination. *Journal of Cognitive Neuroscience, 16,* 53–64.

Barnet, A. B. (1975). Auditory evoked potentials during sleep in normal children from ten days to three years of age. *Electroencephalography and Clinical Neurophysiology, 39,* 29–41.

Bastien, C. H., Crowley, K. E., & Colrain, I. M. (2002). Evoked potential components unique to non-REM sleep: relationship to evoked K-complexes and vertex sharp waves. *International Journal of Psychophysiology, 46,* 257–274.

Beagley, H. A., & Kellogg, S. E. (1969). A comparison of evoked response and subjective auditory thresholds. *International Audiology, 8,* 345–353.

Billings, C. J., Tremblay, K. L., Souza, P. E., & Binns, M. A. (2007). Effects of hearing aid amplification and stimulus intensity on cortical auditory evoked potentials. *Audiology and Neurotology, 12,* 234–246.

Billings, C. J., Tremblay, K. L., Stecker, G. C., & Tolin, W. M. (2009). Human evoked cortical activity to signal-to-noise ratio and absolute signal level. *Hearing Research, 254,* 15–24.

Bishop, D. V. (2007). Using mismatch negativity to study central auditory processing in developmental language and literacy impairments: Where are we, and where should we be going? *Psychological Bulletin, 133,* 651–672.

Brattico, E., Tervaniemi, M., & Picton, T. W. (2003). Effects of brief discrimination-training on the auditory N1 wave. *NeuroReport, 14,* 2489–2492.

Bregman, A. S. (1990). *Auditory scene analysis: The perceptual organization of sound.* Cambridge, MA: Bradford Books.

Bruneau, N., Roux, S., Guérin, P., Barthélémy, C., & Lelord, G. (1997). Temporal prominence of auditory evoked potentials (N1 wave) in 4–8 year-old children. *Psychophysiology, 34,* 32–38.

Budd, T. W., Barry, R. J., Gordon, E., Rennie, C., & Michie, P. T. (1998). Decrement of the N1 auditory event-related potential with stimulus repetition: Habituation vs. refractoriness. *International Journal of Psychophysiology, 31,* 51–68.

Budd, T. W., & Michie, P. T. (1994). Facilitation of the N1 peak of the auditory ERP at short stimulus intervals. *NeuroReport, 5,* 2513–2516.

Butler, R.A. (1968). Effect of changes in stimulus frequency and intensity on habituation of the human vertex potential. *Journal of the Acoustical Society of America, 44,* 945–950.

Butler, R. A., Spreng, M., & Keidel, W. D. (1969). Stimulus repetition rate factors which influence the auditory evoked potential in man. *Psychophysiology, 5,* 665–672.

Cacace, A. T., & McFarland, D. J. (2003). Quantifying signal-to-noise ratio of mismatch negativity in humans. *Neuroscience Letters, 341,* 251–255.

Campbell, K. B. (2000). Information processing during sleep. onset and sleep. *Canadian Journal of Experimental Psychology, 54,* 209–218.

Campbell, K. B., & Colrain, I. M. (2002). Event-related potential measures of the inhibition of information. Processing: II. The sleep onset period. *International Journal of Psychophysiology, 46,* 197–214

Clynes, M. (1969). Dynamics of vertex evoked potentials: The R-M brain function. In E. Donchin & D. B. Lindsley (Eds.), *Average evoked potentials: Methods, results and evaluations.* (pp. 363–374). Washington, DC: National Aeronautics and Space Administration.

Colrain, I. M., & Campbell, K. B. (2007). The use of evoked potentials in sleep research. *Sleep Medicine Reviews, 11,* 277–293.

Colrain, I. M., Di Parsia, P., & Gora, J. (2000). The impact of prestimulus EEG frequency on auditory evoked potentials during sleep onset. *Canadian Journal of Experimental Psychology, 54,* 243–254.

Coles, R. R. A., & Mason, S. M. (1984). The results of cortical electrical response audiometry in medico-legal investigations. *British Journal of Audiology, 18,* 71–78.

Cowan, N., Winkler, I., Teder, W., & Näätänen, R. (1993). Memory pre-requisites of mismatch negativity in the auditory even-related potential (ERP). *Journal of Experimental Psychology. Learning, Memory and Cognition, 19,* 909–921

Davis, H., Bowers, C., & Hirsh, S. K. (1968). Relations of the human vertex potential to acoustic input: Loudness and masking. *Journal of the Acoustical Society of America, 43,* 431–438.

Davis, H., Hirsh, S. K., Shelnutt, J., & Bowers, C. (1967). Further validation of evoked response audiometry (ERA). *Journal of Speech and Hearing Research, 10,* 717–732.

Davis, H., Mast, T., Yoshie, N., & Zerlin, S. (1966). The slow response of the human cortex to auditory stimuli: Recovery process. *Electroencephalography and Clinical Neurophysiology, 21,* 105–113.

Dehaene-Lambertz, G., & Gliga, T. (2004). Common neural basis for phoneme processing in infants and adults. *Journal of Cognitive Neuroscience 16,* 1375–1387.

Deouell, L., & Bentin, S. (1998). Variable cerebral responses to equally distinct deviance in four auditory dimensions: A mismatch negativity study. *Psychophysiology, 35,* 745–754.

Derbyshire, A. J., Fraser, A. A., McDermott, M., & Bridge, A. (1956). Audiometric measurements by electroencephalography. *Electroencephalography and Clinical Neurophysiology, 8,* 467–478.

Friederici, A. D., Friedrich, M., & Weber, C. (2002). Neural manifestation of cognitive and precognitive mismatch detection in early infancy. *NeuroReport, 13,* 1251–1254.

Fruhstorfer, H., Soveri, P., Järvilehto, T. (1970). Short-term habituation of the auditory evoked response in man. *Electroencephalography and Clinical Neurophysiology, 28,* 153–161.

Fujioka, T., Ross, B., Okamoto, H., Takeshima, Y., Kakigi, R., & Pantev, C. (2003). Tonotopic representation of missing fundamental complex sounds in the human auditory cortex. *European Journal of Neuroscience, 18,* 432–440.

Fujioka, T., Trainor, L. J., Ross, B., Kakigi, R., & Pantev, C. (2005). Automatic encoding of polyphonic melodies in musicians and non-musicians. *Journal of Cognitive Neuroscience, 17,* 1578–1592.

Gabriel, D., Veuillet, E., Ragot, R., Schwartz, D., Ducorps, A., Norena, A., . . . Collet, L. (2004). Effect of stimulus frequency and stimulation site on the N1m response of the human auditory cortex. *Hearing Research, 197,* 55–64.

Gaeta, H., Friedman, D., Ritter, W., & Cheng, J. (1998). An event-related potential study of age-related changes in sensitivity to stimulus deviance. *Neurobiology of Aging, 19,* 447–459.

Garrido, M. I., Friston, K. J., Kiebel, S. J., Stephan, K. E., Baldeweg, T., & Kilner, J. M. (2008). The functional anatomy of the MMN: A DCM study of the roving paradigm. *NeuroImage, 42,* 936–944.

Garrido, M. I., Kilner, J. M., Stephan, K. E., & Friston, K. J. (2009). The mismatch negativity: A review of underlying mechanisms. *Clinical Neurophysiology, 120,* 453–463.

Giard, M. H., Lavikainen, J., Reinikainen, K., Bertrand, O., Pernier, J., & Näätänen, R. (1995). Separate representation of stimulus frequency, intensity, and duration in auditory sensory memory: An event-related potential and dipole-model study. *Journal of Cognitive Neuroscience, 7,* 133–143.

Giard, M. H., Perrin, F., Pernier, J., & Bouchet, P. (1990). Brain generators implicated in the processing of auditory stimulus deviance: A topographic event-related potential study. *Psychophysiology, 27,* 627–40.

Gilley, P. M., Sharma, A., Dorman, M., & Martin, K. (2005). Developmental changes in refractoriness of the cortical auditory evoked potential. *Clinical Neurophysiology, 116,* 648–657.

Godey, B., Schwartz, D., de Graaf, J. B., Chauvel, P., & Liégeois-Chauvel, C. (2001). Neuromagnetic source localization of auditory evoked fields and intracerebral evoked potentials: A comparison of data in the same patients. *Clinical Neurophysiology, 112,* 1850–1859.

Golding, M., Pearce, W., Seymore, J., Cooper, A., Ching, T., & Dillon, H. (2007). The relationship between obligatory cortical auditory evoked potentials (CAEPs) and functional measures in young infants. *Journal of the American Academy of Audiology, 18,* 117–125.

Goodin, D. S., Squires, K. C., Henderson, B. H., & Starr, A. (1978). Age-related variations in evoked potentials to auditory stimuli in normal human subjects. *Electroencephalography and Clinical Neurophysiology, 44,* 447–458.

Gutschalk, A., Micheyl, C., Melcher, J. R., Rupp, A., Scherg, M., & Oxenham, A. J. (2005). Neuromagnetic correlates of streaming in human auditory cortex. *Journal of Neuroscience, 25,* 5382–5388.

Hari, R., Kaila, K., Katila, T., Tuomisto, T., & Varpula, T. (1982). Interstimulus interval dependence of the auditory vertex response and its magnetic counterpart: Implications for their neural generation. *Electroencephalography and Clinical Neurophysiology, 54,* 561–569.

Hari, R., Pelizzone, M., Mäkelä, J. P., Hällström, J., Leinonen, L., & Lounasmaa, O. V. (1987). Neuromagnetic responses of the human auditory cortex to on- and offsets of noise bursts. *Audiology, 26,* 31–43.

Hillyard, S. A., & Picton, T. W. (1978). ON and OFF components in the auditory evoked potential. *Perception and Psychophysics, 24,* 391–398.

Hillyard, S. A., Picton, T. W., & Regan, D. B. (1978). Sensation, perception, attention: Analysis using ERPs. In E. Callaway, P.

Tueting, & S. H. Koslow (Eds.), *Event-related brain potentials in man* (pp. 223–321). New York, NY: Academic Press.

Hone, S. W., Norman, G., Keogh, I. & Kelly, V. (2003). The use of cortical evoked response audiometry in the assessment of noise-induced hearing loss. *Otolaryngology-Head and Neck Surgery, 128,* 257–262.

Horváth, J., Czigler, I., Jacobsen, T., Maess, B., Schröger, E., & Winkler, I. (2008). MMN or no MMN: No magnitude of deviance effect on the MMN amplitude. *Psychophysiology, 45,* 60–69.

Huotilainen, M., Kujala, A., & Alku, P. (2001). Long-term memory traces facilitate short-term memory trace formation in audition. *Neuroscience Letters, 310,* 133–136.

Hyde, M. (1993). The slow vertex potential: properties and clinical applications. In J. T. Jacobson (Ed.), *Principles and applications of auditory evoked potentials* (pp. 179–218). New York, NY: Allyn & Bacon.

Hyde, M., Alberti, P., Matsumoto, N., & Li, Y. L. (1986). Auditory evoked potentials in audiometric assessment of compensation and medicolegal patients. *Annals of Otology, Rhinology and Laryngology. 95,* 514–519.

Iragui, V. J., Kutas, M., Mitchiner, M. R., & Hillyard, S. A. (1993). Effects of aging on event-related brain potentials and reaction times in an auditory oddball task. *Psychophysiology, 30,* 10–22.

Jääskeläinen, I. P., Ahveninen, J., Bonmassar, G., Dale, A. M., Ilmoniemi, R. J., Levänen, S., . . . Belliveau, J. W. (2004). Human posterior auditory cortex gates novel sounds to consciousness. *Proceedings of the National Academy of Sciences, USA, 101,* 6809–6814.

Jacobsen, T., Schröger, E., Horenkamp, T., & Winkler, I. (2003). Mismatch negativity to pitch change: Varied stimulus proportions in controlling effects of neural refractoriness on human auditory event-related brain potentials. *Neuroscience Letters, 344,* 79–82.

Jacobson, G. P., Lombardi, D. M., Gibbens, N. D., Ahmad, B. K., & Newman, C. W. (1992). The effects of stimulus frequency and recording site on the amplitude and latency of multichannel cortical auditory evoked potential (CAEP) component N1. *Ear and Hearing, 13,* 300–306.

Javitt, D. C., Steinschneider, M., Schroeder, C. E. & Arezzo, J. C. (1996). Role of cortical N-methyl-D-aspartate receptors in auditory sensory memory and mismatch negativity generation: Implications for schizophrenia. *Proceedings of the National Academy of Sciences, USA, 93,* 11962–11967.

Jones, S. J., & Perez, N. (2001). The auditory "C-process": Analysing the spectral envelope of complex sounds. *Clinical Neurophysiology, 112,* 965–975.

Knight, R. T., Scabini, D., Woods, D. L., & Clayworth, C. (1988). The effects of lesions of superior temporal gyrus and inferior parietal lobe on temporal and vertex components of the human AEP. *Electroencephalography and Clinical Neurophysiology, 70,* 499–509.

Koelsch, S., Gunter, T. C., Schröger, E., Tervaniemi, M., Sammler, D., & Friederici, A. D. (2001). Differentiating ERAN and MMN: An ERP study. *NeuroReport, 12,* 1385–1389.

Koelsch, S., Schmidt, B. H., & Kansok, J. (2002). Effects of musical expertise on the early right anterior negativity: An event-related brain potential study. *Psychophysiology. 39,* 657–663.

Kohn, M., Lifshitz, K., & Litchfield, D. (1978). Averaged evoked potentials and frequency modulation. *Electroencephalography and Clinical Neurophysiology, 45,* 236–243.

Kohn, M., Lifshitz, K., & Litchfield, D. (1980). Averaged evoked potentials and amplitude modulation. *Electroencephalography and Clinical Neurophysiology, 50,* 134–140.

Kraus, N., McGee, T. J., Carrell, T. D., Zecker, S. G., Nicol, T. G., & Koch, D. B. (1996). Auditory neurophysiologic responses and discrimination deficits in children with learning problems. *Science, 273,* 971–973.

Kuriki, S., Kanda, S., & Hirata, Y. (2006). Effects of musical experience on different components of MEG responses elicited by sequential piano-tones and chords. *Journal of Neuroscience, 26,* 4046–4053.

Kushnerenko, E., Ceponiené, R., Balan, P., Fellman, V., Huotilainen, M., & Näätänen R. (2002). Maturation of the auditory event-related potentials during the first year of life. *NeuroReport, 13,* 47–51.

Lavikainen, J., Huotilainen, M., Ilmoniemi, R. J., Simola, J. T, & Näätänen, R. (1995). Pitch change of a continuous tone activates two distinct processes in human auditory cortex: A study with whole-head magnetometer. *Electroencephalography and Clinical Neurophysiology, 96,* 93–96.

Lightfoot, G., & Kennedy, V. (2006). Cortical electric response audiometry hearing threshold estimation: Accuracy, speed, and the effects of stimulus presentation features. *Ear and Hearing, 27,* 443–456.

Loveless, N., Hari, R., Hamalainen, M., & Tiihonen, J (1989). Evoked responses of human auditory cortex may be enhanced by preceding stimuli. *Electroencephalography and Clinical Neurophysiology, 74,* 217–227.

Loveless, N., Levanen, S., Jousmaki, V., Sams, M., & Hari, R. (1996). Temporal integration in the auditory sensory memory: Neuromagnetic evidence. *Electroencephalography and Clinical Neurophysiology, 100,* 220–228.

Lovio, R., Pakarinen, S., Huotilainen, M., Alku, P., Silvennoinen, S., Näätänen, R., & Kujala, T. (2009). Auditory discrimination profiles of speech sound changes in 6–year-old children as determined with the multi-feature MMN paradigm. *Clinical Neurophysiology, 120,* 916–921.

Lü, Z. L., Williamson, S. J., & Kaufman, L. (1992). Human auditory primary and association cortex have differing lifetimes for activation traces. *Brain Research, 572,* 236–241.

Lütkenhöner, B., Seither-Preisler, A., & Seither, S. (2006). Piano tones evoke stronger magnetic fields than pure tones or noise, both in musicians and non-musicians. *NeuroImage, 30,* 927–937.

Martin, B. A., & Boothroyd, A. (2000). Cortical auditory evoked potentials in response to changes of spectrum and amplitude. *Journal of the Acoustical Society of America, 107,* 2155–2161.

May, P. J., & Tiitinen, H. (2009). Mismatch negativity (MMN), the deviance-elicited auditory deflection, explained. *Psychophysiology, 47,* 66–122.

May, P., Tiitinen, H., Ilmoniemi, R. J., Nyman, G., Taylor, J. G., & Näätänen, R. (1999). Frequency change detection in human auditory cortex. *Journal of Computational Neuroscience, 6,* 99–120.

McCallum, W. C., & Curry, S. H. (1979). Hemispheric differences in event related potentials and CNVs associated with monaural stimuli and lateralized motor responses. In D. Lehmann & E. Callaway (Eds.), *Human evoked potentials: Applications and problems* (pp. 235–250). New York, NY: Plenum.

McEvoy, L., Levanen, S., & Loveless, N. (1997) Temporal characteristics of auditory sensory memory: Neuromagnetic evidence. *Psychophysiology, 34,* 308–316

McEvoy, L. K., Picton, T. W., Champagne, S. C., Kellett, A. J. C., & Kelly, J. B. (1990). Human evoked potentials to shifts in the lateralization of a noise. *Audiology, 29,* 163–180.

Mendel, M. I., Hosick, E. C., Windman, T. R., Davis, H., Hirsh, S. K., & Dinges, D. F. (1975). Audiometric comparison of the middle and late components of the adult auditory evoked potentials awake and asleep. *Electroencephalography and Clinical Neurophysiology, 38,* 27–33.

Micheyl, C., Carlyon, R. P., Gutschalk, A., Melcher, J. R., Oxenham, A. J., Rauschecker, J. P., . . . Courtenay-Wilson, E. (2007). The role of auditory cortex in the formation of auditory streams. *Hearing Research, 229,* 116–131.

Milner, B. A. (1969). Evaluation of auditory function by computer techniques. *International Audiology, 8,* 361–370.

Molholm, S., Martinez, A., Ritter, W., Javitt, D. C., & Foxe, J. J. (2005). The neural circuitry of pre-attentive auditory change-detection: An fMRI study of pitch and duration mismatch negativity generators. *Cerebral Cortex, 15,* 545–551.

Moore, J. K., & Guan, Y. L. (2001). Cytoarchitectural and axonal maturation in human auditory cortex. *Journal of the Association for Research in Otolaryngology, 2,* 297–311.

Moss, F., Ward, L. M., & Sannita, W. G. (2004). Stochastic resonance and sensory information processing: A tutorial and review of application. *Clinical Neurophysiology, 115,* 267–281.

Müller, D.,& Schröger, E. (2007). Temporal grouping affects the automatic processing of deviant sounds. *Biological Psychology, 74,* 358–364.

Muller-Gass, A., Marcoux, A., Jamshidi, P., & Campbell, K. (2008). The effects of very slow rates of stimulus presentation on event-related potential estimates of hearing threshold. *International Journal of Audiology, 47,* 34–43.

Näätänen, R. (1992). *Attention and brain function.* Hillsdale, NJ: Erlbaum.

Näätänen, R., & Alho, K. (1995). Mismatch negativity—a unique measure of sensory processing in audition. *International Journal of Neuroscience, 80,* 317–337.

Näätänen, R., Jacobsen, T., & Winkler, I. (2005). Memory-based or afferent process in mismatch negativity (MMN): A review of the evidence. *Psychophysiology, 42,* 25–32.

Näätänen, R., Lehtokoski, A., Lennes, M., Cheour, M., Huotilainen, M., Iivonen, A., . . . Alho, K. (1997). Language-specific phoneme representations revealed by electric and magnetic brain responses. *Nature, 385,* 432–434.

Näätänen, R., Paavilainen, P., Alho, K., Reinikainen, K., & Sams, M. (1987a). Interstimulus interval and the mismatch negativity. In C. Barber & T. Blum (Eds.), *Evoked potentials III* (pp. 392–397). Boston, MA: Butterworth.

Näätänen, R., Paavilainen, P., Alho, K., Reinikainen, K., & Sams, M. (1987b). The mismatch negativity to intensity changes in an auditory stimulus sequence. *Electroencephalography and Clinical Neurophysiology, (Suppl. 40),* 125–131.

Näätänen, R., Paavilainen, P., & Reinikainen, K. (1989). Do event-related potentials to infrequent decrements in duration of auditory stimuli demonstrate a memory trace in man? *Neuroscience Letters, 107,* 347–352.

Näätänen, R., Paavilainen, P., Rinne, T., & Alho, K. (2007). The mismatch negativity (MMN) in basic research of central auditory processing: A review. *Clinical Neurophysiology, 118,* 2544–2590.

Näätänen, R., Pakarinen, S., Rinne, T., & Takegata R. (2004). The mismatch negativity (MMN): Towards the optimal paradigm. *Clinical Neurophysiology, 115*, 140–144.

Näätänen, R., & Picton, T. W. (1987). The N1 wave of the human electric and magnetic response to sound: A review and an analysis of the component structure. *Psychophysiology, 24*, 375–425.

Näätänen, R., Sams, M., Alho, K., Paavilainen, P., Reinikainen, K., & Sokolov, E. N. (1988). Frequency and location specificity of the human vertex N1 wave. *Electroencephalography and Clinical Neurophysiology, 69*, 523–531.

Näätänen, R. Schröger, E., Karakas, S., Tervaniemi, M., & Paavilainen, P. (1993). Development of a memory trace for a complex sound in the human brain. *NeuroReport, 4*, 503–506.

Näätänen, R., Tervaniemi, M., Sussman, E., Paavilainen, P., & Winkler, I. (2001). "Primitive intelligence" in the auditory cortex. *Trends in Neurosciences, 24*, 283–288.

Näätänen, R., & Winkler, I. (1999). The concept of auditory stimulus representation in cognitive neuroscience. *Psychological Bulletin, 125*, 826–859.

Nelson, D. A., & Lassman, F. M. (1968). Effects of intersignal interval on the human auditory evoked response. *Journal of the Acoustical Society of America, 44*, 1529–1532.

Nordby, H., Roth, W.T., & Pfefferbaum, A. (1988). Event-related potentials to breaks in sequences of alternating pitches or interstimulus intervals. *Psychophysiology, 25*, 262–268.

Onishi, S., & Davis, H. (1968). Effects of duration and rise time of tone bursts on evoked V potentials. *Journal of the Acoustical Society of America, 44*, 582–591.

Osterhammel, P. A., Davis, H., Wier, C. C., & Hirsh, S. K. (1973). Adult auditory evoked vertex potentials in sleep. *Audiology, 12*, 116–128.

Otten, L. J., Alain, C., & Picton, T. W. (2000). Effects of visual attentional load on auditory processing. *NeuroReport, 11*, 875–880.

Ozaki, I., Suzuki, Y., Jin, C. Y., Baba, M., Matsunaga, M., & Hashimoto, I. (2003). Dynamic movement of N100m dipoles in evoked magnetic field reflects sequential activation of isofrequency bands in human auditory cortex. *Clinical Neurophysiology, 114*, 1681–1688.

Paavilainen, P., Cammann, R., Alho, K., Reinikainen, K., Sams, M., & Näätänen, R. (1987). Event-related potentials to pitch change in an auditory stimulus sequence during sleep. In: R. Johnson, J. W. Rohrbaugh, & R. Parasuraman (Eds.), *Current trends in event-related brain potential research. Electroencephalography and Clinical Neurophysiology. Supplement 40*, 246–255. Amsterdam, The Netherlands: Elsevier.

Pakarinen, S., Huotilainen, M., & Näätänen, R. (2010). The mismatch negativity (MMN) with no standard stimulus. *Clinical Neurophysiology, 121*, 1043–1050..

Pakarinen, S., Lovio, R., Huotilainen, M., Alku, P., Näätänen, R., & Kujala, T. (2009). Fast multi-feature paradigm for recording several mismatch negativities (MMNs) to phonetic and acoustic changes in speech sounds. *Biological Psychology, 82*, 219–226.

Pakarinen, S., Takegata, R., Rinne, T., Huotilainen, M., & Näätänen, R. (2007). Measurement of extensive auditory discrimination profiles using the mismatch negativity (MMN) of the auditory event-related potential (ERP). *Clinical Neurophysiology, 118*, 177–185.

Pang, E. W., & Taylor, M. J. (2000). Tracking the development of the N1 from age 3 to adulthood: An examination of speech and non-speech stimuli. *Clinical Neurophysiology, 111*, 388–397.

Pantev, C., Bertrand, O., Eulitz, C., Verkindt, C., Hampson, S., Schuierer, G., & Elbert, T. (1995). Specific tonotopic organizations of different areas of the human auditory cortex revealed by simultaneous magnetic and electric recordings. *Electroencephalography and Clinical Neurophysiology, 94*, 26–40.

Pantev, C., Eulitz, C., Hampson, S., Ross, B., & Roberts, L. E. (1996). The auditory evoked "off" response: Sources and comparison with the "on" and the "sustained" responses. *Ear and Hearing, 17*, 255–265.

Pantev, C., Hoke, M., Lehnertz, K., Lütkenhöner, B., Anogianakis, G., & Wittkowski, W. (1988). Tonotopic organization of the human auditory cortex revealed by transient auditory evoked magnetic fields. *Electroencephalography and Clinical Neurophysiology, 69,* 160–170.

Pantev, C., Hoke, M., Lütkenhöner, B., & Lehnertz, K. (1989). Tonotopic organization of the auditory cortex: Pitch versus frequency representation. *Science, 246,* 486–488.

Pekkonen, E., Jousmäki, V., Partanen, J., & Karhu, J. (1993). Mismatch negativity area and age-related auditory memory. *Electroencephalography and Clinical Neurophysiology, 87,* 321–325.

Picton, T. W., Alain, C., Otten, L., Ritter, W., & Achim, A. (2000). Mismatch negativity: Different water in the same river. *Audiology and Neuro-Otology, 5,* 111–139.

Picton, T. W., Goodman, W. S., & Bryce, D. P. (1970). Amplitude of evoked responses to tones of high intensity. *Acta Otolaryngologica, 70,* 77–82.

Picton, T. W., Hillyard, S. A., & Galambos, R. (1976). Habituation and attention in the auditory system. In W. D. Keidel & W. D. Neff (Eds.), *Handbook of sensory physiology. Vol. V/3. Auditory system. Clinical and special topics* (pp. 343–389). Berlin, Germany: Springer-Verlag.

Picton, T. W., Stuss, D. T., Champagne, S. C., & Nelson, R. F. (1984). The effects of age on human event-related potentials. *Psychophysiology, 21,* 312–325.

Picton, T. W., & Taylor, M. J. (2007). Electrophysiological evaluation of human brain development. *Developmental Neuropsychology, 31,* 251–280.

Picton, T. W., Woods, D. L., Baribeau-Braun, J., & Healey, T. M. G. (1977). Evoked potential audiometry. *Journal of Otolaryngology, 6,* 90–119.

Picton, T. W., Woods, D. L., & Proulx, G. B. (1978a). Human auditory sustained potentials. I. The nature of the response. *Electroencephalography and Clinical Neurophysiology, 45,* 186–197.

Picton, T. W., Woods, D. L., & Proulx, G. B. (1978b). Human auditory sustained potentials. II. Stimulus relationships. *Electroen-*

cephalography and Clinical Neurophysiology, 45,* 198–210.

Pincze, Z., Lakatos, P., Rajkai, C., Ulbert, I., & Karmos, G. (2002). Effect of deviant probability and interstimulus/interdeviant interval on the auditory N1 and mismatch negativity in the cat auditory cortex. *Cognitive Brain Research, 13,* 249–253.

Polich J. (1997). EEG and ERP assessment of normal aging. *Electroencephalography and Clinical Neurophysiology, 104,* 244–256.

Ponton, C. W., Eggermont, J. J., Khosla, D., Kwong, B., & Don, M. (2002). Maturation of human central auditory system activity: Separating auditory evoked potentials by dipole source modeling. *Clinical Neurophysiology, 113,* 407–420.

Ponton, C. W., Eggermont, J. J., Kwong, B., & Don, M. (2000). Maturation of human central auditory system activity: Evidence from multi-channel evoked potentials. *Clinical Neurophysiology, 111,* 220–236.

Poulsen, C., Picton, T. W., & Paus, T. (2009). Age-related changes in transient and oscillatory brain responses to auditory stimulation during early adolescence. *Developmental Science, 12,* 220–235.

Prasher, D. K. (1980). The influence of stimulus spectral content on rise time effects in cortical-evoked responses. *Audiology, 19,* 355–362.

Prasher, D., Mula, M., & Luxon, L. (1993). Cortical evoked potential criteria in the objective assessment of auditory threshold: A comparison of noise induced hearing loss with Ménière's disease. *Journal of Laryngology and Otology, 107,* 780–786.

Prescott, J., Connolly, J. F., & Gruzelier, J. H. (1984). The augmenting/reducing phenomenon in the auditory evoked potential. *Biological Psychology, 19,* 31–44.

Rauschecker, J. P., & Tian, B. (2000). Mechanisms and streams for processing of "what" and "where" in auditory cortex. *Proceedings of the National Academy of Sciences, USA, 97,* 11800–11806.

Reinke, K. S. He, Y., Wang, C., & Alain, C. (2003). Perceptual learning modulates sensory evoked response during vowel segregation. *Cognitive Brain Research, 17,* 781–791.

Reneau, J. P., & Hnatiow, G. Z. (1975). *Evoked response audiometry: A topical and historical review.* Baltimore, MD: University Park Press.

Ritter, W., Sussman, E., Molholm, S., & Foxe, J. J. (2002). Memory reactivation or reinstatement and the mismatch negativity. *Psychophysiology, 39,* 158–165.

Ritter, W., Vaughan, H. G., Jr, & Costa, L. D. (1968). Orienting and habituation to auditory stimuli: A study of short term changes in average evoked responses. *Electroencephalography and Clinical Neurophysiology, 25,* 550–556.

Roberts, T. P., & Poeppel, D. (1996). Latency of auditory evoked M100 as a function of tone frequency. *NeuroReport, 7,* 1138–1140.

Rosburg, T., Haueisen, J., & Kreitschmann-Andermahr, I. (2004). The dipole location shift within the auditory evoked neuromagnetic field components N100m and mismatch negativity (MMNm). *Clinical Neurophysiology, 115,* 906–913.

Ross, B., Fujioka, T., Tremblay, K.L., & Picton, T. W. (2007). Aging in binaural hearing begins in mid-life: Evidence from cortical auditory evoked responses to changes in interaural phase. *Journal of Neuroscience, 27,* 11172–11178.

Ross, B., Lütkenhöner, B., Pantev, C., & Hoke, M. (1999). Frequency-specific threshold determination with the CERAgram method: Basic principle and retrospective evaluation of data. *Audiology and Neuro-Otology, 4,* 12–27.

Saarinen, J., Paavilainen, P., Schöger, E., Tervaniemi, M., & Näätänen, R. (1992). Representation of abstract attributes of auditory stimuli in the human brain. *NeuroReport, 3,* 1149–1151.

Sable, J. J., Low, K. A., Maclin, E. L., Fabiani, M., & Gratton, G. (2004). Latent inhibition mediates N1 attenuation to repeating sounds. *Psychophysiology, 41,* 636–642.

Sabri, M., & Campbell, K. B. (2001). Effects of sequential and temporal probability of deviant occurrence on mismatch negativity. *Cognitive Brain Research, 12,* 171–180.

Sabri, M., & Campbell, K.B. (2005). Is the failure to detect stimulus deviance during sleep due to a rapid fading of sensory memory or a degradation of stimulus encoding? *Journal of Sleep Research, 14,* 113–122.

Sams, M., Alho, K., & Näätänen, R. (1984). Short-term habituation and dishabituaton of the mismatch negativity of the ERP. *Psychophysiology, 21,* 434–441.

Sams, M., Hari, R., Rif, J., & Knuuttila, J. (1993). The human auditory sensory memory trace persists about 10 s: Neuromagnetic evidence. *Journal of Cognitive Neuroscience, 5,* 363–370.

Sams, M., Kaukoranta, E., Hämäläinen, M., & Näätänen, R. (1991). Cortical activity elicited by changes in auditory stimuli: Different sources for the magnetic N100m and mismatch responses. *Psychophysiology, 28,* 21–29.

Sams, M., Paavilainen, P., Alho, K., & Näätänen, R. (1985). Auditory frequency discrimination and event-related potentials. *Electroencephalography and Clinical Neurophysiology, 62,* 437–448.

Scherg, M., Vajsar, J., & Picton, T. W. (1989). A source analysis of the late human auditory evoked potentials. *Journal of Cognitive Neuroscience, 1,* 336–355.

Sculthorpe, L. D., Ouellet, D. R., & Campbell, K. B. (2009). MMN elicitation during natural sleep to violations of an auditory pattern. *Brain Research, 1290,* 52–62.

Shahin, A., Bosnyak, D. J., Trainor, L. J., & Roberts, L. E. (2003). Enhancement of neuroplastic P2 and N1c auditory evoked potentials in musicians. *Journal of Neuroscience, 23,* 5545–5552.

Shahin, A. J., Roberts, L. E., Miller, L. M., McDonald, K. L., & Alain, C. (2007). Sensitivity of EEG and MEG to the N1 and P2 auditory evoked responses modulated by spectral complexity of sounds. *Brain Topography, 20,* 55–61.

Shahin, A. J., Roberts, L. E., Pantev, C., Aziz, M., & Picton, T. W. (2007). Enhanced anterior-temporal processing for complex tones in musicians. *Clinical Neurophysiology, 118,* 209–220.

Shahin, A., Roberts, L. E., Pantev, C., Trainor, L. J., & Ross, B. (2005). Modulation of P2 auditory-evoked responses by the spectral complexity of musical sounds. *NeuroReport, 16,* 1781–1785.

Sheehan, K. A., McArthur, G. M., & Bishop, D. V. (2005). Is discrimination training necessary to cause changes in the P2 auditory event-related brain potential to speech sounds? *Cognitive Brain Research, 25,* 547–553.

Shtyrov, Y., Kujala, T., Lyytinen, H., Kujala, J., Ilmoniemi, R. J., & Näätänen, R. (2000). Lateralization of speech processing in the brain as indicated by the mismatch negativity and dichotic listening. *Brain and Cognition, 43,* 392–398.

Skinner, P. H., & Jones, H. C. (1968). Effects of signal duration and rise time on the auditory evoked potential. *Journal of Speech and Hearing Research, 11,* 301–306.

Snyder, J. S., & Alain, C. (2007). Toward a neurophysiological theory of auditory stream segregation. *Psychological Bulletin, 133,* 780–799.

Snyder, J. S., Alain, C., & Picton, T.W. (2006). Effects of attention on neuroelectric correlates of auditory stream segregation. *Journal of Cognitive Neuroscience, 18,* 1–13.

Stapells, D. R. (2009). Cortical event-related potentials to auditory stimuli. In J. Katz, L. Medwetsky, R. Burkard & L. Hood (Eds.), *Handbook of clinical audiology* (6th ed., pp. 395–430). Baltimore, MD: Lippincott Williams & Wilkins.

Sussman, E. S. (2005). Integration and segregation in auditory scene analysis. *Journal of the Acoustical Society of America, 117,* 1285–1298.

Sussman, E., Ritter, W., & Vaughan, H. G. (1998). Predictability of stimulus deviance and the mismatch negativity. *NeuroReport, 9,* 4167–4170.

Takegata, R., Paavilainen, P., Näätänen, R., & Winkler, I. (1999). Independent processing of changes in auditory single features and feature conjunctions in humans as indexed by the mismatch negativity (MMN). *Neuroscience Letters, 266,* 109–112.

Tervaniemi, M., Maury, S., & Näätänen, R. (1994). Neural representations of abstract stimulus features in the human brain as reflected by the mismatch negativity. *NeuroReport, 5,* 844–846.

Tervaniemi, M., Rytkönen, M., Schröger, E., Ilmoniemi, R. J., & Näätänen, R. (2001). Superior formation of cortical memory traces for melodic patterns in musicians. *Learning and Memory, 8,* 295–300.

Tiitinen, H., Alho, K., Huotilainen, M., Ilmoniemi, R. J., Simola, J., & Näätänen, R. (1993). Tonotopic auditory cortex and the magnetoencephalographic (MEG) equivalent of the mismatch negativity. *Psychophysiology. 30,* 537–540.

Tiitinen, H., May, P., Reinikainen, K:, & Näätänen, R. (1994). Attentive novelty detection in humans is governed by pre-attentive sensory memory. *Nature, 372,* 90–92.

Tomlin, D., Rance, G., Graydon, K., & Tsialios, I. (2006). A comparison of 40 Hz auditory steady-state response (ASSR) and cortical auditory evoked potential (CAEP) thresholds in awake adult subjects. *International Journal of Audiology, 45,* 580–588.

Tonnquist-Uhlen, I., Borg, E., & Spens, K. E. (1995). Topography of auditory evoked long-latency potentials in normal children, with particular reference to the N1 component. *Electroencephalography and Clinical Neurophysiology, 95,* 34–41.

Tonnquist-Uhlen, I., Ponton, C. W., Eggermont, J. J., Kwong, B., & Don, M. (2003). Maturation of human central auditory system activity: The T-complex. *Clinical Neurophysiology, 114,* 685–701.

Tremblay, K., Kraus, N., Carrell, T. D., & McGee, T. (1997). Central auditory system plasticity: Generalization to novel stimuli following listening training. *Journal of the Acoustical Society of America, 102,* 3762–3773.

Tremblay, K., Kraus, N., McGee, T., Ponton, C., & Otis, B. (2001). Central auditory plasticity: Changes in the N1-P2 complex after speech-sound training. *Ear and Hearing, 22,* 79–90.

Tremblay, K. L., Shahin, A. J., Picton, T., & Ross, B. (2009). Auditory training alters the physiological detection of stimulus-specific cues in humans. *Clinical Neurophysiology, 120,* 128–135.

Umbricht, D., Schmid, L., Koller, R., Vollenweider, F. X., Hell, D., & Javitt, D. C. (2000). Ketamine-induced deficits in auditory and visual context-dependent processing in healthy volunteers. *Archives of General Psychiatry, 57,* 1139–1147.

van Maanen, A., & Stapells, D. R. (2005). Comparison of multiple auditory steady-state responses (80 versus 40 Hz) and slow cortical potentials for threshold estimation in hearing-impaired adults. *International Journal of Audiology, 44,* 613–624.

Verkindt, C., Bertrand, O., Perrin, F., Echallier, J. F., & Pernier, J. (1995). Tonotopic organization of the human auditory cortex: N100 topography and multiple dipole model analysis. *Electroencephalography and Clinical Neurophysiology, 96,* 143–156.

Viemeister, N. F., & Wakefield, G. H. (1991). Temporal integration and multiple looks. *Journal of the Acoustical Society of America, 90,* 858–865.

Wang, A. L., Mouraux, A., Liang, M., & Iannetti, G. D. (2008). The enhancement of the N1 wave elicited by sensory stimuli presented at very short inter-stimulus intervals is a general feature across sensory systems. *PLoS One, 3*(12), e3929.

Wennberg, R. (2010). Intracranial cortical localization of the human K-complex. *Clinical Neurophysiology, 121,* 1176–1186.

Williams, H. L., Tepas, D. I., & Morlock, H. C., Jr. (1962). Evoked responses to clicks and electroencephalographic stages of sleep in man. *Science, 138,* 685–686.

Winkler, I., Kushnerenko, E., Horváth, J., Ceponiené, R., Fellman, V., Huotilainen, M., . . . Sussman, E. (2003). Newborn infants can organize the auditory world. *Proceedings of the National Academy of Sciences, USA, 100,* 11812–11815.

Winkler, I., Paavilainen, P., Alho, K., Reinikainen, K., Sams, M., & Näätänen, R. (1990). The effect of small variation of the frequent auditory stimulus on the event-related brain potential to the infrequent stimulus. *Psychophysiology, 27,* 228–235.

Wolpaw, J. R., & Penry, J. K., 1975. A temporal component of the auditory evoked response. *Electroencephalography and Clinical Neurophysiology, 39*(6), 609–620.

Woods, D. L. (1992). Auditory selective attention in middle-aged and elderly subjects: An event-related brain potential study. *Electroencephalography and Clinical Neurophysiology: Evoked Potentials, 84,* 456–468.

Woods, D. L., Alain, C., Covarrubias, D., & Zaidel, O. (1993) Frequency-related differences in the speed of human auditory processing. *Hearing Research, 66,* 46–52.

Woods, D. L., Clayworth, C. C., Knight, R. T., Simpson, G. V., & Naeser, M. A. (1987). Generators of middle- and long-latency auditory evoked potentials: Implications from studies of patients with bitemporal lesions. *Electroencephalography and Clinical Neurophysiology, 68,* 132–148.

Woods. D. L., Stecker, G. C., Rinne, T., Herron, T. J., Cate, A. D., Yund, E. W., . . . Kang, X. (2009). Functional maps of human auditory cortex: effects of acoustic features and attention. *PLoS One, 4*(4), e5183.

Wunderlich, J. L., & Cone-Wesson, B. K. (2001). Effects of stimulus frequency and complexity on the mismatch negativity and other components of the cortical auditory-evoked potential. *Journal of the Acoustical Society of America, 109,* 1526–1537.

Wunderlich, J. L., & Cone-Wesson, B. K. (2006). Maturation of CAEP in infants and children: A review. *Hearing Research, 212,* 212–223.

Wunderlich, J. L., Cone-Wesson, B. K., & Shepherd, R. (2006). Maturation of the cortical auditory evoked potential in infants and young children. *Hearing Research, 212,* 185–202.

Yabe, H., Tervaniemi, M., Sinkkonen, J., Huotilainen, M., Ilmoniemi, R. J., & Näätänen, R. (1998). Temporal window of integration of auditory information in the human brain. *Psychophysiology, 35,* 615–619.

Yabe, H., Winkler, I., Czigler, I., Koyama, S., Kakigi, R., Sutoh, T., . . . Kaneko S (2001). Organizing sound sequences in the human brain: The interplay of auditory streaming and temporal integration. *Brain Research, 897*, 222–227.

Yeung, K. N. K., & Wong, L. L. N. (2007). Prediction of hearing thresholds: Comparison of cortical evoked response audiometry and auditory steady state response audiometry techniques. *International Journal of Audiology, 46*, 17–25.

Zeng, F-G., Fu, Q-J., & Morse, R. (2000). Human hearing enhanced by noise. *Brain Research, 869*, 251–255.

Zouridakis, G., Simos, P. G., & Papanicolaou, A. C. (1998). Multiple bilaterally asymmetric cortical sources account for the auditory N1m component. *Brain Topography, 10*, 183–189.

12

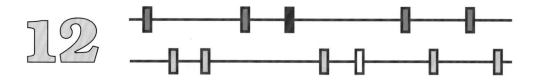

Endogenous Auditory Evoked Potentials: Attention Must Be Paid

> I don't say he's a great man. Willy Loman never made a lot of money. His name was never in the paper. He's not the finest character that ever lived. But he's a human being, and a terrible thing is happening to him. So attention must be paid.
>
> Arthur Miller, *Death of a Salesman*, 1949

The endogenous event-related potentials represent the interpretation of incoming sensory information in the context of an individual perceiver. Attention is the process whereby such interpretation occurs. Attention has several dimensions. The amount of attention given to incoming information—the depth of processing—determines whether something is simply noticed or fully understood. The usual metaphors for this are economic: attention is paid, resources are allocated, and work is done. The direction of attention controls what is processed and what is ignored. Here, we often use the metaphor of a spotlight focused on what is attended and relegating the rest to darkness. Attention also takes place along an internal to external continuum. This idea typically revolves around what controls our attention. We can be prepared to respond something that we expect to happen (active attention), or something unexpected can grab our attention and demand response (passive attention). Sometimes, we imagine what might happen without regard to reality; at other times, we attend to the real world but understand it only according to what we want to perceive. A final dimension of attention is the strategy that determines how attention is allocated over time. Attention can be sustained or divided.

The temporal metaphor is a switching system that directs the flow of information over time and monitors its effectiveness.

Attention is crucial to the mental processes that we consider human. Language is created and understood under the control of attention. What we attend to becomes what we might remember. Recalling our past and predicting our future occur when we attend to internal rather than external information. Being conscious is the exercise of attention.

Attention usually changes the late auditory evoked potentials (LAEPs) without affecting earlier responses. Figure 12–1 shows recordings of the auditory brainstem responses (ABRs), middle-latency responses (MLRs), and LAEPs during a simple manipulation of attention (Picton & Hillyard, 1974). In the "attend" condition, the subject attended to a prolonged train of "standard" clicks in order to detect an occasional "target" of slightly lower intensity. In the "ignore" condition, the subject read a book and paid little if any attention to the clicks. The only significant physiologic differences were that the N1 and P2 waves were larger when the subject was paying attention to the clicks. Under certain situations, as we have seen, attention can affect the earlier components of the response. However, it exerts its main effect on the LAEPs.

Figure 12–1 considers only the responses to the standard stimuli. Figure 12–2 compares the responses to the targets and the standards. When the subject is attending to the task, the LAEPs evoked by the targets differ from those evoked by the standards. In particular, the LAEP contains a large late positive wave, called the P3 wave as it follows the P2. This wave also is known as the P300 from its peak-latency in milliseconds when the task is simple and the subject is a young adult. In the experiment illustrated in Figure 12–2, the task of detecting the targets was difficult and the P300 wave occurred with a latency near 400 ms.

This simple experiment brings up two basic principles that we need to consider prior to further examining the endogenous responses. The first is the need to control "subject option" (Sutton, 1969). The second is the need to distinguish different components of the waveforms.

BASIC PRINCIPLES

Subject Option

The clarity of the results in Figures 12–1 and 12–2 does not always occur when studying the effects of attention on the auditory evoked potentials (EPs). Often, we can find no definite changes in the LAEPs when comparing attend and ignore conditions. One possible explanation is that the subject may not be doing exactly what she or he has been instructed to do. In the attend condition, the subject may be more concerned with when the experiment will end than whether the auditory stimuli are loud or soft. In the ignore condition, the subject may continue to listen to the stimuli and not pay much attention to the book he or she is supposed to be reading. This is subject option. Even when we do find differences, we need to be sure that they are related to attention and not to some other factor. If the subject is wide awake when attending to the clicks and drowsy when trying to read a book, the differences in the auditory EPs may be related to changes in the state of arousal rather than the direction of attention.

Setting up a paradigm to ensure that we can record the effects of attention and isolate these effects from other processes

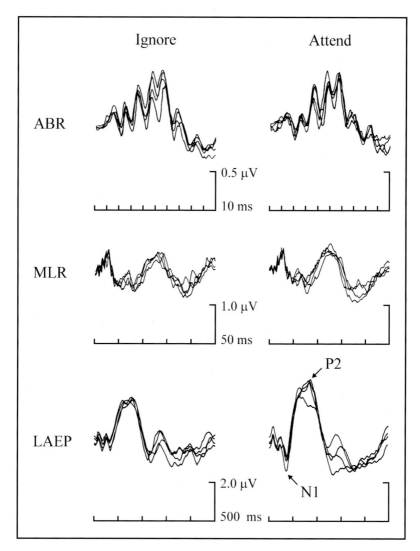

Figure 12–1. *Effects of attention on the auditory EPs. Auditory EPs were evoked by 60-dB SL clicks presented at a rate of 1/s. In the "attend" condition, the subject listened closely to the clicks and counted the number of target clicks (1–5 dB lower in intensity) that occurred with a probability of 0.1. In the "ignore" condition, the subject read a book and ignored the clicks. The responses to the standard clicks were recorded using three different time scales and amplifications. The only EPs to change significantly with attention were the N1 and P2 waves. Data from Picton and Hillyard (1974).*

requires empathy between experimenter and subject. We need to understand what the subject might be doing, and we need to design the experiment so that the subject can only do what we ask. As an example, we can consider the issues in setting up a paradigm for evaluating selective attention (Hillyard & Picton, 1987; Näätänen,

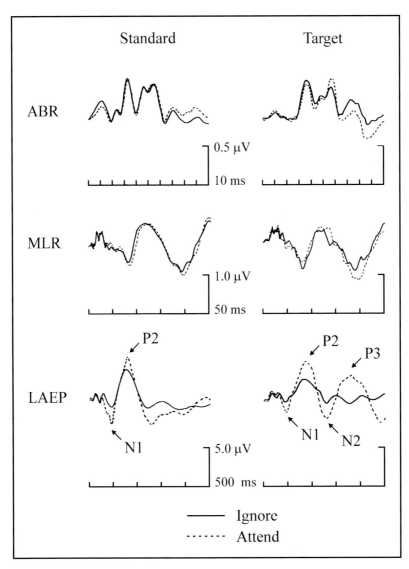

Figure 12–2. *Auditory EPs during the discrimination of targets. The paradigm was the same as that described for Figure 12–1 with the exception that the targets occurred more frequently (p = 0.2). The responses to the target stimulus were averaged over fewer trials than the responses to the targets. The ABR and MLR show small changes between target and standard (and between attend and ignore) that are within the range of what might be expected from the residual background noise (compare the replicated individual waveforms in the preceding figure). The LAEPs to the standards and targets are both changed significantly by attention. As well as the enhancement of the N1 and P2, the target EP shows additional N2 and P3 waves. Data from Picton and Hillyard (1974).*

1967, 1975). One way to control for differences in general arousal between attend and ignore conditions is to present two concomitant trains of stimuli and have the subject attend to one and ignore the other. Early studies alternated auditory and visual stimuli and required the subject to attend to one modality (e.g., Spong, Haider, & Lindsley, 1965). The LAEP was increased when the subject attended to the auditory stimuli. However, because stimulus-modality alternated regularly, the subject knew which stimulus was coming next and could differentially prepare to respond to those that she or he had been asked to attend to. Any effect of attention might then be caused by the subject's level of arousal waxing and waning in time with the attended stimuli.

To remove this subject option, the occurrence of the stimuli in the attended or ignored trains could be randomized. Smith, Donchin, Cohen, and Starr (1970) used a dichotic listening task, one set of stimuli were presented to the right ear and a different set to the left ear, with the subject unable to predict in which ear the stimuli would occur. The paradigm derived from studies of Cherry (1953) on the "cocktail party problem"—how we can nod occasionally in response to the boring speaker before us while following a much more interesting conversation at some other location in the room. Smith et al. (1970) had the subjects follow a train of spoken numbers or letters in one ear and ignore a similar train in the other ear, while recording the LAEPs to clicks occasionally intermixed with the spoken stimuli.

These initial studies with the selective dichotic listening task found no effect of attention on the LAEPs before 200 ms. However, the stimuli occurred infrequently and the subject may have been attending to all stimuli despite the instructions to attend to some and ignore the others. The stimuli evoking the LAEPs were occasional clicks intermixed with more frequent spoken stimuli (letters in one ear and numbers in the other). The subjects may have found it easier or more interesting to switch their attention between the ears, processing the clicks in either ear. Hillyard, Hink, Schwent, and Picton (1973) removed this possibility by presenting stimuli at a faster rate; the overall stimulus onset asynchrony (SOA) for the stimuli varied between 100 and 800 ms compared to the average SOA of 2.5 s in the Smith et al. study. This rate made it impossible to switch between the two ears and still perform the assigned task of detecting an occasional change in the attended ear. The paradigm clearly demonstrated that the N1 wave of the response was significantly enhanced when the subject was attending to the stimuli. Some of the original data were shown in Figure 1–8. A similar stimulus paradigm is illustrated Figure 12–3.

In addition to experimentally controlling what the subject does, wherever possible we should monitor what the subject is actually doing. Performance can be measured by having the subject count or press a button in response to the targets. Debriefing the subject after an experiment is always helpful. The subject may tell us about strategies that we had not imagined when we set up our control conditions.

Component Structure

In their binaural study, Smith et al. (1970) did find effects of attention on later waves in the LAEP, with the P300 being enhanced when the subjects counted the clicks in the attended ear. Hillyard et al. (1973) found the occasional target in the attended ear—the stimulus that the subject was required

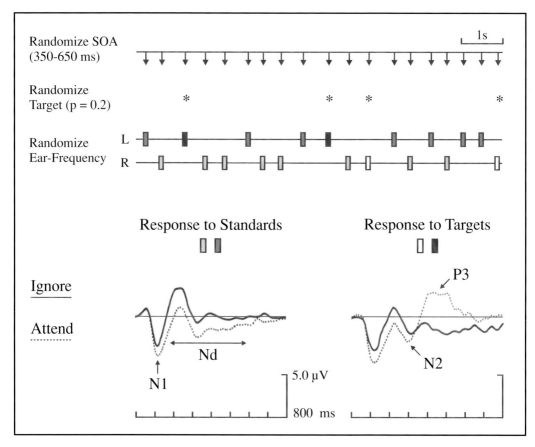

Figure 12–3. Paradigm for studying selective attention. The upper section of this figure shows how the stimulus presentation is programmed. Initially we set up the random timing of the stimuli. An average rate of 2 stimuli/s makes it extremely difficult to attend to the stimuli in both ears. The second step is to choose the unpredictable and improbable target stimuli. In this particular paradigm, the targets had a different tonal frequency than the standard stimuli. The final step is to create the stimuli and to allocate them randomly into two channels. (This step can occur before the target selection.) In this particular paradigm, the channels were defined both by the left or right earphone and by the tonal frequency (1000-Hz standard and 1200-Hz target in the left ear, 500-Hz standard and 400-Hz target in the right ear). In different conditions, the ears could be reversed to obviate any ear-frequency effects. The lower section of the figure shows the LAEPs (recorded from the vertex) combined across ears to show the effects of attention on the standard and target responses. Attention causes an enhanced N1 wave and a later sustained negativity, the Nd or processing negativity. The LAEP to the targets in the attended channel contains an N2-P3 complex. The general concept of the paradigm derives from Hillyard et al. (1973). The particular SOA and frequency parameters are from Maiste and Picton (1987).

to count—elicited a P3 or P300 wave. The N1 and P3 are both affected by attention but they represent different "components" of the psychophysiologic response. Hillyard et al. (1973) attributed different perceptual processes to each of these components, using a distinction proposed by Broadbent (1971). The enhanced N1 to all stimuli in the attended ear was related to "stimulus-set" attention, and the P3 wave to the detected targets was related to "response-set" attention.

Deciding how to separate the recorded waveform into different components is difficult. We considered different types of component analysis in Chapters 1, 2, 4, and 11. One approach is to consider components in terms of variance (what parts of the waveform behaved similarly in terms of the experimental manipulations); another approach considers them in terms of sources (activities occurring in specific regions of the brain). With the LAEPs, we generally use a combination of both approaches to decide how a specific region of the brain contributes to the processing of sensory information. Dissecting the N1 from the P3 is relatively easy; they are affected differently by the experimental manipulations. Early studies of the scalp distribution of the responses also showed that they have different intracerebral sources. The N1 is maximally recorded from the frontal regions of the scalp in keeping with a major source on the superior surface of the temporal lobe (see Chapters 4 and 11), whereas the P3 is maximally recorded from parieto-central scalp suggesting a source in parietotemporal cortex (Vaughan & Ritter, 1970). However, as we found with the N1 and soon will find with the P3, scalp waves likely do not come solely from one brain region. Other waves in the LAEP are even more complex than the N1 and the P3.

The N2 wave, the second negative wave in the vertex potential, is perhaps the most protean of the auditory EPs (see discussion in Näätänen & Picton, 1986, and in Novak, Ritter, Vaughan, & Wiznitzer, 1990). A simple listing of the different processes that might manifest themselves in the N2 wave gives us some flavor of the complex structure of the LAEPs. The N2 wave is dramatically enhanced during sleep, becoming the vertex sharp wave that can be seen in the ongoing electroencephalogram (EEG). However, we do not know whether this large wave represents the same or different processes from the normal waking N2. If the stimulus lasts longer than a few milliseconds, a sustained potential (SP) should occur; this can sometimes appear as an N2 wave. In the temporal regions, an N1c wave occurs about 40 ms later than the N1b wave at the vertex and 70 ms later than an N1a wave in frontotemporal regions. In response to a deviant stimulus, two additional N2s can be recognized: a mismatch negativity (MMN) and an N2b wave. The N2b wave occurs only when the subject is actively detecting the deviance, whereas the MMN can occur when the subject is not attending to the stimuli. An N2a wave was initially reported as a ramp-like precursor of the N2b when a subject detected an occasional omission in a train of stimuli. Attention also evokes an Nd (negative difference) wave, isolated by subtracting the response to an ignored stimulus from the response to the same stimulus when it is attended. Distinguishing all these different components of the "N2 wave" requires the patience to evaluate controls for arousal, stimulus deviance, attention, and task-relevance.

SELECTIVE ATTENTION

N1 and Nd

The paradigm illustrated in Figure 11–3 allowed extensive investigations into the neurophysiologic processes underlying selective attention. Schwent, Snyder, and Hillyard (1976) showed that the N1 enhancement occurred for stimuli within an attended channel that could be defined by location (left ear, right ear, or binaural), frequency (low, middle, or high pitch) or both location and frequency. The P3 enhancement occurred only for the detected targets within the attended channel. Hink and Hillyard (1976) found that the N1 was increased in response to probe stimuli in a channel of attended speech, provided the probes (vowel sounds) were similar to the speech. This study differed from that of Smith et al. (1970) by having the subjects attend to continuous speech rather than isolated letters and numbers and by using probes that were similar to the speech they were following (although not meaningfully related to its actual import). The enhanced N1-responsiveness occurred for all stimuli that were within an attended channel, regardless of whether they were meaningful or not. Hink, Van Voorhis, Hillyard, and Smith (1977) showed that, when attention was divided between the two ears, the N1 responses were enhanced compared to when the stimuli were ignored but not as much as when the attention was focused on one ear. The performance of the subjects in detecting targets also decreased when the attention was divided. Attentional resources are limited, and when attention is divided between channels, performance may deteriorate. Thus, the N1 effect was related to the allocation of attention.

However, some controversy soon arose. Using a constant SOA of 800 ms rather than the faster randomized SOA used by Hillyard et al., Näätänen, Gaillard, and Mantysalo (1978) found no N1 enhancement for stimuli in the attended ear, but demonstrated a later slow negative shift superimposed on the LAEPs. They suggested that this represented the same attention-related effect seen by Hillyard et al., but that this effect could be distinguished from the N1 by its more prolonged time course. Näätänen et al. proposed that the negative shift represented extra processing of stimuli chosen on the basis of a preceding selection, and called it the "processing negativity." In the same paper, they described a "mismatch negativity" (MMN) that was related to the discrimination of the targets, and that occurred even when the targets were in the unattended channel. The MMN was associated with passive attention and the processing negativity with active attention. Näätänen and Michie (1979) reinterpreted the N1-enhancement observed by Hillyard and his colleagues as the superposition of the processing negativity on the LAEP waveform. When the stimuli occurred very rapidly, the processing negativity could begin during the N1 and thus make it appear as though this wave was enhanced.

Resolution to this controversy came from the work of Hansen and Hillyard (1980). They examined the LAEPs during selective attention to frequency with very rapidly occurring stimuli. All tones were presented binaurally and the two channels of stimuli were defined by the frequency of the tones (cf. Schwent et al., 1976). The attend-ignore difference waveforms showed a negative shift that began during the N1 but lasted several hundred milliseconds longer than the N1 and obscured the P2 wave. (The LAEP waveforms were similar to those shown in Figure 12–3.) They called this the negative difference wave or Nd. When the frequency separation between the two channels was decreased (making the discrimination between the channels more difficult), the Nd began later. The early Nd showed a scalp topography that was similar to that of the N1 but the later part of the Nd was much more frontal in its topography (see also Giard, Perrin, Pernier, & Peronnet, 1988; Novak, Ritter, & Vaughan, 1992; Woldorff & Hillyard, 1991). Further work with channels involving both frequency and location showed a hierarchy of Nd processes, with the more easily discriminable channel parameter being processed earlier than the less easily discriminable parameter (Hansen & Hillyard, 1983).

Therefore, the Nd demonstrates two overlapping processes: the early selection of stimuli within an attended channel on the basis of easily discriminable sensory attributes, and the further processing these stimuli to refine the selection and to distinguish those that require response. Both processes likely involve interactions between frontal and temporal cortices, with the frontal contribution being greater for the late Nd component. The early part of the Nd may reflect a true enhancement of the N1 wave, and at rapid rates, the P2 also can be enhanced (Woldorff & Hillyard, 1991). Lesions of the temporoparietal regions decrease the amplitude of the Nd (Woods, Knight, & Scabini, 1993). Unilateral lesions of the frontal lobe decreased the Nd but this decrease was not asymmetrical, indicating that the contribution of the frontal lobe involves a modulation of temporal lobe processing rather than a specific generator in the frontal lobe (Knight, Hillyard, Woods, & Neville, 1981). The Nd associated with selection by location shows a different scalp topography to the Nd associated with selection by frequency (Dagerman, Rinne, Särkkä, Salmi, & Alho, 2008; Woods, Alho, & Algazi, 1994). These findings might indicate separate attention-related processes in the "what" and "where" regions of the auditory cortex of the temporal lobe and their connections.

The timing of the Nd is determined by various parameters. The onset depends on both the ease at which the stimuli in an attended channel can be discriminated and the urgency with which the selection must be performed. Urgency is itself determined by both the rate of stimulation and the motivation of the subject to perform quickly and accurately. The duration likely reflects the time needed to make whatever further discriminations are required and to monitor task-performance. When the subject finds the task easy, the Nd lasts only a brief time. Figure 12–4 shows the Nd to standards and to target stimuli when the target was rapidly discriminated from the standard.

Exactly what is represented by the Nd wave is not known. The original formulation of Hillyard et al. (1973) was that it represented the operation of a filter tuned to the channel of information that needed to be attended to—the instantiation of "stimulus set." Näätänen (1992) suggested that it represented the comparison between the incoming stimulus and an attentional template of what the subject was listening for. The later part of the Nd wave might also represent the refinement of the attentional template so that subsequent stimuli might be more efficiently evaluated. Alain and Arnott (2002) proposed that the Nd might represent the process of putting together an auditory object out of the various features (e.g., location and pitch) that are being analyzed. This concept could explain the effects of signal clustering on the allocation of Nd to attended and ignored stimuli. Kauramäki, Jääskeläinen, and Sams (2007) suggested that the enhanced N1 (early Nd) is more related to adjusting the tuning of cortical neurons than to simply enhancing their response. Attention to

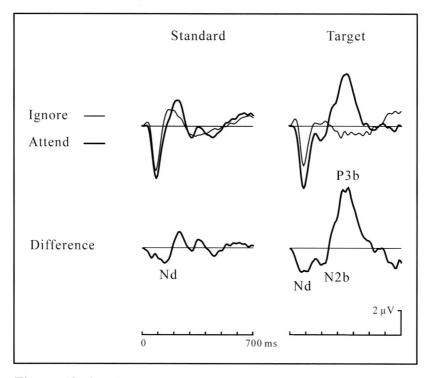

Figure 12–4. *Selective auditory attention.* *This figure shows LAEPs recorded from the vertex of a single subject in the paradigm described in the preceding figure (Maiste & Picton, 1987). This figure shows the effects of attention on the LAEPs. The difference waveforms are calculated by subtracting the ignore response from the attend response. The difference waveform shows the Nd to both kinds of stimuli and the N2b-P3b complex to the target.*

particular frequencies then would involve tuning the cortical neurons to respond preferentially to those frequencies.

The stimuli in an unattended channel may be actively rejected rather than just passively ignored. The LAEPs to the stimuli in the unattended auditory channel are less negative than the responses to the same stimuli in neutral conditions such as dividing the attention between the two channels or paying attention to visual stimuli. The responses to unattended stimuli thus may show a positive wave in the difference waveform calculated by subtracting the responses in the neutral condition from those in the unattended condition (Alho, Woods, & Algazi, 1994; Donald, 1987; Michie, Bearpark, Crawford, & Glue, 1990; Münte, Spring, Szycik, & Noesselt, 2010). This positivity occurs only when attended and unattended channels are easily distinguishable (Alain & Woods 1994). The positive deflection has gone by various names, among them the "Pd wave" and the "rejection positivity." Like the Nd, there may be different positive waves occurring at short and long latencies. What these results indicate is not clear. They may indicate some active inhibition of unattended information. Woods (1990) suggested the idea of an attentional parasol (as opposed to a spotlight). Another interpretation is that the positivity may indicate the cessation of processing once sufficient information has been received (Alho, Töttölä, Reinikainen, Sams, & Näätänen, 1987). Figure 12–5 shows some negative and positive difference waveforms.

Recent studies using fMRI have shown that selective attention mainly affects the more lateral regions of the auditory cor-

tices (Ahveninen et al., 2006; Petkov et al., 2004; Woods et al., 2009). The more medial core regions process specific features of the stimuli independently of whether they are relevant or not, whereas the more lateral belt and parabelt regions integrate the features to fit with the ongoing cognitive task. In particular, attention to location modulates the posterior activity and attention to phonetic content modulates anterior

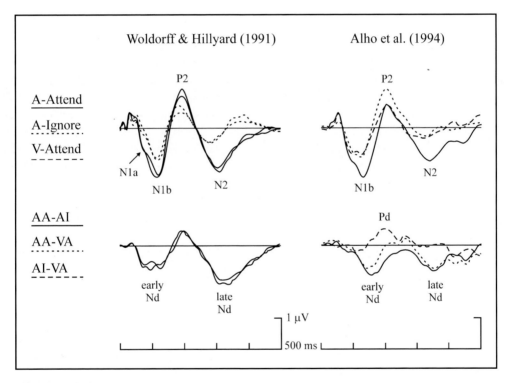

Figure 12–5. Negative and positive difference waveforms. Data from two different studies (Alho et al., 1994; Woldorff & Hillyard, 1991) are shown in this figure. The Woldorff and Hillyard data are for a dichotic selective attention task with the stimuli presented at a very rapid rate (SOA of 120–320 ms). Responses were compared for the standard stimuli in the attended ear (A-Attend) and in the ignored ear (A-Ignore). The two tracings represent the data for the left-ear and right-ear stimuli. The Alho et al. study used a slower rate (SOA 200–400 ms) and included another condition wherein the subjects attended to visual stimuli (V-attend). The difference between the attended and ignored auditory stimuli (AA-AI) shows early and late Nd components in both studies. In the Alho et al. study the early Nd begins later and continues into the latency of the P2 wave. When the responses to the ignored auditory stimuli in the dichotic task are compared to those during visual attention (AI-VA) a positive difference wave can be seen (Pd).

activity (Ahveninen et al., 2006). We can relate these findings to the electrophysiologic recordings: the Nd waves (or at least those parts that originate in the temporal lobe) likely arise from these belt and parabelt regions of the auditory cortex.

The auditory cortices on the superior surface of the temporal lobe have reciprocal connections with many other regions. During attention to auditory stimuli, activation occurs in multiple regions of the temporal, parietal, and frontal lobes. Available evidence suggests that the Nd recorded from the scalp reflects the activation of these areas in addition to those in the auditory cortices, the opening of the networks responsible for perceiving and responding to the stimuli. Attention to "what" involves anterior connections in the temporal lobe and projections to inferior frontal regions, whereas attention to "where" involves temporoparietal activation and projections to more dorsal regions of the frontal lobe (Alain, Arnott, Hevenor, Graham, & Grady, 2001). Most of these connections have been evaluated using hemodynamic recordings, although new developments in source analysis with magnetoencephalography (MEG) have allowed us to map the connections active during auditory attention and to specify their timing (Ross, Hillyard, & Picton, 2010).

Attention and the MMN

In the original reports, the MMN to a deviant stimulus occurred whether or not the subject was paying attention to the stimuli (Näätänen et al., 1978). This is clearly shown in Figure 12–6, which compares the LAEPs to standard and target stimuli in the attended and ignored channels. In the ignore condition, the target is more appropriately called a deviant stimulus as it only becomes a target when it is attended to. Most studies showed that the MMN is unaffected by whether the deviant stimuli are attended or ignored (e.g., Alho, K., Sams, Paavilainen, Reinikainen, & Näätänen, 1989; Alho et al., 1994; Maiste & Picton, 1987). This led to the concept that the MMN represents a completely automatic process to detect changes in the world (Näätänen, 1992; Näätänen, Paavilainen, Rinne, & Alho, 2007). Sensory information is analyzed in a bottom-up manner independently of top-down control.

One purpose of this automatic process would be to notify the perceptual system of changes that need further attention. Although the MMN is generated mainly on the superior surface of the temporal lobe, other brain regions contribute to the scalp-recorded wave. Giard, Perrin, Pernier, and Bouchet (1990) demonstrated that frontal activation, particularly on the right, occurs simultaneously with the temporal MMN. Alain, Woods, and Knight (1998) showed that the MMN was affected by lesions to either frontal or temporal lobes. Rinne, Degerman, and Alho (2005) found fMRI activation in both the superior temporal cortex and the inferior frontal cortex when comparing periods in which an MMN occurred to control periods without an MMN. Like the N1, the MMN reflects the activation of a network of brain regions. The role of the frontal regions in the MMN is not known. The frontal activity might represent further evaluation of the detected deviance, or index some inhibitory process preventing any such further evaluation. Schönwiesner et al. (2007) suggested that the frontal activation was involved in judging whether the deviant was of sufficient novelty to require allocating attentional resources to its further processing.

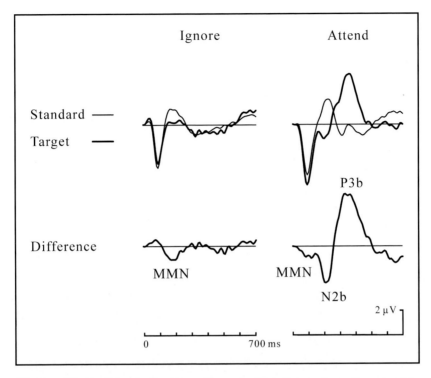

Figure 12–6. Discrimination of targets. This figure shows the same data as in Figure 12–4, but arranged to show the difference between the responses to targets and standards. The difference waveforms (calculated by subtracting the standard response from the target response) show a MMN in both attend and ignore conditions. When the stimuli are attended, the MMN leads to the N2b-P3b complex. The N2b is superimposed on the later part of the MMN.

In this regard, the MMN often is linked to a late positive wave (P3a) that occurs earlier than the usual late positive wave (P3b) associated with the active detection of a target stimulus (Snyder & Hillyard, 1976; Squires, Squires, & Hillyard, 1975). The P3a is maximal frontally whereas the P3b is maximal parietally. As illustrated in the left section of Figure 12–7, both waves occur when a target is detected, the larger P3b beginning during the P3a. The MMN and P3a often coexist, although when the difference between deviant and standard is small, the MMN can occur without any P3a. The P3a therefore may represent the

noticing of an automatically detected deviance. For example, the P3a may occur when the deviance is an intensity increment but not when it is an intensity decrement (Rinne, Särkkä, Degerman, Schröger, & Alho, 2006). However, this differentiation is not always the case; Squires et al. (1975) recorded a P3a to both increments and decrements of intensity.

A completely novel stimulus—a dog barking or a bell ringing during in a simple oddball task involving two tones of different frequency—evokes a large frontal positive wave (Knight, 1984). This wave is decreased by lesions to the dorsofrontal

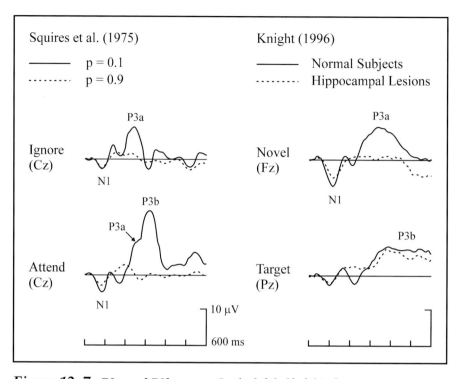

Figure 12–7. **P3a and P3b waves.** *In the left half of this figure are shown some LAEP waveforms from Squires et al. (1975). In their experiment, loud and soft tones occurred with probabilities of 0.1 or 0.9 and the subjects either ignored the stimuli (and read a book) or counted the number of improbable tones. The waveforms show the responses for the loud tones. When the tones were ignored, the LAEP to the improbable tone showed a P3a wave with a latency near 250 ms. When the subject counted the improbable tones, there was an additional P3b wave with a peak latency near 330 ms. These LAEPs are for a single representative subject. In the right half of the figure are shown LAEPs to novel stimuli (barks and bells) and to improbable target tones in two groups: normal subjects and patients with hippocampal lesions. The LAEP to the novel stimulus is shown at the midfrontal electrode (Fz) to accentuate the P3a response. This wave is not present in patients with hippocampal lesions. The LAEP to the improbable target tone is shown at the midparietal electrode to accentuate the P3b. The patients with hippocampal lesions still show a normal P3b response.*

cortex (Knight, 1984) and can be severely attenuated by lesions to the hippocampus (Knight, 1996). These results (illustrated in the right section of Figure 12–7) suggest that novelty is processed in a network connecting the hippocampus to the prefrontal cortex. The novelty P3 likely is a larger and later version of the P3a recorded to

simple deviances in tonal frequency. Barks and bells require more processing than beeps and boops.

The automaticity of the MMN (the lack of any effect of attention or other cognitive process) was questioned by the findings of Woldorff, Hackley, and Hillyard (1991). Using a demanding attentional task with very rapid stimulus rates, they found that the MMN in the attended channel was significantly larger than that in the unattended channel. Näätänen (1991) pointed out the difficulty in distinguishing the MMN from the N2b wave (associated with the P3b) that occurred when an attended deviant (target) was detected. The deviants in the attended channel may have evoked a similar MMN to those in the unattended channel, but the recorded MMN would appear larger because of the N2b. The right section of Figure 12–6 shows the N2b wave, which normally occurs toward the end of the MMN when the deviant is a target to be attended to. At rapid rates, the subject is forced to discriminate the targets very quickly and the N2b might occur even earlier and override the MMN. Oades and Dittmann-Balcar (1995) reported an enhancement of the MMN to an irrelevant deviant stimulus in a task where the subject was responding to one deviant (relevant) and not to another (irrelevant) compared to when the subject was passively listening to the stimuli. However, the waveforms in their paper certainly look like an N2b is superimposed on an earlier MMN unaffected by attention.

The N2b can be distinguished from the MMN in terms of its topography; the N2b is more central than the frontal MMN and it does nor invert below the lateral cerebral sulcus. This topography indicates that much or all of the wave is generated somewhere else in the brain than the superior temporal cortex (Novak et al., 1990). The main sources of the N2b are likely radial and therefore invisible to MEG evaluation. Sources might involve simultaneous activity in areas of the frontal lobe and in lateral temporal cortex.

Data soon began to accumulate showing that the MMN that was enhanced by attention could be distinguished from the N2b wave. Alain and Woods (1997) showed that the attentional enhancement of the MMN to a deviance in stimulus pattern inverted below the lateral cerebral sulcus and differed from the later N2b which did not. Sussman, Ritter, and Vaughan (1998) found that a deviant sequence of high- and low-pitch tones did not elicit an MMN when subjects passively listened to the stimuli but did elicit a clear MMN when the sequences were "segregated" by asking the subjects to attend to the sequencing of either the high- or low-pitch tones. Woldorff, Hillyard, Gallen, Hampson, and Bloom (1998) found that the attentional enhancement of the MMN could be measured using MEG, which showed sources in the superior temporal cortex. Arnott and Alain (2002) had subjects attend to a particular location in space and found that the MMN to deviants in unattended channels varied with the angular distance of the channel from that being attended. They suggested that spatial attention acted as a spotlight and that the MMN varied with the stimulus location relative to the center of the spotlight. The MMN clearly can be modulated by attention.

How this modulation occurs is not known. Ritter, Sussman, Deacon, Cowan, and Vaughan (1999) suggested that the MMN system still functions in an automatic bottom-up fashion, with attention simply gating more sensory information into cortex, for example, by facilitating thalamocortical afferents. This would fit with the findings of Woldorff and Hillyard (1991) showing an attentional enhancement of an early positive wave from 30 to 50 ms in the same paradigm that demonstrated the attentional modulation of the MMN. In less demanding tasks, where there is no effect of attention on the auditory MLR, the MMN is insensitive to the direction of attention. Ritter et al. (1999) also demonstrated the difference between the auditory MMN system and a multimodal cognitive system by providing subjects with visual information about the nature of an upcoming auditory stimulus. A deviant auditory stimulus (as determined by the preceding sequence of auditory stimuli) elicited a MMN even when its occurrence was completely predicted by the visual information. The MMN system therefore operates on the basis on bottom-up information and is unaffected by any top-down predictions from a multimodal cognitive system.

However, the MMN is not immune to information presented in the visual modality. Multimodal interactions can occur very early in the analysis of auditory information. The perception of a phoneme can be altered by linking its sound with a visual stimulus that shows the mouth making a different sound. The phoneme occurring with the incongruent visual stimulus evokes an MMN even though it does not differ from the other stimuli in terms of its sound (Sams et al., 1991). When presenting simultaneous tones and flashes, the MMN is evoked when the flash comes from a different location, even though the tone is exactly the same as the preceding tones (Stekelenburg, Vroomen, & de Gelder, 2004). In this paradigm, the tones are heard as coming from a different locations depending on the location of the flash—a "ventriloquism" effect. These experiments indicate that multimodal interactions occur very early in the processing of sounds by the auditory cortex. Furthermore, although the processes underlying the MMN are not affected by top-down effects of cognitive context, they are sensitive to multimodal interactions that occur in a bottom-up manner.

The Cocktail Party Problem

Before we leave this section on selective auditory attention, we should return to the basic questions that spurred this research. How is it that we can attend to one conversation at cocktail party and ignore others? One important characteristic is the ability to follow a particular person's voice. Woods, Hillyard, and Hansen (1984) found that the Nd to probes in speech during selective listening to dichotic spoken messages was larger for probes that matched the speaker's voice than pure-tone probes. This depends greatly on the fundamental frequency but other features also are important. The physiologic processing of these voice characteristics needs further evaluation.

The ability to focus our attention on a particular location in space also is essential to selective listening. We localize much better with two ears than with one. We normally never hear sounds at one ear and not at the other, as is possible with earphones. The basic idea of attending to one ear and ignoring the other is not related to normal listening experience. Attending to a location in space requires attention to both ears.

Selective attention to real spatial locations involves both early and late selection mechanisms. Teder-Sälejärvi, Hillyard, Röder, and Neville (1999) showed that Nd effects could provide preferential processing for broad regions of auditory space but that P3 selectivity was needed to make more precise distinctions. Both mechanisms can be enhanced in patients with blindness, the congenitally blind having better Nd selectivity (Röder et al.,1999) and the late-onset blind having more precise P3 tuning (Fieger, Röder, Teder-Sälejärvi, Hillyard, & Neville, 2006).

Clearly, there is continuous interplay between incoming information and our ongoing expectancies; these act together to allow us to follow one of many messages arriving at our ears. Although very difficult, following one of two superimposed messages spoken by the same speaker is possible (Cherry, 1953). This involves using the highest levels of analysis and expectancy—from voice dynamics to syntactic transitions.

EXPECTANT ATTENTION

Preparation and Anticipation

While we are expecting a stimulus that we need to discriminate, a slow negative wave develops, the "expectancy-wave." This often occurs in a paradigm wherein a "warning" stimulus (S1) notifies the subject of an upcoming "imperative" stimulus (S2) to which the subject must respond. In this classic paradigm, a "contingent negative variation" (CNV) develops between the warning and imperative stimuli (Walter, Cooper, Aldridge, McCallum, & Winter, 1964). Rohrbaugh and Gaillard (1983) proposed that the CNV consists mainly of a slow negative "orienting" wave in response to the warning stimulus and a later Bereitschaftspotential or "readiness potential" (RP) that reflects the preparation of the motor system for the response (Kornhuber & Deecke, 1965; Shibasaki & Hallett, 2006). As discussed in Hillyard and Picton (1987), the CNV also can contain a sensory anticipation wave that primes the necessary areas of cortex for the discrimination of the second stimulus. When a perceptual task is required at S2, the CNV is frontal prior to an auditory stimulus and parieto-occipital prior

to a visual stimulus (Picton, Hillyard, & Galambos, 1976). A parietal negative wave precedes an auditory stimulus when it provides feedback about performance on a prior task (Brunia & van Boxtel, 2004; Stuss & Picton, 1978). Negative waves preceding both perceptual tasks and feedback stimuli are illustrated in Figure 12–8. The various negative waves that occur when sensory stimuli are anticipated have been called "stimulus-preceding negativities" (SPNs) by Brunia (1988). In addition, the baseline shift between S1 and S2 likely also contains a negative wave that monitors the association between the two stimuli and reflects the amount of effort devoted to the task. This might represent the true CNV in the way it was originally conceived. Such a sustained negative frontal shift probably also occurs during any task that requires attention (e.g., McCallum, 1988; Picton, Campbell, Baribeau-Braun, & Proulx, 1978), but this very slow change in the EEG baseline cannot be measured unless recordings are obtained using either direct-coupled amplifiers or a very long time constant.

Expectancy and Predictability

What happens to the LAEPs when an earlier warning stimulus prepares the subject to process the auditory stimulus? Depending on the context, the LAEPs may be larger or smaller. If the nature of the stimulus is known, for example, if the stimulus merely serves to indicate when the motor response should be given, then the LAEP will be smaller than if subject does not know what stimulus to expect. When measuring the LAEP in this situation, we have to account for the falloff in the CNV

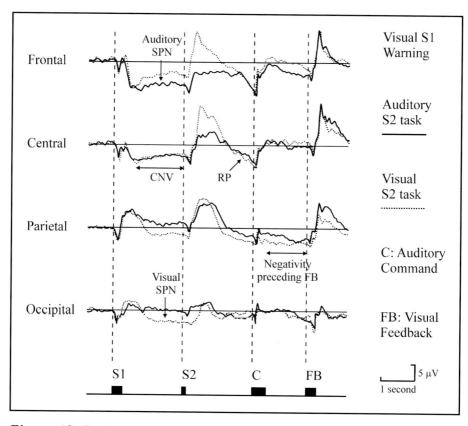

Figure 12–8. *Slow cortical waves associated with motor preparation and sensory anticipation. In this experiment a visual warning stimulus (S1) informed the subject on each trial whether an auditory or visual task was to be performed at S2. The visual task was to recognize a tachistoscopically presented number and the auditory task was to determine the frequency of a brief tone. The subject then responded at an auditory command signal (C) and received visual feedback about the correctness of the response. Only correct trials were averaged. The scalp topography (midline electrodes referred to a chest reference) of the negativity preceding S2—the auditory and visual stimulus-preceding negativities (SPN)—varied with the task modality. The negativity was larger over frontal regions for the auditory stimulus (likely because of activation of the superior surface of the temporal lobe) and larger over the occipital regions for the visual stimulus. The contingent negative variation (CNV) is the negative shift recorded between S1 and S2; this comprises an orientation response to S1 and the SPN preceding S2. A readiness potential (RP) precedes the motor response. The negativity preceding feedback is prominent in parietal regions (cf. Stuss & Picton, 1978). Data from Picton et al. (1976).*

that occurs at the same time as the stimulus is processed. Depending on its timing, this could decrease the N1 or add to the P2. On the other hand, if the subject must make some discrimination when the stimulus occurs and does not know exactly which of two or more possible stimuli will occur, the LAEP may be increased by the preparation (e.g., Davis, 1964). The subject has been able to focus attention on the stimuli and the usual attention effects, N1-enhancement and Nd waves, should occur. Lange, Rösler, and Röder (2003) had subjects attend at either one of two moments in time following an initial stimulus in order to detect a slight increase in the intensity of a brief noise burst. At the moment of attention, the stimuli were preceded by a larger negative slow wave and their LAEP showed a larger N1 wave than at the unattended moment.

When the timing and nature of the stimulus is predictable, the LAEP generally is reduced in amplitude. Schafer, Amochaev, and Russell (1981) had subjects respond to a tone in two conditions. In one condition, the timing of the tone was predictable on the basis of concomitantly presented visual numbers; the tone occurred whenever the counter reached 10. In the control condition, the tone (occurring at the same rate) was not temporally related to the numbers. The N1 and P2 waves in the LAEPs to the tones were smaller when the tone was predictable than when it was unpredictable.

The clearest way for the stimuli to become predictable is to make them self-initiated. In these paradigms, the subject hears a tone when he or she presses a button. Schafer and Marcus (1973) recorded LAEPs in response to self-initiated clicks, machine-initiated clicks (presented at the same intervals as those that occurred during self-stimulation), and periodic clicks. The N1 and P2 components of the LAEP were largest for the machine-initiated and smallest for the self-initiated clicks. These results were confirmed by McCarthy and Donchin (1976) who added conditions wherein the stimulus was one of two possibilities; thus both the timing and the nature of the stimulus could be made

unpredictable. Both temporal and event predictability decreased the amplitude of the N1 wave (see also Bäss, Jacobsen, & Schröger, 2008). A P300 wave occurred for the improbable stimulus when the stimulus was made unpredictable, and its amplitude was decreased when stimuli were self-initiated. When the stimuli are triggered by a motor act such as a button press, we must be concerned with overlapping potentials generated in motor and somatosensory cortex in relation to the behavioral response. However, Maritkainen, Kaneko, and Hari (2005) showed that the decrease in the LAEPs with self-initiation clearly occurred in auditory cortex by using MEG dipole analysis.

The results of these self-initiation experiments show that the brain carries a forward model of what is expected in response to behavior. This forward model likely is instantiated by activation of the networks needed to process what is expected prior to its occurrence. When the event then occurs, these networks need only be reminded rather than recreated.

This forward modeling harkens back to the "corollary discharge" and "efference copy" of basic neurophysiology (reviewed by Crapse & Sommer, 2008). The initiation of a motor act also activates the sensory systems that will be affected by the act by means of a corollary discharge, the parallel activation (or inhibition) of sensory neurons. A simple example is that we do not perceive the world as moving during an ocular saccade, even though the image on the retina is moving. The eye-movement system sends the necessary information about the saccade (an efference copy) to the visual system so that it can compensate.

An important set of forward models are involved in hearing speech. Under normal conditions, we pay little attention to the sounds of what we are saying. Our attention is invoked only if what we are saying sounds wrong—if the incoming sounds do not fit the forward model. Vowel sounds evoke much smaller N1 responses when they are spoken by the subject than when they are played back from tape (Curio, Neuloh, Numminen, Jousmaki, & Hari, 2000; Houde, Nagarajan, Sekihara, & Merzenich, 2002) The effects of this forward modeling are very precise; the N1 is more reduced when subjects hear themselves talking normally than when they hear themselves talking with a pitch that has been altered using online computer software (Heinks-Maldonado, Mathalon, Gray, & Ford, 2005).

LATE POSITIVE WAVES

Uncertainty and Information Processing

We briefly reviewed the early studies of the late positive wave in Chapter 1. These studies proposed the main theoretical constructs that have since been used to evaluate these late endogenous waves. The first paper (Sutton, Braren, & Zubin, 1965) showed that the LAEP to a stimulus about which the subject was uncertain contained a large late positive wave (see Figure 1–7), which was larger the more improbable the stimulus. The second paper (Sutton, Tueting, Zubin, & John, 1967) showed that this late positive wave occurred when uncertainty was resolved, whether this resolution occurred with a particular stimulus or at a time when a stimulus might have occurred but did not. The subject guessed whether the upcoming stimulus would consist of a single or a double click. The late positive wave peaked about 300 ms after the second click or after the point in time when the second click would have

occurred if the stimulus was a single click. The fact that this late positive wave occurred without any evoking stimulus led to the classification of the EPs as exogenous (determined by the external world) and endogenous (determined by the perceptual significance).

The late positive wave has assumed many different names. The most common are the P3 from its location in the sequence of negative and positive waves in the LAEP and the P300 from its typical latency in milliseconds, although this latency occurs only when an easy discrimination is made by a young adult. We use both names according to the preference of the papers we review.

The various findings in the two initial papers on the P300 could be integrated using basic concepts of information theory. First, the amount of information delivered by a stimulus is equivalent to the amount of uncertainty that it resolves in the perceiver. Second, the amount of information that a stimulus can provide is inversely proportional to the logarithm of its probability—the more improbable a stimulus, the more information it provides when it occurs. A completely predictable stimulus is uninformative, whereas one that surprises us can be highly informative. Information is related to knowledge, but the amount of new knowledge provided by an improbable stimulus depends on what the perceiver already knows.

Probability

The simplest way to manipulate the information content of a stimulus is to change its probability. The effect of probability on the late positive wave has been studied extensively using the oddball paradigm. This is the same as the paradigm used to evaluate deviance-detection except that the improbable deviant stimulus occurring in a train of standards is called the "target" or "oddball." In the typical paradigm, the stimuli are presented at an SOA of between 1and 2 seconds and the target occurs with a probability of between 0.1 and 0.2. The LAEPs are recorded from multiple scalp electrodes using a bandpass of 0.1 to 30 Hz, trials contaminated by blinks or eye-movements are rejected, and averaging occurs over at least 30 targets. Further details are provided by Duncan et al. (2009).

Duncan-Johnson and Donchin (1977) recorded the LAEPs as subjects listened to a random sequence of two tones and counted one of them. They found that the amplitude of the P300 was inversely proportional to the probability of each tone. The P300 was slightly larger when the tone was counted but this difference was much smaller than the effect of probability. Some of the results are shown in the upper left section of Figure 12–9.

The probability of a stimulus will depend on how the perceiver classifies the stimuli. When only one of several equiprobable stimuli is considered a target, only this stimulus will evoke a P300 even though its actual probability is no different from that of the other stimuli. For example, Johnson and Donchin (1980) presented three equiprobable tones, and had their subjects respond to only one. The designated target elicited a large P300 but neither of the other stimuli evoked more than a suggestion of a P300. Some results are shown in the upper right section of Figure 12–9. The P300 is determined by subjective probability—based on the way in which the subject categorizes the stimuli—rather than the objective probability of the stimulus. However, categorization is controlled by both bottom-up and top-down processes. If the subject is asked to respond to only one of two improbable stimuli (each occurring on 14% of trials) in a train of more probable standards (72% of trials), the improbable stimulus that it is not responded to still elicits a robust P300 although this is slightly smaller and later than the P300 to the designated target stimulus (Pfefferbaum, Ford, Wenegrat, Roth, & Kopell, 1984). In this paradigm, the subject uses three categories (target, nontarget, and standard), even though the experimental design uses two (those to be responded to and those not). Mecklinger and Ullsperger (1994) discuss how categorization can be determined by both stimulus characteristics and response requirements. The way in which the subject categorizes the stimuli may or may not correspond to the way the experimenter wishes; such is subject option.

Squires, Wicken, Squires, and Donchin (1976) maintained the global probability of a target constant over a block of stimuli and examined the effects of the sequence of stimuli immediately preceding the target to determine how the P300 varied with local probability. The P300 in response to a target was larger when the target followed a series of standard stimuli than when it followed a series of other targets. These results are illustrated in the lower right section of Figure 12–9.

Fitzgerald and Picton (1981) considered the P300 wave in terms of temporal probability. Temporal probability, which is the number of targets within an amount of time, differs from the stimulus probability, which is the number of targets in a set of stimuli. Changing the stimulus onset asynchrony (SOA) changes the temporal probability without affecting the stimulus probability. When the stimulus probability of the target is 1/10, the temporal probability of the target is 1/10s when the SOA is 1 s and 1/20s when the SOA is 2 s. Fitzgerald and Picton (1981) found that the P300 increased with increasing SOA.

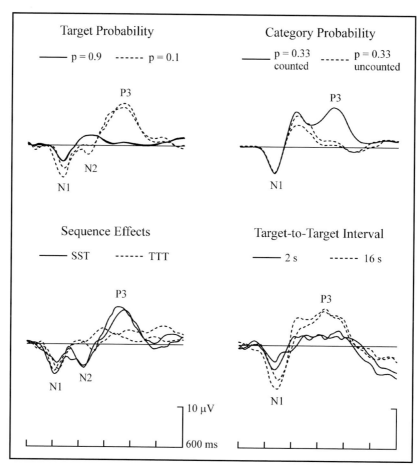

Figure 12–9. Effects of probability on the late positive wave of the LAEP. Four different aspects of probability are considered. The LAEPs in the upper left (from Duncan-Johnson & Johnson, 1977) show the effects of simple stimulus probability. The subject is asked to count the improbable (p = 0.1) stimuli in an auditory oddball paradigm. The responses at each probability are replicated. The LAEPs in the upper right (from Johnson & Donchin, 1980) show the effects of categorizing the stimuli. Three equiprobable (p = 0.33) stimuli occur and the subject is asked to count one of them. The LAEPs in the lower left (from Squires et al., 1976) show the effects of the preceding sequence of stimuli when the overall probabilities of standard (S) and target (T) are equal. The P3 wave is larger when the target is preceded by standards (SST) than when it follows other targets (TTT). The LAEPs in the lower right (from Gonsalvez et al. 2007) are from a simple target detection task when there were no standards. Both the N1 and the P3 wave vary with the interval from the preceding target. All LAEPs were recorded from the vertex and have been replotted to be on the same scale.

These results are illustrated in Figure 12–10. By varying both the temporal and stimulus probabilities, they were able to show that the P300 is related mainly to the temporal probability of the target. Polich (1990) found that there may be limits to this effect

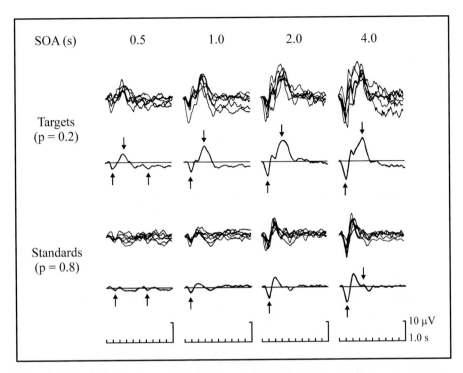

Figure 12–10. Effects of stimulus onset asynchrony (SOA) on the LAEPs in the oddball paradigm. In this study six subjects counted the number of target tones occurring with a probability of 0.2 in a train of standard tones. The SOA was varied from 0.5 to 4.0 seconds, with the SOA constant in each recording block. The figure shows the superimposed LAEPs for the six subjects and the average LAEP for both targets and standards. The upgoing arrows indicate the N1 wave. At the 0.5 s SOA, there are two responses within the recording sweep. The downgoing arrows indicate the P3 wave. This gets larger at longer SOAs, which also mean a longer average target-to-target interval. At the longest SOA, there is also a small P3 in the response to the standard. These data are from Fitzgerald and Picton (1981).

when the SOA is increased; at an SOA of 10 s, there is little difference between the P300s evoked by stimuli occurring with a probability of 80 or 20%. In reviewing these and related studies, Picton (1992) suggested that, when the time was 10 s or less, the P300 varied with the time since the last target.

Gonsalvez et al. (1999) used an oddball paradigm in which the SOA varied and separately averaged target responses on the basis of the time since the previous stimulus and the time since the previous target. The time from the preceding stimulus was the main determinant of the N1 amplitude and the target-to-target interval was the main determinant of the P3 amplitude. Data from Gonsalvez and Polich (2002) suggest that the P3 amplitude begins to asymptote at target-to-target intervals above 10 seconds (cf. Picton, 1992). Croft, Gonsalvez, Gabriel, and Barry (2003) found a similar dependence of the P3 on the target-to-target interval in an oddball task with constant SOA. The P3 was similar when the standards were omitted, indicating the that the need to discriminate between stimuli had little effect on the response. Sample results are shown in the lower right section of Figure 12–9. However, at long intertarget intervals (40–90 seconds), the P3 was larger when the standard stimulus was omitted indicating an effect of the time from the preceding stimulus at these long intervals (Sambeth, Maes, & Brankack, 2004). Also, when the target stimuli occurred alone, the P3 was larger for more intense stimuli (Gonsalvez, Barry, Rushby, & Polich, 2007). Both effects may indicate that some part of the P3 is sensitive to exogenous rather than endogenous parameters; the louder and more infrequent a stimulus, the more likely it will grab our attention.

Another finding that needs to be considered in the context of target-to-target intervals is that, in certain paradigms, large P3 waves occur at very short intervals. Woods and Courchesne (1986) used a task wherein subjects had to decide whether one, two, or three tones occurred in a period of 1200 ms. When three targets occurred, they all evoked large P300 waves. Verleger and Berg (1991) had subjects count the number of times three targets occurred in a row—the "waltzing oddball"—when the probability of an individual target was 0.5. The P300 increased in amplitude over the sequence of three targets. In both these experiments, the subject likely set up different categories for the different targets. The occurrence of two (or three) targets in a row would be a different category from a single target. Each category then would involve a separate P300 system with its own temporal parameters.

Difficulty and Equivocation

As the task of detecting a stimulus is made more difficult, the P3 wave increases in latency and decreases in amplitude. This initially was found when stimuli were presented at intensities near threshold (Hillyard, Squires, Bauer, & Lindsay, 1971). When LAEPS were averaged on the basis of whether stimuli were detected or not, a P3 occurred only with stimuli that were detected and not with those that were missed. The amplitude of the P3 to the detected stimuli decreased with decreasing intensity. The decreased amplitude and increased latency of the P3 also occur in the oddball task when the difficulty of discriminating target from standard (rather than signal from noise) is increased (Ritter, Simson, & Vaughan, 1972). This is illustrated in Figure 12–11. In this experiment (Fitzgerald & Picton, 1983), four different targets were used, each with a probability of 5%. The task was to detect all of the targets and to press a button as quickly as possible when the target was recognized. The P3 wave was smaller and later when the frequency difference between the target and standard decreased.

The amplitude results usually are interpreted using the concept of equivocation (Ruchkin & Sutton, 1978). The more difficult the discrimination, the less information is transferred from the stimulus to the perceiver. Information may be obscured by noise anywhere in the processing. Noise can occur with the acoustic stimulus, in the transduction mechanisms of the cochlea, and during the neuronal processes needed to make the final perceptual discrimination. The perceiver's uncertainty about the decision is reflected in the decreased amplitude of the P300. Consistent with the idea that the P300 reflects the amount of task relevant information processed from a stimulus was the finding of Squires, Hillyard, and Lindsay (1973) that the P300 amplitude to faint auditory targets varied with the confidence with which the targets were detected. The amplitude of the P300 therefore reflects the information content of the stimulus less the information lost

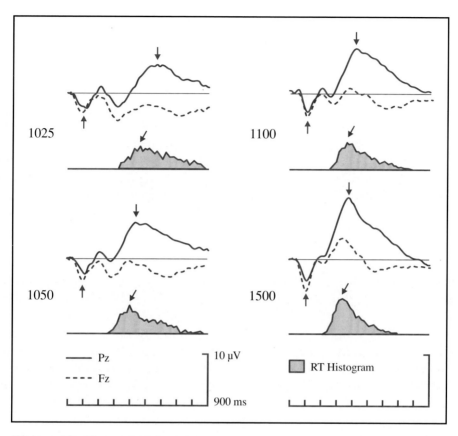

Figure 12–11. *Task-difficulty and the P3 wave. In this paradigm, 1000-Hz standards occurred with a probability of 0.8 and four different targets (1025, 1050, 1100, and 1500 Hz) occurred with a probability of 0.05 each. The subject's task was to press a button in response to the targets. This figure plots the LAEPs to each target together with the histogram of the reaction time (RT). LAEPs are plotted for the Fz (dashed line) and Pz (continuous line) electrode locations. The upward arrow indicates the N1 wave. This is larger at Fz than at Pz and larger for the higher frequency target. The downward arrow indicates the P3 peak. This is larger at Pz and becomes larger and earlier as the tonal frequency of the target becomes higher (and the discrimination easier). The peak latency of the P3 wave follows the modal reaction time (indicated by the diagonal arrow), with the difference being larger for the more difficult target. These data are from Fitzgerald and Picton (1983).*

in its processing. The lost information is known as equivocation, the amount of information that points to either answer (target or standard, signal or noise) rather than to the correct one.

The latency of the button press to the different targets in the experiment shown in Figure 12–10 increases with increasing task difficulty. Determining that the target really differs from the standard takes longer when the frequency difference between them is less. The mean reaction time (RT) in this particular experiment occurred about 50 ms later than the peak of the P3 wave (measured at Cz). However, the modal RT, probably a better measure than the mean in the skewed distribution of the reaction times, occurs just before the P3 peak. In experiments measuring the latencies on a single-trial basis (Kutas, McCarthy, & Donchin, 1977; Ritter et al., 1972), the RT typically occurs several tens of milliseconds earlier than the peak of the P3 wave. The time involved in transmitting impulses from cortex to nerve, from nerve to muscle and from muscle to button is probably of the order of 90 ms. The cerebral decision that initiates the response occurs well before the peak of the P3 wave. Therefore, the P3 wave must represent a process occurring after the decision to respond. Ritter, Simson, Vaughan, and Friedman (1979) suggested that the N2 might represent the decision process. However, Goodin, Aminoff, and Mantle (1986) recorded the EMG activity associated with the response and found that even the N2 can sometimes follow the decision process.

In more complex tasks involving decisions about both stimulus and response, the P3 latency is related mainly to the completion of stimulus evaluation and is relatively independent of the time required to select the appropriate motor response. These studies have been performed in the visual modality where it is simpler to adjust stimulus evaluation and response selection independently (e.g., McCarthy & Donchin, 1981). However, some data have suggested that the P3 latency also can be affected by response selection (e.g., Verleger, 1997). We return to this issue when we evaluate the nature of the P3 wave.

Audibility and Discriminability

Oates, Kurtzberg, and Stapells (2002) and Korczak, Kurtzberg, and Stapells (2005) have recorded the LAEPs in hearing-impaired patients using an oddball task with /ba/ and /da/ stimuli. The N1, P2, MMN, N2b, and P3 waves of the LAEPS increased in amplitude when hearing aids were used. In addition, the latency of the N2b wave decreased. Clearly, the LAEPs vary with the amount of auditory information available to the subject and this is increased by amplification when there is a hearing impairment. We are tempted to interpret the increase in the early waves of the LAEP (N1 in particular) as an increase in audibility of the sound in keeping with the results of Hillyard et al. (1971). The increase in the N2b and P3 waves therefore might indicate an increase in the discriminability of the sounds. The auditory information being processed then is sufficiently free of noise (or equivocation) to allow the subject to distinguish the different speech sounds with some degree of confidence, which is in keeping with the results of Squires et al. (1973). Additional studies with different stimuli might allow us to evaluate more precisely the effects of hearing aids on the audibility and discriminability of various sounds. Measuring the P3 waves can provide evidence concerning the timing of the subject's sensory discrimination and the confidence with which the discrimination is made.

Attention, Task-Relevance, and Meaning

As we have reviewed (see Figures 12–2 and 12–4), a large P3b wave occurs in the response to a target only when the subject is attending to the stimuli and responding to the targets in some way. The small early P3a occurs when targets occur in an unattended channel and the target is sufficiently discriminable to be noticed even without paying much attention.

If the stimulus is particularly noticeable, a P3b can occur (in addition to the P3a) even when the subject is not instructed to pay attention to the stimuli (Polich, 1989). This is particularly evident when the stimuli are more intense (Roth, Blowers, Doyle, & Kopell, 1982). These effects may be due to stimulus "salience," the way in which some stimuli naturally stand out from the background (and demand our attention).

The P3b amplitude varies with the task-relevance of the improbable stimulus —whether it requires some cognitive or motor response or whether it can be ignored. In addition, the P3 gets larger the more meaningful the target stimulus, the more cognitive and motor responses that it entails. Johnson (1986) proposed that the P300 amplitude is related to the sum of the effects of stimulus probability and stimulus meaning multiplied by a transmission factor that considers the amount of information lost in the processing. Nowhere is the effect of stimulus meaning more evident than when stimuli provide feedback about performance on a preceding task (Campbell, Courchesne, Picton, & Squires, 1979; Chwilla & Brunia, 1991: Picton et al., 1976; Stuss & Picton, 1978). As clearly illustrated in Figure 12–12, the P3 wave is much larger when the stimuli provide feedback than when they are simply counted. In general, feedback telling the subject that performance was incorrect gives a larger P3 and a more prominent N2 wave than feedback confirming correct performance. Campbell et al. (1979) found that the amplitude of the feedback P3 was linearly related to "contingent probability," the probability of the feedback given the behavioral response made on the task. This relates the P3 to the subject's expectancy that she or he will be right or wrong. Contingent probability also is known as conditional or Bayesian

probability and its relationship to the P3 wave has been more extensively considered by Kopp (2006).

Many other LAEP components can occur in association with the P3, particularly as the task becomes more complicated. Stuss and Picton (1978) demonstrated an extra large posterior positive wave in the feedback response when it signified a necessary change in cognitive strategy during a conceptual learning task. This P4 wave, so-called because it occurred after the P3 wave, may have been related to the positive slow wave (SW) occurring in other paradigms (Squires et al., 1975). Frontal negative slow waves occur at about the same time as the posterior SW but are distinguishable in terms of the effect of SOA (Fitzgerald & Picton, 1981). Exactly what these different SWs represent in terms of cognitive processing remains unknown. They probably are related to various postperceptual processes that update our memory and world model after we have finished responding to a particular stimulus.

When, usually because of responding too quickly, a subject makes an error and knows it, a negative-positive complex can be recorded in LAEP (Falkenstein, Hohnsbein, Hoormann, & Blanke, 1991; Gehring, Goss, Coles, Meyer, & Donchin, 1993). The clearest way to evaluate this response is to synchronize the averaging to the behavioral response rather than to the stimulus. This recording gives an "error-related" negativity and positivity—Ne and Pe. These also are called the "oops!" or "awshit!" waves after the common utterances associated with recognized errors. The main source for these responses is in the region of the anterior cingulate (Dehaene, Posner, & Tucker, 1994; Kiehl, Liddle, & Hopfinger, 2000). The response probably is related more to monitoring conflict than to processing the error, to

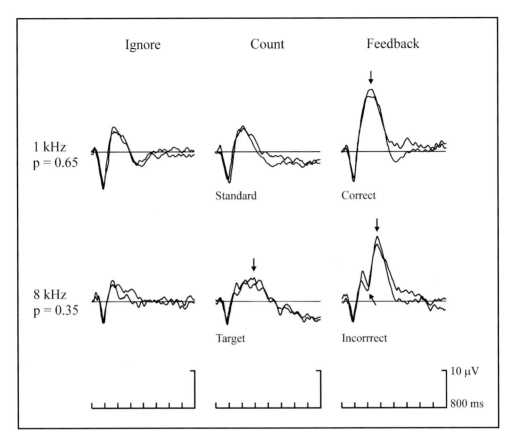

Figure 12–12. *Effects of task relevance and meaning on the P3 wave. In this experiment, an initial pair of tone pips and then a brief light preceded a tone burst of either 1 or 8 kHz occurring with probabilities of about 0.65 and 0.35. In the "Ignore" condition the subjects read a book and ignored all the stimuli. In the "Count" condition the subject counted the number of 8-kHz stimuli (considered as targets) while ignoring the other stimuli. In the "Feedback" condition, the subject made a difficult discrimination between the initial two tone pips, responded at the light and then received feedback about whether the response was "correct" (1 kHz) or "incorrect" (8 kHz). Counting enhances the P3 wave to less probable targets. However, the P3 wave (*downward arrow*) becomes much larger when the stimuli provide feedback about prior performance (which was about 65% correct). The feedback denoting correct performance has a large early P3 wave. The P3 is delayed when the stimulus denotes incorrect performance and a prominent N2 wave occurs (*diagonal arrow*). These recordings are from Picton et al. (1976).*

noticing that the actual response does not fit with the task instructions rather than to doing something about it (see review by Mathalon, Whitfield, & Ford, 2003). The large N2 waves associated with negative feedback (Miltner, Braun, & Coles, 1997) and with inhibiting responses in a No-Go task (Nieuwenhuis, Yeung, & Cohen, 2004) likely are similar in nature to the error-related negativity.

Nature of the P3 Wave

Many studies have indicated that the P3 wave contains multiple components. As Dien, Spencer, and Donchin (2004) suggest, this region of the LAEP is a "neighborhood" with many dwellings. Several distinct subcomponents of the late positive wave have been identified in different studies. For example, Falkenstein, Hohnsbein, and Hoorman (1994) proposed that the LAEP contained a frontocentral response associated with making simple responses and a parietal response related to response selection. These components have been reinterpreted by Dien et al. (2004) as representing the P3a and P3b waves, the P3a associated with novelty-detection and the P3b associated with stimulus-categorization. Key to this interpretation is the idea that the P3b is independent of response selection and provides a chronometric index for the end of stimulus evaluation. On the other hand, Verleger, Jaśkowskis, and Wascher (2005) found that the P3b is affected by both stimulus evaluation and response selection. They suggest that the P3b represents a system that links stimulus to response and monitors how well this occurs.

Physiologic and pathologic studies of the late positive wave in human subjects clearly support at least two sources. We have already reviewed the evidence suggesting the P3a depends on interactions between hippocampus and prefrontal cortex. Lesion studies indicate the temporoparietal regions of the cerebral cortex as the main source of the scalp-recorded P3b (reviewed by Soltani & Knight 2000). Functional MRI studies of auditory oddball paradigms (e.g. Kiehl & Liddle, 2003; Linden et al., 1999; Menon, Ford, Lim, Glover, & Pfefferbaum,. 1997) and studies combining functional MRI and EPs (Opitz, Mecklinger, von Cramon, & Kruggel, 1999; Shahin, Alain, & Picton, 2006) also have implicated the temporoparietal regions in the generation of the P3b. Intracerebral recordings have demonstrated activity in the hippocampus during the P3, but also have indicated the simultaneous involvement of many other regions of the brain (Halgren, Marinkovic, & Chauvel, 1998).

What the P3 represents in terms of cerebral or psychologic processing remains unknown. Many theorists have dissociated the P3a and P3b, relating the P3a to an automatic orientation system that reacts to novel events and the P3b to the controlled processing of task-relevant events (e.g., Dien et al., 2004; Polich, 2007; Squires et al., 1975). Different neurotransmitter systems (dopamine for the P3a and norepinephrine for the P3b) may underlie the two processes (Polich, 2007). However, both transmitters are widely distributed and it is difficult to relate them to specific electrophysiologic events, or to determine whether general transmitter activation contributes to or results from the physiologic event. Although everyone agrees that the P3a system is related to novelty detection, exactly what the P3b represents is disputed.

Two main theories of the P3b have been proposed. Both account for the fact that the P3 can occur after a decision is made about the stimulus. One is that the P3b represents the resolution of the expectancy when the expected event occurs (Verleger, 1988). A related theory involves the "closure" of perceptual processing (Desmedt, 1980). The second theory is that the P3b represents the context-updating necessary when an improbable event occurs (Donchin & Coles, 1988). This can be quite general, but a particular type of updating necessary in the oddball paradigm concerns the local probabilities of the stimuli. We need to know how often each event is occurring and whether these relative probabilities are changing. Because context updating involves working memory, and because this is hypothesized to be the location of conscious or controlled processing, this theory also is related to the idea that the P3b reflects access to consciousness (Picton 1992). Similar to the psychologic theories, physiologic theories divide into those postulating activation of the consequences of target recognition and those postulating inhibition of other activity to allow further attention to the present stimulus (see Polich, 2007, for further support of the inhibitory interpretation). While dealing with one target (and generating a P3 wave), a subject often will miss the occurrence of another. This has been called the "attentional blink" (Shen & Alain, 2010).

Many cerebral processes are occurring during the P3 even when the task is simple. Stimuli have to be categorized; appropriate responses have to be selected and initiated; performance has to be monitored; perceptual analyzers have to be retuned to detect upcoming stimuli; motor systems have to be recharged for subsequent responses; working memory has to be updated; long-term memory has to be revised; and consciousness has to become aware of what is happening. All these processes may contribute to what is recorded in the late positive wave of the LAEP.

Stuss, Shallice, Alexander, and Picton (1995) described controlled attention in terms of a supervisory system setting up, maintaining, organizing, and monitoring perceptuomotor "schemata" that link incoming sensory information to appropriate response (see Norman & Shallice, 1986, and Shallice, Stuss, Picton, Alexander, & Gillingham, 2008, for earlier and later formulations of this concept). A simplified version of this system is shown in Figure 12–13. The supervisory (or executive) system depends on networks that involve the prefrontal cortex. A schema is the neuronal basis for the performance of tasks that require attention, but the nature and location of schemata are not known. One possibility is that they are instantiated in neuronal networks connected through nodes in the temporoparietal regions. Activation of the schemata by incoming information would then initiate the appropriate behavioral responses, activate or inhibit other schemata, and provide feedback to the supervisory system. The P3b then might represent the activation of a schema and its connections, thus entailing the consequences of a particular stimulus being recognized. If the stimulus occurred infrequently, the schema and its connections would require more activation than if the stimulus were frequent and the schema residually active from previous stimuli. This might explain the dependence of the P3b on target-to-target intervals. These ideas of schema activation are similar in some ways to recent formulations of Verleger et al. (2005) who have associated the P3b with linking stimulus to response and monitoring the appropriateness of the linkage.

POSSIBLE CLINICAL USES OF THE LAEPS

As the electrophysiologic manifestations of cognition, the late EPs in auditory and other sensory modalities have long been investigated in patients with disorders of higher nervous functions. Guidelines for using the MMN and P300 in clinical research have been published recently

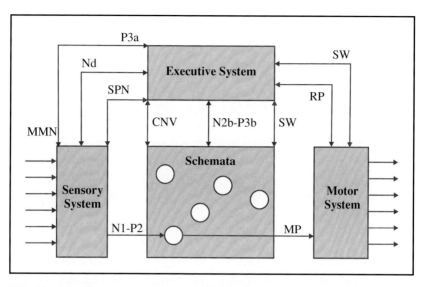

Figure 12–13. Architecture of attention. *This diagram is based on proposals for the supervisory attention system of Norman and Shallice (1986). Schemata are temporary processes set up to handle expected sensory information and to initiate appropriate responses. Possible associations with the different components of the LAEP have been mapped on the diagram. The processes represented all are described in the text except for the motor potentials (MP) related to initiating the behavioral responses. Several processes occur prior to the stimulus, most notably the tuning of the sensory analyzers (perhaps through the stimulus preceding negativity or SPN), the activation of the schemata necessary for performing the task (through the contingent negative variation or CNV), and the preparation of the motor responses (through the readiness potential or RP). These were illustrated in Figure 12–8. The slow waves (SW) that follow stimulus processing probably represent feedback processes between the executive system and the perceptual and motor systems. Attention works through networks of interconnected brain regions (through the lines rather than the boxes). Sensory analysis for the auditory system is focused in the temporal lobe, the executive in the prefrontal cortex, the schemata in temporoparietal regions and motor action in the medial and posterior regions of the frontal lobe. For simplicity, the diagram does not consider the relation of ongoing processing to long-term memory.*

(Duncan et al., 2009). The main goal has been to understand what is not functioning correctly in the brains of these patients. An even greater goal would be to find some physiologic measurement that can help to diagnose their disorders and to follow their response to treatment. More recently, we have become interested in

defining some genetic liability for particular disorders of cognition so that we may possibly act to prevent or attenuate the development of the disorder.

Our goals for the LAEPs in patients with cognitive disorders have not been realized for four main reasons. First is the variability of the recordings in normal subjects. The large overlap in the measurements between patients and controls does not prevent us from using group differences to understand physiologic differences between patients and normal subjects. However, it does make it difficult to use the measurements in the diagnosis of individual subjects. The variability of the response can be reduced by accounting for normal factors known to affect the response. Polich and Herbst (2000) review many parameters, from time of day to body temperature, that can affect the P3 in normal subjects.

Second is our incomplete understanding of what cerebral processes are related to the different physiologic measurements. For example, we do not really know what it means to have a malfunctioning P3 system. We know that the system is involved in linking stimulus to response but this can go wrong in many ways and each type of malfunction may lead to different symptoms. Perhaps it might be more helpful to determine the specific situations in which a particular EP component is abnormal. Evaluating the MMN or P3 under various experimental paradigms might allow us to distinguish between different cognitive abnormalities that become manifest in different contexts.

Third is that abnormal measurements lack specificity. Small MMNs or small P3 waves can occur in many different clinical situations—learning disorders, psychoses, aphasia, alcoholism, and dementia, to name just a few. Pfefferbaum, Wenegrat, Ford, Roth, and Kopell (1984) found that the P3 amplitude was reduced and the P3 latency prolonged in patients with dementia, depression, and schizophrenia. The patterns of abnormality were slightly different (e.g., the demented patients tended to have more prolonged latencies than the other patients) but the overlap was such that differential diagnosis was impossible. An abnormal P3 therefore had little meaning beyond showing that something was wrong with cognition. Long lists of disorders where an electrophysiologic measurement may be abnormal (e.g., for the MMN by Näätänen & Escera, 2000) illustrate both how the measurement may index cognitive dysfunction and how it still remains nonspecific in terms of diagnosis. This lack of specificity may be decreased if the measurement is only abnormal in certain paradigms (e.g., abnormal duration MMN but not abnormal pitch MMN) or in a certain way (e.g., small but not delayed, or delayed but not small) and if these paradigms and patterns are specific for to particular disorders.

Fourth is the question of whether the abnormal EP measurement is the cause or the result of abnormal brain processing. A small P3 wave can occur when attention is distracted from the task in a normal subject. If a patient shows a small P3, is the disorder caused by an abnormality in the brain system that generates the P3 or is the disorder an abnormality in some other brain system that makes the patient more easily distractible? The MMN to a duration deviant is abnormally small in chronic schizophrenic patients but not in patients at the time of their first psychotic episode (Magno et al., 2008). These results suggest that the abnormality is not related to the etiology of the disorder but occurs as one of its consequences.

The LAEPs have been examined in many different cognitive disorders. In this chapter, we consider the LAEPs in dementia and in schizophrenia. These examples illustrate how to consider the LAEPs in patients with cognitive disorder. To begin with, however, we consider the LAEP effects of aging (and the age-related cognitive changes we all inevitably experience).

Aging

The endogenous components of the LAEP change significantly with age. The latencies of all the peaks in the adult LAEP waveform increase with age but the earlier more exogenous waves N1 and P2 show only small changes that often do not reach significance. On the other hand, the N2 and P3 waves in the response to detected oddball stimuli increase in latency quite regularly beyond the age of 15 years. The rate of change for the P3 latency is between 0.5 and 2.0 ms per year and the rate for the N2 latency about half that. Table 12–1 presents the results from several representative studies that have examined the effects of age on the P3 wave

(Goodin, Squires, & Starr, 1978; Iraqui, Kutas, Mitchiner, & Hillyard, 1993; Pfefferbaum, Ford, Wenegrat, Roth, & Kopell, 1984; Picton, Stuss, Champagne, & Nelson, 1984; Polich, 1996). The right section of Figure 12–14 graphs some sample data. Polich (1996) provides an extensive meta-analysis of published results. He found many experimental variables significantly affected the age-related latency change, most particularly whether the subject counted the targets or pressed a button in response to the targets. The slope was greater when the subjects counted. In childhood, the N2 and P3 latencies decrease with increasing ages, reaching their minimum at around age 15 years and then increase regularly with increasing age

Table 12–1. Age Effects on P3 Latency

Study	Stimuli	Resp[a]	Target Prob.	SOA (s)	b (ms)	m (ms/yr)	r	SE[b] (ms)
Goodin, Squires, and Starr, 1978	1 vs. 2 kHz	C	0.15	1.5	285	1.64	0.81	21
Picton et al., 1984	1 vs. 2 kHz	C	0.10	1.1	273	1.36	0.55	35[c]
Pfefferbaum et al., 1984a	1 vs. 0.5/ 2 kHz[d]	R	0.14	1.0	325	0.94	0.32	51
Iragui et al., 1993	1 vs. 1.5 kHz	R	0.20	1.5	294	0.88	0.36	44
Polich, 1996[e]	1 vs. 2 kHz	R	0.20	1.0	304	0.92	0.46	32

Data are regressed according to the formula $y = mx + b$ where y is the latency of the P3 peak in ms, m is the slope of the regression, and b is the y-intercept (the hypothetical latency at age 0 years).

[a]Response to target: Count (C) or press a button (R).

[b]Standard error of the regression estimate.

[c]The original paper tabulated the standard error of the slope rather than the standard error of the regression estimate.

[d]Subjects pressed a button to one improbable stimulus (target) and not to another equally improbable.

[e]Data from an unpublished 1995 study reported in the 1996 review.

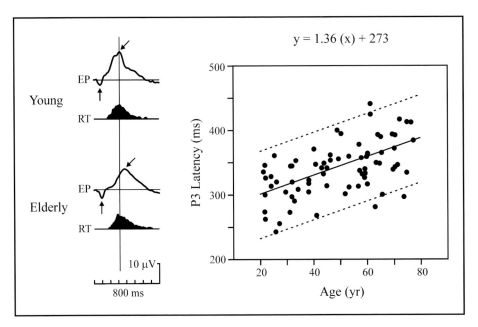

Figure 12–14. **Effects of age on the LAEPs.** *The left section of the figure shows the grand mean LAEPs from 10 young female subjects (mean age 23years) and 10 elderly female subjects (mean age 69 years). The responses were evoked by the counting of 2000-Hz tones occurring with a probability of 0.20 in a train of standard 500-Hz tones occurring at a rate of 1/s. The N1 peak (upgoing arrow) does not change in amplitude or latency with age, whereas the P3 wave (diagonal arrow) decreases in amplitude and increases in latency. The reaction time (RT) histograms show no clear effect of age. The vertical line is located at the peak latency of the P3 wave in the young subjects. These data are from Picton et al. (1986). The right section of the figure shows the regression line for the increase in P3 latency with age. These responses were recorded in response to a 2000-Hz target presented with a probability of 0.10 in a train of standard 1000-Hz tones occurring at a rate of 1/s. The dashed lines represent the ±2 standard errors of the regression estimate. These data are adapted from Picton et al. (1984).*

above 15 years (Goodin, Squires, Henderson, & Starr, 1978).

The amplitudes of the N2 and P3 waves generally decrease with age but these changes are more variable than the latency changes and do not always show up as significant on the age regressions. The P3 wave is larger in female subjects but this difference does not interact significantly with age (Picton et al., 1984). Part of the age-related amplitude change may be related to an increased variability in the timing of the P3 peak latency on single

trials, although Pfefferbaum, Ford, Wenegrat, Roth, and Kopell, (1984) found that the age-related decrease in the P3 amplitude still occurred after the LAEPs had been latency-compensated using adaptive filtering.

The age-related changes in the P3 wave—increasing latency and decreasing amplitude—are similar to those that occur when the perceptual discrimination is made more difficult. However, the age-related changes occur independently of the changes associated with discrimination-difficulty (Picton, Cerri, Champagne, Stuss, & Nelson, 1986).

The scalp topography of the P3 wave changes with age. In general, the peak amplitude becomes more evenly recorded from frontal to parietal regions and less prominent in the midline centroparietal areas with increasing age (Pfefferbaum, Ford, Wenegrat, Roth, & Kopell, 1984; Picton et al., 1984; Polich, 1997). Friedman, Simpson, and Hamberger (1993) found that both the target and novelty P3 showed relatively greater frontal scalp distribution with increasing age. It is difficult to determine the meaning of these topographic changes because what is measured at the scalp reflects the overlapping fields of multiple generators. One possibility is that the P3b activity generated in the temporoparietal regions decreases more with aging than the P3a activity generated in frontal and hippocampal circuits.

Age often has little effect on the reaction time (RT) recorded simultaneously with the P3 wave (e.g., Iragui et al., 1993; Pfefferbaum, Ford, Wenegrat, Roth, & Kopell, 1984; Picton et al., 1984). Typically, there is a slight age-related increase in modal and mean RT but these changes often are not significant on statistical testing and show no clear correlations with the P3 latency. The older subjects who volunteered for these studies may have been more motivated to perform quickly than the normal elderly population; they may have wanted to demonstrate to the scientists that they were just as fast as their younger colleagues. However, the results still show a clear dissociation between the effects of age on the P3 wave and the RT. In young subjects performing a simple choice reaction time task, the P3 latency peaks at about the same time as the RT. In older subjects, the P3 wave occurs significantly later than the RT. These findings can be seen in the left section of Figure 12–14. These results therefore indicate that aging does not just cause a uniform slowing of cerebral processing, but that some brain processes (those underlying the P3) are slowed more by aging than others (those leading to the RT). These ideas are discussed at greater length by Bashore, Osman, and Heffley (1989).

The age-related changes in the P3 wave became particularly clear to me as the years went by. In my youth, I made a point of participating in all the EP studies in the laboratory. As I became older, the latency of my P3 wave started to drift away from that of the younger subjects, even though I was able to perform the tasks as quickly and as accurately as they could. Although I continued as a subject in the studies of early auditory EPs, I stopped participating in LAEP studies unless age was included as an independent variable. Otherwise, the longer P3 latency related to my increasing worldly wisdom (or my accumulating mental lethargy) would have jeopardized the experimental variance.

Dementia

Patients with Alzheimer's disease often show abnormally late P3 waves when examined in a simple auditory oddball paradigm (Goodin, Squires, & Starr, 1978). Polich and Corey-Bloom (2005) review the extensive literature comparing patients with Alzheimer's disease to age-matched control subjects as well as documenting their own results. The latency of the P3 wave usually is delayed and its amplitude often is decreased in demented patients. However, there is a large overlap in the results between the normal and the demented subjects and it is difficult to use P3 measurements as a diagnostic test for dementia independently of other findings. When comparing patients with Alzheimer's disease to normal controls, the sensitivity for the P3 latency is variously reported as 91% (Bennys, Portet, Touchon, & Rondouin, 2007) and 53% (Gironell, Garcia-Sanchez, Estevez-Gonzalez, Boltes, & Kulisevsky, 2005), with specificities of 100% and 77%, respectively. Polich and Corey-Bloom (2005) found that recording the P3 in either an auditory or visual task was similarly effective in discriminating subjects with Alzheimer's disease from normal controls, and that easy perceptual tasks were better than more difficult tasks. Combining the latency and amplitude and measurements might provide a more effective discrimination of the subject groups, but even then there would be more overlap between the groups than we would like. Sample measurements of the P3 latency and amplitude are shown in Figure 12–15.

Separating the scalp-recorded P3 wave into different source waveforms (for P3a and P3b components) also may increase the ability to distinguish subjects with dementia from normal control subjects

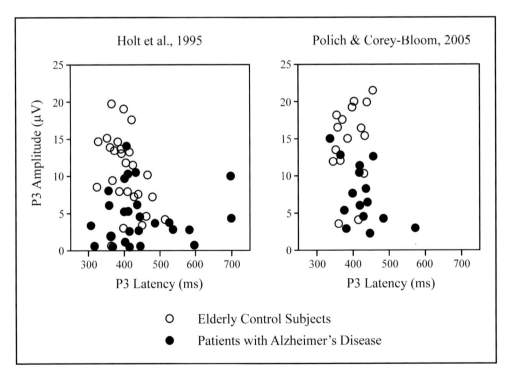

Figure 12–15. *P3 measurements in patients with Alzheimer's disease. Measurements of the amplitude and latency of the P3 wave measured at the Pz electrode are compared between patients with Alzheimer's disease* (filled circles) *and age-matched controls* (empty circles) *in two representative studies. In both studies the P3 wave was measured in an easy oddball task (discriminating 2000-Hz targets occurring with a probability of 0.2 in a train of 1000-Hz standards with an SOA of 2 s). For the Holt et al. (1995) study, P3 amplitudes that were measured as slightly negative are arbitrarily plotted at zero.*

(Frodl et al., 2002; Juckel et al., 2008). The P3b deriving from the posterior temporal regions of the brain decreases in amplitude and the more frontotemporal P3a increases in latency in patients with dementia. Combining these source measurements gives a sensitivity of 81% and a specificity of 83% (Juckel et al., 2008).

LAEP recordings in patients with mild cognitive impairment show complex effects. The P3 amplitude and latency can distinguish groups of these patients from normal controls but there is even greater overlap than when comparing patients with Alzheimer's to controls (Bennys et al., 2007; Golob, Irimajiri, & Starr, 2007; Golob, Johnson, & Starr, 2002). The P3 wave does not clearly differ between patients who remain with a stable mild cognitive impairment and those who convert to Alzheimer's disease, although, as reviewed in Chapter 9, some measurements of the P50 wave may have predictive significance (Golob et al., 2007). Patients who are carriers of the genetic abnormalities associated with a familial Alzheimer's disease show longer latency P3 waves than noncarrier family members even before any clinical manifestations of dementia (Golob et al., 2009).

Although they do not indicate clear diagnoses, the LAEPs recorded in oddball paradigms do provide useful information that can be used together with other clinical findings to evaluate patients with dementia (Aminoff & Goodin, 2008; Golub & Starr, 2007). Considering different patterns of abnormality in the LAEP waveform can be more informative than focusing on one wave of the response. Goodin and Aminoff (1986) found that the P3 wave was delayed in dementia caused by Alzheimer's disease, Parkinson's disease, and Huntington's disease. However, earlier waves of

the LAEP were differentially affected by the different disorders, with the N1 showing prolongation in both Parkinson's and Huntington's disease and the P2 being particularly prolonged in Huntington's disease. Yamaguchi, Tsuchiya, Yamagata, Yoyoda, and Kobayashi (2000) found that patients with either vascular dementia or Alzheimer's disease both showed prolongation of the P3 latency and reduction in P3 amplitude in the target LAEP. However, only the patients with vascular dementia showed an abnormally small and delayed P3 to novel stimuli such as bells and barks.

Human cognition is a highly complex process. Disorders of cognition have complicated presentations. To evaluate these disorders, we must integrate information from many sources. Electrophysiologic recordings will remain important. Even if we can diagnose a disease by a blood test, we need to see how the disease manifests itself in the brain as it processes information.

Schizophrenia

Early studies of the LAEPs in patients with schizophrenia found that the N1 (Saletu, Itil, & Saletu, 1971) and the P3 (Roth & Cannon, 1982) were smaller than in normal subjects. Because it was difficult to determine if these effects were related to the patients paying less attention to the stimuli than normal subjects, Baribeau-Braün, Picton, and Gosselin (1983) evaluated the LAEPs in a selective listening task. In general, the N1 was significantly smaller in schizophrenic subjects than in normal control subjects. However, at fast stimulus rates, the N1 was significantly increased by attention in schizophrenic subjects, indicating that they could selectively attend to one ear and ignore the other. At slower rates, the schizophrenic subjects showed no effect of attention on the N1. The P3 wave to the target was reduced in amplitude significantly in the schizophrenic subjects, but did occur appropriately for targets and not for standards. These findings suggested that the basic mechanisms of attention were intact in schizophrenic subjects but that they were not able to set up and maintain appropriate attentional strategies. Some of the results are shown in Figure 12–16. Michie, Fox, Ward, Catts, and McConaghy (1990) also studied the effects of selective attention on the LAEPs in schizophrenic subjects. They found that the schizophrenic subjects showed early Nd effects but these were not organized appropriately when the

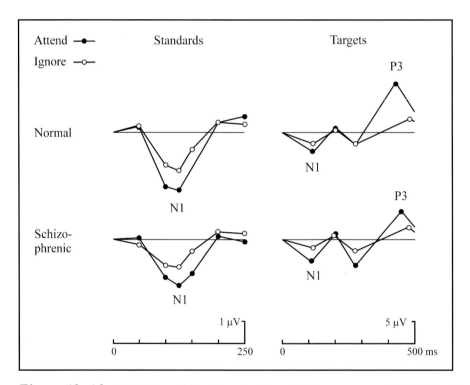

Figure 12–16. **LAEPs in schizophrenia.** *These findings compare the LAEPs of schizophrenic subjects to normal subjects while they performed a selective dichotic listening task with the stimuli presented at a rapid rate. In the left half of the figure are shown the responses to the standard stimuli. These were measured at set latencies during the initial 250 ms of the response. The schizophrenic subjects show a smaller N1 wave than the normal subjects but both groups show a significant increase in the N1 when the stimuli were in the attended ear. In the right half of the figure are shown the responses to the target stimuli. These were measured at the peaks and troughs of the waveform. Both subjects show enhanced N1 and P3 waves when the targets occurred in the attended ear. The P3 wave of the schizophrenic subjects was significantly smaller and later than in the normal subjects. Data from Baribeau-Braün et al. (1983).*

subjects had to select stimuli on the basis of pitch and location. In addition, the parietal P300 was substantially reduced. Mathalon, Heinks, and Ford (2004) confirmed that schizophrenic subjects could implement an early attentional filter during cross-modal selective attention but found that this could not be sustained. All of these studies suggest that the main deficit in schizophrenia resides in the executive control of attention.

As already discussed, the N1 to one's own voice is significantly reduced in normal subjects. This does not occur in schizophrenic subjects (Ford et al., 2001; Ford, Gray, Faustman, Roach, & Mathalon, 2007) and this decreased ability to tune out one's own voice correlates with auditory hallucination (Heinks-Maldonado, Mathalon, Houde, Gray, & Ford, 2007). Perhaps the typical auditory hallucinations that occur in schizophrenia are caused by an inability to distinguish between one's own subvocal thoughts and external sounds.

The extensive literature on the LAEPs in schizophrenia has been subjected to meta-analyses. Rosburg, Boutros, and Ford (2008) found that the N1 was reduced in schizophrenia but that this effect was only weakly related to psychophathology. The relationship between schizophrenia and the P300 (both the decrease in amplitude and the increase in latency) is more consistent, with the auditory oddball paradigm giving the most reproducible results (Jeon & Polich, 2003). An abnormal P300 is present in first-episode schizophrenics (e.g., Wang et al., 2010) and in first-degree relatives (Bramon et al., 2005), suggesting that it might be related to a genetic predisposition to develop the disorder. However, this is not always the case; de Wilde et al. (2008) found a small P300 in first-episode patients but not in healthy siblings.

CONCLUSION

Over this and the preceding chapter, we examined many different aspects of the LAEPs. We followed the roving standard and danced with the waltzing oddball. In some ways, we know a lot about how the brain processes auditory information, but in other ways we understand very little. Any model that we make of auditory perception (e.g., Figure 12–13) is an incomplete version of reality. Like a sketch, it may capture some aspects well, but it may miss others completely. Several authors have attempted to map auditory perception to the brain using the LAEPs (e.g., Dien et al., 2004; Näätänen, Kujala, & Winkler, in press). The different regions of the human brain are all connected and the processing of sounds involves extensive interacting networks (e.g., Ross et al., 2010). These networks are activated both by bottom-up sensory information and top-down cognitive expectancies.

Among the cortical networks operating during the LAEPs, we can distinguish four particular processes. First is the activation of the various regions of the auditory cortex on the superior surface of the temporal lobe. The N1 and P2 waves are related to this activation. Second is the relatively automatic detection of unexpected events. This involves an MMN and P3a system that is manifest in auditory cortex, hippocampus, and frontal lobes. Third is the selective processing of attended information manifest in the Nd (for stimulus selection) and N2 (for target discrimination) and involving interactions between frontal lobes and temporal cortex. Fourth is the putting together of appropriate responses (motor and cognitive) to the perceived world. This is manifest in the P3b wave generated with a focus in the temporoparietal regions and with connections to many other brain regions. The activity of these connections represents the working of our consciousness.

Because we began the previous chapter with a reference to Marcus Aurelius, we might end the present chapter with another quotation from the emperor. We have found that the LAEPs represent the interaction of bottom-up sensory information with top-down expectancies. Hearing is an interaction between sound waves and brain waves. The world is constantly changing and we must continue to interpret it as best we can. In the words of Marcus Aurelius (*Meditations*, IV-3, translation by George Long), "The universe is transformation: life is opinion."

ABBREVIATIONS

ABR	Auditory brainstem response
CNV	Contingent negative variation
EEG	Electroencephalography
EP	Evoked potential
LAEP	Late auditory evoked potential
MEG	Magnetoencephalography
MLR	Middle-latency response
MMN	Mismatch negativity
MRI	Magnetic resonance imaging
MP	Motor potential
Nd/Pd	Negative/positive difference wave
Ne/Pe	Error-related negativity/positivity
nHL	Normal hearing level
RP	Readiness potential
SOA	Stimulus onset asynchrony
RT	Reaction time
SP	Sustained potential
SPN	Stimulus preceding negativity
SW	Slow wave

REFERENCES

Ahveninen, J., Jääskeläinen, I. P., Raij, T., Bonmassar, G., Devore, S., Hämäläinen, M., . . . Belliveau, J. W. (2006). Task-modulated "what" and "where" pathways in human auditory cortex. *Proceedings of the National Academy of Sciences, USA, 103,* 14608–14613.

Alain, C., & Arnott, S. R. (2000). Selectively attending to auditory objects. *Frontiers in Bioscience, 5,* 202–212.

Alain, C., Arnott, S. R., Hevenor, S., Graham, S. & Grady, C. L. (2001) "What" and "where" in the human auditory system. *Proceedings of the National Academy of Sciences, USA, 98,* 12301–12306.

Alain, C., & Woods, D. L. (1994). Signal clustering modulates auditory cortical activity in humans. *Perception and Psychophysics, 56,* 501–516.

Alain, C., & Woods, D. L. (1997). Attention modulates auditory pattern memory as indexed by event-related brain potentials. *Psychophysiology, 34,* 534–546.

Alain, C., Woods, D. L., & Knight, R. T. (1998). A distributed cortical network for auditory sensory memory in humans. *Brain Research, 812,* 23–37.

Alho, K., Sams, M., Paavilainen, P., Reinikainen, K., & Näätänen, R. (1989). Event-related brain potentials reflecting processing of relevant and irrelevant stimuli during selective listening. *Psychophysiology, 26,* 514–528.

Alho, K., Töttölä, K., Reinikainen, K., Sams, M., & Näätänen, R., (1987). Brain mechanism of selective listening reflected by event-related potentials. *Electroencephalography and Clinical Neurophysiology, 68*, 458–470.

Alho, K., Woods, D.L. & Algazi, A. (1994) Processing of auditory stimuli during auditory and visual attention as revealed by event-related potentials. *Psychophysiology, 31*, 469–479.

Aminoff, M. J., & Goodin, D. S. (2008). Electrophysiological evaluation of dementia. In C. Duyckaerts & I. Litvan (Eds.), *Handbook of clinical neurology. Vol. 89. Dementias* (pp. 63–74). Amsterdam, The Netherlands: Elsevier.

Arnott, S. R., & Alain, C. (2002). Stepping out of the spotlight: MMN attenuation as a function of distance from the attended location. *NeuroReport, 13*, 2209–2212.

Baribeau-Braün, J., Picton, T. W., & Gosselin, J. Y. (1983). Schizophrenia: A neurophysiological evaluation of abnormal information processing. *Science, 219*, 874–876.

Bashore, T. R., Osman, A., & Heffley, E. F. (1989). Mental slowing in elderly persons: A cognitive psychophysiological analysis. *Psychology and Aging, 4*, 235–244.

Bäss, P., Jacobsen, T., & Schröger E. (2008). Suppression of the auditory N1 event-related potential component with unpredictable self-initiated tones: Evidence for internal forward models with dynamic stimulation. *International Journal of Psychophysiology, 70*, 137–143.

Bennys, K., Portet, F., Touchon, J., & Rondouin, G. (2007). Diagnostic value of event related evoked potentials N200 and P300 subcomponents in early diagnosis of Alzheimer's disease and mild cognitive impairment. *Journal of Clinical Neurophysiology, 24*, 405–412.

Bramon, E., McDonald, C., Croft, R. J., Landau, S., Filbey, F., Gruzelier, J. H., . . . Murray, R. M. (2005). Is the P300 wave an endophenotype for schizophrenia? A meta-analysis and a family study. *NeuroImage, 27*, 960–968.

Broadbent, D. E. (1971). Stimulus set and response set. In *Decision and stress* (pp. 177–190). London, UK: Academic Press.

Brunia, C. H. M. (1988). Movement and stimulus preceding negativity. *Biological Psychology, 26*, 165–178.

Brunia, C. H. M., & van Boxtel, G. J. M. (2004). Anticipatory attention to verbal and nonverbal stimuli is reflected in a modality-specific SPN. *Experimental Brain Research, 156*, 231–239.

Campbell, K. B., Courchesne, E., Picton, T. W., & Squires, K. C. (1979). Evoked potential correlates of human information processing. *Biological Psychology, 8*, 45–68.

Cherry, E. C. 1953. Some experiments on the recognition of speech with one and with two ears. *Journal of the Acoustical Society of America, 25*, 975–979.

Chwilla, D. J., & Brunia, C. H. (1991). Event-related potentials to different feedback stimuli. *Psychophysiology, 28*, 123–132.

Crapse, T. B., & Sommer, M. A. (2008). Corollary discharge across the animal kingdom. *Nature Reviews. Neuroscience, 9*, 587–600.

Croft, R. C., Gonsalvez, C. J., Gabriel, C., & Barry, R. J. (2003). Target-to-target interval versus probability effects on P300 in one- and two-tone tasks. *Psychophysiology, 40*, 322–328.

Curio, G., Neuloh, G., Numminen, J., Jousmaki, V., & Hari, R. (2000). Speaking modifies voice-evoked activity in the human auditory cortex. *Human Brain Mapping, 9*, 183–191.

Davis, H. (1964). Enhancement of evoked cortical potentials in humans related to a task requiring a decision. *Science, 145*, 182–183.

Degerman, A., Rinne, T., Särkkä, A. K., Salmi, J., & Alho, K. (2008). Selective attention to sound location or pitch studied with event-related brain potentials and magnetic fields. *European Journal of Neuroscience, 27*, 3329–3341.

Dehaene, S., Posner, M. I., & Tucker, D. M. (1994). Localization of a neural system for error detection and compensation. *Psychological Science, 5*, 303–305.

Desmedt, J. E. (1980). P300 in serial tasks: An essential post-decision closure mechanism. In H. H. Kornhuber & L. Deecke (Eds.),

Progress in brain research Vol. 54. Motivation, motor and sensory processes of the brain: Electric potentials, behaviour and clinical use (pp. 682–686). Amsterdam, The Netherlands: Elsevier.

de Wilde, O. M., Bour, L. J., Dingemans, P. M., Koelman, J. H., Boerée, T., & Linszen, D. H. (2008). P300 deficits are present in young first-episode patients with schizophrenia and not in their healthy young siblings. *Clinical Neurophysiology, 119,* 2721–2726.

Dien, J., Spencer, K. M., & Donchin, E. (2004). Parsing the "late positive complex": Mental chronometry and the ERP components that inhabit the neighborhood of the P300, *Psychophysiology, 41,* 665–678.

Donald, M. W. (1987). The timing and polarity of different attention-related ERP changes inside and outside of the attentional focus. In R. Johnson, Jr., J. W. Rohrbaugh, & R. Parasuraman (Eds.), *Current trends in event-related potential research* (pp. 81–86). Amsterdam, The Netherlands: Elsevier.

Donchin, E., & Coles, M. G. H. (1988). Is the P300 component a manifestation of context updating? *Behavioral and Brain Sciences, 11,* 357–374.

Duncan, C. C., Barry, R. J., Connolly, J. F., Fischer, C., Michie, P. T., Näätänen, R., . . . Van Petten, C. (2009). Event-related potentials in clinical research: Guidelines for eliciting, recording, and quantifying mismatch negativity, P300, and N400. *Clinical Neurophysiology, 120,* 1883–1908.

Duncan-Johnson, C. C., & Donchin, E. (1977). On quantifying surprise: The variation of event-related potentials with subjective probability. *Psychophysiology, 14,* 456–467.

Falkenstein, M., Hohnsbein, J., & Hoorman, J. (1994). Effects of choice complexity on different subcomponents of the late positive complex of the event-related potential. *Electroencephalography and Clinical Neurophysiology, 92,* 148–160.

Falkenstein, M., Hohnsbein, J., Hoormann, J., & Blanke, L. (1991). Effects of crossmodal divided attention on late ERP components. 2. Error processing in choice reaction tasks.

Electroencephalography and Clinical Neurophysiology, 78, 447–455

Fieger, A., Röder, B., Teder-Sälejärvi, W., Hillyard, S. A., & Neville, H. J. (2006). Auditory spatial tuning in late-onset blindness in humans. *Journal of Cognitive Neuroscience, 18,* 149–157.

Fitzgerald, P. G., & Picton, T. W. (1981). Temporal and sequential probability in evoked potential studies. *Canadian Journal of Psychology, 35,* 188–200.

Fitzgerald, P. G., & Picton, T. W. (1983). Event-related potentials during the discrimination of improbable stimuli. *Biological Psychology, 17,* 241–276,

Ford, J. M., Gray, M., Faustman, W. O., Roach, B. J., & Mathalon, D. H. (2007). Dissecting corollary discharge dysfunction in schizophrenia. *Psychophysiology, 44,* 522–529.

Ford, J. M., Mathalon, D. H., Kalba, S., Whitfield, S., Faustman, W. O., & Roth, W. T. (2001). Cortical responsiveness during talking and listening in schizophrenia: An event-related brain potential study. *Biological Psychiatry, 50,* 540–549.

Friedman, D., Simpson, G. V., & Hamberger, M. (1993). Age-related changes in scalp topography to novel and target stimuli. *Psychophysiology, 30,* 383–396.

Frodl, T., Hampel, H., Juckel, G., Bürger, K., Padberg, F., Engel, R. R., Möller, H. J., & Hegerl, U. (2002). Value of event-related P300 subcomponents in the clinical diagnosis of mild cognitive impairment and Alzheimer's disease. *Psychophysiology, 39,* 175–181

Gehring, W. J., Goss, B., Coles, M. G. H., Meyer, D. E., & Donchin, E. (1993). A neural system for error detection and compensation. *Psychological Science, 4,* 385–390.

Giard, M. H., Perrin, F., Pernier, J., & Bouchet, P. (1990). Brain generators implicated in processing of auditory stimulus deviance: A topographic event-related potential study. *Psychophysiology, 27,* 627–640.

Giard, M. H., Perrin, F., Pernier, J., & Peronnet, F. (1988). Several attention-related wave forms in auditory areas: A topographic study.

Electroencephalography and Clinical Neurophysiology, 69, 371–384.

Gironell, A., García-Sánchez, C., Estévez-González, A., Boltes, A., & Kulisevsky, J. (2005). Usefulness of P300 in subjective memory complaints: A prospective study. *Journal of Clinical Neurophysiology, 22,* 279–284.

Golob, E. J., Irimajiri, R., & Starr, A. (2007). Auditory cortical activity in amnestic mild cognitive impairment: relationship to subtype and conversion to dementia. *Brain, 130,* 740–752.

Golob, E. J., Johnson, J. K., & Starr, A. (2002). Auditory event-related potentials during target detection are abnormal in mild cognitive impairment. *Clinical Neurophysiology, 113,* 151–161.

Golob, E. J., Ringman, J. M., Irimajiri, R., Bright, S., Schaffer, B., Medina, L. D., & Starr, A. (2009). Cortical event-related potentials in preclinical familial Alzheimer disease. *Neurology, 73,* 1649–1655.

Golob, E. J., & Starr, A. (2007). Cognitive factors modulating auditory cortical evoked potentials. In R. F. Burkard, M. Don, & J. J. Eggermont (Eds.), *Auditory evoked potentials: Basic principles and clinical applications* (pp. 508–524). Baltimore, MD: Lippincott Williams & Wilkins.

Gonsalvez, C. J., Barry, R. J., Rushby, J. A., & Polich J. (2007). Target-to-target interval, intensity, and P300 from an auditory single-stimulus task. *Psychophysiology, 44,* 245–250.

Gonsalvez, C. J., Gordon, E., Grayson, S., Barry, R. J., Lazzaro, I., & Bahramali, H. (1999). Is the target-to-target interval a critical determinant of P3 amplitude? *Psychophysiology, 36,* 643–654.

Gonsalvez, C. J., & Polich, J. (2002). The target-to-target interval is the critical determinant of the P3. *Psychophysiology, 39,* 388–396.

Goodin, D. S., & Aminoff, M. J. (1986). Electrophysiological differences between subtypes of dementia. *Brain, 109,* 1103–1113.

Goodin, D. S., Aminoff, M. J., & Mantle, M. M. (1986). Subclasses of event-related potentials: response-locked and stimulus-locked components. *Annals of Neurology, 20,* 603–609.

Goodin, D. S., Squires, K. C., Henderson, B. H., & Starr, A. (1978). Age-related variations in evoked potentials to auditory stimuli in normal human subjects. *Electroencephalography and Clinical Neurophysiology, 44,* 447–458.

Goodin, D. S., Squires, K. C., & Starr A. (1978). Long latency event-related components of the auditory evoked potential in dementia. *Brain, 101,* 635–648.

Halgren, E., Marinkovic, K., & Chauvel, P. (1998). Generators of the late cognitive potentials in auditory and visual oddball tasks. *Electroencephalography and Clinical Neurophysiology, 106,* 156–164.

Hansen, J. C., & Hillyard, S. A. (1980). Endogenous brain potentials associated with selective auditory attention. *Electroencephalography and Clinical Neurophysiology, 49,* 277–290.

Hansen, J. C., & Hillyard, S. A. (1983). Selective attention to multidimensional auditory stimuli in man. *Journal of Experimental Psychology: Human Perception and Performance, 9,* 1–19.

Heinks-Maldonado, T. H., Mathalon, D. H., Gray, M., & Ford, J. M. (2005). Fine-tuning of auditory cortex during speech production. *Psychophysiology, 42,* 180–190.

Heinks-Maldonado, T. H., Mathalon, D. H., Houde, J. F., Gray, M., Faustman, W. O., & Ford, J. (2007). Relationship of imprecise corollary discharge in schizophrenia to auditory hallucinations. *Archives of General Psychiatry, 64,* 286–296.

Hillyard, S. A., Hink, R. F., Schwent, V. L., & Picton, T. W. (1973). Electrical signs of selective attention in the human brain. *Science, 182,* 177–180.

Hillyard, S. A., & Picton, T. W. (1987). Electrophysiology of cognition. In F. Plum (Ed.), *Handbook of physiology. Section 1 The nervous system Vol. V. Higher functions of the nervous system* (pp. 519–584). Bethesda, MD: American Physiological Society.

Hillyard, S. A., Squires, K. C., Bauer, J. W., & Lindsay, P. H. (1971). Evoked potential correlates of auditory signal detection. *Science, 172,* 1357–1360.

Hink, R. F., & Hillyard, S. A. (1976). Auditory evoked potentials during selective listening to dichotic speech messages. *Perception and Psychophysics, 20,* 236–242.

Hink, R. F., Van Voorhis, S. T., Hillyard, S. A., & Smith, T. S. (1977). The division of attention and the human auditory evoked potential. *Neuropsychologia, 15,* 597–605.

Holt, L. E., Raine, A., Pa, G., Schneider, L. S., Henderson, V. W., & Pollock, V. E. (1995). P300 topography in Alzheimer's disease. *Psychophysiology, 32,* 257–265.

Houde, J. F., Nagarajan, S. S., Sekihara, K., & Merzenich, M. M. (2002). Modulation of the auditory cortex during speech: an MEG study. *Journal of Cognitive Neuroscience, 14,* 1125–1138.

Iragui, V. J., Kutas, M., Mitchiner, M. R., & Hillyard, S. A. (1993). Effects of aging on event-related brain potentials and reaction times in an auditory oddball task. *Psychophysiology, 30,* 10–22.

Jeon, Y.-W., & Polich, J. (2003). Meta-analysis of P300 and schizophrenia: Patients, paradigms, and practical implications. *Psychophysiology, 40,* 684–701.

Johnson, R., Jr. (1986). A triarchic model of P300 amplitude. *Psychophysiology, 23,* 367–384.

Johnson, R., Jr., & Donchin, E. (1980). P300 and stimulus categorization: Two plus one is not so different from one plus one. *Psychophysiology, 17,* 167–178.

Juckel, G., Clotz, F., Frodl, T., Kawohl, W., Hampel, H., Pogarell, O., & Hegerl, U. (2008). Diagnostic usefulness of cognitive auditory event-related p300 subcomponents in patients with Alzheimer's disease? *Journal of Clinical Neurophysiology, 25,* 147–152.

Kauramäki, J., Jääskeläinen, I. P., & Sams, M., (2007). Selective attention increases both gain and feature selectivity of the human auditory cortex. *PLoS ONE, 2,* e909.

Kiehl, K. A., & Liddle, P. F. (2003). Reproducibility of the hemodynamic response to auditory oddball stimuli: A six-week test-retest study. *Human Brain Mapping, 18,* 42–52.

Kiehl, K. A., Liddle, P. F., & Hopfinger, J. B. (2000). Error processing and the rostral anterior cingulate: An event-related fMRI study. *Psychophysiology, 37,* 216–223.

Knight, R. T. (1984). Decreased response to novel stimuli after prefrontal lesions in man. *Electroencephalography and Clinical Neurophysiology, 59,* 9–20.

Knight, R. T. (1996). Contribution of human hippocampal region to novelty detection. *Nature, 383,* 256–259.

Knight, R. T., Hillyard, S. A., Woods, D. L., & Neville, H. J. (1981). The effects of frontal cortex lesions on event-related potentials during auditory selective attention. *Electroencephalography and Clinical Neurophysiology, 52,* 571–582.

Kopp, B. (2006). The P300 component of the event-related brain potential and Bayes' theorem. *Cognitive Sciences, 2,* 113–125.

Korczak, P. A., Kurtzberg, D., & Stapells, D. R. (2005). Effects of sensorineural hearing loss and personal hearing aids on cortical event-related potential and behavioral measures of speech-sound processing. *Ear and Hearing, 26,* 165–185.

Kornhuber, H. H., & Deecke, L. (1965). Hirnpotentialänderungen bei Willkurbewegungen und passiven Bewegungen des Menschen: Bereitschaftspotential und reafferente Potentiale. *Pflügers Archiv für die gesamte Physiologie des Menschen und der Tiere, 284,* 1–17.

Kutas, M., McCarthy, G., & Donchin, E. (1977). Augmenting mental chronometry: The P300 as a measure of stimulus evaluation time. *Science, 197,* 792–795.

Lange, K., Rösler, F., & Roder, B. (2003). Early processing stages are modulated when auditory stimuli are presented at an attended moment in time: An event-related potential study. *Psychophysiology, 40,* 806–817.

Linden, D. E. J., Prvulovic, D., Formisano, E., Völlinger, M., Zanella, F., Goebel, R. & Dierks, T. (1999). The functional neuroanatomy of target detection: An fMRI study of visual and auditory oddball tasks. *Cerebral Cortex, 9,* 815–823.

Magno, E., Yeap, S., Thakore, J. H., Garavan, H., De Sanctis, P., & Foxe, J. J. (2008). Are auditory-evoked frequency and duration mismatch negativity deficits endophenotypic for schizophrenia? High-density electrical mapping in clinically unaffected first-degree relatives and first-episode and chronic schizophrenia. *Biological Psychiatry, 64*, 385–391.

Maiste, A. C., & Picton, T. W. (1987). Auditory evoked potentials during selective attention. In C. Barber & T. Blum (Eds.), *Evoked potentials III* (pp. 385–391). Boston, MA: Butterworth.

Martikainen, M. H., Kaneko, K., & Hari, R. (2005). Suppressed responses to self-triggered sounds in the human auditory cortex. *Cerebral Cortex, 15*, 299–302.

Mathalon, D. H. Heinks, T., & Ford J. M. (2004). Selective attention in schizophrenia: Sparing and loss of executive control. *American Journal of Psychiatry, 161*, 872–881.

Mathalon, D. H., Whitfield, S. L., & Ford, J. M. (2003). Anatomy of an error: ERP and fMRI. *Biological Psychology, 64*, 119–141.

McCallum, W. C. (1988). Potentials related to expectancy, preparation and motor activity. In T. W. Picton (Ed.), *Handbook of electroencephalography and clinical neurophysiology. (Revised series) Volume 3. Human event-related potentials* (pp. 427–534). Amsterdam, The Netherlands: Elsevier.

McCarthy, G., & Donchin, E. (1976). The effects of temporal and event uncertainty in determining the waveforms of the auditory event related potential (ERP). *Psychophysiology, 13*, 581–590.

McCarthy, G., & Donchin E. (1981). A metric for thought: a comparison of P300 latency and reaction time. *Science, 211*, 77–80.

Mecklinger, A., & Ullsperger, P. (1993). P3 varies with stimulus categorization rather than probability. *Electroencephalography and Clinical Neurophysiology, 86*, 395–407.

Menon, V., Ford, J. M., Lim, K. O., Glover, G. H., & Pfefferbaum, A. (1997). Combined event-related fMRI and EEG evidence for temporal-parietal cortex activation during target detection. *NeuroReport, 8*, 3029–3037.

Michie, P. T., Bearpark, H. M., Crawford, J. M., & Glue, L. C. (1990). The nature of selective attention effects on auditory event-related potentials. *Biological Psychology, 30*, 219–250.

Michie, P. T., Fox, A. M., Ward, P. B., Catts V. S., & McConaghy, N. (1990). Event-related potential indices of selective attention and cortical lateralization in schizophrenia. *Psychophysiology, 27*, 209–227.

Miltner, W. H. R., Braun, C. H., & Coles, M.G.H. (1997). Event-related brain potentials following incorrect feedback in a time-production task: Evidence for a "generic" neural system for error detection. *Journal of Cognitive Neuroscience, 9*, 788–798.

Münte, T. F., Spring, D. K., Szycik, G. R., & Noesselt, T. (2010). Electrophysiological attention effects in a virtual cocktail-party setting. *Brain Research, 1307*, 78–88.

Näätänen, R. (1967). Selective attention and evoked potentials. *Annales Academiae Scientiarum Fennicae B, 151*, 1–226.

Näätänen, R. (1975). Selective attention and evoked potentials in humans—a critical review. *Biological Psychology, 2*, 237–307.

Näätänen, R. (1991). Mismatch negativity (MMN) outside strong attentional focus: A commentary on Woldorff et al. *Psychophysiology, 28*, 478–484.

Näätänen, R. (1992). *Attention and brain function*. Hillsdale, NJ: Lawrence Erlbaum.

Näätänen, R., & Escera, C. (2000). Mismatch negativity: Clinical and other applications. *Audiology and Neuro-Otology, 5*, 105–110.

Näätänen, R., Gaillard, A. W, & Mäntysalo, S. (1978). Early selective-attention effect on evoked potential reinterpreted. *Acta Psychologica, 42*, 313–329.

Näätänen,. R., Kujala, T., & Winkler, I. (in press). Mechanisms underlying conscious perception in audition: A unique window to central auditory processing opened by the mismatch negativity (MMN) and related responses. *Psychophysiology.*

Näätänen, R., & Michie, P. T. (1979). Early selective-attention effects on the evoked potential: A critical review and reinterpretation. *Biological Psychology, 8*, 81–136.

Näätänen, R., Paavilainen, P., Rinne, T., & Alho, K. (2007). The mismatch negativity (MMN) in basic research of central auditory processing: A review. *Clinical Neurophysiology, 118*, 2544–2590.

Näätänen, R., & Picton, T.W. (1986). N2 and automatic versus controlled processes. In W. C. McCallum, R. Zappoli, & F. Denoth, (Eds.), *Cerebral psychophysiology: Studies in event-related potentials of the brain. Electroencephalography and Clinical Neurophysiology Supplement 38* (pp. 171–188) Amsterdam, The Netherlands: Elsevier.

Näätänen, R., & Picton, T. W. (1987). The N1 wave of the human electric and magnetic response to sound: A review and an analysis of the component structure. *Psychophysiology, 24,* 375–425.

Nieuwenhuis, S., Yeung, N., & Cohen, J. D. (2004). Stimulus modality, perceptual overlap, and the go/no-go N2. *Psychophysiology, 41,* 157–160.

Norman, D. A., & Shallice, T. (1986). Attention to action: Willed and automatic control of behaviour. In R. J. Davidson, G. E. Schwartz, & D. Shapiro (Eds.), *Consciousness and self-regulation: Advances in research and theory* (Vol. 4, pp. 1–18). New York, NY: Plenum Press.

Novak, G., Ritter, W., & Vaughan, H. G., Jr. (1992). Mismatch detection and the latency of temporal judgements. *Psychophysiology, 29,* 398–411.

Novak, G., Ritter, W., Vaughan, H. G., Jr., & Wiznitzer, M. L. (1990). Differentiation of negative event-related potentials in an auditory discrimination task. *Electroencephalography and Clinical Neurophysiology, 75,* 255–275.

Oades, R. D., & Dittmann-Balcar, A. (1995). Mismatch negativity (MMN) is altered by directing attention. *NeuroReport, 6,* 1187–1190.

Oates, P. A., Kurtzberg, D., & Stapells, D. R. (2002). Effects of sensorineural hearing loss on cortical event-related potential and behavioral measures of speech-sound processing. *Ear and Hearing, 23,* 399–415.

Opitz, B., Mecklinger, A., von Cramon, D.Y., & Kruggel, F. (1999). Combining electrophysiological and hemodynamic measures of the auditory oddball. *Psychophysiology, 36,* 142–147.

Petkov, C.I., Kang, X., Alho, K., Bertranc, O., Yund, E. W., & Woods, D. L. (2004) Attentional modulation of human auditory cortex. *Nature Neuroscience, 7,* 658–663.

Pfefferbaum, A., Ford, J. M., Wenegrat, B. G., Roth, W. T., & Kopell, B. S. (1984). Clinical application of the P3 component of event-related potentials. I. Normal aging. *Electroencephalography and Clinical Neurophysiology, 59,* 85–103.

Pfefferbaum, A., Wenegrat, B. G., Ford, J. M., Roth, W. T., & Kopell, B. S. (1984). Clinical application of the P3 component of event-related potentials. II. Dementia, depression and schizophrenia. *Electroencephalography and Clinical Neurophysiology, 59,* 104–124.

Picton, T. W. (1992). The P300 wave of the human event-related potential. *Journal of Clinical Neurophysiology, 9,* 456–479.

Picton, T. W., Campbell, K. B., Baribeau-Braun, J., & Proulx, G.B. (1978). The neurophysiology of human attention: A tutorial review. In J. Requin (Ed.), *Attention and performance VII* (pp. 429–467). Hillsdale, NJ: Lawrence Erlbaum.

Picton, T. W., Cerri, A. M., Champagne, S. C., Stuss, D. T., & Nelson, R. F. (1986). The effects of age and task difficulty on the late positive component of the auditory evoked potentials. In W. C. McCallum, R. Zappoli, & F. Denoth (Eds.), *Cerebral psychophysiology: Studies in event-related potentials of the brain. Electroencephalography and Clinical Neurophysiology Supplement 38,* 132–133.

Picton, T. W., & Hillyard, S.A. (1974). Human auditory evoked potentials. II. Effects of attention. *Electroencephalography and Clinical Neurophysiology, 36,* 191–200,

Picton, T. W., Hillyard, S. A. & Galambos, R. (1976). Habituation and attention in the auditory system. In W. D. Keidel & W. D. Neff (Eds.), *Handbook of sensory physiology Vol. V/3. Auditory system. Clinical and special topics* (pp. 343–389). Berlin, Germany: Springer-Verlag.

Picton, T. W., Hillyard, S. A., Krausz, H. I., & Galambos, R. (1974). Human auditory evoked potentials. I. Evaluation of components. *Electroencephalography and Clinical Neurophysiology, 36,* 179–190.

Picton, T. W., Stuss, D. T., Champagne, S. C., & Nelson, R. F. (1984). The effects of age on human event-related potentials. *Psychophysiology, 21*, 312–325.

Polich, J. (1989). P300 from a passive auditory paradigm. *Electroencephalography and Clinical Neurophysiology, 74*, 312–320.

Polich, J. (1990). P300, probability, and interstimulus interval. *Psychophysiology, 27*, 396–403.

Polich, J. (1996). Meta-analysis of P300 normative aging studies. *Psychophysiology, 33*, 334–353.

Polich J. (1997). EEG and ERP assessment of normal aging. *Electroencephalography and Clinical Neurophysiology, 104*, 244–256.

Polich, J. (2007). Updating P300: An integrative theory of P3a and P3b. *Clinical Neurophysiology. 118*, 2128–2148.

Polich, J., & Corey-Bloom, J. (2005). Alzheimer's disease and P300: Review and evaluation of task and modality. *Current Alzheimer Research, 2*, 515–525.

Polich, J., & Herbst, K. (2000). P300 as a clinical assay: Rationale, evaluation, and findings. *International Journal of Psychophysiology, 38*, 3–19.

Rinne, T., Degerman, A., & Alho, K. (2005). Superior temporal and inferior frontal cortices are activated by infrequent sound duration decrements: An fMRI study. *NeuroImage, 26*, 66–72.

Rinne, T., Särkkä, A., Degerman, A., Schröger, E., & Alhof, K. (2006). Two separate mechanisms underlie auditory change detection and involuntary control of attention. *Brain Research, 1077*, 135–143.

Ritter, W., Simson, R., & Vaughan, H. G., Jr. (1972). Association cortex potentials and reaction time in auditory discrimination. *Electroencephalography and Clinical Neurophysiology, 33*, 547–555.

Ritter, W., Simson, R., Vaughan, H. G., Jr., & Friedman, D. (1979). A brain event related to the making of a sensory discrimination. *Science, 203*, 1358–1361.

Ritter, W., Sussman, E., Deacon, D., Cowan, N., & Vaughan, H. G., Jr. (1999). Two cognitive systems simultaneously prepared for opposite events. *Psychophysiology, 36*, 835–838.

Röder, B., Teder-Sälejärvi, W., Sterr, A., Rösler, F., Hillyard, S. A., &. Neville, H. J. (1999). Improved auditory spatial tuning in blind humans. *Nature, 400*, 162–166.

Rohrbaugh, J. W., & Gaillard, A. W. K. (1983). Sensory and motor aspects of the contingent negative variation. In A. W. K. Gaillard & W. Ritter (Eds.), *Tutorials in event-related potential research: Endogenous components* (pp. 269–310). Amsterdam, The Netherlands: North Holland.

Rosburg, T., Boutros, N. N., & Ford, J. M. (2008). Reduced auditory evoked potential component N100 in schizophrenia—a critical review. *Psychiatry Research, 161*, 259–274.

Ross, B., Hillyard, S. A., & Picton, T. W. (2010). Temporal dynamics of selective attention during dichotic listening. *Cerebral Cortex, 20*, 1360–1371.

Roth, W. T., Blowers, G. H., Doyle, C. M., & Kopell, B. S. (1982). Auditory stimulus intensity effects on components of the late positive complex. *Electroencephalography and Clinical Neurophysiology, 54*, 132–146.

Roth, W. T., & Cannon, E. H. (1972). Some features of the auditory evoked response in schizophrenics. *Archives of General Psychiatry, 27*, 466–471.

Ruchkin, D. S., & Sutton, S. (1978). Equivocation and P300 amplitude. In D. Otto (Ed.), *Multidisciplinary perspectives in event-related potential research* (pp. 175–177). Washington, DC: EPS 600/9-77-043, Government Printing Office.

Saletu, B., Itil, T. M., & Saletu, M. (1971). Auditory evoked response, EEG, and thought process in schizophrenics. *American Journal of Psychiatry, 128*, 336–344.

Sambeth, A., Maes, J. H., & Brankack, J. (2004). With long intervals, inter-stimulus interval is the critical determinant of the human P300 amplitude. *Neuroscience Letters, 359*, 143–146.

Sams, M., Aulanko, R., Hämäläinen, M., Hari, R., Lounasmaa, O. V., Lu, S.-T., & Simola, J. (1991). Seeing speech: visual information from lip movements modifies activity in the human auditory cortex. *Neuroscience Letters, 127*, 141–145.

Schafer, E. W., Amochaev, A., & Russell, M. J. (1981). Knowledge of stimulus timing attenuates human evoked cortical potentials. *Electroencephalography and Clinical Neurophysiology, 52*, 9–17.

Schafer, E. W., & Marcus, M. M. (1973). Self-stimulation alters human sensory brain responses. *Science, 181*, 175–177.

Schönwiesner, M., Novitski, N., Pakarinen, S., Carlson, S., Tervaniemi, M., & Näätänen, R. (2007). Heschl's gyrus, posterior superior temporal gyrus, and mid-ventrolateral prefrontal cortex have different roles in the detection of acoustic changes. *Journal of Neurophysiology, 97*, 2075–2082.

Schwent, V. L., Snyder, E., & Hillyard, S. A. (1976). Auditory evoked potentials during multichannel selective listening: Role of pitch and localization cues. *Journal of Experimental Psychology: Human Perception and Performance, 2*, 313–325.

Shahin, A. J., Alain, C., & Picton, T. W. (2006). Scalp topography and intracerebral sources for ERPs recorded during auditory target detection. *Brain Topography, 19*, 89–105,

Shallice, T., Stuss, D. T., Picton, T. W., Alexander, M. P., & Gillingham, S. (2008). Mapping task switching in frontal cortex through neuropsychological group studies. *Frontiers in Neuroscience, 2*, 79–85.

Shen, D., & Alain, C. (2010). Neuroelectric correlates of auditory attentional blink. *Psychophysiology, 47*, 184–191.

Shibasaki, H., & Hallett, M. (2006). What is the Bereitschaftspotential? *Clinical Neurophysiology, 117*, 2341–2356.

Smith, D. B., Donchin, E., Cohen, L., & Starr, A. (1970). Auditory averaged evoked potentials in man during selective binaural listening. *Electroencephalography and Clinical Neurophysiology, 28*, 146–152.

Snyder, E., & Hillyard, S. A. (1976). Long-latency evoked potentials to irrelevant, deviant stimuli. *Behavioral Biology, 16*, 319–331.

Soltani, M. & Knight, R.T. (2000). Neural origins of the P300. *Critical Reviews in Neurobiology, 14*, 199–224.

Spong, P., Haider, M., & Lindsley, D. B. (1965). Selective attentiveness and cortical evoked responses to visual and auditory stimuli. *Science, 148*, 395–397.

Squires, K. C., Hillyard, S. A., & Lindsay, P. L. (1973). Vertex potentials evoked during auditory signal detection: Relation to decision criteria. *Perception and Psychophysics, 14*, 265–272.

Squires, K. C., Wickens, C., Squires, N. K., & Donchin, E. (1976). The effect of stimulus sequence on the waveform of the cortical event-related potential. *Science, 193*, 1142–1146.

Squires, N. K., Squires, K. C., & Hillyard, S. A. (1975). Two varieties of long-latency positive waves evoked by unpredictable auditory stimuli. *Electroencephalography and Clinical Neurophysiology, 38*, 387–401.

Stekelenburg, J. J., Vroomen, J., & de Gelder, B. (2004). Illusory sound shifts induced by the ventriloquist illusion evoke the mismatch negativity. *Neuroscience Letters, 357*, 163–166.

Stuss, D. T., Shallice, T., Alexander, M. P., & Picton, T. W. (1995). A multidisciplinary approach to anterior attentional functions. *Annals of the New York Academy of Sciences, 769*, 191–211.

Stuss, D. T., & Picton, T. W. (1978). Neurophysiological correlates of human concept formation. *Behavioral Biology, 23*, 135–162.

Sussman, E., Ritter, W., & Vaughan, H. G., Jr. (1998). Attention affects the organization of auditory input associated with the mismatch negativity system. *Brain Research, 789*, 130–138.

Sutton, S. (1969). The specification of psychological variables in an average revoked potential experiment. In E. Donchin & D. B. Lindsley (Eds.), *Average evoked potentials: Methods, results and evaluations* (pp. 237–262). Washington, DC: NASA SP-191, Superintendent of Documents, Government Printing Office.

Sutton, S., Braren, M., & Zubin, J. (1965). Evoked potential correlates of stimulus uncertainty. *Science, 150*, 1187–1188.

Sutton, S., Tueting, P., Zubin, J., & John, E. R. (1967). Information delivery and the sensory evoked potential. *Science, 155*, 1436–1439.

Teder-Sälejärvi, W. A., Hillyard, S. A. Röder, B., & Neville, H. J. (1999). Spatial attention to central and peripheral auditory stimuli as indexed by event-related potentials. *Cognitive Brain Research, 8,* 213–227.

Vaughan, H. G.. Jr., & Ritter, W. (1970). The sources of auditory evoked responses recorded from the human scalp. *Electroencephalography and Clinical Neurophysiology, 28,* 360–367.

Verleger, R. (1988). Event-related potentials and cognition: A critique of the context-updating hypothesis and an alternative interpretation of P3. *Behavioral and Brain Science, 11,* 343–356.

Verleger, R. (1997). On the utility of P3 latency as an index of mental chronometry. *Psychophysiology, 34,* 131–156.

Verleger, R., & Berg, P. (1991). The waltzing odd-ball. *Psychophysiology, 28,* 468–477.

Verleger, R., Jaśkowskis, P., & Wascher, E. (2005). Evidence for an integrative role of P3b in linking reaction to perception. *Journal of Psychophysiology, 19,* 182–194.

Walter, W. G., Cooper, R., Aldridge, V. J., McCallum, W. C., & Winter, A. L. (1964). Contingent negative variation: An electric sign of sensorimotor association and expectancy in the human brain. *Nature, 203,* 380–384.

Wang, J., Tang, Y., Li, C., Mecklinger, A., Xiao, Z., Zhang, M., Hirayasu, Y., & Hokama, H., Li, H. (2010). Decreased P300 current source density in drug-naive first episode schizophrenics revealed by high density recording. *International Journal of Psychophysiology, 75,* 249–257.

Woldorff, M. G., Hackley, S. A., & Hillyard, S. A. (1991). The effects of channel-selective attention on the mismatch negativity wave elicited by deviant tones. *Psychophysiology, 28,* 30–42.

Woldorff, M. G., & Hillyard, S. A. (1991). Modulation of early auditory processing during selective listening to rapidly presented tones. *Electroencephalography and Clinical Neurophysiology, 79,* 170–191.

Woldorff, M. G., Hillyard, S. A., Gallen, C. C., Hampson, S. A., & Bloom, F. E. (1998). Magnetoencephalographic recordings demonstrate attentional modulation of mismatch-related neural activity in human auditory cortex. *Psychophysiology, 35,* 283–292.

Woods, D. L. (1990). The physiological basis of selective attention: Implications of event-related potential studies. In J. W. P. Rohrbaugh & R. Johnson Jr. (Eds.), *Event-related brain potentials: Basic issues and applications* (pp. 178–209). Oxford, UK: Oxford University Press.

Woods, D. L., Alho, K., & Algazi, A. (1994). Stages of auditory feature conjunction: An event-related brain potential study. *Journal of Experimental Psychology: Human Perception and Performance, 22,* 81–94.

Woods, D. L., & Courchesne, E. (1986). The recovery functions of auditory event-related potentials during split-second discriminations. *Electroencephalography and Clinical Neurophysiology, 65,* 304–315.

Woods, D. L., Hillyard, S. A., & Hansen, J. C. (1984). Event-related brain potentials reveal similar attentional mechanisms during selective listening and shadowing. *Journal of Experimental Psychology: Human Perception and Performance, 10,* 761–777.

Woods, D. L., Knight, R. T., & Scabini, D. (1993). Anatomical substrates of auditory selective attention: behavioral and electrophysiological effects of posterior association cortex lesions. *Cognitive Brain Research, 1,* 227–240.

Woods. D. L., Stecker, G. C., Rinne, T., Herron, T. J., Cate, A. D., Yund, E. W., . . . Kang, X. (2009). Functional maps of human auditory cortex: Effects of acoustic features and attention. *PLoS One, 4*(4), e5183.

Yamaguchi, S., Tsuchiya, H., Yamagata, S., Toyoda, G., & Kobayashi, S. (2000). Event-related brain potentials in response to novel sounds in dementia. *Clinical Neurophysiology, 111,* 195–203.

13

Infant Hearing Assessment: Opening Ears

> And straightway his ears were opened, and the string of his tongue was loosed, and he spake plain.
>
> And he charged them that they should tell no man: but the more he charged them, so much the more a great deal they published it;
>
> And were beyond measure astonished, saying, He hath done all things well: he maketh both the deaf to hear and the dumb to speak.
>
> Mark (King James Version), 7: 35–37.

This chapter reviews how physiologic measurements can be used to assess hearing in newborn babies and young infants. Currently, this is the most important application of the auditory evoked potentials (EPs). It is where miracles happen: where hearing impairment is detected and treated so that those once destined to become deaf can begin to hear and learn to speak.

Hearing is necessary for the normal development of speech and language. Children born with hearing impairment begin to babble but, without auditory feedback, they will not develop normal speech. Language still can develop through signing, but usually not as extensively as in the normal child. Because speech and language develop most rapidly during the first few years of life, we must find children who are born with a hearing impairment (or who acquire a hearing loss in infancy) as soon as possible and provide them with hearing and language support during this critical period. In the words of Marion Downs (1976), an indefatigable champion of infant hearing, we must ensure "a bountiful intake of sensory material in the first two years of the child's life."

NEWBORN HEARING SCREENING

Historical Background

Unfortunately, detecting hearing impairment in an infant is not easy. Newborn infants do not raise their fingers when a tone is presented nor do they repeat words when they are spoken. Newborn infants can be startled by loud sounds. However, mild and moderate hearing losses may not be detected by these responses. Startle responses are elicited by high-intensity sounds, and can occur even in the presence of a moderate hearing loss if there is recruitment. Furthermore, infants who are unwell may not respond normally even when the sensory system is working. Procedures measuring heart rate or startle movements were found to be too variable to provide a reliable assessment of hearing status (e.g., Durieux-Smith, Picton, Edwards, Goodman, & MacMurray, 1985). Early recordings of the auditory EPs in infants showed promise, but before the auditory brainstem (ABR) became available, these responses were problematic. Infant middle-latency responses (MLRs) were small and clearly recognizable only at slow rates (Jerger, Chmiel, Glaze, & Frost, 1987) and the late auditory evoked potentials (LAEPs) varied with the infant's state of arousal (e.g., Taguchi, Picton, Orpin, & Goodman, 1969).

The current approach to detecting hearing impairment in infancy required the development of two physiologic tests: the ABR and otoacoustic emissions (OAEs). Recordings of these two responses to sound are illustrated in Figure 13–1. Hecox and Galambos (1974) showed that the ABR could be reliably recorded in infants and that these responses could be used to esti-mate auditory thresholds. Galambos and his colleagues then embarked on a 20-year 5,901 infant study (Galambos, Wilson, & Silva, 1994) of how the ABR could be used to assess hearing in babies in a neonatal intensive care unit. Several studies followed up infants who were tested in this way and demonstrated the sensitivity and specificity of ABR testing (e.g., Durieux-Smith, Picton, Bernard, MacMurray, & Goodman, 1991; Hyde, Riko, & Malizia, 1990). Near the same time, Kemp, Ryan, and Bray (1990) provided OAE techniques that could be used as a rapid test of normal infant hearing, and White and Behrens (1993) completed an extensive study of how the OAEs could be used to screen infants for hearing loss in Rhode Island.

By 1993, the stage was set for important decisions (Gravel & Tocci, 1998). The National Institutes of Health (1993) convened a consensus conference to review the data concerning infant hearing impairment. The conference found the ABR and OAE to be valid and reliable ways to test infant hearing. In addition, the conference reviewed the accumulating epidemiologic data showing that more than half of young children with permanent hearing impairment had no discernible risk factors. Therefore, simply testing those at risk would miss large numbers of children with hearing impairment. The conference therefore recommended universal hearing screening for all infants within the first 3 months of age. A two-stage screening process was proposed: OAEs as the first test and ABRs as a follow-up for those babies failing OAEs. Similar conclusions soon were reached in other countries (e.g., United Kingdom: Davis et al. 1997; Europe: Grandori & Lutman, 1998). By the new millennium, the idea of universal newborn hearing screening was widely accepted and screening programs

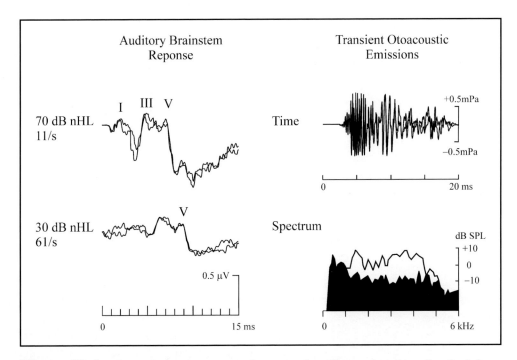

Figure 13–1. *Physiologic measures of neonatal auditory function. On the left are shown the ABRs evoked by clicks. The upper tracings show replicate responses at high intensity and slow rates. These responses clearly show waves I, III, and V. The lower tracings show that wave V of the response is still recognizable when the intensity is decreased to 30 dB nHL. On the right are shown the OAEs evoked by a click at 85 dB pSPL (adapted from Kemp et al., 1990). The upper tracings show the OAE waveforms plotted in the time domain. The early part of the tracing, which would have shown the click stimulus, has been zeroed. The OAE response measured in neonates is about 10 dB larger than in the adult OAE. The lower right shows the spectrum of the response (shaded white) together with the estimated acoustic noise (shaded black). The OAE response is visible above the acoustic noise at frequencies from 1 to 5 kHz.*

soon became available. From 1999 to 2007, the percentage of newborn infants screened for hearing impairment in the United States increased from 47% to 97% (Gaffney, Eichwald, Grosse, & Mason, 2010).

This chapter is mainly concerned with how the auditory EPs contribute to our present programs for hearing-impaired infants. Table 13–1 summarizes the components of a typical program. There are three basic stages: identification, evaluation, and intervention. Auditory EPs play an

essential role in identification and assessment. Once the hearing-impaired infant is detected and assessed, we must determine whether any treatment is needed, decide on a program of management, and begin training in speech and hearing. EPs may help during the initial course of management and training, but subjective behavioral testing soon takes over. The path from detection to training must flow smoothly so that no hearing-impaired infant ever gets lost along the way.

Table 13–1. Role of Physiologic Tests in Neonatal Hearing Screening

	Identification	*Evaluation*	*Intervention*
Process	Screening	Audiometry	Monitoring
Present	OAEs click-ABRs	Tone-ABRs OAEs 1-kHz-Tympanometry	Prescriptive fitting Behavioral testing
Possible	ASSRs to clicks, noise, chirps, or tones OAEs with contralateral suppression	Multiple ASSRs	Suprathreshold ASSRs LAEPs

The Concept of Objective Audiometry

Older infants can be assessed using behavioral responses. After the age of about 6 months, almost all normal infants can be examined using conditioned orientation responses, looking toward the source of a sound in order to see something appealing. By the age of about 2 years, children can be assessed by involving them in hearing games and providing high levels of social reinforcement for their performance—play audiometry. These behavioral techniques are considered "subjective." The subject being tested must decide whether he or she has heard the sound and must then communicate this to the examiner. The decision and the communication may be either reflex (the orientation response) or conscious (playing).

Infants below the age of 6 months and older infants who are unable to cooperate with behavioral testing (such as the developmentally delayed) cannot be accurately assessed using these techniques. These subjects must be tested using measurements that do not require the subject to make a decision or provide a behavioral response. In "objective audiometry," the examiner measures a physiologic response to a sound. This physiologic measurement may be more or less distant from the auditory system. At some distance, we can record a startle reflex by detecting the movements of a baby following a sound or by measuring the change in heart rate. Electrical measurements of the responses of the cochlea or brain to sound are more direct. They are not susceptible to errors caused by abnormalities in the musculoskeletal or cardiovascular systems that might prevent any response to a sound even when it is heard.

As Dobie (1993) has pointed out, fully objective audiometry eliminates the need for subjective response from the examiner as well as the examinee. The assessment should not depend on the examiner's (subjective) interpretations of whether a response is present or whether it is abnormal. Having a computer make these judgments on the basis of strict criteria is better than having the examiner decide on the basis of undefined intuition.

However, nothing is fully objective. The subject examined during evoked potential audiometry must allow the recording electrodes to be placed on the scalp, and must stay reasonably still and quiet during the recording. No matter how sophisticated the computer assessment of the responses, the initial decisions about which test to use and the final estimations of behavioral hearing thresholds from physiologic thresholds always remain with the examiner.

Evoked potential audiometry is essential during early infancy. There is no other way to assess the hearing of young infants with sufficient accuracy to decide about management. The thresholds obtained with evoked potential audiometry can be used to determine how powerful a hearing aid to use. If the thresholds indicate a profound hearing loss, they can become part of an extensive set of clinical findings that may make us consider a cochlear implant (when the child's age is 1 year or older). Evoked potential audiometry also is important in other situations where subjective responses to sound are not available or unreliable: mentally challenged or emotionally disturbed patients, subjects with a nonorganic hearing loss, patients in coma or under anesthesia, and elderly subjects. This chapter is concerned with infants but many of the principles we review also apply in these other contexts.

Justification for Newborn Hearing Screening

We first consider the evidence that justifies newborn hearing screening and its protocols: Why and how should we identify hearing impaired infants? Screening is worthwhile if the benefits that accrue from detecting a disorder are greater than the costs incurred during the screening process (Porter, Neely, & Gorga, 2009).

Screening therefore is justifiable only if the patient detected by screening can be treated or managed effectively. Unfortunately, it is not clear how the management of hearing-impairment should be evaluated. The simple ability to hear sounds may be the most powerful of all justifications; better hearing is clearly sufficient reason for the treatment of adults with hearing impairment (Hyde, 2005). Management with a hearing aid or a cochlear implant makes the world more clearly audible. Given the assumption that all infants should have access to sound, all that is needed to justify neonatal hearing screening is to show that it leads to earlier detection and provision of hearing aids. The effect of screening on the age of detection must be disentangled from the confounding factor that the age of detection for unscreened infants varies with the degree of hearing-impairment with more severe impairments being noticed earlier. With due consideration to these confounding factors, newborn screening definitely decreases the age when a hearing loss is diagnosed and therefore increases the time that an infant can experience sound (Durieux-Smith, Fitzpatrick, & Whittingham, 2008; Sininger, Grimes, & Christensen, 2009).

Because infants with hearing impairment can be treated or managed in many different ways, other measurements of the efficacy of early management are complex. Age-appropriate development of speech and language often is considered an important criterion, but this will vary with the type of training and the degree of hearing loss. Infants with hearing impairment who are detected and managed with hearing aids before the age of 6 months (and if necessary later provided with cochlear implants) develop spoken language more rapidly than infants who are not detected until later. At the age of 2 or 3 years, oral language scores of hearing-impaired infants who are provided with amplification before the age of 6 months generally are within the lower limits of the scores of normal-hearing children, whereas the scores of infants for whom intervention occurred later are lower than normal (reviewed by Yoshinaga-Itano, 2003). However, these studies are difficult to evaluate because other variables are correlated with the age at which an infant's hearing impairment is detected (Thompson et al., 2001). Recent evidence is more convincing: hearing-impaired children whose management began before the age of 9 months showed significantly better language scores at ages 5 to 11 years than an equivalent group of hearing-impaired children whose management began later (Kennedy et al., 2006; Watkin et al., 2007). A recent review of such studies (Nelson, Bougatsos, & Nygren, 2008) led the U.S. Preventive Services Task Force (2008) to recommend that all newborn infants be screened for hearing loss. Sininger et al. (2009, 2010) recently demonstrated that early detection decreases the age at which intervention is provided to a hearing-impaired infant and that this increases the ability of the child to communicate orally and aurally.

Given that early detection is beneficial, we then must consider the costs of screening. Because screening a population costs about the same regardless of the prevalence of the detected disorder (as all of the population must be screened), the cost-benefit ratio of screening varies inversely with the prevalence of the disorder (because each detection leads to a benefit). An important reason for newborn hearing screening therefore is that the prevalence of hearing loss in newborn infants is high relative to other disorders for which screening is used. The actual prevalence will depend on the criteria for what is con-

sidered a significant hearing loss. These usually include the characteristics "permanent" and "bilateral." The prevalence generally is about 1.5 per 1000 for a permanent bilateral hearing loss with the better ear having a pure tone average threshold greater than 40 dB HL (hearing level). Figure 13–2 presents the prevalence data reviewed by Fortnum (2003) as well as more recent data presented by Bamford et al. (2007). About one third of the infants identified with significant hearing loss have a loss of severe or profound degree.

Many risk factors are related to hearing loss in the newborn period. The most common is a family history of hearing loss. Other important etiologic factors are craniofacial abnormalities, intrauterine infections, prematurity, perinatal anoxia, and ototoxic drugs. Table 13–2 presents the incidence of these risk factors (derived from Fortnum, 2003). Because most of the risk factors (except the family history) occur in infants admitted to a neonatal intensive care unit, the initial approach to newborn screening combined screening babies in the neonatal intensive care unit with tracking down infants with a family history of congenital hearing loss. It soon became apparent that about three quarters of the children born with a significant hearing loss had not been treated in the neonatal intensive care unit. Therefore, to be effective, a screening program would have to check all infants not just those admitted to a neonatal intensive care unit.

As we have seen, these facts led the Joint Committee on Infant Hearing (2000) to recommend universal newborn hearing screening using physiologic measurements for the identification of infants, and a subsequent extensive follow-up evaluation of infants not passing the initial screen. More recent recommendations of the Joint Committee (2007) are quite specific for

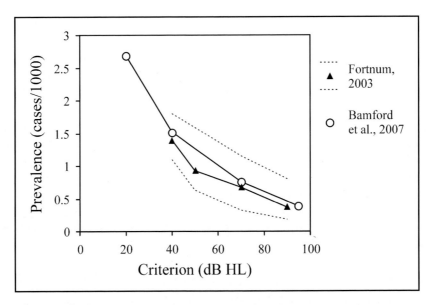

Figure 13–2. *Prevalence of permanent bilateral sensorineural hearing loss in childhood. Data from the 17 studies reviewed in Table 1 of Fortnum (2003) are plotted as weighted means (triangles) together with range of values reported in the different studies (dashed lines). In addition, more recent data from Appendix 3 of Bamford et al. (2007) are plotted (circles), as these also estimate the prevalence of mild hearing loss. The criterion is the pure tone average threshold in the best ear.*

Table 13–2. Risk Factors for Permanent Childhood Hearing Impairment

Risk Factor	Percentage (Range)[a]	Weighted Average[b]
Family history	14–40	29
Neonatal intensive care unit >48 hours	11–35	28
Craniofacial abnormality	2–24	10
Ototoxic medication	2–21	9
Congenital infection (TORCH[c])	1–7	5
Mechanical ventilation (>5 days)	0–10	4
Prematurity (<1500 g)	0–8	4
Hyperbilirubinemia	0–9	3
No known risk factors	19–61	41

[a]Incidence is % of hearing-impaired infants with risk factor. Data were taken from Table 4 of Fortnum (2003). Note that infants can have multiple risk factors and that these percentages therefore do not add to 100.

[b]Obtained by weighting available data by number of hearing-impaired children evaluated in each study.

[c]TORCH is an antibody test that evaluates whether there is or has been an infection with toxoplasmosis, rubella, cytomegalovirus, or herpes simplex. The test often checks for other infectious agents as well.

screening: ABRs must be recorded in infants in the neonatal intensive care unit, but either the OAEs or the ABR can be used for screening other infants. The guidelines also propose that a battery of tests be used in the follow-up assessment of infants identified by the screening procedure. ABRs to air- and bone-conducted tones, OAEs, and 1000-Hz tympanometry are recommended. The joint committee considered the evidence insufficient at the time of their report to justify using other techniques such as electrocochleography (ECochG), ASSRs, or middle-ear muscle reflexes in the assessment of infant hearing impairment. Furthermore, the committee did not provide guidance on how electrophysiologic measurements could play a role in the fitting of hearing aids or in the decision to provide a cochlear implant.

SCREENING PROTOCOLS

Newborn hearing screening can be effectively and efficiently performed using either the OAEs or the ABRs. Each approach has its advantages and disadvantages. Spivak (1998) and Norton et al. (2000) provide details about the methods and results of different screening procedures.

OAE Screening

The rationale behind the OAE screen is that the presence of emissions in response to sounds of moderate intensity indicates normal external hair cells in the cochlea. We then can conclude that the hearing threshold will be within 30 dB of normal provided that there is no dysfunction in the inner hair cell, auditory nerve, or central nervous system. The test is susceptible to increased acoustic noise in the environment, which can be a problem if the

testing is carried out in an active intensive care unit. The most common technical problem during OAE recordings is an inability to maintain an effective seal for the probe in the external auditory meatus. OAE tests are particularly compromised by conductive hearing loss. This is not as much because the stimulus is attenuated when reaching the cochlea as because the emissions are attenuated when leaving the cochlea. An attenuation of 20 dB in the outgoing OAE signal can render it undetectable when the signal-to-noise ratio (SNR) of the recorded OAE typically is 10 to 15 dB.

Two kinds of OAEs can be evaluated during screening. Transient OAEs are generated in response to a brief stimulus such as a click. Screening with transient OAEs typically is based on the total response over all recorded frequencies, although the higher frequencies will contribute more to the measurement than the low. Distortion-product OAEs are responses generated at the frequency 2f1-f2 by the nonlinear processing of a simultaneously presented pair of tones f1 and f2. Because distortion-product OAEs in the neonatal period can be recorded only at higher frequencies, screening systems typically check for responses between 2000 and 5000 Hz.

ABR Screening

ABR-screening can be performed in two contexts. In automatic ABR recordings, the response is evoked by a click presented at an intensity of 35 dB nHL (normal hearing level) and a relatively rapid rate (generally 30 or more clicks/s). The response is assessed as present or absent by means of computer algorithms that compare the recorded waveform to a template for the normal response in newborn infants. Typically, the template weights most strongly at the latencies of wave V and the aftergoing vertex-negative wave. In conventional ABR recordings, the response is recorded (often to clicks presented at a slower rate than in the automatic recordings) and the waveform is interpreted by the examiner, usually with the help of some SNR measurement such as the F-ratio at a single point (Fsp: Sininger, 2007).

Because ABR recordings require electrodes to be attached to the scalp, ABR testing takes a little longer time than that required for OAEs. Although not as susceptible to conductive hearing loss as OAEs, ABRs require the infant to be quietly asleep to decrease the level of the electrical noise generated by the muscles. Technical problems that occur with ABR recordings usually involve the placement of the electrodes or the presence of high levels of nonphysiologic electrical noise generated by the machinery in the neonatal intensive care unit. The main advantage of ABR screening is that it can detect the presence of abnormalities in auditory processing proximal to the hair cell. Auditory neuropathy will not be detected by OAE screening. Because many of the risk factors for auditory neuropathy (such as hyperbilirubinemia) are criteria for admission to a neonatal intensive care unit, ABR screening is recommended for infants who are treated in a neonatal intensive care unit (Joint Committee, 2007).

Sample protocols for neonatal hearing screening are given in Figure 13–3. Automatic ABR testing is recommended for the neonatal intensive care unit. For infants seen in well-baby nurseries, some programs use the same protocol but most programs use OAEs (either transient or distortion products) as a first screening test. In the protocols shown in the figure, a repeat testing before discharge is provided for the newborn infant who fails the first screening assessment. This formal rescreening (at about 1 month of age) is most commonly done using the automatic ABR (although some programs also repeat the OAE testing).

Referral Rates from Screening Protocols

The expense of screening is relatively low compared to the expense of a full hearing evaluation by a pediatric audiologist. Therefore, every effort is made to reduce the rate of referral for further testing as much as possible without decreasing the sensitivity of the screening. The sensitivity and specificity of screening usually are assessed on the presence or absence of a permanent hearing loss of 40 dB or more. The sensitivity of screening (the percentage of hearing-impaired infants detected as impaired) is high, somewhere between 95 and 100%. The specificity of screening (the percentage of normal-hearing infants detected as normal) also is very high. However, specificity is not quite 100%. Because normal hearing is much more common than hearing impairment, many infants who will later be determined to have normal hearing are still referred for further testing. If only one test is performed, the referral rate from screening might be anywhere between 5 and 20%. If the initial test is abnormal, repeating the test at a later time in the neonatal stay decreases the referral rate, perhaps because of better recording-conditions for the second test or because of the increased age of the infant at the time of the second test (and the resolution of any conductive loss). Finally, a confirmatory screening test at a later time (even at a month after discharge) also can be used to decrease the rate of referral for a full audiologic evaluation. With protocols for repeated

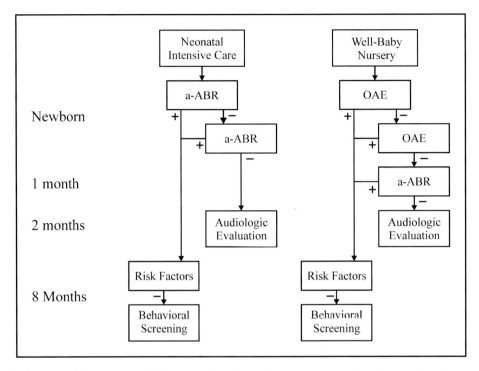

Figure 13–3. Protocols for newborn hearing screening. These two protocols are representative of the great variety presently being used. The protocol on the left, based on automatic ABR screening, is appropriate for screening babies in a neonatal intensive care unit, but can also be used for well babies. The protocol on the right, based on OAEs, is the most commonly used but this is not appropriate for babies in a neonatal intensive care unit, because of the possibility of auditory neuropathy. The risk register and behavioral testing suggested at 8 months is to catch those babies with postnatal hearing loss. Exactly how this should be done is not presently clear. Risk factors for postnatal hearing loss are given in Table 13–3.

testing (both in hospital and after discharge), the referral rate can be reduced to the benchmark of 4% recommended by the Joint Committee on Infant Hearing (2007). Although both types of screening (OAE and ABR) can provide referral rates close to this benchmark, slightly higher numbers tend to occur for the OAE screening (Vohr et al., 2001: ABR 3.2%, two-step OAE-ABR 4.7%, click-OAE 6.4%). The higher rate for the click-OAE screening protocols may be related to mild transient conductive hearing losses occurring in the neonatal period (which can affect the OAE more than the ABR). As more experience has been gained, the referral rates from screening programs have decreased. Johnson et al. (2005) found that a two-stage screening process with initial OAE testing followed by automatic ABR testing gave average referral rates of 4.8% after the initial OAE stage and 1.0% after the ABR follow-up.

New Developments in Newborn Screening

ASSRs may become helpful in screening for hearing impairment in infancy. Savio and Perez-Abalo (2008) have investigated the possibility of using ASSRs to 500- and 2000-Hz tones as a newborn screening tool and found it promising. However, the ASSRs evoked by tones in newborns are small (John, Brown, Muir, & Picton, 2004) and demonstrating reliable responses might take too long for screening. ASSRs evoked by rapidly presented clicks (Stürzebecher, Cebulla, & Neumann, 2003), chirps (Elberling, Don, Cebulla, & Stürzebecher, 2007), or amplitude-modulated white noise (Picton, 2007) can be quickly recorded and objectively recognized. These approaches may make it easier to record ASSRs in the newborn period. Figure 13–4 shows some responses to amplitude-modulated white noise in the newborn period.

One of the disadvantages of ABR recording is the time taken to affix the electrodes to the scalp. A new system, the BERA-Phone, combines the electrodes and the auditory stimulator in one handheld device (Melagrana, Casale, Calevo, & Tarantino,

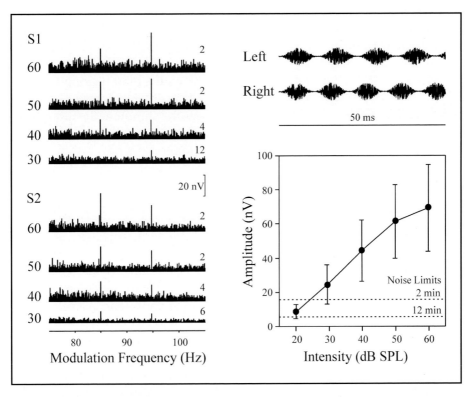

Figure 13–4. Responses to amplitude-modulated white noise in newborn infants. The stimuli are shown in the upper right of the figure; the modulation frequency was 85 Hz for the left ear and 95 Hz for the right ear. On the left are shown the responses of two newborn infants (S1 and S2) at different stimulus levels (dB SPL). Normal behavioral thresholds in an adult are near 18 dB SPL. S1 responses are clearly seen to 40 dB and the response is still recognizable in the right ear at 30 dB SPL. S2 responses are clearly seen down to 30 dB SPL in both ears. The numbers to the right of the responses represent the duration of the recording in minutes. The graph in the lower right shows the mean amplitudes for 51 infants. The horizontal dotted lines show mean p <0.05 confidence limits for the noise after 2 and 12 minutes of recording.

2007). The electrodes are covered with conductive paste and held in place on the scalp while the testing is performed.

A main disadvantage of using the OAEs in screening is that they do not test the function of the auditory nerve. However, measuring the suppression of emissions by contralateral noise assesses the auditory nerves as well as reflex connections in the brainstem (James, Harrison, Pienkowski, Dajani, & Mount, 2005). Thus, we might conceive of an OAE testing procedure that evaluates the cochlea by the OAEs recorded in response to ipsilateral stimuli and evaluates the contralateral auditory nerve by the response of these OAEs to contralateral noise.

ISSUES FOR NEWBORN HEARING SCREENING

Mild Hearing Loss

Screening protocols are designed to detect hearing impairments of 40 dB HL or greater and will miss mild hearing losses or hearing losses at some frequencies and not others (J. L. Johnson et al., 2005). OAE screening presents stimuli at moderate intensity and, if emissions are present, concludes that the external hair cells are functioning correctly and that the hearing thresholds should therefore be below 30 dB HL. However, mild hearing losses may still show OAEs, and the OAEs related to the frequencies of 1500 Hz or lower are difficult to assess in newborns because of the higher levels of acoustic noise at these frequencies. ABR screening will miss infants with mild hearing loss or infants with hearing loss that spares some range of frequencies (Durieux-Smith et al., 1991). This is illustrated in Figure 13–5. Children with a hearing loss that is mild or restricted to

certain frequencies should still be detected at some time. Exactly how this is best done remains unclear.

Stimulus and Calibration Issues

The click is the stimulus most commonly used to screen for hearing with the ABR. Although most of the initial work was done using a screening level of 30 dB (e.g., Galambos et al., 1994; Norton et al., 2000), most present screening procedures use a level of 35 dB nHL (normal hearing level). This level decreases the number of infants referred for subsequent evaluation, but also may cause the screening to miss more infants with a mild hearing loss.

Many different transducers are used to present the stimuli to the infant and there is no clear consensus as to how they should be calibrated (Durrant, Sabo, & Delgado, 2007; Lightfoot, Sininger, Burkard, & Lodwig, 2007). Insert earphones were originally designed for adults to provide sound levels in the external ear canal similar to those occurring with supra-aural earphones. Because the ear canals of infants are much smaller than those of adults, sound levels using insert earphones are significantly higher in infants than in adults. Some data are presented in Figure 13–6.

Interestingly, the sound levels in the infant canal measured during bone-conduction simulation are significantly higher than in adults (Cone-Wesson & Ramirez, 1997). Part of the difference is related to the smaller size of the ear canal. Another factor may be the lack of fusion of the bones of the infant skull, which results in less energy being transmitted away from the temporal bone. Thus, more energy might be transmitted out to the canal through the middle ear. However, the mechanisms of

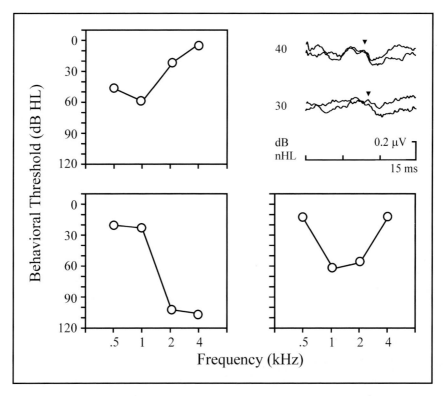

Figure 13–5. **Hearing impairments missed by click-ABR screening.** *The upper left of the figure shows the audiogram of an infant (taken at age 3 years) who was passed on click-ABR screening at birth. The ABR waveforms at birth are shown on the upper right. The normal hearing thresholds at high frequencies generated an ABR with normal thresholds (Durieux-Smith et al., 1991). The lower half of the figure shows other audiograms that would allow an infant to pass a click-ABR screening test (see Stapells, 2000b, for further discussion).*

bone-conduction hearing in infants are complex and further research in needed.

What should we do about the infant calibration issues? In a little while, there probably will be some age-related standards. We also might wish for a simple insert system with an extra microphone tube to allow the measurement of the sound level in the ear canal while the ABRs or ASSRs are recorded. In the best of all possible worlds, there might be a single insert for recording OAEs, EPs, and tympanometry and for measuring sound levels. In the meantime, we should use adult norms for sound level calibration because these levels were used to gather the normative data in infants and these are the only norms we have. Then we have to use an additional correction to compensate for the adult-infant differences (cf. Figure 13–6). However, we must be aware of differences between transducers. Most of the early normative data in infants were obtained with supra-aural earphones rather than inserts. Compared to inserts, supra-aural earphones would show less difference between infants and adults in the sound levels in the external auditory canal.

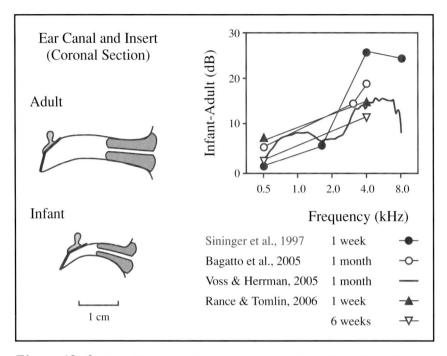

Figure 13–6. Sound levels in the infant ear canal. On the left are diagrammatic coronal sections through representative adult and infant external ear canals with inserts in place. The volume of air in ear canal between the insert and the tympanic membrane is much less for the infant than the adult. For the same intensity settings, the sound level at the tympanic membrane is therefore larger in the infant. The infant-adult level difference will vary with the intersubject variability in ear canal size and with the placement of the insert. Infant-adult differences as reported by several authors are presented in the graph on the right.

Sound levels are much less an issue with OAE screening. The decision that the hearing is normal is based on the presence of the OAEs in response to a stimulus of moderate sound level, rather than on the level of sound that elicits the OAE. This is a decided advantage of the technique, although the disadvantage is that there is no information about threshold levels when the OAEs are absent.

We do not use a click to assess hearing in adults; we use pure tones. As we have seen, some infants with significant hearing loss may pass the screening test with a click because they have hearing within normal limits at some frequencies (see Figure 13–5). The possibility of using frequency-specific stimuli for infant screening might be considered. Because screening has to be done rapidly, the test would likely be some variant of the multiple steady-state responses (where multiple frequencies are assessed simultaneously). Van Maanen and Stapells (2009) have found that normal physiologic thresholds in most infants can be determined using multiple steady state responses (both ears, four frequencies per ear) in about 5 minutes. This depends a little on what is considered normal in terms of physiologic thresholds: infant ASSR thresholds are higher than those in adults. Van Maanen and

Stapells suggest that an ASSR evaluation might be used as an initial assessment in infants for normal hearing when they are referred for audiologic evaluation after the initial neonatal screening. How such a test might work at the initial neonatal screening (instead of ABR or OAE) might also be considered (cf. Savio & Perez-Abalo, 2008), although the cost of validating such a protocol would be high.

Postnatal Hearing Loss

Some children will have a hearing impairment that develops after birth. This could be caused by an adventitious event such as meningitis, or a congenital hearing loss that was originally within screening limits but has become progressively worse. Identifying these infants requires continuing surveillance.

In Fortnum's extensive review (2003), the causes of permanent childhood hearing impairment were considered postnatal in 2 to 19% of the identified cases of hearing loss. However, these numbers are based on retrospective diagnoses. The data may be different when universal hearing screening is in place and we know when a child has passed the screening. Weichbold, Nekahm-Heis, and Welzl-Mueller (2006) reviewed the incidence of permanent bilateral hearing loss in children age 4 to 9 years who had been screened at birth. They estimated that, by age 9 years, approximately 25% of those with hearing impairment had normal hearing at birth. Bamford et al. (2007) found that the total prevalence of permanent bilateral hearing loss with thresholds equal to or greater than 40 dB HL (hearing level) at school entry (age 6 years) was 1.49 per 1000 and that 0.22 per 1000 (15%) had a postnatal cause. The percentage of hearing-impair-

ment detected postnatally was higher if the criterion allowed mild and/or unilateral losses. Using these criteria, the prevalence of hearing loss was 3.47 per 1000, and of these only 1.56 (46%) were identified during the neonatal screening. Most of the children were identified following concerns of the parent or physician.

The most common causes of postnatal hearing loss in the Weichbold et al. (2006) study were meningitis, hereditary hearing loss, and ototoxic medications (for bacterial infection or cancer). Any child with meningitis must be fully evaluated audiologically prior to final discharge from hospital, and should be followed up after discharge because a hearing loss may develop after the resolution of the acute infection. Any child who is treated with ototoxic medication also should also be followed audiologically.

We might consider a second hearing screening at a later age for any infant who passes the initial screening protocol but has risk factors for postnatal hearing impairment. The Joint Committee (2007) flagged several risk factors that should be considered risk factors for postnatal hearing loss (Table 13–3). In addition, the committee added parental concern about a baby's hearing as an indication for postnatal hearing evaluation. However, the best means of this later screening procedure—OAEs, ABR, or behavioral testing—is not known. The time at which this screening should be performed also is not known. Optimum timing will depend on the effectiveness of the testing procedures and the temporal incidence of postnatal hearing loss. The protocols illustrated in Figure 13–2 suggest a behavioral screening at age 8 to 12 months (Parry, Hacking, Bamford, & Day, 2003; Widen et al., 2000). A final question about postnatal hearing loss is whether the secondary screening

Table 13–3. Risk Factors for Postnatal Hearing Loss

Caregiver concern regarding hearing, speech, language, or developmental delay

Family history of childhood hereditary hearing disorders

Extracorporeal membrane oxygenation

Congenital infections, particularly cytomegalovirus

Syndromes associated with late onset or progressive hearing loss such as neurofibromatosis, osteopetrosis, and Usher's syndrome

Neurodegenerative disorders such as Hunter's syndrome, Friedrich's ataxia, and Charcot-Marie-Tooth disorder

Meningitis, either bacterial or viral

Head trauma requiring hospitalization, particularly if associated with skull fracture

Chemotherapy and other ototoxic medication

Source: Adapted from Joint Committee (2007).

should be based on risk factors or universal. Weichbold et al. (2006) could not find a clear risk factor in 26% of their children. Bamford et al. (2007) found no risk factors in 20%. Perhaps, a reasonable approach would combine an early (8–12 month) screen for infants at risk, a mandatory audiologic evaluation for any child with meningitis or when parents are concerned about their child's hearing, and a universal school-entry screening.

Auditory Neuropathy

OAE screening will not detect auditory neuropathy. Auditory neuropathy is more prevalent in infants in the neonatal intensive care units (Berg, Spitzer, Towers, Bartosiewicz, & Diamond, 2005), but a significant number of infants with auditory neuropathy may never be admitted to these units (e.g., Dunkley, Farnsworth, Mason, Dodd, & Gibbin, 2003). Should we therefore screen all newborns with ABR? Or use an OAE measurement such as contralateral suppression (James et al., 2005) that will evaluate the nerve as well as the hair cells? A related issue is that some newborn infants may show abnormal or distorted ABRs that then mature into normal responses within a few months (e.g., Psarommatis et al., 2006). Infants who were born prematurely or who have experienced some degree of anoxia in the perinatal period may be more likely than others to show this delayed maturation. These issues are discussed in greater detail in Chapter 15.

Conductive Hearing Loss

Conductive hearing loss in infancy needs to be considered more extensively. A child might be as impaired by a conductive hearing loss as by a sensorineural loss. How is it best detected? How accurate are the thresholds for tone-ABRs and ASSRs when bone-conducted stimuli are used? How should a detected conductive loss be treated? Conductive hearing loss can be considered the major cause of false positives in the screening process for permanent sensorineural hearing loss. However, such findings can be true positives for middle-ear problems, which might require further evaluation and treatment. Furthermore, the presence of a conductive hearing loss in the newborn period may be a warning sign for later chronic middle ear effusions.

Otitis media is particularly common between the ages of 6 month and 3 years.

Almost every child may have a transient otitis during this period. In 5 to 10% of all children, the disorder becomes chronic with middle-ear effusions ("glue ear") causing a more persistent conductive hearing loss (e.g., Paradise et al., 2005). The diagnosis of middle-ear effusions is best made by pneumatic otoscopy, with tympanometry as a confirmatory (but not primary) test (American Academy of Pediatrics, 2004). Recent studies (e.g., McCormick, Johnson, & Baldwin, 2006; Paradise et al., 2005) have found that middle-ear effusions do not cause significant deterioration of later school performance or language ability. Conservative treatment ("watchful waiting") is therefore recommended (American Academy of Pediatrics, 2004). If the disorder is bilateral and persists for more than 4 months with more than a mild conductive hearing loss, or if there are concomitant disorders that are associated with developmental delay, surgery with tympanostomy tubes might be considered. A particular problem in infancy is the combination of a permanent sensorineural and a transient or intermittent conductive hearing loss.

Unilateral Hearing Loss

The prevalence of unilateral hearing loss in young children appears to be approximately one half that of bilateral loss: Pastorino et al. (2005) 48%; Bamford et al. (2007) 54%; De Capua et al. (2007) 25%; Declau, Boudewyns, Van den Ende, Peeters, & van den Heyning (2008) 70%. Current screening procedures evaluate each ear separately and therefore will detect unilateral as well as bilateral hearing impairments. We need to work out the optimum management of infants with unilateral impairment (Holstrum, Gaffney, Gravel, Oyler, & Ross, 2008). An important out-

come of universal screening is that parents and teachers become aware of children with a unilateral loss. They should be informed that the infant will detect sounds normally through the normal ear but will have difficulty localizing sounds and understanding speech when there is background noise. The role of hearing aids and FM hearing devices needs to be determined. Continuing surveillance is necessary because a transient otitis in the good ear will affect hearing more significantly than in a child with normal hearing in both ears.

Genetic Screening

Targeted genetic screening is becoming available for assessing infants for a variety of disorders. Morton and Nance (2006) have pointed out that genetic abnormalities cause approximately 60% of permanent childhood hearing loss. Of these, abnormalities of the GJB2 (gap junction protein beta 2) gene, which encodes the protein connexin, are by far the most common cause of nonsyndromic sensorineural hearing loss, accounting for approximately 20% of hearing-impaired newborn infants (e.g., 25% in Schimmenti et al., 2008). We need to work out the role of genetic testing in relation to hearing screening.

AUDIOLOGIC EVALUATION OF THE INFANT REFERRED AS POSSIBLY HEARING IMPAIRED

Protocols for newborn hearing screening are designed to identify hearing-impaired infants. Because screening is not 100% specific, some infants with normal hearing also will be identified by the screening procedure. Moreover, current screening tests do not indicate either the severity or frequency-pattern of the hearing loss in infants who are truly impaired. Therefore, the next step is to evaluate the audiologic status of the referred infant, determining which infants have normal hearing and obtaining sufficient threshold information for those who have an impairment to support intervention. Recommendations concerning how to assess infants referred from screening (ASHA, 2004; Joint Committee on Infant Hearing, 2007) indicate that physiologic testing is essential.

For ABR and ASSR testing, young infants need to be asleep in order to reduce the background electrical noise. Young infants usually fall asleep after feeding and typically sleep for about an hour. As much information as possible must be obtained before the sleeping infant wakes up. Janssen, Usher, and Stapells (2010) have found that a young infant will sleep on average for about 55 minutes for testing; young infants slept without sedation and older infants were sedated with chloral hydrate. This amount of time is sufficient for about seven audiologic measurements, essentially seven threshold estimations, such as tone-ABR threshold-estimations at a particular frequency, click ABR measurements, ASSRs at multiple frequencies, and so on.

Therefore, the audiologist must proceed in an organized and time-efficient way. Recording electrodes must be placed before the infant falls asleep so that the infant's sleep is not disturbed by these manipulations. We might try to obtain OAE or tympanometric measurements before the infant falls asleep; even if the infant is upset, we often can get a minute or so of quiet testing time. Wherever possible, we should use acoustic transducers that do not interfere with the infant's sleep. Transducers that can be comfortably affixed to both ears are good. Another approach is to use a handheld earphone that can be held over the ear of an infant asleep in the parent's arms. Bilateral inserts are the most acoustically reliable transducers provided the infant does not dislodge them.

Several factors need to be considered so that threshold information is collected efficiently. We should dispense with the mantra of 10 dB down and 5 dB up, even though this is deeply engrained in our audiologic psyches. Unfortunately, it takes much longer to determine whether an infant's auditory EP is present than to detect an adult's button press. Given the accuracy of the testing procedures, we should probably not decrease our step size below 10 dB. Thresholds are most efficiently bracketed using a binary search procedure. According to this protocol, we initially test at the halfway point between the range of possible thresholds. Once a decision is made about the response at this intensity, we then jump halfway toward the upper limit if there is no response or toward the lower limit if a response is reliably recognized.

When deciding on the initial intensity, we should be aware that most infants referred from the screening protocols will have normal thresholds. We might expect that about 2% of newborn infants are referred for follow-up evaluation after screening. This will depend on the type of screening procedure; if we repeat ABR testing the referral rate will be lower. Because only 0.5% of infants have a hearing loss (accepting that there will be transient conductive losses as well as bilateral or unilateral sensorineural losses of mild or greater degree), about 75% of those referred for audiologic testing will be normal. Karzon and Lieu (2006) found that

72% of the infants referred from screening had normal hearing. Given these probabilities, much more information is obtained by starting threshold testing at 30 dB nHL rather than at 60 dB nHL. As shown diagrammatically in Figure 13–7, this is just above the median point in the distribution of expected thresholds—half of the infants have higher thresholds and half lower. As well as being more efficient, this approach also decreases the possibility that the louder stimuli will wake up the infant and render impossible further testing at low intensity.

Recording Click ABRs in Infants

The click-ABR has been studied extensively in infants (Picton, Durieux-Smith, & Moran,

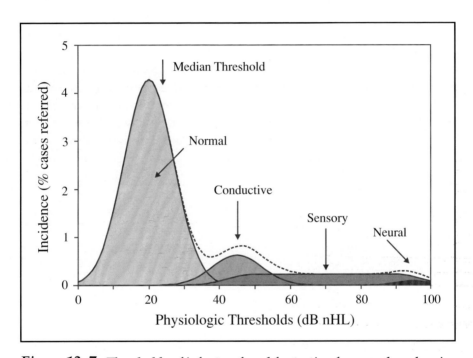

Figure 13–7. *Thresholds of infants referred for testing from newborn hearing screening. This graph is an estimate of what thresholds might be expected during the audiologic evaluation of referred infants. Thresholds are determined on the basis of tone-ABR thresholds. The incidence (75% normal, 11% conductive, 12% sensory, and 2% neural [auditory neuropathy]) is based roughly on the results of Karzon and Lieu (2006) although mixed hearing losses have been included with the sensory losses, and the incidence of auditory neuropathy (neural loss) has been increased a little in keeping with other studies. The neural hearing loss group has been plotted as showing thresholds (e.g., for the CM) at high intensity. The dotted line shows the sum of the different incidences. Half of the referred infants show thresholds below the "Median Threshold." The y-axis is plotted based on a resolution of 1 dB on the x-axis. If we were to estimate thresholds in 10-dB steps, the incidence should be multiplied by 10. For example, about 40% of infants referred for testing will show thresholds of 20 dB nHL.*

1994). The response differs from the adult response in many ways. As shown in Figure 13–8, the infant response generally is smaller and the waves occur at a longer latency. The infant response also differs from that of the adult in its waveform: wave II is less prominent, wave III is less distinct, often running into the IV-V complex, wave V is smaller relative to wave I, and the negative wave that follows wave V is more pronounced.

The infant ABR is quite asymmetric. Myelination of the auditory pathways occurs in the contralateral brainstem pathways more rapidly than in the ispsilateral pathways. This, together with the different geometry of the infant brain, can cause significant asymmetries in the scalp topography of the evoked potentials. As illustrated in Figure 13–9, the infant ABR can be almost invisible when using a contralateral mastoid reference (e.g., Edwards, Durieux-Smith, & Picton, 1985a). We must be sure that we are recording the ABR between vertex and ipsilateral mastoid by checking and documenting the electrodes in any infant whose thresholds are elevated. Sometimes, when the baby rolls over onto one side, we might forget to switch the reference electrodes. In this regard, it is much safer to record using two channels, making it unnecessary to switch electrodes.

The click-ABR allows the examiner to measure absolute and interpeak latencies and compare these to developmental norms. Therefore, although the click-ABR has been largely superseded by more frequency-specific techniques in the audiologic evaluation, there remain four areas

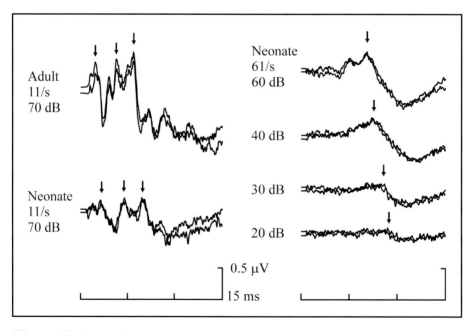

Figure 13–8. *Click-ABRs in newborn infants. On the left, the typical ABR of an adult in response to a 70 dB nHL click is compared to that of a neonate. Waves I, III, and V are indicated by arrows. On the right is shown a typical neonatal intensity series recorded at rapid click rates. Wave V (arrows) is clearly recognizable down to 20 dB. All intensities are relative to nHL.*

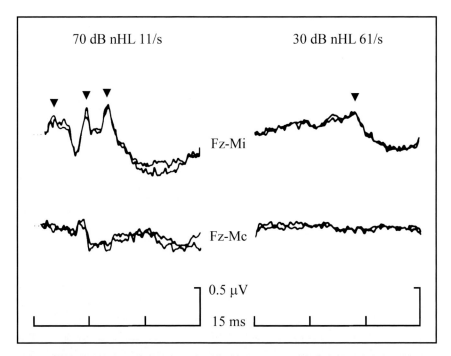

Figure 13–9. **Ipsilateral and contralateral recordings of the click-ABR in neonates.** *Responses were recorded simultaneously between an electrode anterior to the anterior fontanelle (Fz) and a reference either on the ispsilateral (Mi) or contralateral (Mc) mastoid. At high intensities, there was an ABR with clearly recognizable waves I, III, and V (triangles) on the ipsilateral recording. The morphology of the response was quite different on the contralateral recording and no clear wave V was seen. At low intensities, wave V was clearly recognizable on the ipsilateral recording but there was no response on the contralateral recording. Data from Edwards, Durieux-Smith, and Picton (1985a).*

in which the click ABR is important. First, infants with auditory neuropathy show absent or abnormal ABRs in the presence of demonstrable OAEs or CMs. To demonstrate clearly the absent or abnormal ABR, a loud click stimulus is better than tones. If at the time of the audiologic evaluation the OAEs are normal in the sense that all frequencies are clearly recognizable in the spectrum of the click-OAE or the distortion-product OAEs, we can be sure that the infant has good outer hair cell function. Then a click-ABR will show whether or not the auditory nerve is functioning correctly as well. Second, the click

ABR is useful in assessing the neurologic integrity of the auditory brainstem (Picton, Taylor, & Durieux-Smith, 2005). Some infants may not show a clear wave V in response to sounds because of dysfunction in the brainstem rather than the ear. In these infants, a click response recorded at slow click rates (near 10/s) may show a wave I and absent or abnormal later waves. Some idea of the hearing thresholds then may be gained by evaluating the thresholds for wave I (Figure 13–10). Third, the click ABR can demonstrate normal neurologic development in an infant. Showing normal amplitudes and latencies

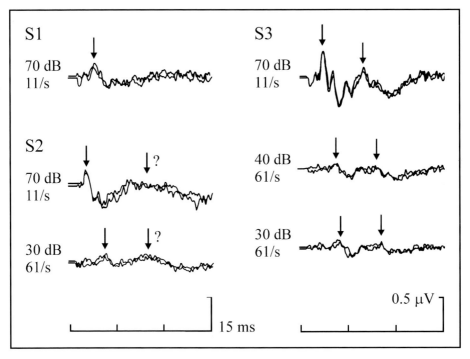

Figure 13–10. *Click ABRs in infants with hydrocephalus.* The responses of three different subjects (S1, S2, and S3) are shown. The response of S1 shows a clear wave I but no recognizable later waves. S2 shows a clear wave I but the rest of the response is small and distorted. The wave I is recognizable at 30 dB. S3 shows all components of the ABR but wave V is small. At low intensities, wave I is just as recognizable as wave V. All intensities are relative to dB nHL. Data from Edwards, Durieux-Smith, and Picton (1985b).

for the age of the infant provides a simple (although far from complete) check for normal brain development. Fourth, because the click ABR is much larger and easier to record than the tone-ABR, it usually is the test of last resort when trying to demonstrate any sound-evoked responses in a profoundly deaf infant. In all of the applications except the first (normal OAEs), the click ABR likely best follows the recording of tone-evoked ABRs or ASSRs. The click intensity should be 60 or 70 dB nHL for infants who have shown normal OAEs or normal thresholds on frequency-specific testing, and 90 dB nHL for infants in whom no clear tone-ABRs have been evoked, or in whom there was no response to lower intensity clicks. Even in these situations, clicks should not be presented for periods lasting longer than 3 minutes at this high level—perhaps just two separate averages of 1000 trials each.

Tone-ABRs

The most widely used technique for assessing frequency-specific thresholds in infants is the tone-ABR (Stapells & Oates, 1997; Stapells, Picton, & Durieux-Smith, 1993). The stimulus is a brief tone, most typically the 2-1-2 tone (2 cycles rise, 1 cycle plateau, and 2 cycles fall) recommended by Davis, Hirsh, Popelka, and Formby (1984). Typically, we use tones of alternating polarity (or random phase) to remove any stimulus artifact (although this is not necessary if the tone is brief (see Ribeiro & Carvallo, 2008).

Notched noise masking can render the responses more frequency-specific (Hyde, 1987; Picton, Ouellette, Hamel, & Smith, 1979; Stapells, Gravel, & Martin, 1995). The spectrum of a brief tone contains energy in frequency-regions (often called "skirts") away from the nominal frequency. Notched noise masking prevents the ear from responding to the energy in the skirts while allowing a response to the nominal frequency. However, because notched noise is not available in commercial systems, most tone-ABRs currently are recorded without masking. If the audiogram estimated from these thresholds shows an interoctave slope 20 dB or more, we must consider the possibility that the lower thresholds are underestimated. For example, if tone-ABR thresholds are 20 dB nHL at 1000 Hz and 50 dB at 2000 Hz, the behavioral thresholds at 2000 Hz might be 80 dB or more. The response to 2000-Hz tones of 50-dB or more nHL could be mediated through the 500-Hz region of the cochlea, activated by energy in skirts of the spectrum of the brief 2000-Hz tone.

When we record infant tone-ABRs, we need to change several recording parameters from those used to assess click-ABRs in adults. The infant tone-ABR is later than the adult click-ABR for several reasons: conduction speeds are slower in infants; low-frequency tones are delayed by the increased time taken by the traveling wave to reach the responsive area of the basilar membrane, and the rise-time of the stimulus is slower than for a click. The sweep duration for recording the infant tone-ABRs therefore should be signifi-cantly longer than that used for the adult click-ABR: at least 15 ms for tones of 2000 or 4000 Hz and 20 or even 25 ms for 1000 and 500 Hz tones. In addition, the frequency bandpass of the amplifier should be broadened to allow frequencies below 100 Hz to be recorded without attenuation. Reasonable bandpasses for recording tone-ABRs are between 30 and 3000 Hz or between 30 and 1000 Hz. The more slowly changing waveform can be difficult to recognize. Eyes used to the sharp peaks evoked by clicks must be adjusted to identify the rolling hills evoked by a 500-Hz tone. Figure 13–11 illustrates the tone-ABRs of a newborn infant.

When recording ABRs for audiologic purposes, we should make the rate of stimulus presentation as rapid as possible. Thresholds are based on the recognition of wave V, and the amplitude of this component is little affected when stimulus presentation is increased to rates of 80/s or more. Components earlier than wave V are much more susceptible to increasing rate, but we typically do not use these for threshold estimation. Therefore, when recording the tone-ABRs, we should use the fastest rates that are allowed by the sweep duration we have chosen—up to 39/s for sweeps of 25 ms and up to 65/s for sweeps of 15 ms. If available, other techniques such as those based on maximum length sequences can be used to record at even faster rates. Certain infants, particularly those who have suffered from perinatal asphyxia, may show an abnormal sensitivity to increasing stimulus rate (e.g., Jiang, Brosi, Shao, & Wilkinson, 2008). Thus, if the thresholds are elevated after testing at rapid rates, we should confirm some of these thresholds using stimuli presented more slowly to show that the cause of the elevated thresholds is audiologic rather than neurologic.

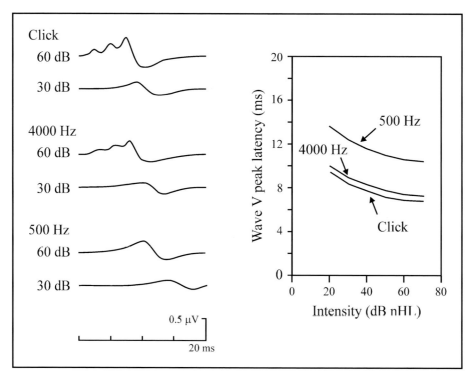

Figure 13–11. *Tone-ABRs in infants. The left side of this figure shows template-waveforms for the tone-ABRs in newborn infants to clicks and tones presented at rates between 40 and 50 Hz. These are diagrammatic templates rather than real waveforms. These are based on the data presented in Sininger et al. (1997), Ribeiro and Carvallo (2008), and Vander Werff et al. (2009). On the right are the expected wave V peak latencies for the different stimuli.*

Table 13–4 shows the average thresholds for tone-ABRs in normal infants obtained in a meta-analysis (Stapells, 2000a). Because many of the studies included in the meta-analysis involved infants that were several months of age, the table also includes data from other studies that studied newborn infants (e.g., Sininger, Abdala, & Cone-Wesson, 1997). The physiologic-behavioral differences for tone-ABR thresholds in infants with a sensorineural hearing impairment are smaller than those in normal infants (see Table 8–5) but most of these studies were done with older infants and need to be evaluated further in the first few months of life.

Recording Auditory Steady-State Responses in Infants

Steady-state responses are relatively new in the clinic. They have several advantages over the transient responses. One is the ease by which they can be assessed, a simple statistical comparison of the response at the frequency of stimulation to the electrical noise at adjacent frequencies in the spectrum. Another advantage is the possibility of recording responses to multiple simultaneous tones. Each tone is modulated at a particular frequency and then the specific response to the tone can be seen at that frequency in the response spectrum.

Table 13–4. Normal Physiological Thresholds for Air-Conducted Tone-ABRs in Infants (means ± SD in dB peSPL)

	Frequency (Hz)			
	500	**1000**	**2000**	**4000**
ABR Thresholds				
Stapells (2000a)[a]	43 ± 10	37 ± 12	38 ± 10	43 ± 13
Sininger et al. (1997)[b]	42 ± 9	38 ± 8		40 ± 10
Rance et al. (2006)[c]	53 ± 4			42 ± 4
Lee et al., (2007)[d]	44 ± 5	38 ± 8	35 ± 7	39 ± 7
Vander Werff et al. (2009)[e]	48 ± 8		31 ± 6	31 ± 6
nHL Thresholds (TDH39)				
Fedtke and Richter (2007)	23	20	25	28

[a]Data from the meta-analysis were converted from nHL to peSPL using the normal nHL values for adults for 20 Hz brief tones as provided by Fedtke and Richter (2007) for TDH 39 earphones. The standard deviations were calculated from the standard errors in the meta-analysis. More complete data from the meta-analysis are presented in Table 8–5 (which gives the nHL thresholds rather than the peSPL thresholds).

[b]Data were taken from Figure 4 for frequencies 500, 1500, and 4000 Hz.

[c]Data for newborns (Table 2) were converted to peSPL using the nHL values provided in the paper (Table 1).

[d]Data for infants 3 to 12 months old, converted from nHL as per note a.

[e]Converted to peSPL using the nHL measurements provided in the paper.

ASSRs recorded in infants are smaller than those recorded in adults. Figure 13–12 shows ASSRs in a normal newborn infant. Like the ABR, the ASSR also is best seen when recording from the vertex to the ipsilateral mastoid (Small & Stapells, 2008a; van Maanen & Stapells, 2009' van der Reijden, Mens, & Snik, 2005).

Several different types of stimuli have been used to evoke the ASSRs: amplitude and frequency-modulated tones (e.g., Rickards et al., 1994); sinusoidally amplitude-modulated tones (Lins et al., 1996); exponentially amplitude-modulated tones (John et al., 2004); tones amplitude-modulated using a half-wave rectified sinusoid (Riquelme, Kuwada, Filipovic, Hartung, & Leonard, 2006); and repeating brief tones (van Maanen & Stapells 2009, 2010). Exponential tones evoked larger responses than sinusoidally modulated tones.

Tables 13–5 and 13–6 show the normal thresholds for the ASSRs in infants and children. Some of the studies were obtained in less than optimal recording conditions (in terms of the ambient acoustic noise or the duration of recordings). Figure 13–13 shows the cumulative detectability of the responses at different stimulus intensities in several studies. We must be aware that ASSR thresholds decrease over the first few weeks of life (e.g., Rance & Tomlin, 2006) and that more normative data are necessary, particularly for the ASSRs

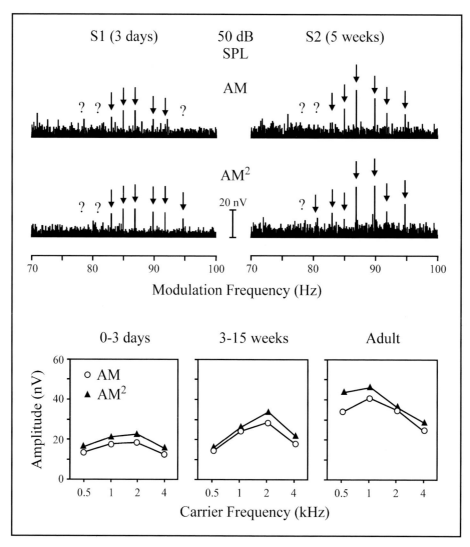

Figure 13–12. ASSRs in infants. *The upper half of the figure shows ASSR recordings in an newborn infant (S1) and in a 5-week-old infant (S2). Responses are to eight stimuli (four in each ear) with 500 Hz tones modulated at 78 and 80 Hz (in the right and left ears), 1 kHz at 83 and 85 Hz, 2 kHz at 87 and 90 Hz, and the 4-kHz tones at 92 and 95 Hz. All stimuli were presented at 50 dB SPL. The upper responses were evoked by sinusoidally amplitude-modulated tones and the lower responses by exponentially modulated tones. Responses to the 500-Hz tones were not consistent and only occurred in the older infant and then only for the exponentially modulated tones in the left ear. The responses to the 4-kHz tones were also small. The lower half of the figure shows average amplitudes for newborn and older infants, and for adults. The infant data are from John et al. (2004) and the adult data from John, Dimitrijevic, and Picton (2002).*

Table 13–5. Normal Physiologic Thresholds for Tone-ASSRs in Infants (Means ± SD in dB SPL)

	Frequency (Hz)			
	500	1000	2000	4000
Long recording time, quiet environment				
Lins et al. (1996)[a]	45 ± 13	29 ± 10	26 ± 8	29 ± 10
Luts et al. (2006)[b]	42 ± 10	35 ± 10	32 ± 10	36 ± 9
van Maanen and Stapells (2009)[c]	39 ± 7	33 ± 5	29 ± 7	24 ± 10
Ribeiro et al. (2010)[d]	43 ± 10	27 ± 7	26 ± 6	31 ± 7
Alaerts et al. (2010)	45 ± 13	38 ± 13	33 ± 11	38 ± 11
Qian et al. (2010)[e]	39 ± 5	29 ± 3	23 ± 3	36 ± 5
Short recording time				
Rickards et al. (1994)[f]	41 ± 10	24 ± 9		35 ± 11
Rance and Tomlin (2006)[g]	50 ± 11			43 ± 11
High-Noise Environment				
Savio et al. (2001)[h]	63 ± 11	55 ± 12	54 ± 12	54 ± 13
Pure Tone HL (Insert Earphones)	5.5	0.0	3.0	5.5

[a]Only data from the Ottawa cohort (age 1 to 10 mo, tested in quiet environment) are presented.
[b]Data are for newborns –23 to 70 days corrected age.
[c]Data are from the younger subjects (<6 mos).
[d]Data for term infants as determined using p <0.05 criterion.
[e]nHL thresholds for newborn subjects converted to SPL using adult HL conversions.
[f]Data are for newborns; 500, 1500, and 4000 Hz.
[g]Data are presented for newborns, dB HL converted to SPL.
[h]Data from the young subjects (<1 mo)

evoked with bone-conduction stimuli and in young infants with sensorineural hearing loss (Stapells, 2010). .

The most important aspect of recording ASSRs in infants is that the residual EEG noise must be reduced below levels necessary to recognize the small infant ASSR. ASSRs that are obtained using a brief recording time (e.g., in the studies of the Melbourne group such as those summarized by Rance and Rickards, 2002, and Rance et al., 2005) can accurately determine elevated thresholds but do not perform well when assessing hearing thresholds that are normal or only mildly elevated (Luts & Wouters, 2005; Rance, 2008). Regression formulae can be used to compensate for the elevation of ASSR thresholds in these cases but the estimated behavioral thresholds remain quite variable.

The ASSR thresholds measured relative to HL for pure tones in normal infants

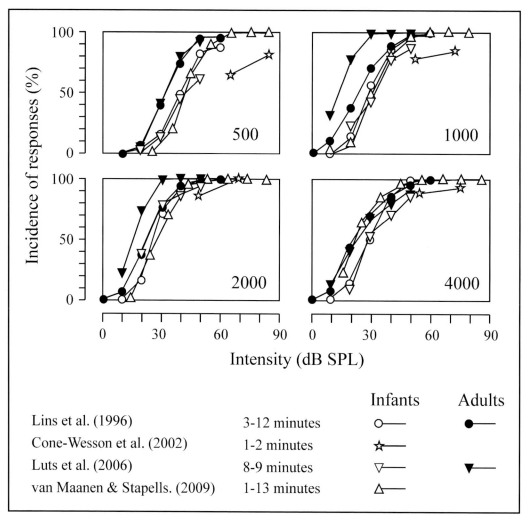

Figure 13–13. **Detectability of ASSR responses in infancy.** *The data are plotted as the percentage of responses detected at each intensity. Open symbols show infant data and filled symbols show adult data. The data are plotted for each carrier frequency (noted at the bottom right of each graph). The data from van Maanen and Stapells (2009) have been converted from HL to SPL. The data from Cone-Wesson, Parker, Swiderski, and Rickards (2002) are derived from their Figure 1.*

and young children are approximately 5 to 15 dB higher than the tone-ABR thresholds measured relative to nHL for brief tones. This comparison is between the tone-ABR thresholds in Table 13–4 less the nHL thresholds at the bottom of the table and the ASSR-thresholds in Table 13–5 less the HL thresholds at the bottom of that table. For example, the average 500-Hz threshold for the Stapells (2000a) meta-analysis of the tone-ABR data is 43 less 23 or 20 dB nHL, whereas in the van Maanan and Stapells (2009) data the average ASSR threshold at 500 Hz thresholds is 39 less 5.5 or 33.5 dB—13.5 dB higher. Van Maanen and Stapells (2010) have compared the

Table 13–6. Normal Physiologic Thresholds for Bone Conduction Stimuli in Infants (Means ± SD in dB re 1 μN)

	Frequency (Hz)			
	500	**1000**	**2000**	**4000**
Tone-ABR				
Foxe and Stapells (1993)	61 ± 10		45 ± 7	
Cone-Wesson & Ramirez (1997)[a]	52 ± 10			53 ± 10
Vander Werff et al. (2009)	74 ± 8		57 ± 7	
ASSR				
Small and Stapells (2006)[b]	72 ± 13	45 ± 7	57 ± 6	58 ± 8
Normal HL	58	43	31	36

[a]Newborn infants. Standard deviations estimated from Figure 2 of the paper.
[b]Data for "post-term" infants (0–6 months).

two tests in infants with normal hearing and in infants with hearing impairment. The difference is greater for 500 Hz than for 4000 Hz (13 vs. 8 dB) and about 5 dB greater in the normal hearing infants than in the hearing-impaired infants. Similar results were reported by Qian et al. (2010).

Why the ASSRs should have thresholds in infants that are not as close to tone-ABR thresholds as those recorded in adults is not clear. In adults and older children, the ASSR reported thresholds relative to HL are close to the tone-ABR thresholds relative to nHL. Perhaps, the infant auditory system is less sensitive to the slower rise time of a modulated tone than to the rapid onset of a brief tone. In this regard, Han, Mo, Lui, Chen, and Huang (2006) found that the ASSR thresholds for brief tones presented at rapid rates were only 8 to 15 dB above behavioral thresholds in a group of normal and hearing-impaired children age 6 months to 5 years. These results may be related partly to age and partly to using brief tones instead of modulated continuous tones.

Both ASSRs and tone-ABRs can be used to estimate behavioral thresholds by subtracting from the physiologic threshold a correction factor equal to the mean physiologic-behavioral difference. As discussed in Chapter 6, the key determinant of the accuracy of the estimation is the inter-subject variability as seen in the standard deviation (SD). This variability measure is similar for tone-ABRs and ASSRs (as seen in Tables 13–4 to 13–6). Another important source of variability is the age of the infant; the correction factors change with age. More data about the development of both ABRs and ASSRs over the first few years of life are needed.

Tympanometry in Infants

Tympanometric measurements of middle-ear function in infants recently have been widely evaluated. The most important finding is that the frequency at which reflectance is optimally measured in infants differs from adults. Probe frequencies should be 600 or 1000 Hz rather than the 226 Hz used in adults (Alaerts, Luts, & Wouters, 2007; Margolis, Bass-Ringdahl, Hanks, Holte, & Zapala, 2003). Nevertheless, the middle ear changes significantly with the infant's age and there is a great need for more normative data (Mazlan et al. 2007).

An underlying problem with tympanometric measurements is that, although they can indicate a conductive problem, they do not indicate the severity of any associated conductive hearing loss. ABR or ASSR thresholds to bone-conducted tones are more informative. Tympanometric studies can be performed in a short time provided we obtain a good seal for the probe. Such recordings therefore might be obtained before the infant falls asleep for threshold ABR studies.

OAEs in Infants

Recording the OAEs in infants referred from screening provides a rapid demonstration of cochlear function if it is normal. Some protocols record OAEs at the beginning of the examination of the referred infant. One definite advantage of the OAEs is that they are independent of the state of the infant (Gorga et al., 2000). Provided the infant is not crying, the response can be recorded reliably. If the OAEs are present, we have quickly checked for normal cochlear function and then can assess the function of the auditory nerve using click-ABRs. DPOAEs are particularly helpful as they directly assess the cochlear responsiveness at different frequencies. Figure 13–14 shows normative DPOAE data from infants. What is displayed when recording

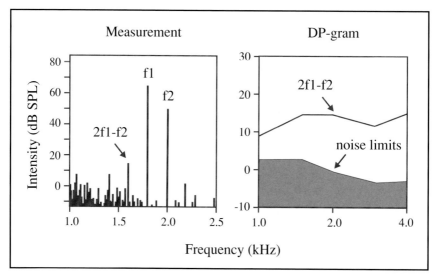

Figure 13–14. **Distortion product otoacoustic emissions (DPOAEs).** *The diagram on the left shows the measurement that is made for one pair of stimuli at f1 and f2. A distortion product emission is recognizable at 2f1-f2 with an amplitude that is much smaller than the amplitude of the two stimuli but larger than the amplitude of the acoustic noise at nearby frequencies. This can then be plotted at the frequency of f2 on a DP-gram as illustrated on the right. In the DP-gram, the values plotted are the modal values for the perinatal DPOAE and the noise limits as documented in Gorga et al. (2000).*

the DPOAEs is a DP-gram showing the 2f1-f2 response relative to noise at each f2. The DP-gram is not an audiogram, as it indicates only when the hair cells are normal and cannot tell you how elevated the threshold might be when the hair cells are abnormal and the DPOAE is absent. In infants, the low-frequency acoustic noise levels are sufficiently high that we often cannot consider the responses at 1500 Hz or below. Furthermore, isolated frequency regions may not show clear responses even in normal hearing infants.

Strategies for the Audiologic Evaluation

The number of different strategies for evaluating the infant referred for testing after newborn screening probably approaches the number of audiologists who perform the testing. Many different protocols have been described, but few have been assessed in terms of questions such as: What are the goals of the testing? How effective is the protocol in attaining these goals? and How long does the testing take? A possible strategy for the audiologic examination is illustrated in Figure 13–15. Several other protocols have been presented in detail on Web sites (e.g., British Columbia Early Hearing Program, 2008; National Health Service Newborn Hearing Screening Programme, 2008), and one particular protocol has been formally evaluated with respect to its effectiveness in obtaining thresholds (Karzon & Lieu, 2006; Lieu, Karzon, & Mange, 2006). Stapells (2010) provides an excellent review and justification of the strategies used in British Columbia to assess infants referred from newborn hearing screening programs.

The first goal of the audiologic evaluation is to determine if there is a significant hearing impairment. The second goal is to obtain frequency-specific threshold information that can be used to determine management. Specific thresholds can be used to fit hearing aids. Thresholds indicating a profound hearing loss can contribute along with other clinical assessments to a consideration of cochlear implants. A third goal is to determine the type of hearing loss that is causing the elevated thresholds—conductive or mixed, cochlear, and neural. Given these goals the following are suggestions.

The caregivers or parents should be instructed on the importance of having the baby sleep through much of the testing. This might be facilitated by keeping the baby awake before the test—not letting him or her sleep in the car—and then feeding the baby after the electrodes are applied for the EP recordings. The typical baby then falls asleep and we can follow the sequence of tests outlined in Figure 13–15.

If the OAEs are not normal on the initial evaluation or if the baby has already gone to sleep, testing should proceed to a frequency-specific EP assessment like that described in Figure 13–15. There are two possible approaches: tone ABR or ASSR. If we use the tone-ABRs, we have to decide which frequency to start with. If the baby wakes up and we are limited in the number of threshold assessments, we would like the most informative thresholds to have been obtained. The response at 2 kHz is likely the most important in terms of how much it might tell us about the hearing loss. This would be followed by 500 Hz, and then the other ear at 2 kHz and 500 Hz. Testing at 1 and 4 kHz can be added if time permits. If the thresholds are elevated, thresholds with bone-conduction must be measured. A handheld bone conduction transducer is gentle enough not to wake the baby (Small, Hatton, & Stapells, 2007; Small & Stapells, 2006, 2008b).

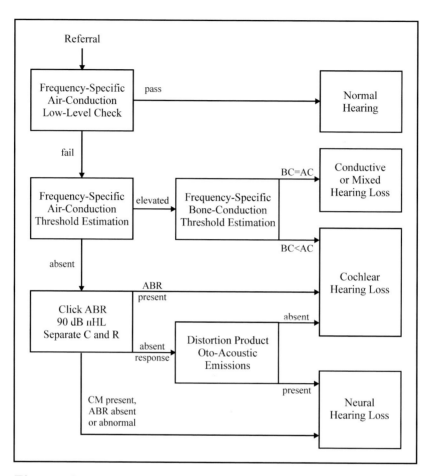

Figure 13–15. *Strategy for the audiologic evaluation of the infant referred from screening. These sequences are appropriate for a sleeping baby. The strategy mainly focuses on obtaining thresholds using auditory EPs. Either tone-ABRs or ASSRs can be used for the initial low-level check or later threshold estimation. Recommended low-level assessment levels are 30 dB (35 at 500 Hz) nHL for tone-ABRs, and 50, 45, 40, and 40 dB HL for ASSRs at 500, 1000, 2000, and 4000 Hz, respectively (see van Maanen & Stapells, 2009). If single stimuli are used, we should probably follow the order: 2000 Hz then 500 Hz, then the other ear, then 1000 and 4000 Hz as time allows. If ASSRs are used, some confirmation at one frequency with tone-ABRs is required. Other tests such as pneumatic otoscopy and tympanometry are helpful adjuncts, particularly when there is a conductive loss. Although in this diagram the OAEs are shown late into the diagnostic logic, they also can be performed early in the testing session (e.g., before the infant falls asleep), and provide confirmatory evidence in cases of hearing impairment.*

The ASSRs, when tested using multiple stimulation techniques, do not require decisions about what frequency to start with, as all audiometric frequencies can be tested simultaneously. Although both ears can be tested simultaneously, it might be more comfortable for the baby if one ear is tested at a time. Because the ASSRs have not been evaluated in infancy as extensively as the tone-ABRs, we should confirm these results by repeating one of the thresholds using tone-ABRs. Present guidelines (e.g., Joint Committee on Infant Hearing, 2007) do not support the use of ASSRs in the audiometric assessment of infants. Recent research with these responses (e.g., van Mannen & Stapells, 2009, 2010), nevertheless, indicates that they may provide reasonable estimates of hearing threshold in infants. Further research is warranted, particularly concerning how well these responses can assess infants with various kinds of hearing loss. This chapter proposes that they can be used for the audiometric evaluation of infants, provided some thresholds are confirmed with tone-ABR.

As indicated earlier, it is better for both tone ABRs and ASSRs to begin at low intensities and then to narrow in on the possible threshold. Starting at low intensities is important because it will not wake the infant. Thus, we could begin the test at a low level where most normal infants should show a response (see Figure 13–15). For tone-ABRs, this level would be at 30 dB nHL for tones of 1 to 4 kHz and 35 dB nHL for 500 Hz (British Columbia Early Hearing Program, 2008). The intensities at which to start the ASSRs would be 50, 45, 40, and 40 dB HL for ASSRs at 500, 1000, 2000, and 4000 Hz, respectively (Stapells, 2010; van Maanen & Stapells, 2009).

If the baby shows good responses at all frequencies on this low-level check, the evaluation can be completed. If the baby is still sleeping, however, it is always a good idea to obtain some other confirmatory information. For example, if ASSRs were used it would be nice to confirm that thresholds are normal with low-level tone-ABRs. A click-ABR at slow rates would

also demonstrate integrity of the brainstem auditory pathways.

If the baby does not quickly fall asleep, the following tests can be performed while the baby is still awake: OAEs, either transient or distortion products, and tympanometry. These tests can be done in brief periods of relative quiet. If the baby insists on staying awake after these tests, we also can consider evaluating the postauricular muscle (PAM) reflexes. As reviewed in Chapter 9, these responses can be recorded in young infants and do indicate auditory function. We can record PAM reflexes using the same setup as for the tone-ABR and simply increasing the duration of the recording sweep. Current data are not sufficient to provide threshold estimates in infants, but the presence of a clear muscle reflex can indicate that the sound at that level has been processed in the ear and brainstem.

If the OAEs in an awake baby show completely normal findings, the next examination might be the ABR to clicks at moderate intensity presented at rates of 10 or 20/s. The combination of normal OAEs and normal click ABR means that the infant has hearing that can be considered normal. Because OAEs do not give an accurate assessment at frequencies of 1500 Hz or below, an assessment of the tone-ABR using 500 Hz tones either with bone- or air-conduction might be a helpful addendum. If the ABRs show normal responses, the caregivers should be counseled about the possibility of a progressive or late-onset hearing loss and told to return if there is any concern about the child's hearing.

If a permanent hearing loss is documented with the EPs, an additional testing session should be scheduled to confirm the data from the first assessment, to fill in missing thresholds and to begin hearing aid selection.

Any infant with elevated thresholds should be referred for otologic examination, which will include pneumatic otoscopy. This requires an otolaryngologist or someone with similar skills and experience. Pneumatic otoscopy is the primary method for diagnosing otitis media (American Academy of Pediatrics, 2004). Further referrals are necessary to check on other aspects of the hearing loss, such as genetics and psychology. These are described more fully in the report of the Joint Committee on Infant Hearing (2007).

Care and sensitivity must be exercised throughout the evaluation of the infant suspected of a hearing loss. We must be as certain as we can be about the findings, and we must present these to the infant's family with gentleness and empathy. When there is a hearing loss, we must ensure that the family has access to programs that can manage the impairment and provide support during this management.

Fitting Hearing Aids

When an infant identified as hearing-impaired is followed up with audiologic testing that indicates a permanent hearing loss, the next step is to use the audiogram estimated from the physiologic tests to fit a hearing aid. Even if the hearing loss is severe or profound, hearing aids will be tried before cochlear implants are considered. Fitting procedures are based on measurements of real-ear-to-coupler differences (e.g., Bagatto, Seewald, Scollie, & Tharpe, 2006; Scollie & Seewald, 2002). Fitting the hearing aid requires setting the amount of amplification at each frequency to compensate for the elevated thresholds. To do this, we combine the amplification factor of the aid (measured using a coupler) with a measurement of the real-ear-to-coupler

difference measured in the individual infant (or failing that, an age-appropriate estimate). Compression is then adjusted so that the amplified sound does not exceed some estimate of the levels at which saturation likely occurs (usually extrapolated from adult maximum loudness levels, but possibly related in some way to acoustic reflexes if they are present). Because of the variability in getting accurate estimates of hearing thresholds from the physiologic thresholds, this fitting is never perfect and we must find ways to live with uncertainty. A fuzzy perception of the world is better than not seeing anything. As the infant grows older, the fuzziness will give way to clarity: we will get better physiologic thresholds and then obtain more and more accurate behavioral thresholds.

The general goal of fitting hearing aids is illustrated in Figure 13–16. The ver-

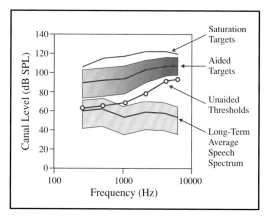

Figure 13–16. *Fitting hearing aids. The goal is to amplify the sounds of speech (represented by the long-term average speech spectrum) so that they fit between the unaided thresholds and the saturation target. This entails both amplification (moving the sounds upward on the graph) and compression (decreasing the intensity range of the sounds as illustrated by the darker shading of the aided targets). This figure is derived from the work of Scollie and Seewald (2002).*

tical axis is in dB SPL in the canal. The prerequisites are the top and bottom levels of audibility and the range of the speech signal that must be made audible. The aid then is adjusted to amplify and compress the signal so that speech is audible. In the diagram, the amount of compression is shown by the depth of shading.

Thresholds for recognizing a physiologic response are almost always higher than behavioral thresholds. Therefore, we often estimate the behavioral thresholds by subtracting a compensation factor from the physiologic thresholds. This can be a constant or it can vary with the level of the physiologic threshold. Whatever technique we use, we must always be clear that we are using estimated behavioral thresholds rather than physiologic thresholds when we are fitting hearing aids.

Now we must consider the main problem of the estimated thresholds—how accurate they are. The most important measure here is the intersubject variability. Behavioral thresholds as measured using conventional audiometric techniques (down 10 dB, up 5 dB) are a little variable. Within a subject, the thresholds may depend on how much attention the subject is paying, or on the variability of concomitant physiologic acoustic noise (blood-flow, breathing, etc.). The variability in threshold among normal subjects depends on their different levels of experience with hearing tests, and the variability of the external ear and its fit to the transducer. We usually do not expect more than ±5 dB of variability within a subject or more than ±10 dB of variability across subjects (using ±2 standard deviations, which include 95% of the subjects). These estimates are for adults; they are higher in children and higher still in infants.

Physiologic thresholds are more variable from subject to subject than the behavioral thresholds. The extra variability will depend on the size of the response, the amplitude of the background EEG, and the amount of time spent averaging. We can compensate out the mean physiologic-behavioral difference to get an estimated behavioral threshold but we are then left with the intersubject variability. In some subjects, we will underestimate behavioral threshold and in others we will overestimate.

The standard deviation of physiologic thresholds, for tone-ABR or for ASSR, is usually about 10 dB (see Tables 13–4 and 13–5). This means that the actual thresholds for 95% of the subjects will be anywhere in the range ±20 dB from the mean. One in 20 subjects will be outside this range. This degree of variability allows a wide range of behavioral audiograms to be associated with any given set of physiologic thresholds. This issue is discussed at greater length in Chapter 6 (see Figure 6–15). The actual behavioral audiogram associated with any given set of physiologic thresholds may show very distinct patterns (such as flat or steep high frequency) that require very different fittings for a hearing aid. We need to have more data on whether the pattern of the physiologic audiogram can be better predicted from the pattern of estimated thresholds. If a particular subject shows elevated thresholds at one frequency, will there be a similar elevation at another? There is some evidence that this is true (Perez-Abalo et al., 2001). We can handle some uncertainty by using convergent information. We can bring to bear our knowledge concerning the relative incidence of different audiometric patterns. A steep high-frequency loss is less common than a gently sloping loss. If there are acoustic reflexes at 90 dB, the behavioral thresholds are likely at least 15 dB below that.

Nevertheless, convergent information will not resolve everything. We must learn to "satisfice," (a term used by Herbert Simon, who received the Nobel Prize in Economics). Make the most of what we know, take our best guess, and act on this. Better to act and worry about being wrong than to refuse to act until we are completely sure. Once we have fit the aid, we must monitor the infant's response and adjust the aid if the infant's behavior clearly indicates that the sounds are too loud.

Once the hearing aid is fitted, we can check that the sounds previously unheard are now activating the brain by recording auditory EPs when the subject hears sounds through the hearing aid. EPs to transient stimuli may not be optimal in this regard as hearing aids respond preferentially to slowly changing sounds. Early ideas that we might be able to adjust the hearing aid to normalize the latency of the click ABR (e.g., Hecox, 1983) have not really gained much acceptance clinically. ASSRs may be more effective (Picton et al., 1998) as they are less distorted by the amplification of the aid. We may be able to fit the amplitude, compression, and maximum output of the aid by evaluating the threshold, slope, and upper limits of the amplitude-intensity function of the ASSR. These possibilities are discussed more fully by Zenker-Castro and Barajas de Prat (2008). Figure 13–17 illustrates these possibilities.

A final area of uncertainty about hearing aid fitting concerns the discriminability of the amplified sounds. Although we can make sounds audible, we do not know whether the subject can perceive them clearly. To assess this, we have to evaluate responses to aided sounds and show that the brain is discriminating them. Dimitrijevic, John, and Picton (2004) recorded ASSRs to sounds that varied in both their amplitude and frequency over the ranges that occur in normal speech sounds. The actual stimuli do not sound much like speech but they might assess the brain's ability to discriminate speech-like changes.

What would be really helpful would be to speak directly to the subject and to record the physiologic responses to real speech sounds. Several researchers (Aiken & Picton, 2008a, 2008b; Johnson, Nicol, & Kraus, 2005; Krishnan, 2007) have been looking at brainstem responses to speech sounds. We briefly described these responses to speech in Chapter 5. Cortical responses in infants also might be helpful in demonstrating the response to speech sounds (Golding et al., 2007; Wunderlich & Cone-Wesson, 2006). This type of research is just beginning, but it is fun to speculate that one day we might be able to fit an aid to an infant, talk to her, and watch her brain respond to our talking.

CONCLUDING COMMENTS

Testing the hearing of infants is the most important application of the auditory EPs. We have developed tests that can identify hearing-impaired infants, assess the hearing thresholds in these subjects, and even monitor how well their hearing aids might work. Universal newborn hearing screening has been an exciting development, allowing us to provide auditory assistance to those who need it at a time when they need it most. The miracle of the deaf becoming able to hear is now possible. However, much further work must still be done. We need more research on the best way to assess the hearing impairment and to decide on what therapies can be provided to the hearing-impaired infant. Miracles are wonderful. They provide answers to our questions but often demonstrate further mysteries to be investigated.

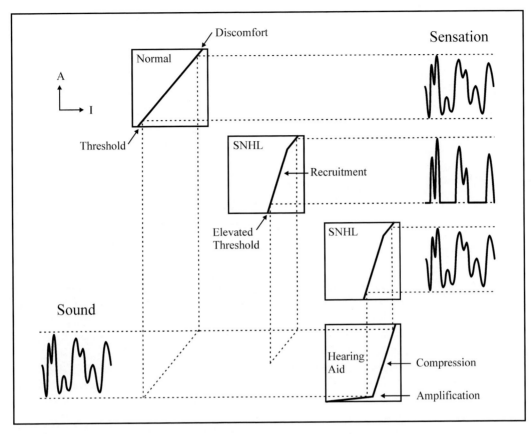

Figure 13–17. *Amplification and compression. This diagram shows how one might fit a hearing aid on the basis of the amplitude-intensity (A-I) function of the ASSR (e.g., as shown in the right half of Figure 13–4). Sound (such as the waveform in the lower left, a plot of the root-mean square amplitude over time, or the envelope of the sound) is converted to a physiologic response according to these amplitude-intensity functions. In a normal subject, the function is linear between threshold and discomfort levels and the physiologic response therefore replicates the stimulus envelope* (upper right). *In the subject with a sensorineural loss, the threshold is elevated and the slope of the function is increased so that more intense sounds are perceived at the same loudness level as in the normal subject (recruitment). However, lower intensity sounds are not processed, gaps occur and the sensation is distorted. This is illustrated in the second response on the right. If a hearing aid amplifies the sound and compresses its range to fit within the range of audibility of the hearing-impaired subject, the sensory response may more accurately represent the sound (third response on the right). These procedures depend on the concept that the amplitude of the physiologic response is a valid representation of sensory magnitude.*

ABBREVIATIONS

ABR	Auditory brainstem response
DPOAE	Distortion product otoacoustic emissions
ECochG	Electrocochleogram
EP	Evoked potential
Fsp	F-ratio at a single point
GJB2	Gap junction protein beta 2
HL	Hearing level

LAEP   Late auditory evoked potential

MLR   Middle-latency response

nHL   Normal hearing level

OAE   Otoacoustic emission

SD   Standard deviation

SNR   Signal-to-noise ratio

TORCH   Toxoplasmosis, Rubella, Cytomegalovirus, Herpes

REFERENCES

Aiken, S. J., & Picton, T. W. (2008a). Human cortical responses to the speech envelope. *Ear and Hearing, 29,* 139–157.

Aiken, S. J., & Picton, T. W. (2008b). Envelope and spectral frequency-following responses to vowel sounds. *Hearing Research, 245,* 35–47.

Alaerts, J., Luts, H., Van Dun, B., Desloovre, C., & Wouters, J. (2010). Latencies of auditory steady-state responses recorded in early infancy. *Audiology & Neurootology, 15,* 116–127.

Alaerts, J., Luts, H., & Woulters, J. (2007). Evaluation of middle ear function in young children: Clinical guidelines for the use of 226- and 1,000-Hz tympanometry. *Otology & Neurotology, 28,* 727–732.

American Academy of Pediatrics. (2004). Clinical Practice Guideline: Otitis media with effusion. *Pediatrics, 113,* 1412–1429.

American Speech-Language-Hearing Association (ASHA). (2004). Guidelines for the audiologic assessment of children from birth to 5 years of age. Available from http://www.asha.org/docs/pdf/GL2004-00002.pdf

Bagatto, M. P., Seewald, R. C., Scollie, S. D., & Tharpe, A. M. (2006). Evaluation of a probe-tube insertion technique for measuring the real-ear-to-coupler difference (RECD) in young infants. *Journal of the American Academy of Audiology, 17,* 573–581.

Bamford, J., Fortnum, H., Bristow, K., Smith, J., Vamvakas, G., Davies, L., . . . Hind, S. (2007). Current practice, accuracy, effectiveness and cost-effectiveness of the school entry hearing screen. *Health Technology Assessment, 11*(32), 1–168.

Berg, A. L., Spitzer, J. B., Towers, H. M., Bartosiewicz, C., & Diamond, B. E. (2005). Newborn hearing screening in the NICU: Profile of failed auditory brainstem response/passed otoacoustic emission. *Pediatrics, 116,* 933–938.

British Columbia Early Hearing Program. (2008). Diagnostic audiology protocol. Available from: http://www.phsa.ca/NR/rdonlyres/06D79FEB-D187-43E9-91E4-8C09959F38D8/40115/aDAAGProtocols1.pdf

Cone-Wesson, B., Parker, J., Swiderski, N., & Rickards, F. (2002). The auditory steady-state response: Full term and premature infants. *Journal of the American Academy of Audiology, 13,* 260–269.

Cone-Wesson, B., & Ramirez, G. M. (1997). Hearing sensitivity in newborns estimated from ABRs to bone-conducted sounds. *Journal of the American Academy of Audiology, 8,* 299–307.

Davis, A., Bamford, J., Wilson, I., Ramkalawan, T., Forshaw, M., & Wright, S. (1997). A critical review of the role of neonatal hearing screening in the detection of congenital hearing impairment. *Health Technology Assessment, 1*(10), 1–176.

Davis, H., Hirsh, S. K., Popelka, G. R., & Formby, C. (1984). Frequency selectivity and thresholds of brief stimuli suitable for electric response audiometry. *Audiology, 23,* 59–74.

De Capua, B., Costantini, D., Martufi, C., Latini, G., Gentile, M., & De Felice, C. (2007). Universal neonatal hearing screening: The Siena (Italy) experience on 19,700 newborns. *Early Human Development, 83,* 601–606.

Declau, F., Boudewyns, A., Van den Ende, J., Peeters, A., & van den Heyning, P. (2008). Etiologic and audiologic evaluations after universal neonatal hearing screening: Analysis of 170 referred neonates. *Pediatrics, 121,* 1119–1126.

Dimitrijevic, A., John, M. S., & Picton, T. W. (2004). Auditory steady-state responses and word recognition scores in normal hearing and hearing-impaired adults. *Ear and Hearing, 25,* 68–84.

Dobie, R. A. (1993). Objective response detection. *Ear and Hearing, 14,* 31–35.

Downs, M. P. (1976). Early identification of hearing loss: Where are we? Where do we go from here? In G. T. Mencher (Ed.), *Early identification of hearing loss* (pp. 14–22). Basel, Switzerland: Karger.

Dunkley, C., Farnsworth, A., Mason, S., Dodd, M., & Gibbin, K. (2003). Screening and follow up assessment in three cases of auditory neuropathy. *Archives of Disease in Childhood, 88,* 25–26.

Durieux-Smith, A., Fitzpatrick, E., & Whittingham, J. (2008). Universal newborn hearing screening: A question of evidence. *International Journal of Audiology, 47,* 1–10.

Durieux-Smith, A., Picton, T. W., Bernard, P., MacMurray, B., & Goodman, J. T. (1991). Prognostic validity of brainstem electric response audiometry in infants of a neonatal intensive care unit. *Audiology, 30,* 249–265.

Durieux-Smith, A., Picton, T., Edwards, C., Goodman, J. T., & MacMurray, B. (1985). The Crib-O-Gram in the NICU: An evaluation based on brain stem electric response audiometry. *Ear and Hearing, 6,* 20–24.

Durrant, J. D., Sabo, D. L., & Delgado, R. E. (2007). Call for calibration standard for newborn screening using auditory brainstem responses. *International Journal of Audiology, 46,* 686–691.

Edwards, C. G., Durieux-Smith, A., & Picton, T. W. (1985a). Neonatal auditory brainstem responses from ipsilateral and contralateral recording montages. *Ear and Hearing, 6,* 175–178.

Edwards, C. G., Durieux-Smith, A., & Picton, T. W. (1985b). Auditory brainstem response audiometry in neonatal hydrocephalus. *Journal of Otolaryngology,14*(Suppl. 14), 40–46.

Elberling, C., Don, M., Cebulla, M., & Stürzebecher, E. (2007). Auditory steady-state responses to chirp stimuli based on cochlear traveling wave delay. *Journal of the Acoustical Society of America, 122,* 2772–2785.

Fedtke, T., & Richter, U. (2007). Reference zero for the calibration of air-conduction audiometric equipment using "tone bursts" as test signals. *International Journal of Audiology, 46,* 1–10.

Fortnum, H. (2003). Epidemiology of permanent childhood hearing impairment: Implications for neonatal hearing screening. *Audiological Medicine, 1,* 155–164.

Foxe, J. J., & Stapells, D. R. (1993). Normal infant and adult auditory brainstem responses to bone-conducted tones. *Audiology, 32,* 95–109.

Gaffney, M., Eichwald, J., Grosse, S. D., & Mason, C. A. (2010). Identifying infants with hearing loss—United States, 1999–2007. *Centers for Disease Control and Prevention Morbidity and Mortality Weekly Report, 59*(8), 220–223. (Erratum in *Morbidity and Mortality Weekly Report, 59*(15), 460).

Galambos, R., Wilson, M. J., & Silva, P. D. (1994). Identifying hearing loss in the intensive care nursery: A 20-year summary. *Journal of the American Academy of Audiology, 5,* 151–162.

Golding, M., Pearce, W., Seymour, J., Cooper, A., Ching, T., & Dillon, H. (2007). The relationship between obligatory cortical auditory evoked potentials (CAEPs) and functional measures in young infants. *Journal of the American Academy of Audiology, 18,* 117–125.

Gorga, M. P., Norton, S. J., Sininger, Y. S., Cone-Wesson, B ., Folsom, R. C., Vohr, B. R., . . . Neely, S. T. (2000). Identification of neonatal hearing impairment: distortion product otoacoustic emissions during the perinatal period. *Ear and Hearing, 21,* 400–424.

Grandori, F., & Lutman, M. E. (1998). European Consensus Statement on Neonatal Hearing Screening. *International Journal of Pediatric Otorhinolaryngology, 44,* 309–310.

Gravel, J. S., & Tocci, L. A. (1998). Setting the stage for universal newborn hearing screening. In L. G. Spivak (Ed.), *Universal newborn hearing screening* (pp. 1–27). New York, NY: Thieme.

Han, D., Mo, L., Lui, H., Chen, J., & Huang, L. (2006) Threshold estimation in children using auditory steady-state responses to multiple simultaneous stimuli. *ORL—Journal of Oto-Rhino-Laryngology and Related Specialties, 68,* 64–68.

Hecox, K. (1983). Role of auditory brain stem response in the selection of hearing aids. *Ear and Hearing, 4,* 51–55.

Hecox, K., & Galambos, R. (1974). Brain stem auditory evoked responses in human infants and adults. *Archives of Otolaryngology, 99,* 30–33.

Holstrum, W. J., Gaffney, M., Gravel, J. S., Oyler, R. F., & Ross, D. S. (2008). Early intervention for children with unilateral and mild bilateral degrees of hearing loss. *Trends in Amplification, 12,* 35–41.

Hyde, M. L. (1987). Frequency-specific BERA in infants. *Journal of Otolaryngology, 14* (Suppl. 14), 19–27.

Hyde, M. L. (2005). Newborn hearing screening programs: Overview. *Journal of Otolaryngology, 34*(Suppl. 2), S70–S78.

Hyde, M. L., Riko, K., & Malizia, K. (1990). Audiometric accuracy of the click ABR in infants at risk for hearing loss. *Journal of the American Academy of Audiology, 1,* 59–66.

James, A. L., Harrison, R. V., Pienkowski, M., Dajani, H. R., & Mount, R. J. (2005). Dynamics of real time DPOAE contralateral suppression in chinchillas and humans. *International Journal of Audiology, 44,* 118–129.

Janssen, R. M., Usher, L., & Stapells, D. R. (2010). The British Columbia's Children's Hospital tone-evoked ABR protocol: How long do infants sleep, and how much information can be obtained in one appointment? *Ear and Hearing,* in press.

Jerger, J., Chmiel, R., Glaze, D., & Frost, J. D., Jr. (1987). Rate and filter dependence of the middle-latency response in infants. *Audiology, 26,* 269–283.

Jiang, Z. D., Brosi, D. M., Shao, X. M., & Wilkinson, A. R. (2008). Sustained depression of brainstem auditory electrophysiology during the first months in term infants after perinatal asphyxia. *Clinical Neurophysiology, 119,* 1496–1505.

John, M. S., Brown, D. K., Muir, P. J., & Picton, T. W. (2004). Recording auditory steady-state responses in young infants. *Ear and Hearing, 25,* 539–553.

John, M. S., Dimitrijevic, A., & Picton, T. W. (2002). Auditory steady-state responses to exponential modulation envelopes. *Ear and Hearing, 23,* 106–117.

Johnson, J. L., White, K. R., Widen, J. E., Gravel, J. S., James, M., Kennalley, T., . . . Holstrum, J. (2005). A multicenter evaluation of how many infants with permanent hearing loss pass a two-stage otoacoustic emissions/automated auditory brainstem response newborn hearing screening protocol. *Pediatrics, 116,* 663–672.

Johnson, K. L., Nicol, T. G., & Kraus, N. (2005). Brain stem response to speech: a biological marker of auditory processing. *Ear and Hearing, 26,* 424–434.

Joint Committee on Infant Hearing. (2000). Year 2000 position statement: Principles and guidelines for early hearing detection and intervention programs. *Pediatrics, 106,* 798–817.

Joint Committee on Infant Hearing. (2007). Year 2007 position statement: Principles and guidelines for early hearing detection and intervention programs. *Pediatrics, 120,* 898–921. Also available from: http://www.asha.org/docs/html/PS2007-00281.html or http://www.pediatrics.org/cgi/content/full/120/4/898

Karzon, R. K., & Lieu, J. E. (2006). Initial audiologic assessment of infants referred from well baby, special care, and neonatal intensive care unit nurseries. *American Journal of Audiology, 15,* 14–24.

Kemp, D. T., Ryan, S., & Bray, P. (1990). A guide to the effective use of otoacoustic emissions. *Ear and Hearing, 11,* 93–105.

Kennedy, C. R., McCann, D. C., Campbell, M. J., Law, C. M., Mullee, M., Petrou, S., . . . Stevenson, J. (2006). Language ability after early detection of permanent childhood hearing impairment. *New England Journal of Medicine, 354,* 2131–2141.

Krishnan, A. (2007). Frequency following response. In R. F. Burkard, M. Don, & J. J.

Eggermont (Eds.), *Auditory evoked potentials: Basic principles and clinical applications* (pp. 313–333). Baltimore, MD: Lippincott Williams & Wilkins.

Lee, C. Y., Hsieh, T. H., Pan, S. L., & Hsu, C. J. (2007). Thresholds of tone burst auditory brainstem responses for infants and young children with normal hearing in Taiwan. *Journal of the Formosan Medical Association, 106*, 847–853.

Lieu, J. E., Karzon, R. K., & Mange, C. C. (2006). Hearing screening in the neonatal intensive care unit: Follow-up of referrals. *American Journal of Audiology, 15*, 66–74.

Lightfoot, G., Sininger, Y., Burkard, R., & Lodwig, A. (2007). Stimulus repetition rate and the reference levels for clicks and short tone bursts: A warning to audiologists, researchers, calibration laboratories, and equipment manufacturers. *American Journal of Audiology, 16*, 94–95.

Lins, O. G., Picton, T. W., Boucher, B. L., Durieux-Smith, A., Champagne, S. C., Moran, L. M., . . . Savio, G. (1996). Frequency-specific audiometry using steady-state responses. *Ear and Hearing, 17*, 81–96.

Luts, H., Desloovere, C., & Wouters, J. (2006). Clinical application of dichotic multiple-stimulus auditory steady-state responses in high-risk newborns and young children. *Audiology & Neurotology, 11*, 24–37.

Luts, H., & Wouters, J. (2005). Comparison of MASTER and AUDERA for measurement of auditory steady-state responses. *International Journal of Audiology, 44*, 244–253.

Margolis, R. H., Bass-Ringdahl, S., Hanks, W. D., Holte, L., & Zapala, D. A. (2003). Tympanometry in newborn infants—1 kHz norms. *Journal of the American Academy of Audiology, 14*, 383–392.

Mazlan, R., Kei, J., Hickson, L., Stapleton, C., Grant, S., Lim, S., Linning, R., & Gavranich, J. (2007). High frequency immittance findings: Newborn versus six-week-old infants. *International Journal of Audiology, 46*, 711–717.

McCormick, D. P., Johnson, D. L., & Baldwin, C. D. (2006). Early middle ear effusion and school achievement at age seven years. *Ambulatory Pediatrics, 6*, 280–287.

Melagrana, A., Casale, S., Calevo, M. G., & Tarantino, V. (2007). MB11 BERAphone and auditory brainstem response in newborns at audiologic risk: Comparison of results. *International Journal of Pediatric Otorhinolaryngology, 71*, 1175–1180.

Morton, C. C., & Nance, W. E. (2006). Newborn hearing screening—a silent revolution. *New England Journal of Medicine, 354*, 2151–2164.

National Institutes of Health. (1993). Early Identification of Hearing Impairment in Infants and Young Children. *NIH Consensus Statement, 11*(1), 1–24.

National Health Service Newborn Hearing Screening Programme. (2007). Guidelines for the early audiological assessment and management of babies referred from the newborn hearing screening programme. Version 1.1. Available by choosing protocol at http://hearing.screening.nhs.uk/audiologicalassessment

Nelson, H. D., Bougatsos, C., & Nygren, P. (2008). Universal newborn hearing screening: Systematic review to update the 2001 U.S. Preventive Services Task Force Recommendation. *Pediatrics, 122*, e266–e276.

Norton, S. J., Gorga, M. P., Widen, J. E., Folsom, R. C., Sininger, Y., Cone-Wesson, B., . . . Fletcher, K. A. (2000). Identification of neonatal hearing impairment: Summary and recommendations. *Ear and Hearing, 21*, 529–535. (Special issue of journal is devoted to papers on this topic.)

Paradise, J. L., Campbell, T. F., Dollaghan, C. A., Feldman, H. M,. Bernard, B. S., Colborn, D. K., . . . Smith, C. G. (2005). Developmental outcomes after early or delayed insertion of tympanostomy tubes. *New England Journal of Medicine, 353*, 576–586.

Parry, G., Hacking, C., Bamford, J., & Day, J. (2003). Minimal response levels for visual reinforcement audiometry in infants. *International Journal of Audiology, 42*, 413–417.

Pastorino, G., Sergi, P., Mastrangelo, M., Ravazzani, P., Tognola, G., Parazzini, M., . . . Grandori, F. (2005). The Milan Project: A newborn hearing screening programme. *Acta Paediatrica, 94*, 458–463.

Perez-Abalo, M. C., Savio, G., Torres, A., Martín, V., Rodríguez, E., & Galán, L. (2001). Steady state responses to multiple amplitude-modulated tones: An optimized method to test frequency-specific thresholds in hearing-impaired children and normal-hearing subjects. *Ear and Hearing, 22*, 200–211.

Picton, T. W. (2007). Audiometry using auditory steady-state responses. In R. F. Burkard, M. Don, & J. J. Eggermont (Eds.), *Auditory evoked potentials: Basic principles and clinical applications* (pp. 441–462). Baltimore, MD: Lippincott Williams & Wilkins.

Picton, T. W., Durieux-Smith, A. , Champagne, S. C., Whittingham, J., Moran, L. M., Giguère, C., & Beauregard, Y. (1998). Objective evaluation of aided thresholds using auditory steady-state responses. *Journal of the American Academy of Audiology, 9*, 315–331.

Picton, T. W., Durieux-Smith, A., & Moran, L. M. (1994). Recording auditory brainstem responses from infants. *International Journal of Pediatric Otorhinolaryngology, 28*, 93–110.

Picton, T. W., Ouellette, J., Hamel, G., & Smith, A. D. (1979). Brainstem evoked potentials to tonepips in notched noise. *Journal of Otolaryngology, 8*, 289–314.

Picton, T. W., Taylor, M. J., & Durieux-Smith, A. (2005). Brainstem auditory evoked potentials in pediatrics. In M. J. Aminoff (Ed.), *Electrodiagnosis in clinical neurology* (5th ed., pp. 525–552). Philadelphia, PA: Elsevier Churchill Livingstone.

Porter, H. L., Neely, S. T., & Gorga, M. P. (2009). Using benefit-cost ratio to select Universal Newborn Hearing Screening test criteria. *Ear and Hearing, 30*, 447–457.

Psarommatis, I., Riga, M., Douros, K., Koltsidopoulos, P., Douniadakis, D., Kapetanakis, I., & Apostolopoulos, N. (2006). Transient infantile auditory neuropathy and its clinical implications. *International Journal of Pediatric Otorhinolaryngology, 70*, 1629–1637.

Qian, L., Yi, W., Xingqi, L., Yinsheng, C., Wenying, N., Lili, X., & Yinghui, L. (2010). Development of tone-pip auditory brainstem responses and auditory steady-state responses in infants aged 0–6 months. *Acta Otolaryngologica*, in press.

Rance, G. (2008). Auditory steady-state responses in neonates and infants. In G. Rance (Ed.), *Auditory steady-state response: Generation, recording, and clinical applications* (pp. 161–184). San Diego, CA: Plural Publishing.

Rance, G., & Rickards, F. (2002). Prediction of hearing threshold in infants using auditory steady-state evoked potentials. *Journal of the American Academy of Audiology, 13*, 236–245.

Rance, G., Roper, R. A., Symons, L., Moody, L. J., Poulis, C., & Kelly, T. (2005). Hearing threshold estimation in infants using auditory steady-state responses. *Journal of the American Academy of Audiology, 16*, 291–300.

Rance, G., & Tomlin, D. (2006). Maturation of auditory steady-state responses in normal babies. *Ear and Hearing, 27*, 20–29.

Ribeiro, F. M., & Carvallo, R. M. (2008). Tone-evoked ABR in full-term and preterm neonates with normal hearing. *International Journal of Audiology, 47*, 21–29.

Ribeiro, F. M., Carvallo, R. M., & Marcoux, A. M. (2010). Auditory steady state responses for preterm and term neonates. *Audiology and Neurotology, 15*, 97–110.

Rickards, F. W., Tan, L. E., Cohen, L. T., Wilson, O. J., Drew, J. H., & Clark, G. M. (1994). Auditory steady-state evoked potential in newborns. *British Journal of Audiology, 28*, 327–337.

Riquelme, R., Kuwada, S., Filipovic, B., Hartung, K., & Leonard, G. (2006). Optimizing the stimuli to evoke the amplitude modulation following response (AMFR) in neonates. *Ear and Hearing, 27*, 104–119.

Savio, G., Cárdenas, J., Pérez Abalo, M., González, A., & Valdés, J. (2001). The low and high frequency auditory steady state responses mature at different rates. *Audiology & Neuro-Otology, 6*, 279–287.

Savio, G., & Perez-Abalo, M. C. (2008). Auditory steady-state responses and hearing screening. In G. Rance (Ed.), *The auditory steady-state response: Generation, recording, and clinical application* (pp. 185–199). San Diego, CA: Plural Publishing.

Schimmenti, L. A., Martinez, A., Telatar, M., Lai, C. H., Shapiro, N., Fox, M., . . . Palmer,

C. G. (2008). Infant hearing loss and connexin testing in a diverse population. *Genetics in Medicine, 10,* 517–524.

Scollie, S., & Seewald, R. (2002). Hearing aid fitting and verification procedures for children. In J. Katz, R. F. Burkard, & L. Medwetsky (Eds.), *Handbook of clinical audiology* (5th ed.). Philadelphia, PA: Lippincott Williams & Wilkins.

Sininger, Y. S. (2007). The use of auditory brainstem response in screening for hearing loss and audiometric threshold prediction. In R. F. Burkard, M. Don, & J. J. Eggermont (Eds.), *Auditory evoked potentials: Basic principles and clinical applications* (pp. 254–274). Baltimore, MD: Lippincott Williams & Wilkins.

Sininger, Y. S., Abdala, C., & Cone-Wesson, B. (1997). Auditory threshold sensitivity of the human neonate as measured by auditory brainstem response. *Hearing Research, 104,* 27–38.

Sininger, Y. S., Grimes, A., & Christensen, E. (2010). Auditory development in early amplified children: Factors influencing auditory-based communication outcomes in children with hearing loss. *Ear and Hearing, 31,* 166–185

Sininger, Y. S., Martinez, A., Eisenberg, L., Christensen, E., Grimes, A., & Hu, J. (2009). Newborn hearing screening speeds diagnosis and access to intervention by 20–25 months. *Journal of the American Academy of Audiology, 20,* 49–57.

Small, S. A., Hatton, J. L., & Stapells, D. R. (2007). Effects of bone oscillator coupling method, placement location, and occlusion on bone-conduction auditory steady-state responses in infants. *Ear and Hearing, 28,* 83–98.

Small, S. A., & Stapells, D. R. (2006). Multiple auditory steady-state response thresholds to bone-conduction stimuli in young infants with normal hearing. *Ear and Hearing, 27,* 219–228.

Small, S. A., & Stapells, D. R. (2008a). Normal ipsilateral/contralateral asymmetries in infant multiple auditory steady-state responses to air- and bone-conduction stimuli. *Ear and Hearing, 29,* 185–198.

Small, S. A. & Stapells, D. R. (2008b). Maturation of bone-conduction multiple auditory steady-state responses. *International Journal of Audiology, 47,* 476–488.

Spivak, L. G. (1998). *Universal newborn hearing screening.* New York, NY: Thieme.

Stapells, D. R. (2000a). Threshold estimation by the tone-evoked auditory brainstem response: A literature meta-analysis. *Journal of Speech-Language Pathology and Audiology, 24,* 74–83.

Stapells, D. R. (2000b). Frequency-specific evoked potential audiometry in infants. In R. C. Seewald (Ed.), *A sound foundation through early amplification* (pp. 13–31). Basel, Switzerland: Phonak.

Stapells, D. R. (2010). Frequency-specific threshold assessment in young infants using the transient ABR and the brainstem ASSR. In R. C. Seewald & A. M. Tharpe, (Eds.), *Comprehensive handbook of pediatric audiology.* San Diego, CA: Plural Publishing.

Stapells, D. R., Gravel, J. S., & Martin, B. A. (1995). Thresholds for auditory brainstem responses to tones in notched noise from infants and young children with normal hearing or sensorineural hearing loss. *Ear and Hearing, 16,* 361–371.

Stapells, D. R., & Oates, P. (1997). Estimation of the pure-tone audiogram by the auditory brainstem response: A review. *Audiology & Neuro-Otology, 2,* 257–280.

Stapells, D., Picton, T., & Durieux-Smith, A. (1993). Electrophysiologic measures of frequency-specific auditory function. In J. T. Jacobson (Ed.), *Principles and applications of auditory evoked potentials* (pp. 251–283). New York, NY: Allyn & Bacon.

Stürzebecher, E., Cebulla, M., & Neumann, K. (2003). Click-evoked ABR at high stimulus repetition rates for neonatal hearing screening. *International Journal of Audiology, 42,* 59–70.

Taguchi, K., Picton, T. W., Orpin, J. A., & Goodman, W. S. (1969). Evoked response audiometry in newborn infants. *Acta Otolaryngologica Supplementum, 252,* 5–17.

Thompson, D. C., McPhillips, H., Davis, R. L., Lieu, T. L., Homer, C. J., & Helfand, M. (2001). Universal newborn hearing screening: Summary of evidence. *Journal of the American Medical Association, 286,* 2000–2010.

U.S. Preventive Services Task Force. (2008). Universal screening for hearing loss in newborns: U.S. Preventive Services Task Force recommendation statement. *Pediatrics, 122,* 143–148.

Van Maanen, A., & Stapells, D. R. (2009). Normal multiple auditory steady-state response thresholds to air-conducted stimuli in infants. *Journal of the American Academy of Audiology, 20,* 196–207.

Van Maanen, A., & Stapells, D. R. (2010). Multiple-ASSR thresholds in infants and young children with hearing loss. *Journal of the American Academy of Audiology, 21,* in press.

van der Reijden, C. S., Mens, L. H. M., & Snik, A. F. (2005). EEG derivations providing auditory steady-state responses with high signal-to-noise ratios in infants. *Ear and Hearing, 26,* 299–309.

Vander Werff, K. R., Prieve, B. A., & Georgantas, L. M. (2009). Infant air and bone conduction tone burst auditory brain stem responses for classification of hearing loss and the relationship to behavioral thresholds. *Ear and Hearing, 30,* 350–368. (Erratum in *Ear and Hearing, 31,* 379).

Vohr, B. R., Oh, W., Stewart, E. J., Bentkover, J. D., Gabbard, S., Lemons, J., Papile, L. A., & Pye, R. (2001). Comparison of costs and referral rates of 3 universal newborn hearing screening protocols. *Journal of Pediatrics, 139,* 238–244.

Voss, S. E., & Herrmann, B. S. (2005). How does the sound pressure generated by circumaural, supra-aural, and insert earphones differ for adult and infant ears? *Ear and Hearing, 26,* 636–650.

Watkin, P., McCann, D., Law, C., Mullee, M., Petrou, S., Stevenson, J., . . . Kennedy, C. (2007). Language ability in children with permanent hearing impairment: The influence of early management and family participation. *Pediatrics, 120,* e694–e701.

Weichbold, V., Nekahm-Heis, D., & Welzl-Mueller, K. (2006). Universal newborn hearing screening and postnatal hearing loss. *Pediatrics, 117,* e631–e636.

White, K. R., & Behrens, T. R. (1993). The Rhode Island hearing assessment project: Implications for universal newborn hearing screening. *Seminars in Hearing, 14,* 1–122.

Widen, J. E., Folsom, R. C., Cone-Wesson, B., Carty, L., Dunnell, J. J., Koebsell, K., . . . Norton, S. J. (2000). Identification of neonatal hearing impairment: Hearing status at 8 to 12 months corrected age using a visual reinforcement audiometry protocol. *Ear and Hearing, 21,* 471–487.

Wunderlich, J. L., & Cone-Wesson, B. K. (2006). Maturation of the cortical auditory evoked potential in infants and young children. *Hearing Research, 212,* 185–202.

Yoshinaga-Itano, C. (2003). Universal newborn hearing screening programs and developmental outcomes. *Audiological Medicine, 1,* 199–206.

Zenker-Castro, F., & Barajas de Prat, J. (2008). The role of auditory steady-state responses in fitting hearing aids. In G. Rance (Ed.), *The auditory steady-state response. Generation, recording and clinical application* (pp. 241–258). San Diego, CA: Plural Publishing.

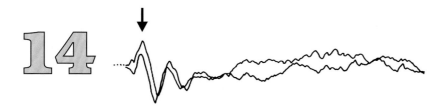

14

Neurotology and Neurology: From Cochlea to Cortex

Toute évidence est donc énigmatique: elle est abîme et fondement. L'honneur de l'homme n'est pas d'être meilleur, plus véridique, ou plus beau: il est d'envisager son évidence, d'y reconnaître sa question, et d'y répondre par un acte intégral—par l'être. L'honneur de l'homme est d'atteindre à ce centre où la certitude se fait vertige et le vertige certitude.

(All evidence is thus enigmatic: both bottomless abyss and solid ground. The greatness of man is not to be better, more truthful or more beautiful: it is to examine the evidence, to recognize the questions therein and to answer them with integrity—by being. The greatness of man is to reach the point where certainty becomes vertigo and vertigo certainty.)

Pierre Emmanuel, *Versant de l'Âge*, Preface, 1958

Neurotology is the study of the ear in relation to the brain. In this complex field at the intersection of neurology and otology, diagnosis is often uncertain. The clinician must combine an astute analysis of the patient's history with an extensive battery of tests to evaluate anatomy and function. Each test by itself may not be diagnostic but, when all the evidence is collected, some reasonable certainty can be attained. In this chapter, we consider several neurotologic disorders and evaluate the role

that the auditory evoked potentials (EPs) might play in their diagnosis. This is a selective rather than exhaustive review of neurotology, which is covered in much more detail by Baloh (1997) and by Lustig, Niparko, Minor, and Zee (2003). Because of its extensive recent literature, auditory neuropathy is covered separately in the following chapter.

This chapter also considers the use of auditory EPs in neurology. Before the auditory brainstem response (ABR), the evaluation of hearing played little role in neurological examination. The ABR gave a precise timing to abnormalities in the transmission of auditory information through the brainstem and showed that localizing lesions in the auditory pathways could be an important adjunct to patient assessment. Here again, this review is selective and the reader can refer to Chiappa (1997) for a more comprehensive treatment.

MÉNIÈRE'S DISEASE

Ménière's disease is characterized by four main symptoms: vertigo, hearing loss, tinnitus, and aural fullness (Beasley & Jones, 1996; Committee on Hearing and Equilibrium, 1995). The vertigo comes in spells that typically last between 20 minutes and 24 hours. The spells usually are associated with nausea and often cause vomiting, and the patient is prostrated by the vertigo but does not lose consciousness. After the vertigo passes, the patient can suffer from disequilibrium for several days. When examined during the attack, the patient always shows nystagmus. The tinnitus is most commonly described as low- or mid-frequency ("roaring"). Audiometric examination during the attack shows a sensorineural hearing loss. At the beginning of the disorder, the hearing loss only occurs during the spells of vertigo. With repeated attacks, the hearing loss can persist during the periods when there is no vertigo.

The disease is caused by endolymphatic hydrops, an overaccumulation of endolymph in the cochlear and vestibular labyrinth (Sajjadi & Paparella, 2008). In the cochlea, this causes Reissner's membrane to balloon out, and exerts severe pressure on the basilar membrane. In the vestibular system, the hydrops causes outpouchings and ruptures of the membranous labyrinth. The cause of the increased endolymph is not known—there may be decreased resorption through the endolymphatic sac and/or increased production through the stria vascularis. Both processes may be related to an accumulation of proteins in the endolymph, which can increase production by osmosis and decrease resorption by blocking membrane channels.

The diagnosis of Ménière's disease is based mainly on the patient's history. The differential diagnosis includes disorders of the eighth nerve or brainstem, perilymphatic fistula, and migraine. The most important tests in the evaluation of the patient with intermittent vertigo are audiometry and electronystagmography with caloric testing of semicircular canal function. The audiogram may show greater loss at the low and mid frequencies, be flat across all frequencies, or show a loss in both low and high frequencies with near-normal thresholds at 2000 Hz (the "tent" or "peak" pattern). Caloric testing typically shows unilateral hypofunction of the vestibular end-organ, although the results may be within normal limits between attacks or even during the attacks early in the disease. Recent developments in magnetic resonance imaging (MRI) can provide a visual demonstration of endolymphatic hydrops: intratympanically injected gadolinium is taken up through the round window and outlines the perilymphatic spaces in the inner ear (Naganawa et al., 2008; Nakashima et al., 2009). Several electrophysiologic tests provide confirmatory evidence for Ménière's disease. They are not diagnostic by themselves although they may bolster an uncertain diagnosis.

Electrochochleography (ECochG)

The ECochG shows two main findings in Ménière's disease (Abbas & Brown, 2009;

Ferraro & Durrant, 2006; Schoonhoven, 2007). First, the summating potential (SP) evoked by clicks or by middle-frequency tones is increased in amplitude. The tone-SP effects can be further examined in relation to glycerol administration or in relation to biasing the basilar membrane with low-frequency tones. Second, the peak latency of the N1 wave of the compound action potential (CAP) shows a greater difference between condensation and rarefaction than in normal subjects. Figure 14–1 summarizes the ECochG findings in patients with Ménière's disease.

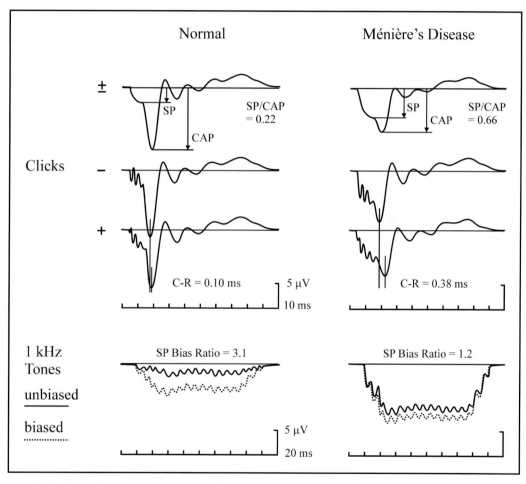

Figure 14–1. ECochG findings in patients with Ménière's disease. *This figure represents diagrammatically the typical changes in transtympanic ECochG recordings in Ménière's disease (right) compared to normal subjects (left). The click-evoked response shows an increased SP/CAP ratio (above the normal limits of about 0.4), and an increased latency difference between the CAP peak latency between condensation and rarefaction clicks (above the normal limits of about 0.13 ms). The lower section of the figure shows the responses to 16-ms 1-kHz tones. The response in a patient with Ménière's disease is larger than normal (normal upper limits of about –6 μV) and shows little effect of biasing with a concomitant low-frequency tone (normal limit for the bias ratio is greater than 1.4).*

As reviewed in Chapter 7, the normal SP/CAP ratio of the click-evoked ECochG is generally below 0.4. The actual limits of normal will depend on stimulus parameters, such as intensity and rate, and recording parameters, such as the location of the electrode. Using laboratory-specific limits of normal for the SP/CAP ratio gives a sensitivity of about 70% and a specificity of about 95% in the investigation of patients with possible Ménière's disease (see Table 9.1 of Schoonhoven, 2007). If the response is abnormal, we can be reasonably sure that there is endolymphatic hydrops. However, the response is within normal limits in about a third of patients who actually have the disease, either because the disease is quiescent at the time of the examination or because of the inherent variance of the measurements.

The SP to a tone varies with the tonal frequency (Eggermont, 1976; Sass, Densert, & Arlinger, 1998). Although tones with frequencies of 1000 or 2000 Hz give consistently negative SP measurements, higher frequency tones can elicit SPs that are near zero or positive. Therefore, clinical testing typically uses the response to 1000 or 2000 Hz tones. The SP amplitude in the tone response is measured in absolute terms and not in relation to the CAP. The SP is larger (more negative) in patients with Ménière's disease. The actual SP amplitude will vary with the stimulus intensity and with the location of the electrode, and the limits of normal therefore are specific to a particular laboratory and its procedures. Conlon and Gibson (2000) found that measuring the SP to a 1000 Hz tone gave a higher level of sensitivity (for similar specificities) than the click SP/CAP ratio. This means that measuring the 1000-Hz SP may be better able to identify the patient with Ménière's disease than the SP/CAP ratio. A review of the find-

ings in transtympanic ECochG in 2717 patients referred for possible Ménière's disease, Gibson (2009) found that measuring the amplitude of the SP to a 1000 Hz tone was a far better indicator of the final diagnosis of Ménière's disease than the SP/CAP ratio for a click. Given a specificity of about 90%, the sensitivity of the 1000-Hz SP-amplitude was between 41 and 94%, depending on the level of hearing loss, and the sensitivity of the click SP/CAP was between 12 and 21%. The SP/CAP results in this particular study were less sensitive than in other studies.

Iseli and Gibson (2010) have evaluated a measurement of SP biasing as a diagnostic tool in Ménière's disease. The changes in the tone-SP as a result of the changing polarity of a 30-Hz biasing sound were measured as a ratio of largest to smallest amplitude. Patients with Ménière's disease showed little or no change. Using a lower normal limit of 1.4, the test showed a sensitivity of 81% with a specificity level of 85%. They suggested that a combination of tests—the click SP/CAP ratio, the 1000 Hz SP, and the biasing ratio—might provide the best diagnostic approach to Ménière's disease.

The increased SP in Ménière's disease can be reduced by the administration of glycerol (Coats & Alford, 1981; Dauman, Aran, Charlet de Sauvage, & Portmann, 1988). The glycerol acts as an osmotic diuretic decreasing the amount of fluid in the body, and thereby reducing the endolymphatic pressure. The glycerol may be administered orally or intravenously, but the intravenous method is more consistent (Aso, Watanabe, & Mizukoshi, 1991). The glycerol procedure is not used much these days. It may be helpful when the SP measurements are abnormal and the history inconclusive. Other causes of vertigo do not make the SP sensitive to glycerol.

A final ECochG measurement that can be added to the armamentarium is the latency difference between the peak of the N1 wave in the CAP for condensation and rarefaction clicks. This measurement requires separately averaging the responses to clicks of opposite polarity. The latency for condensation clicks is slightly longer. The difference is normally less than 0.2 ms, but in Ménière's disease the difference may reach levels of a millisecond (Sass, Densert, Magnusson, & Whitaker, 1998). The laboratories that have used this measurement indicate that it can increase the diagnostic accuracy for Ménière's disease, when taken in combination with measurements of the SP amplitude (Ge & Shea, 2002; Margolis, Rieks, Fournier, & Levine, 1995; Ohashi, Nishino, Arai, Hyodo, & Takatsu, 2009; Orchik, Ge, & Shea, 1998).

Auditory Brainstem Response (ABR)

The ABR to clicks presented at intensities above hearing threshold typically is normal in Ménière's disease. As the click intensity is reduced to threshold levels, the response typically disappears. This sudden transition between a normal waveform and an absent response is related to recruitment. Thus, the click-ABR is a helpful test in the evaluation of a unilateral sensorineural hearing loss, as the waveform is normal in cochlear disorders such as Ménière's disease and abnormal in neural disorders such as acoustic neuroma.

As noted in Chapter 5, high-pass masking of the click ABR can be used to evaluate derived responses to narrow band regions of the spectrum. By measuring the latencies of either the high-pass masked response, or the derived responses, we can estimate the traveling wave velocity in the cochlea. In patients with Ménière's disease, the latencies can show a decreased travel time between the high and low frequency regions of the cochlea (Thornton & Farrell, 1991). The pressure of the endolymphatic hydrops increases the stiffness of the basilar membrane and might thereby speed up the traveling wave. However, measurements of the traveling wave velocity using tone-ABRs did not reveal any difference between normal subjects and patients with Ménière's disease (Murray, Cohn, Harker, & Gorga, 1998). Some patients with Ménière's disease do have a shorter delay between high- and low-frequency regions when measured using high-pass masking techniques, but this is not common and does not correlate well with the severity of their disease (Claes et al., 2008; Donaldson & Ruth, 1996).

Don, Kwong, and Tanaka (2005) proposed a technique that is similar to these traveling wave studies, the cochlear hydrops analysis masking procedure (CHAMP). The click-ABR is recorded alone and in the presence of high-pass masking noise. In normal-hearing subjects, the latency of the wave V increased by more than 0.3 ms when the high-pass masking is extended to 500 Hz. In patients with Ménière's disease, the latency change was essentially zero and never exceeded 0.2 ms. They found no overlap in the measurements between the patients, who showed three of the four hallmark symptoms (tinnitus, hearing loss, vertigo, aural fullness) at the time of testing, and control subjects—a sensitivity and specificity of 100%. Figure 14–2 shows the results in a patient with unilateral Ménière's disease.

Rather than changes in traveling-wave velocity, Don, Kwong, and Tanaka (2005) proposed a different explanation for their results. They interpreted the

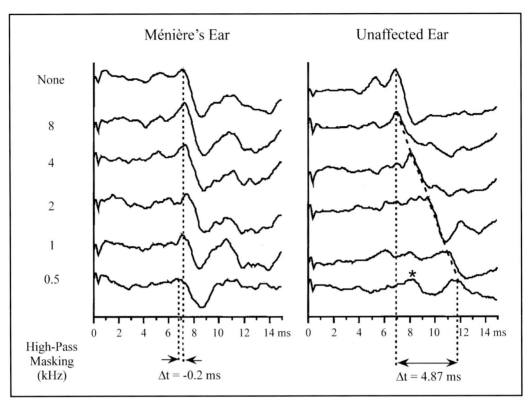

Figure 14–2. Cochlear hydrops analysis masking procedure. This figure plots the ABRs to clicks presented in high-pass masking noise for a subject with unilateral Ménière's disease. ABRs from the affected ear (left) in a patient show virtually no wave V latency shifts. ABRs from the unaffected ear (right) show the large wave V latency shifts similar to those observed in the normal-hearing population. Figure adapted from Don et al. (2005). The asterisk indicates a possible undermasked earlier wave V in the 500-Hz masked response in the normal ear.

early wave V recorded with the 500-Hz high-pass noise as coming from the high-frequency regions of the cochlea. They proposed that mechanical effects of the endolymphatic hydrops reduced the effect of the high-pass masking, thus "under-masking" the high-frequency response. The masking noise used in these studies was pink noise, also known as 1/f noise because the power is inversely proportional to the frequency (making the power equivalent across octaves or across third-octaves). This has less power in the high

frequencies than white noise. The intensity of the noise is adjusted to a level that just masks the detection of a recognizable ABR in normal hearing subjects. Thus, it is not surprising that undermasking of high-frequency regions might occur. Indeed, the authors noted that, in some normal subjects a small undermasked response may occur in addition to the delayed wave V. This can perhaps be recognized (indicated by an asterisk) in Figure 14–2.

An additional difficulty is that the wave V in the 500-Hz masked response may be small and difficult to measure, particularly in patients with a low-frequency hearing loss. Although the original study was able to make definite measurements in all patients, other groups have found the test uninterpretable in 50% (De Valck, Claes, Wuyts, & Van de Heyning, 2007) or 29% (Ordóñez-Ordóñez et al., 2009) of patients with definite Ménière's disease.

A second paper (Don, Kwong, & Tanaka, 2007) therefore proposed some additional measurements to distinguish the patients with Ménière's disease. Amplitudes of wave V were measured between the peak and the succeeding trough. The best discriminant between the patients and the normal controls was a "complex amplitude ratio." The amplitude of wave V was measured in the waveform obtained by subtracting the 0.5-kHz high-pass response from the response to clicks alone. This amplitude was then divided by the amplitude of wave V in the click alone response. In essence, this measures the relative size of the unmasked wave V in the 500-Hz masked response relative to the size of wave V in the click-alone ABR, with the ratio being close to 1 when there is no undermasking (normal finding) and lower than 1 when undermasking occurs (Ménière's disease). This ratio can provide 100% sensitivity with about 75% specificity.

Evaluating the Patient with Ménière's Disease

The diagnosis of Ménière's disease depends mainly on the history, audiometry, and electronystagmography. The simple click-ABR is a useful test to argue against retrocochlear abnormalities. Some measurement of the SP is helpful—an increased size will help confirm the diagnosis of Ménière's disease and distinguish it from cochlear hair cell loss, which will show a reduced SP. The best test appears to be to measure the amplitude of the SP to a 1000-Hz tone in the transtympanic ECochG. This is more sensitive than the SP/CAP ratio. Other electrophysiologic tests such as biasing the SP and measuring ABR undermasking can further bolster the clinical impression. As reviewed in Chapter 9, the vestibular evoked myogenic potential (VEMP) can serve as an adjunct to electronystagmography in evaluating vestibular function by assessing saccular function. This response is discussed later in this chapter. It is uncertain whether the new MRI tests may become diagnostic of hydrops. Even if they do, the problem will remain that the disorder is intermittent, and may not be present at the time of imaging.

The main need is to evaluate the electrophysiologic (and MRI) tests in patients who have possible (or probable) but not definite Ménière's disease. Patients classified as "definite" (Committee on Hearing and Equilibrium, 1995) do not really need further testing. Can the new tests distinguish patients who will later become definite from those who have other disorders of the inner ear or brainstem?

The electrophysiologic tests remain interesting because we have little idea why they present the way that they do. Much of the pathophysiology proposed to explain the test results is speculative. Is the increased size of the SP simply related to distortion of the basilar membrane? The SP is generated by several different processes—is one of them particularly sensitive to the pressure exerted by the hydrops? As the hearing loss progresses are there different effects on the SP—when does distortion of the hair cells lead to loss of hair cells? How much of the

SP/CAP ratio effect is related to increased SP and how much to decreased CAP? What causes the undermasking—is it a mechanical effect or is it related to decreased suppression (or both)? Further evaluation of the electrophysiologic tests therefore may increase our understanding of what might be going wrong in Ménière's disease.

PERILYMPHATIC FISTULA

Patients with a perilymphatic fistula often present with symptoms similar to those of Ménière's disease (Maitland, 2001). The disorder is caused by leakage of perilymph from either the round or oval window. The damage can be caused by sudden changes in the middle ear pressure, by head trauma, or by surgery in the middle ear (e.g., stapedectomy). The SP can be normal or enlarged, just as in Ménière's disease (Meyerhoff & Yellin, 1990). We can surmise that the mechanical distortion of the organ of Corti is similar in the two disorders. The basilar membrane moves down under pressure of the endolymphatic hydrops in Ménière's disease or from a lack of supporting pressure in the scala tympani when there is a perilymphatic fistula.

Clinically, we can check for changes in symptoms or a change in nystagmus when high or low pressure is exerted in the external auditory meatus using a pneumatic otoscope or impedance meter. When this test is clearly positive, the patient likely has a fistula. However, a negative test cannot rule out the disorder, and if the history is suggestive (symptoms coming on after head- or barotrauma), middle-ear exploration is recommended.

ECochG may help in the diagnosis by showing significant changes with changes in the thoracic pressure (Gibson, 1992; Sass, Densert, & Magnusson, 1997) or with changes in posture from upright sitting to lying down (Campbell & Abbas, 1993). Raising the thoracic pressure by forced expiration against a closed glottis or simply lying down will raise the intracranial pressure. This in turn will raise the perilymphatic pressure and therefore change the ECochG toward normal—the SP will decrease and the CAP will increase. In patients with Ménière's disease, these measurements should not change. Measuring the effect of changing the intrathoracic pressure clearly is easier with transtympanic ECochG than with measurements in the external auditory meatus, as the recording time is much less. Expiration against a closed glottis can only be done for short periods of time.

ACOUSTIC NEUROMAS AND OTHER TUMORS

Despite being called "acoustic neuromas," most of the tumors that impinge on the intracranial eighth cranial nerve are actually vestibular schwannomas. These typically arise at the level of the internal auditory canal and expand into the cerebellopontine angle. Although benign and slow growing, the tumors cause significant symptoms by exerting pressure on structures in the internal auditory canal: the eighth nerve, the blood vessels going to the inner ear, and the facial nerve. The patient typically presents with hearing loss, tinnitus, vertigo, disequilibrium, and headache. The hearing loss usually involves the high frequencies more than the low. Speech perception often is decreased more than might be predicted from the pure tone audiogram. Studies of the stapedius reflex show significant decay. The tinnitus is usually high pitched and continuous. The main physical findings are ataxia, nystagmus, and a decreased corneal reflex. The diagnosis should be considered in anyone with a unilateral sensorineural hearing loss. Patients with Type 2 neurofibromatosis can present with bilateral acoustic neuromas.

ABR

The click-ABR was first proposed as a way to screen for an acoustic neuroma by Selters and Brackmann (1977). Almost all patients with acoustic neuromas were found to have an abnormal click-ABR. The ABR is recorded using a loud click—70 db or more relative to normal hearing level (nHL)—presented at slow rates (typically near 10/s). The response is recorded separately for each ear using electrodes on the vertex and ipsilateral earlobe or mastoid. Initially, the focus was on the difference in wave V latency between the two ears, but this soon led to more precise measurements of the I–III and I–V interpeak latencies (Antonelli, Bellotto, & Grandori, 1987). The normal upper limits for the I-III and I-V interpeak latencies are near 2.6 and 4.5 ms, and the normal inter-ear difference in wave V latency is less than 0.3 ms. Further details about normative data for the click-ABR are presented in Chapter 8 (Tables 8–1, 8–2, and 8–3). The different patterns of abnormality seen in patients with an acoustic neuroma are shown in Figure 14–3. The incidence of the different patterns will vary with the referral population, and the percentages provided in Figure 14–3 are approximations (see Picton & Durieux-Smith, 1988).

The pattern that is most specific diagnostically is one in which there is a significant delay between wave I and wave III

of the ABR (top left pattern in Figure 14–3). This indicates dysfunction between the cochlea and the cochlear nucleus. The cause of the slowing could be a reduction in the conduction velocity of the nerve fibers due to the pressure of the tumor. However, it could also be due to the tumor specifically affecting the high-frequency fibers (Eggermont & Don, 1986; see discussion in Picton, 1991). Desynchronizing or blocking these fibers causes the brainstem wave V to be evoked by activity coming from the low-frequency region of the cochlea, whereas in normal subjects the wave V is mainly related to the high-frequency region. Thus, we have wave I generated by the high-frequency region and wave V activated by connections from the low-frequency regions. This causes the I–V interval to be prolonged by the cochlear delay between high- and low frequency regions of the basilar membrane.

Another common pattern is a prolonged wave V with a normal wave I and no clearly recognizable wave III (second pattern in the left column of Figure 14–3). This can be caused by a lesion in either the auditory nerve or the lateral pons. A lesion in the pons rather than nerve might be demonstrated by the presence of clinical signs involving the ascending and descending fibers that pass through the pons or by abnormalities of the contralateral ABR.

Often, the patient has a high-frequency hearing loss and it is difficult to measure a clear wave I. The detectability of wave I can be improved by an electrode in the external auditory canal and slow click rates. Even with these procedures, however, we often are left with a delayed wave V but no clearly recognizable earlier waves (bottom left pattern in Figure 14–3). This may be caused by a cochlear hearing loss or a retrocochlear disorder. Several techniques have been proposed to compensate for a

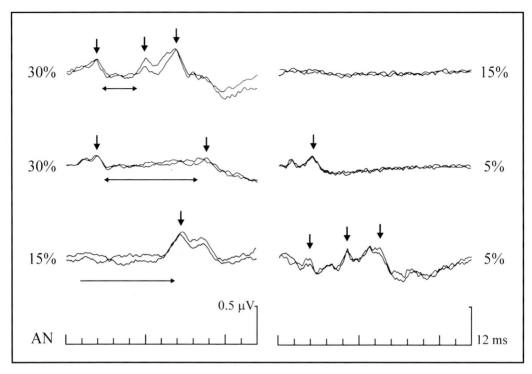

Figure 14–3. ***ABR patterns seen in patients with acoustic neuroma.*** *This figure illustrates the different kinds of ABR waveforms that can be recorded in patients with tumors of the cerebellopontine angle, together with their approximate incidences. These incidences are based on the experience of several laboratories. The arrows point to waves I, III, and V (where they are recognizable). The top left pattern shows a delayed wave I–III interval. The middle left recording shows a delayed I–V interval with no recognizable wave III. In the lower left pattern there is a delayed wave V but no recognizable earlier components. It often is impossible to determine whether this is related to a high-frequency cochlear hearing loss or to a retrocochlear problem. The upper right ABR shows no recognizable response. In the middle right ABR, only wave I is recognizable. The bottom right pattern shows an ABR with normal latencies. In this patient, both the I–III and I–V latencies are just within the upper limits of normal.*

cochlear high-frequency hearing loss, but they do not always work.

Sometimes, there is no recognizable ABR (upper right pattern in Figure 14–3). This could be due to a severe cochlear hearing loss or a retrocochlear hearing loss. If the patient has measurable hearing with thresholds below 80 dB HL, the absence of any ABR to 90 dB nHL clicks suggests the hearing loss is most likely retrocochlear in origin. The presence of wave I with no later components (middle right pattern in Figure 14–3) clearly indicates a retrocochlear abnormality, but is nonspecific as to the etiology.

The major problem with using the click-ABR to rule out an acoustic neuroma is the fact that the ABR may be normal in patients with definite tumors (bottom right pattern in Figure 14–3). This is particularly true if the tumor is small. For the purpose of this discussion, we are not differentiating between the types of cerebel-lopontine angle lesions, but just listing them all under the rubric of acoustic neu-roma. The sensitivity of the ABR screen-ing test typically is based on the criterion that the test is positive if there is any abnormality of the ABR. The sensitivity of the click-ABR is then about 100% for tumors larger than 2 cm, about 90% for tumors between 1 and 2 cm, and about 70% for tumors less than 1 cm (Gordon & Cohen, 1995; Levine, Antonelli, Le, & Haines, 1991; Robinette, Bauch, Olsen, & Cevette, 2000; Schmidt, Sataloff, New-man, Spiegel, & Myers, 2001). The overall incidence of false negatives in screening for an acoustic neuroma with the simple click-ABR therefore varies with the distri-bution of tumor sizes in the screened pop-ulation. If most of the tumors are large, the sensitivity of the ABR is close to 100% (Rupa, Job, George, & Rajshekhar, 2003). In recent years, the size of the acoustic neuromas being detected and operated on has decreased, mainly because of the availability of MRI evaluations. The smaller the tumor, the more likely it is that hear-ing and facial function can be preserved when the tumor is removed.

The specificity of the click-ABR in patients referred for possible acoustic neuroma is difficult to estimate, as it depends how the referral population is selected. Are only patients with asymmet-ric hearing loss evaluated, or do all patients with undiagnosed vertigo and tinnitus get referred for testing? If many patients with cochlear hearing loss are referred for test-ing and if many of them have an abnor-mal ABR, then the specificity will be far lower than if the referral population con-tains only normal subjects and patients with acoustic neuroma. For typical referral contexts, ABR-screening shows a specificity of about 60%. Even if we are just screen-ing those with an asymmetric hearing loss, the specificity is only about 75% (e.g., Cueva, 2004). Thus, between 25% and 40% of the patients without an acoustic neuroma will show false positive findings on the ABR screening test. This is not unreasonable if all subjects failing the test then receive an MRI to determine defini-tively whether or not there is an acoustic neuroma.

When the expense of the MRI was high, it was cost-effective to use an initial ABR to decide which patients should have an MRI. However, recent develop-ments have made the assessment of acoustic neuroma using MRI without contrast rapid, accurate, and inexpensive (e.g., Allen et al.,1996; Daniels et al., 2000). Such MRI techniques are 97 to 100% sen-sitive compared to the gold standard of gadolinium-enhanced MRI. MRI has the further advantage that it can help distin-guish the different types of retrocochlear hearing loss (type of tumor or other pathology), whereas the ABR can only indicate a dysfunction in the auditory nerve and not the etiology. Therefore, the present recommendation (Fortnum et al., 2009) is to use MRI as the primary screen-ing test for an acoustic neuroma, and to use the ABR only in cases where an MRI cannot be performed, such as patients with a cardiac pacemaker, intra-ocular/intracerebral metallic objects, or claustrophobia.

Stacked ABR and Related Techniques

To address the problem that the click-ABR is often normal in patients with small acoustic neuromas, Don, Masuda, Nelson, and Brackmann (1997) proposed a stacked ABR test. This looks at the amplitude of the ABR rather than the latency. The amplitude of the click-ABR generally is smaller in patients with acoustic neuromas than in normal subjects, but the measurement is too variable for clinical use. As reviewed in Chapter 5, the stacked ABR approach calculates derived narrow-band ABRs for each octave between 8 to 0.5 kHz using high-pass masking procedures. The latency of wave V is measured in each of the derived ABRs. The derived ABRs are then latency-compensated to make the wave V latency the same in each and added up to give the stacked ABR. The amplitude of wave V in the stacked ABR is then measured and compared to the mean values for normal subjects of the same gender as the patient. Other possible measurements are the ratio of the stacked ABR to the unmasked ABR wave V (normally around 2 to 4) or comparisons between the normal and the affected ear. Figure 14–4 illustrates the technique.

Patients with acoustic neuromas show stacked-ABR amplitudes that are significantly smaller than those of normal subjects or of subjects with cochlear hearing loss. An extensive evaluation of the test in patients with small acoustic neuromas (Don, Kwong, Tanaka, Brackmann, & Nelson, 2005) showed that the test had 95% sensitivity and 88% specificity for acoustic neuromas less than 1 cm in size. This is better than the simple click-ABR. Nevertheless, to obtain 100% sensitivity the specificity still reduces to 50%. The authors therefore propose that the test (using the criterion for 100% sensitivity) might be a useful initial test to decide who needs MRI. Given the present low costs of MRI screening, however, this may not be more cost-effective than simply screening all referred patients with MRI.

Although the general idea of the stacked ABR technique is reasonable, some concerns need to be considered. Kevanishvili (2000) pointed out that the high-frequency-derived band ABRs might be more specifically affected by acoustic neuromas than the lower frequencies, and that we might actually do better to remove the low-frequency derived responses rather than add them in. The acoustic neuroma exerts its main pressure on the external part of the auditory nerve where the high-frequency fibers are located, and typically spares low-frequency hearing. Another concern with the stacked-ABR procedure is that the technique has only been evaluated against normal hearing subjects. Unfortunately, patients with acoustic neuroma also need to be distinguished from patients with cochlear hearing loss. How does the technique fare when the control group contains patients with asymmetric cochlear hearing loss (particularly if this hearing loss involves the high frequencies)? These patients would be a more representative control group.

Another limitation of the stacked ABR technique is that it is often very difficult to recognize wave V in the derived-band ABRs, especially when the wave actually may not be present because of the pathology. The latency compensation therefore becomes uncertain. Dort et al. (2009) have proposed a modified derived-response technique that does not require any alignment of waveforms and yet promises the same sensitivity—the Power Spectrum ABR. Each of the derived band ABRs is converted to the frequency domain. Because power spectra are relatively insensitive to small delays in the waveforms, adding the power spectra of the derived-band ABRs provides an estimate of the total power present in the neural populations generating the click-ABR. The sum

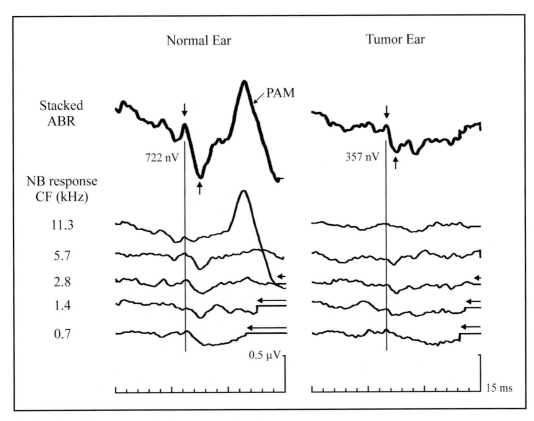

Figure 14–4. Stacked ABR technique in the evaluation of acoustic neuroma. The technique is described in detail in Chapter 5. Sequential subtraction of high-pass noise recordings with decreasing cutoff frequencies gives narrow-band derived responses. These are shown for decreasing center-frequencies (CF). The latencies of these responses are then adjusted to maintain the latency of wave V constant. The horizontal arrows on the right of the tracings show the amount of latency adjustment. The "stacked ABR" is then calculated by adding together the latency-adjusted narrow-band derived responses. In this patient the stacked ABR on the tumor side is about half the amplitude of the response on the normal side—significantly below the normal limits for this comparison. In the normal ear a reflex response in the postauricular muscle (PAM) is evoked by the high-frequency component of the click. Data replotted from Don et al. (1997).

of the power spectra of the derived responses is reduced when there is loss of functioning fibers in the auditory nerve. Dort et al. (2009) found that the Power Spectrum ABR was better able to discriminate patients with small tumors than the stacked ABR or the I–V latency. Dort et al. (2009) also included a no-tumor "referral group" with unilateral audiovestibular symptoms. For these patients, there was definite overlap with the tumor patients on both power spectrum and stacked ABR. The question remains whether screening with power spectrum ABR and subsequent MRI is more cost-effective than simply screening all patients with MRI. This depends on the relative cost and the availability/accessibility of the two tests.

Auditory Nerve Monitoring During Surgery

Intraoperative neurophysiologic monitoring is an important adjunct to surgery for acoustic neuroma and other posterior fossa operations such as microvascular decompression for trigeminal neuralgia or vestibular nerve section for disabling vertigo. As reviewed by Martin and Shi (2007), most retrospective studies comparing the outcome of posterior-fossa surgery with and without neurophysiologic monitoring have shown that hearing is significantly better preserved with monitoring (e.g., Harper et al., 1992; Wilkins, Radtke, & Erwin, 1991). As yet, however, there have not been any prospective randomized control studies, most neurosurgeons being unwilling to forego the perceived benefits of intraoperative monitoring.

Hearing can be disrupted during surgery for acoustic neuroma by two main mechanisms (Legatt, 2002; Ojemann, Levine, Montgomery, & McGaffigan, 1984). First, the vascular supply to the cochlea via the internal auditory artery can be compromised, leading to ischemia and ultimately infarction of the cochlea. Second, the auditory nerve can be damaged during the resection of the tumor, either by direct trauma to the nerve fibers or by occlusion of the small blood vessels supplying the nerve. These two mechanisms of damage must be borne in mind when considering what needs to be monitored during surgery.

Four main responses can be monitored during surgery. First, transtympanic (Morawski et al., 2007; Ojemann et al., 1984) or extratympanic (Attias, Nageris, Ralph, Vajda, & Rappaport, 2008) ECochG can monitor cochlear function. A major advantage of ECochG is that it does not require much averaging and therefore any changes are quickly demonstrated. Its

major disadvantage is that it monitors only functions that occur before the auditory information passes through the location of the resection. The second response that can be monitored is the scalp ABR, which provides information about the brainstem response to auditory stimulation and therefore monitors function beyond the location of resection (Harper et al., 1992; Ojemann et al., 1984). Its main disadvantage is that, because it requires averaging over many trials, it takes a while to be sure that a change has occurred. Third, the cochlear nerve action potential (CNAP) can be directly recorded by placing an electrode, for example, a wet cotton pledget attached to connecting wire (Colletti et al., 2000; Møller, 2006) or a specially designed C-shaped electrode (Cueva, Morris & Prioleau, 1998), on the auditory nerve proximal to the tumor. This is then referred to another electrode placed somewhere else in the surgical field, typically a needle electrode in the exposed neck musculature. The directly recorded CNAP is large and can show changes quickly. Its main disadvantage is when the size or location of the tumor makes it difficult to place the electrode or to maintain it during the resection. A fourth technique is to record the response of the cochlear nucleus (wave III of the ABR) by placing a cotton-wick electrode in the lateral recess of the fourth ventricle, which opens into the cerebellopontine angle through the foramen of Luschka (Kuroki & Møller, 1995; Møller, Jannetta, & Jho, 1994). This may be helpful when placing an electrode on the auditory nerve is difficult. The upper part of Figure 14–5 shows the surgical view of the cerebellopontine angle and the locations where intracranial electrodes can be placed. The lower part of the figure shows the recordings that can be used to monitor the function of the auditory nerve.

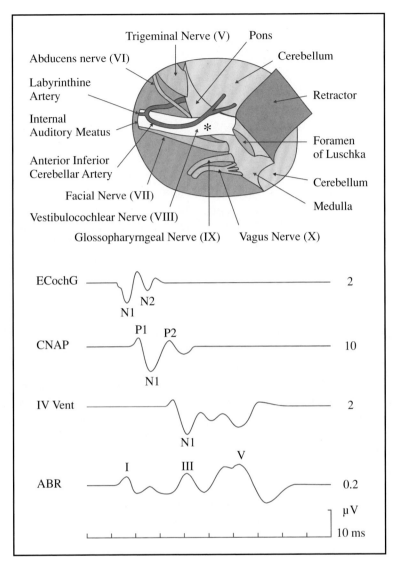

Figure 14–5. *Monitoring auditory function during posterior fossa surgery. The upper part of the figure shows the left cerebellopontine angle from a posteriolateral viewpoint. The cerebellum (including the flocculus) has been retracted to expose the nerves and vessels. The eighth nerve arises from the posterior junction of pons and medulla and courses laterally to the internal auditory meatus together with the seventh nerve. During operations for an acoustic neuroma, auditory potentials can be recorded from the proximal portion of the eighth nerve (asterisk). Recordings can also be obtained from the region of the cochlear nucleus by inserting an electrode into the fourth ventricle through the foramen of Luschka. The vascular supply of the region is variable. The diagram shows the labyrinthine artery coming off a loop of the anterior inferior cerebellar artery. This diagram derives from information in Lang (1985), Kurioki and Møller (1995) and Nowé et al. (2004). The lower part of the figure shows the recordings that can be monitored intra-operatively. These have different amplitudes and are plotted at different scales, as indicated on the right. The EcochG is recorded extratympanically. The cochlear nerve AP (CNAP) is recorded from the location indicated by the asterisk in the upper diagram. The recording from the lateral IV ventricle is close to the cochlear nucleus. Finally, an ABR is recorded from the vertex to the left mastoid. Each of the recordings has different calibration as shown by the numbers at the right. These are representative; the amplitudes will vary with the subject and with the amount of pathology in the eighth nerve.*

The physiologist monitoring the function of the cochlea and auditory nerve must be aware of several nonpathologic changes that can occur during the operation (Legatt, 2002; Martin and Shi, 2007; Møller, 2006). The auditory stimulator may become inoperative, either because the insert falls out of the ear or because it becomes disconnected from the click-generator. Drilling on the temporal bone during the resection may change the physiologic responses through acoustic masking. The anesthetic agents may cause latency delays in the ABR—this effect will occur before the posterior fossa is opened. Opening the dura to enter the posterior fossa can cause ABR delays through two mechanisms: the temperature will go down and the contents of the posterior fossa can shift and stretch the auditory nerve. These effects can cause a delay of up to 1 ms in the latency of the ABR wave V, but typically do not change the amplitude. Irrigation of the acoustic nerve exposing it to the air can cause large changes in the morphology of waves I to III in the ABR and can alter the amplitude and morphology of the directly recorded CNAP (Martin, Pratt, & Schwegler, 1995). Figure 14–6 (lower tracing in left column) shows nonpathologic changes in the ABR prior to the resection of the tumor.

During the resection of the tumor, the physiologist should monitor for pathologic changes in the cochlea and in the auditory nerve. Both pathologies will affect the ABR and the intracranially recorded CNAP. Thus, at least one of these recordings must be monitored. Current practice is to monitor both. Cochlear dysfunction will show up best on the ECochG whereas the cochlear microphonic (CM) and the CAP will decrease in amplitude as the cochlea becomes ischemic. The ECochG provides results quickly and often correlates very well with postoperative hearing thresholds (e.g., Morawski et al., 2007). However, it is possible for the ECochG to be preserved and for the patient to lose all hearing due to disruption in the intracranial auditory nerve at the level of the tumor resection (Attias et al., 2008; Symon et al., 1988). In the patient whose intraoperative ABRs are shown in Figure 14–6, the first abnormality was the loss of waves III and V (likely caused by trauma or ischemia to the nerve during the tumor resection). Only subsequently (perhaps because of later cochlear ischemia) did wave I vanish. It generally makes no sense to monitor only the ECochG without some additional monitor of auditory function beyond the operative site. However, there may be occasional patients who have no clear ABR or intracranial CNAP and yet show some ECochG activity and have some residual hearing.

The physiologist involved in monitoring should follow several principles. First, do not become involved in monitoring as an occasional event. The more experience in the operating room, the easier the recordings will be performed, and the more accurately they will be interpreted. Second, the patient must be evaluated prior to the surgery to determine what the recordings should look like during surgery. Third, as many recordings as possible should be made. ECochG, ABR, and intracranial CNAP are all helpful. In addition, we may wish to monitor other things such as facial nerve function (e.g., Linden et al., 1988). Fourth, the surgeon and the physiologist should agree on clear criteria for when the surgeon is to be notified of changes in the physiologic recordings.

The physiologist will rapidly realize that the monitoring affects the outcome in only a small percentage of the patients

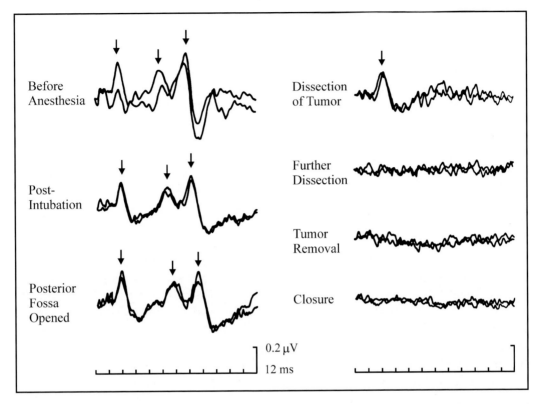

Figure 14–6. *ABRs recorded during removal of an acoustic neuroma. The ABRs recorded before anesthesia showed an increased I–III interpeak latency. After the patient was intubated and anesthetized, waves III and V of the ABR increased in latency slightly. This was caused by the anesthesia. Opening the posterior fossa caused a further increase in the latency of the later waves, related either to cooling or displacement of the brainstem away from the internal auditory canal. During the dissection of the tumor away from the nerve, the late components of the ABR suddenly vanished. Ceasing dissection and relaxing the traction on the cerebellum did not cause any return of function. Likely, there was an infarction of the nerve. A few minutes later wave I vanished as well. This was perhaps due to cochlear infarction. The ABR remained absent through the rest of the operation. The patient had no hearing on the side of the tumor after the operation.*

(Raudzens & Shetter, 1982). In most cases, the resection proceeds well, the physiologic monitors are normal, and hearing is preserved. In some cases, the physiologic recordings change. Many of these changes are due to nonpathologic processes such as acoustic masking or temperature changes. Others are due to pathology. Then, the hope is that the surgeon can do something— stop the drilling, release the traction on the nerve, cease dissection, or irrigate the nerve with warm saline—to reverse the changes. It is difficult to determine how often the pathology will reverse as it depends on both surgical skill and surgical chance. The justification for monitoring is that a significant number of patients will show changes that are reversed because of what the surgeon does following notification of the physiologic changes.

Other Tumors of the Posterior Fossa

Acoustic neuroma (vestibular schwannoma) is the most common tumor of the cerebellopontine angle. Other tumors that arise from or expand into this region include meningioma, paraganglionoma, and cerebellar astrocytoma. The symptoms of these other tumors are similar to those of the acoustic neuroma, although high-frequency hearing tends to be less affected. The ABR generally is abnormal (e.g. Baguley, Beynon, Grey, Hardy, & Moffat, 1997). The ABR can help to localize the lesion, but differential diagnosis will require imaging (Bonneville, Savatovsky, & Chiras, 2007).

The ABR is almost always abnormal in patients with tumors of the brainstem (reviewed by Chiappa, 1997). In the days before modern imaging, the ABR could help to diagnose these lesions and suggest their localization prior to invasive radiologic studies. There are several basic rules that can help interpret ABR abnormalities (e.g., Chiappa, 1997; Picton, 1986). Abnormalities beginning at wave III indicate pontine lesions, and those beginning at wave V indicate lesions of the upper pons or midbrain. If the ABR is affected in both ears, the lesion generally tends to be on the side of the more abnormal ABR. If the ABR is affected in only one ear, the lesion likely involves the ipsilateral pons or auditory nerve. Nowadays, brainstem tumors are definitively identified and evaluated using MRI.

DEMYELINATING LESIONS

Multiple Sclerosis

Multiple sclerosis is a disorder that specifically affects the myelin sheaths of neurons in the central nervous system. The essential clinical characteristic of the disorder is the occurrence of neurologic signs and symptoms that are disseminated in both space and time (McDonald et al., 2001). Separate regions of the nervous system are affected, and the attacks tend to be intermittent. Common symptoms are a transient loss of vision in one eye due to inflammation of the optic nerve behind the eye (retrobulbar neuritis), or loss of feeling and strength in the limbs due to involvement of the pathways in the spinal cord. Each episode is associated with an inflammatory immune response, although exactly what triggers or concludes it is not known. The clinical diagnosis depends on the demonstration of separate lesions in the nervous system by means of MRI and the sensory evoked potentials, and evidence of an abnormal immune response in the cerebrospinal fluid (oligoclonal bands).

The pathophysiology of demyelination is complex (Smith & McDonald, 1999). When the myelin sheath is attacked, the conduction of impulses along the axons is disrupted (Figure 14–7). In a normal myelinated axon, voltage-sensitive sodium channels are located at the nodes of Ranvier. How far the action potential (AP) generated at one node spreads along the axon will depend on the resistance of the myelin sheath. If the myelin is normal and the resistance is high, the AP easily spreads to the next node of Ranvier, and the AP is rapidly regenerated. The AP thus quickly jumps from node to node, leading to rapid "saltatory" conduction. If the myelin is removed by the inflammatory immune response, the decreased membrane resistance short-circuits the spread of the potential along the axon. Whatever potential reaches the next set of voltage-sensitive channels is insufficient to reinitiate the action potential, resulting in conduction block.

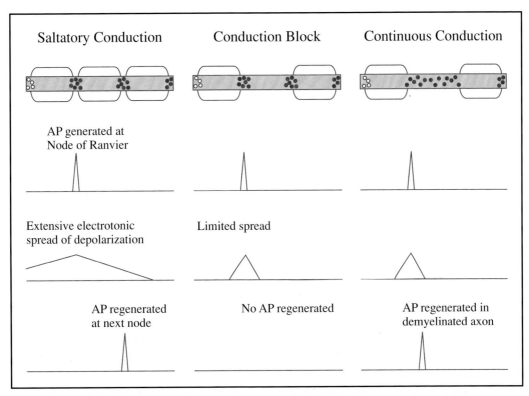

Figure 14–7. Pathophysiologic changes in demyelination. On the left are shown the processes underlying salutatory conduction in a myelinated nerve fiber. At the top is a diagrammatic representation of the axon (gray) with the myelin sheath (white). An action potential (AP) is travelling from left to right and has reached the second node of Ranvier. In the axonal membrane are voltage-sensitive sodium channels which are excitable (black) or refractory (white). Below the representation of the nerve fiber are plots of the membrane potential at three points in time. At the initial time point an AP is generated at a node of Ranvier when the voltage-sensitive channels are excited by the depolarization of the membrane and open. At the next point in time the depolarization of the AP spreads electrotonically along the membrane (in both directions). Because the membrane resistance is high the spread is extensive and reaches the next node with sufficient magnitude to excite the voltage sensitive channels there. This causes the regeneration of an AP as shown at the third point in time. The channels at the node previously activated are refractory from the earlier depolarization and so an AP is not generated there. The AP therefore travels only in one direction (to the right). The central column represents what happens with acute demyelination. The myelin sheath is removed and this decreases the transmembrane resistance. Because the membrane resistance is low, the depolarization from the AP spreads only a limited distance and does not reach the next set of voltage sensitive channels (where the next node of Ranvier was before the demyelination). The AP cannot be regenerated and conduction stops. The right column shows what happens when the voltage sensitive channels diffuse along the membrane into the demyelinated regions during the days to weeks after the acute episode. The demyelinated region then becomes excitable and an AP can be regenerated close to where it initially occurs. Because the distance is much less than the internodal distance, continuous conduction is much slower than saltatory conduction. In multiple sclerosis the patient may experience an acute loss of function due to conduction block during the initial attack of demyelination. After a few weeks, function may return due to the occurrence of continuous conduction in the demyelinated fibers. The diagrams are much simplified. In normal mammalian myelinated fibers, the AP actually jumps across several nodes rather than the one shown here.

As time passes and the inflammatory response declines, one of two things occurs. There may be remyelination of the axons, in which case impulse conduction may be reinstated, although the new myelin sheath is usually not as thick as before and the conduction may intermittently fail (e.g., when the temperature is elevated or when the rate of stimulation is high). The other possibility is that the myelin does not return. In this case, the voltage-sensitive channels previously concentrated at the nodes may diffuse along the axonal membrane and make it possible for the AP in one place to initiate an AP in closely adjacent regions of the axon. Impulses will then be conducted along the axon, although these will travel much more slowly than before. Without the myelin sheath and with repeated inflammation, the axon itself may degenerate, leading to an irreversible loss of function.

The processes illustrated in Figure 14–7 can explain the clinical and electrophysiologic findings in patients with multiple sclerosis. With conduction block, no impulses are transmitted. The patient experiences a loss of function, and the EPs will be absent or reduced in amplitude. If the axons conduct as unmyelinated fibers, the conduction will be slow. The patient may experience a return of many functions since the axons are conducting information. However, some functions may not be normal, particularly those dependent on timing. If all the fibers that are involved in the evoked potentials are similarly affected, the recorded EP is delayed but not decreased in amplitude. If different fibers are demyelinated over different distances, however, the resultant desynchronization of the individual-fiber responses also will decrease the amplitude of the compound response.

The visual EP to a reversing checkerboard stimulus was the first EP to be used in the evaluation of multiple sclerosis (Halliday, McDonald, & Mushin, 1972). In the acute attack of retrobulbar neuritis, the visual EP is absent. After a period of several days to weeks, the visual EP returns but is significantly delayed. The response shows a normal amplitude and morphology but is delayed by several tens of milliseconds. This delay indicates that the visual fibers are functioning but that the conduction is slowed by a region of demyelination. At this time, the visual acuity returns to normal, although color discrimination and motion tracking may remain impaired. A delayed visual EP thus can demonstrate that demyelination has occurred in the optic nerve even after most overt symptoms have subsided. If recorded at the time of another episode presenting with different symptoms, this conduction delay can be used to show that the patient has lesions that are disseminated in time and/or space.

The auditory EPs also can be used to demonstrate subclinical lesions (in the auditory system) in patients with multiple sclerosis who present with visual or somatusensory findings. Various kinds of ABR abnormalities can be seen in patients with multiple sclerosis (Chiappa, 1997; Iragui-Madoz, 1990). These different patterns are illustrated in Figure 14–8, together with some rough estimates of their incidence in patients with definite multiple sclerosis. Despite the fact that demyelination causes a slowing of conduction, the most common abnormalities of the ABR involve a decrease in amplitude rather than increased delays between the waves (Chiappa, 1997). The demyelination causes desynchronization as well as slowing, and this causes the peaks of the ABR to be absent or reduced in amplitude. Very occasionally, a large delayed wave V can be seen (lower right of Figure 14–8). The most common ABR

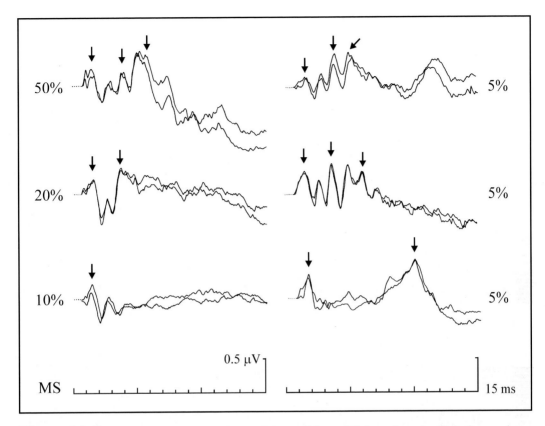

Figure 14–8. ABR patterns seen in patients with multiple sclerosis. This figure shows the different kinds of ABR waveforms that can be recorded in patients with MS together with the approximate incidences of the different patterns based on the results of several laboratories. This incidence is based on the number of ears tested rather than on the number of patients. Half of the patients showing abnormalities will show these only in the response to one ear. The vertical arrows indicate waves I, III, and V where they are recognizable. The top left pattern is a normal ABR. The middle left ABR shows absent waves after wave III, and the bottom response shows absent waves after wave II. The upper right pattern shows preservation of wave IV (diagonal arrow) but an absence of wave V and an attenuation of the negative wave that usually follows V. The middle right ABR pattern shows an abnormally long delay between III and V. The lower right ABR shows a very delayed V with no recognizable wave III. Several other patterns account for the remaining 5%.

abnormality is an absence of waves after wave III (second ABR on the left), likely related to demyelination in the lateral lemniscus.

The incidence of abnormal ABRs in patients with multiple sclerosis occasionally can be increased by presenting clicks at rapid rates (e.g., Jacobson, Murray, & Deppe, 1987; Robinson & Rudge, 1977). Demyelinated fibers are prone to conduc-

tion block when activated at rapid rates (Smith & McDonald, 1999). This would decrease the amplitude of the response more than normal when click rates are increased. Figure 14–9 shows a normal ABR at a click rate of 11/s that becomes unrecognizable with a rates of 81/s. Increasing stimulus rates may also bring out abnormalities in other disorders such as acoustic neuroma (Lightfoot, 1992) and

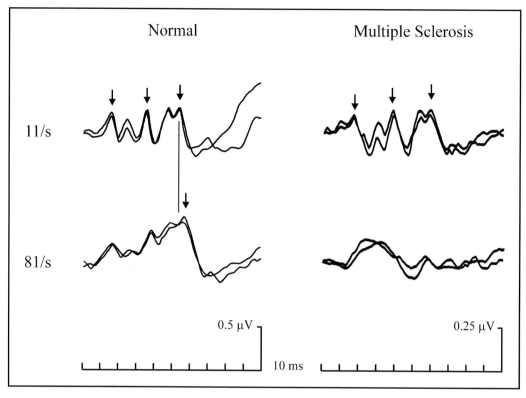

Figure 14–9. *Effects of increasing stimulus rate on the ABR. On the left are shown the results of increasing the rate of stimulus presentation from 11/s to 81/s in a normal subject. The stimuli were 80 dB nHL rarefaction clicks. Waves I and III become smaller. Wave V increases in latency but usually does not change in amplitude. In this particular subject, it actually increases in amplitude. In some patients with multiple sclerosis, the response at 81/s becomes late, small or (as in this case shown on the right) unrecognizable.*

head injury (Podoshin et al., 1990). However, the incidence of this phenomenon when the ABR is completely normal at slow rates is very low (e.g., Chiappa, 1997; Elidan, Sohmer, Gafni, & Kahana, 1982).

The abnormalities in the ABR do not always relate to the clinical symptoms. Figure 14–10 presents a sequence of ABR recordings in a patient who suffered from intermittent hearing loss as part of her relapsing-remitting multiple sclerosis. Normal ABR recordings were obtained when the patient first presented with retrobulbar neuritis. Five years later she presented with hearing loss in the left ear, the ABR showing a complete loss of waves after wave I. The hearing returned to normal within a few weeks and the ABR then showed a wave V that was of normal amplitude but much delayed. Two months later a similar hearing loss occurred in the right ear and it also resolved within a few weeks. In this ear, wave V was present but small and delayed during the period of hearing loss. (It also is possible that this wave may have been a very delayed wave III but this is unlikely.) The wave became more delayed as the hearing returned.

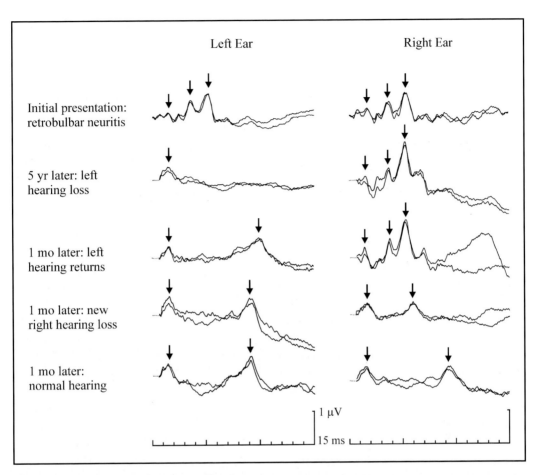

Figure 14–10. Changes in the ABR over the course of relapsing remitting multiple sclerosis. The initial normal ABRs were obtained when this young woman presented with retrobulbar neuritis. The hearing at that time was normal, as were the ABRs. Five years later the patient presented with a severe high-frequency hearing loss in the left ear. The ABR to left ear stimulation showed only wave I. One month later the patient's hearing had returned to normal, the ABR showing a very delayed wave V. Two months later the patient presented with a severe high-frequency hearing loss in the right ear. Wave V to right ear stimulation was attenuated and delayed compared to the earlier recordings. Within a month this hearing impairment had also returned to normal. At this time, wave V to right-ear stimulation was severely delayed. The ABRs in the initial recordings were obtained using alternating clicks at 80 dB nHL. The rest of the recordings were obtained using rarefaction clicks at an intensity of 85 or 90 dB nHL. The filter bandpass was 100 to 3000 Hz for the first recording and 25 to 3000 Hz for subsequent recordings. Stimuli were presented at a rate of 11/sec, and 2000 trials were averaged for each of the superposed tracings.

This may have been due to demyelinated fibers beginning to conduct again but very slowly. Pure tone thresholds and speech discrimination can be normal in patients whose brainstem pathways are affected by multiple sclerosis. However, more precise examination of auditory functions can show definite abnormalities, particularly in binaural tests involving interaural time and intensity differences (Levine et al., 1994; Musiek, Gollegly, Kibbe, & Reeves, 1989).

The incidence of abnormal ABRs in multiple sclerosis is much less than the incidence of abnormal visual EPs. The ABR is abnormal in approximately half of patients with definite multiple sclerosis (e.g., Chiappa, 1997; Japaridze, Shakarishvili, & Kevanishvili, 2002; Picton, 1990). An abnormal ABR could make an important contribution to the diagnosis if there were no other clear symptoms or signs of a lesion in the brainstem. In the days before MRI, such an ABR abnormality could indicate a lesion separate in space from the lesion related to the patient's presenting symptoms. The incidence of such subclinical ABR abnormalities in patients with definite multiple sclerosis is likely about 30% (Chiappa, 1997; Kjaer, 1987; Maurer & Lowitzsch, 1982). In patients presenting with symptoms that may be caused by multiple sclerosis or other disorders, the sensitivity of the ABR is therefore quite low—between 15 and 25%—much less than the visual EP (reviewed by Gronseth & Ashman, 2000)

Today, MRI studies are the main way of demonstrating the disseminated lesions of multiple sclerosis (Bakshi, Hutton, Miller, & Radue, 2004; McDonald et al., 2001; Paty et al., 1988). The role of electrophysiology in the evaluation and management of patients is much reduced. In order to contribute to the diagnosis, the EPs would have to demonstrate a lesion that is not present on MRI examination. The visual EP can do this and is therefore still recommended as essential to the diagnostic workup of a patient who may have multiple sclerosis (Gronseth & Ashman., 2000; McDonald et al., 2001). The incidence of

an abnormal ABR with a normal MRI may be around 10% (Japaridze et al., 2002; Soustiel et al., 1996). The clinical need for recording ABRs in the diagnostic evaluation of patients with suspect multiple sclerosis therefore is not as clearly defined as the visual EP. Nevertheless, in occasional cases, the ABR may demonstrate a lesion that is not visible on MRI and that is separate from the lesion causing the presenting symptoms. Furthermore, because the EPs are functional rather than anatomic, they may help to assess the level of functional disability during the course of the disease (Comi et al., 1999; Jung, Beyerle, & Ziemann, 2008).

Leukodystrophies and Other Degenerative Disorders

The leukodystrophies are genetically determined disorders that affect the oligodendrocytes and the myelin sheath that they create. The disorders manifest as a progressive deterioration in brain function, typically beginning in early childhood. Various types of inheritance occur: adrenoleukodystrophy is usually X-linked (involving male children with the defect carried by the mother), and metachromatic leukodystrophy is autosomal recessive (requiring both parents to have the gene). Children with these disorders initially show slowing of the ABR interpeak latencies and then dropout of the later waves of the response (Markand, Garg, DeMeyer, Warren, & Worth, 1982; Picton, Taylor, & Durieux-Smith, 2005; Shimisu, Moser, & Naidu, 1988). Figure 14–11 shows examples of these recordings. As in multiple sclerosis, the patient may have a significantly abnormal ABR without any hearing symptoms

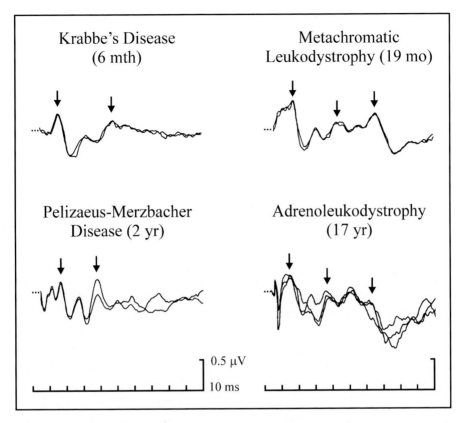

Figure 14–11. *ABR patterns in leukodystrophies. The figure shows recordings from patients with four different kinds of leukodystrophy. Arrows point to recognizable waves I, III and V. The recordings on the left show absent responses after wave III. The recordings on the right show increased interpeak latencies. This slowing is severe for the patient with metachromatic leukodystrophy and mild for the patient with adrenoleukodystrophy. Figure adapted from Picton et al. (2005), based on data from Margot Taylor.*

(Pillion, Kharkar, Mahmood, Moser, & Shimizu, 2006). In adult-onset adrenoleukodystrophy, where the patients can cooperate with psychophysical testing, we can find abnormalities in tests such as the binaural masking level difference (Pillion, Moser, & Raymond, 2008).

A combination of electrophysiologic tests can help differentiate between childhood degenerative disorders caused by abnormalities affecting gray or white matter. Gray matter disorders show a parox-ysmal electroencephalogram (EEG) and normal ABRs, whereas white matter disorders show slowing in the EEG and abnormal ABRs. Today MRI, together with magnetic resonance spectroscopy, is the preferred way to demonstrate the white matter abnormalities (Phelan, Lowe, & Glasier, 2008). Blood chemistry (increased very long chain fatty acids in adrenoleukodystrophy and decreased arylsulfatase activity in metachromatic leukodystrophy) can lead to the definitive diagnosis.

HEAD INJURY, COMA, AND BRAIN DEATH

The sensory EPs can contribute to the assessment of a patient with head injury by demonstrating dysfunction in the afferent pathways. Typically, EPs are evaluated in visual, auditory, and somatosensory modalities to document the extent of lesions (e.g. Guérit, 2005; Narayan et al., 1981). Although CT and MRI are the definitive ways to diagnose structural damage in the nervous system, the EPs may be a helpful adjunct for prognosis, particularly if they are monitored over time. Nevertheless, EP evidence must never be considered in isolation. Although an absent ABR usually is associated with poor prognosis, we must be sure that the cochlea is functioning—"deaf" is not the same as "dead." Patients with head trauma may have cochlear deafness because of temporal lobe fractures, and patients who have been on a respirator often will have a conductive hearing impairment. An absent ABR may occur with desynchronization rather than loss of the discharges and can sometimes occur in a patient who recovers from severe coma (Yamamoto, Katayama, & Tsubokawa, 1994). The evaluation of the patient must take into account all the available information.

Patients with mild traumatic brain injury may develop postconcussion syndrome. The main symptoms are dizziness, headache, and impaired cognition (typically, an inability to maintain attention, concentrate on a task, or plan ahead). Some patients have an abnormality of the ABR, often an increased delay between waves I and III (Noseworthy, Miller, Murray, & Regan, 1981). However, ABR abnormalities do not correlate with the severity of the patient's symptoms (Schoenhuber, Gentilini, & Orlando, 1988). The cognitive abnormalities are likely related to diffuse axonal damage in cerebral neurons related to the sudden shearing forces of the head injury. The evaluation of the patient depends on clinical and neuropsychological assessment (Alexander, 1995). Diffusion tensor imaging, which can assess the extent of diffuse axonal injury, may become a helpful adjunct to the clinical assessment (Inglese et al., 2005).

The EPs can help in the evaluation of a patient presenting with coma (after head injury or from other causes) by documenting dysfunction in sensory pathways (e.g., Picton, Suranyi, Guberman, & Broughton, 1982). Probably the most important contribution of the EPs, however, is to provide information that can be used in coming to a prognosis. Here, repeated testing over time is much more important than a single recording. A deterioration of the EPs, such as illustrated in Figure 14–12, bodes a poor prognosis.

Brain death occurs when the brain is no longer capable of function at even the most basic of levels. Different countries have different diagnostic criteria, which mainly involve the demonstration of brainstem death—a lack of all brainstem reflexes (pupillary, corneal, vestibulo-ocular, gag) and an inability to sustain respiration in the presence of increased blood levels of carbon dioxide. In brain death the EEG is isoelectric (showing no activity other than noncerebral potentials such as the electrocardiogram) and the EPs are absent, although these electrophysiologic findings nowadays are not usually part of the formal evaluation. The ABR in patients with brain death is either absent or shows only waves I and II, compatible with residual function in the cochlea and auditory nerve (Machado et al., 1991; Starr, 1976).

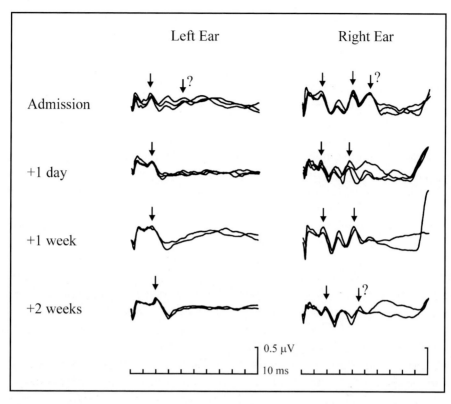

Figure 14–12. *ABR pattern in a comatose patient with a pontine lesion. Dates of testing are relative to admission. This middle-aged alcoholic man was admitted in deep coma. There were no corneal or oculocephalic reflexes, and plantar responses were bilaterally extensor. The cerebrospinal fluid was normal, as were repeated CT scans. The EEG showed diffuse slowing. The ABRs (to 80 dB clicks presented at a rate of 11/s) were severely abnormal for left ear stimulation on the day of admission. Although wave I was clear, wave III was questionable and there was no recognizable wave V. On the succeeding day, the response deteriorated further until only the first component of the response was recognizable. Responses to right ear stimulation were almost normal on the day of admission, although it was not clear whether what was identified as a possible wave V was actually just wave IV. On succeeding days the later components of the right ABR became abnormal and finally vanished. The upgoing wave at the end of the tracing in response to right ear stimulation is the beginning of a postauricular muscle reflex (PAM). The patient died after a 6-week hospital course, and postmortem examination revealed diffuse necrosis of the pons, probably caused by central pontine myelinolysis.*

If a comatose patient does not regain normal consciousness, a persistent vegetative state usually develops. In the vegetative state, the brain is able to control basic functions such as breathing and blood pressure, and typically shows some form of sleep-wake cycling. The main question about these patients is whether their intermittent wakefulness has any conscious content. In some forms of brain damage, the output pathways of the brain may be severely compromised while afferent pathways are preserved. The patient is then conscious of incoming sensory information but unable to communicate normally—the locked-in syndrome. How to assess cognition in patients with disorders of consciousness is an important area of investigation. The main questions are whether a comatose patient will regain consciousness or proceed to an irreversible vegetative state and how much consciousness is actually present in patients who cannot report what they perceive.

Measuring auditory responses probably is an important way to address these issues. It is difficult to present meaningful information through the somatosensory system, and visual input is difficult to control in patients who cannot direct their gaze or maintain their focus. Auditory responses can be measured in two ways: recording cortical EPs (Kotchoubey et al., 2005; Young, Wang, & Connolly, 2004) or measuring changes in cortical blood flow following auditory stimuli using fMRI (Boly et al., 2004; Owen et al., 2005).

The presence of a mismatch negativity (MMN) in a comatose patient is more likely associated with the patient regaining consciousness than not (Fischer et al., 2006; Fischer, Morlet & Giard, 2000; Kane, Butler, & Simpson, 2000), and the same is true concerning recovery from a vegetative state (Wijnen, van Boxtel, Eilander, & de Gelder, 2007). A meta-analysis of the slow auditory EP recordings taken as possible outcome predictors in coma showed that both the MMN and the P300 are reliable indicators of good prognosis (Daltrozzo, Wioland, Mutschler, & Kotchoubey, 2007). Typically, the MMN is recorded

using an oddball paradigm with easily distinguishable tones (e.g., 1000 and 1500 Hz). Using the subject's own name as the deviant stimulus may be the most efficient protocol for evoking a MMN in these patients (Qin et al. 2008).

Kotchoubey et al. (2005) present a reasoned approach to using the slow cognitive EPs to evaluate cognition in patients with disorders of consciousness. The presence of N1-P2 components indicate that the cortex is receiving information; the MMN indicates that the cortex can discriminate between stimuli; the P3 wave indicates that the brain is making some response to the discriminated stimuli; semantic responses like the N400 suggest that the brain is processing meaning. Kotchoubey (2005) also reviews some of the logical and philosophical issues that are raised by these recordings. Of primary concern is that we are not sure of the relationships between neurophysiologic measurements, behavioral states, and first-person consciousness. For example, does the presence of a P3 wave to an oddball stimulus necessarily mean that the subject is conscious that the stimulus changed? The question is even more complicated when we realize that we would have to prove that the P3 wave we record in a sleeping or comatose subject is really the same as the P3 wave we record in a conscious subject (and not just a delayed P2 wave or a part of the K-complex that occurs during sleep).

Another issue, which must be considered, is that the late EPs provide information when they are recognized but not when we fail to demonstrate them. The presence of slow EPs similar to those recorded normally can show that the patient's brain is responding, but their absence does not necessarily mean that it is not responding (Jones et al., 2000). The cerebral neurons may be too desynchronized to generate a clear waveform, the responses may be too variable over time to average, or the brain may be responding in a completely abnormal way.

SOUND-EVOKED VESTIBULAR RESPONSES

Neurotology is as much related to balance as to hearing. Although this book is devoted to the auditory system, the neurotologic evaluation of the patient will evaluate vestibular as well as auditory responses. Physiologic testing of the vestibular system is based largely on the vestibulo-ocular reflex. Movements of the head or fluid movement in the semicircular canals caused by temperature changes in the external auditory canal elicit compensatory eye movements that can be examined using electronystagmography (Baloh, 1997; Brandt & Strupp, 2005). Recently, the battery of tests available for examining the vestibular system has been supplemented by several new physiologic responses that are evoked by loud sounds, but mediated through the saccule.

Early Vestibular Response

Mason, Garnham, and Hudson (1996) reported that children with profound hearing loss can show an unusual early response when examined with very loud clicks or tones. No normal ABR waves were recognized. Instead, the response contained a negative wave peaking at 3 ms. They suggested that this response might be mediated through receptors in the saccule, as this part of the vestibular system is immediately adjacent to the cochlea and could easily be activated by sounds coming through the oval window. The response could be generated by impulses reaching the brainstem; a similar response had been recorded intraoperatively near the vestibular nucleus after electrical stimulation of the vestibular nerve (Häusler, Kasper, & Demierre, 1992). Other investigators also reported a similar early response in profoundly deaf adults as well as children (Kato et al., 1998; Nong, Ura, Kyuna, Owa, & Noda, 2002; Ochi & Ohashi, 2001). This potential also can be recorded in patients with auditory neuropathy who have preserved vestibular function (Picton et al., 1998).

In a normal-hearing subject, the response would be difficult to recognize because it would be overlapped by the ABR. Murofushi, Iwasaki, Takai, and Takegoshi (2005) proposed several techniques to dissociate the responses. First, they used brief tones of 1 kHz (0.5 ms rise and fall, 1 ms plateau) as these might preferentially activate the saccule. The cochlear response to such tones typically does not contain large early waves but only a wave V. Second, they presented the sounds in white noise to mask the ABR. This probably does not affect wave V but would mask earlier waves of the ABR (particularly those related to spread of activation to high-frequency regions of the cochlea). With these techniques, they could demonstrate a distinct early negative wave peaking between 3 and 5 ms for tones with intensities greater than 90 dB nHL. The latency was longer than for clicks, perhaps because of some integration over the duration of the tone. These responses were replicated in normal subjects by Versino et al. (2007). Papathanasiou et al. (2003, 2004) found that recording between the ipsilateral parietal region and the forehead (thus using a montage that is essentially orthogonal to the orientation of the ABR dipoles) also can facilitate the recording of the early vestibular response. These early vestibular responses have been examined in patients with multiple sclerosis and relate to vestibular symptoms experienced during the course of the disease (Papathanasiou et al., 2005). Some of these responses are shown in Figure 14–13.

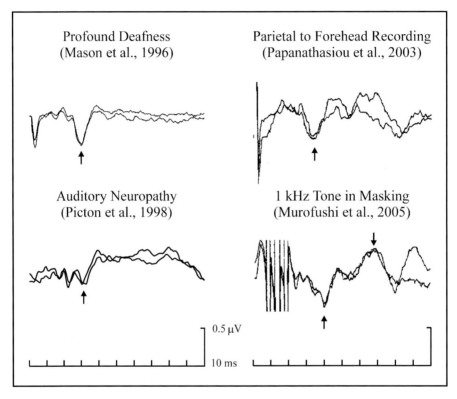

Figure 14–13. *Early neurogenic vestibular evoked potentials. This figure compares different recordings of the N3 wave (indicated by upgoing arrows). Those on the left are from patients without any recognizable ABRs. The stimulus was a click of 105 dB nHL (Mason et al., 1996) or 90 dB nHL (Picton et al., 1998) and both recordings were taken between vertex and mastoid with positivity at the vertex plotted upward. The Picton et al. recordings are presented in greater detail in the next chapter (Figure 15–5). The recordings on the right are from subjects with normal hearing. For the Papathanasiou et al. (2003) recordings, the stimulus was a 105 dB nHL click and the recording was taken from the ipsilateral parietal region using a forehead reference. There are some small later waves but exactly what they represent in this montage is not clear. In the Murofushi et al. (2005) recordings the stimulus was a 95 dB nHL tone lasting 2 ms presented in white noise masking, and the recording was between vertex and mastoid. The response to the tone has a later latency than to the click. A clear wave V is also recognizable (downgoing arrow). For both right-side recordings the tracings have been inverted from those originally published.*

Vestibular Evoked Myogenic Responses

We have already considered the VEMP in Chapter 9. The most easily recorded responses occur in the sternomastoid muscle. Abnormalities of the VEMP can occur in lesions involving the peripheral receptors (in the saccule) or the central vestibular pathways (Welgampola & Colebatch, 2005). Murofushi, Shimizu, Takegoshi, and Cheng (2001) showed that changes in the latency of the response most likely indicate retrolabyrinthine abnormalities such as occur in acoustic neuroma or multiple sclerosis. Another way to distinguish labyrinthine from retrolabyrinthine abnormalities is to record the muscle response to electrical stimulation of the ear (which bypasses the receptors and activates the nerve fibers) and to compare these to the tone-evoked responses. Patients with retrolabyrinthine disorders will show abnormalities with both kinds of stimulation whereas patients with receptor problems should show normal findings with electrical stimulation (Murofushi, Takegoshi, Ohki, & Ozeki, 2002). VEMPs have been used in the evaluation of patients with Ménière's disease (Osei-Lah, Ceranic, & Luxon, 2008; Timmer et al., 2006; Young, Huang, & Cheng, 2003), multiple sclerosis (Patkó, Simó, & Arányi, 2007; Versino et al., 2007), and acoustic neuroma (Ushio et al., 2009). Kim-Lee, Ahn, Kim, and Yoon (2009) have found that, in patients with Ménière's disease, the VEMP elicited by a 1-kHz tone was about the same size as that elicited by a 500-Hz tone. In normal subjects, the 500-Hz response tends to be about twice the 1-kHz response. The abnormal frequency-peak-amplitude ratio may be caused by a change in the mechanical resonance of the saccule brought on by the endolymphatic hydrops.

OVERVIEW

We have covered several clinical disorders where the auditory EPs have been used. The next chapter will consider the syndrome of auditory neuropathy, a relatively new clinical entity with its own burgeoning literature. There is not space to review all of the otologic and neurologic disorders wherein auditory EPs have been recorded. These are covered in more detail in other publications (Chiappa, 1997; Picton et al., 2005). However, we can consider some general statements about the present status of auditory EPs in neurotology, and some tentative speculations about what might happen in the future. The role of the auditory EPs in diagnosis has changed over the years.

Anatomy and Physiology

A common thread through the clinical topics that we have been reviewing is that more and more of our diagnoses are being based on the anatomic evidence provided by the new brain imaging techniques such as MRI. Although physiologic tests can show function, they are never specific about what is causing abnormal function. Imaging procedures accurately demonstrate the etiology of the dysfunction. As time passes, improvements in imaging will extend its role in diagnosis and prognosis.

Physiology is more appropriate when the goal is specifically to assess function. Monitoring the function of the auditory nerves during surgery in the posterior fossa is best done by recording various auditory EPs. Likewise, assessing the degree of hearing impairment in various disorders is generally better done with EPs than with images. Hearing disorders may be subtle and the EPs may show hearing disorders that are not apparent on simple clinical tests. EP abnormalities therefore can make reasonable contributions to our assessment of the burden of disease and how it might change with treatment. In the assessment of prognosis, EP evaluation, particularly when performed sequentially, may help to show improvement or deterioration that is not apparent either clinically or anatomically.

Beyond the Brainstem

Most physiologic assessments of auditory function in clinical patients have used the early auditory EPs—the ECochG and the ABR. A few studies have looked at the later waves such as the MLRs and LAEPs (e.g., in multiple sclerosis: Japaridze et al., 2002; Robinson & Rudge, 1977). Many reasons exist for this concentration on the cochlea and the brainstem to the exclusion of thalamus and cortex. First, the normal limits for the later responses are far broader than for the ABR. Second, the responses vary much more with age and state of arousal. Therefore, it often is hard to determine that a patient is neurologically abnormal and not just immature, inattentive or sleeping. Third, the late responses are generated by multiple overlapping sources and multi-channel recordings usually are needed to disentangle these sources and to demonstrate that one or other of them is abnormal. Trying to dissect out the contributions of each hemisphere (and the different regions of each hemisphere) to the scalp-recorded N1 wave in patients requires proper source analysis (Scherg & von Cramon, 1990). This is much more difficult than simply measuring peaks in a single-channel recording. However, a full analysis of the LAEPs evoked by meaningful sounds might allow us to track the flow of auditory information in the cortex and find

out where it goes awry in disorders such as auditory agnosia, aphasia, and amusia.

More Meaningful Sounds

The auditory EPs typically are evoked by simple stimuli—clicks or tones. More meaningful stimuli probably will lead to more meaningful results if our intent is to evaluate how well a patient's auditory system can process information. Using the subject's own name may be the best way to show residual cognition in patients with disorders of consciousness (Qin et al., 2008). Speech stimuli are perhaps more appropriate than tones when assessing central auditory processing disorders (Johnson, Nicol, & Kraus, 2005).

Uncertainty

The epigraph for this chapter deals with existentialist dilemmas—being unsure of what we know and having to take on faith what we do not know. In philosophy, vertigo is a metaphor for philosophical uncertainty rather than a symptom of Ménière's disease. Nevertheless, a clinician often makes decisions based on uncertain evidence. Auditory EPs can provide information about auditory function that can reduce the clinician's uncertainty, particularly when evaluated together with other findings. The proper management of the patient requires efficient testing and knowledgeable interpretation. Balance is necessary.

ABBREVIATIONS

ABR	Auditory brainstem response
AP	Action potential
CAP	Compound action potential

CHAMP	Cochlear hydrops analysis masking procedure
CM	Cochlear microphonic
CNAP	Cochlear nerve action potential
ECochG	Electrocochleogram
EEG	Electroencephalogram
fMRI	Functional magnetic resonance imaging
HL	Hearing level
MMN	Mismatch negativity
MRI	Magnetic resonance imaging
nHL	Normal hearing level
PAM	Postauricular muscle
SP	Summating potential
VEMP	Vestibular evoked myogenic potential

REFERENCES

Abbas, P. J., & Brown, C. J. (2009). Electrocochleography. In J. Katz (Ed.), *Handbook of clinical audiology* (6th ed., pp. 242–264). Baltimore, MD: Lippincott Williams & Wilkins.

Alexander, M. P. (1995). Mild traumatic brain injury: Pathophysiology, natural history, and clinical management. *Neurology, 45*, 1253–1260.

Allen, R. W., Harnsberger, H. R., Shelton, C., King, B., Bell, D. A., Miller, R., . . . Parker, D. (1996). Low-cost high-resolution fast spin-echo MR of acoustic schwannoma: An alternative to enhanced conventional spin-echo MR? *American Journal of Neuroradiology, 17*, 1205–1210.

Antonelli, A. R., Bellotto, R., & Grandori, F. (1987). Audiologic diagnosis of central versus eighth nerve and cochlear auditory impairment. *Audiology, 26*, 209–226.

Aso, S, Watanabe, Y., & Mizukoshi, K. (1991). A clinical study of electrocochleography in Menière's disease. *Acta Otolaryngologica, 111*, 44–52.

Attias, J., Nageris, B., Ralph, J., Vajda, J., & Rappaport, Z. H. (2008). Hearing preservation using combined monitoring of extratympanic electrocochleography and auditory brainstem responses during acoustic neuroma surgery. *International Journal of Audiology, 47*, 178–184.

Baguley, D. M., Beynon, G. J., Grey, P. L., Hardy, D. G., & Moffat, D. A. (1997). Audiovestibular findings in meningioma of the cerebello-pontine angle: A retrospective review. *Journal of Laryngology and Otology, 111*, 1022–1026.

Bakshi, R., Hutton, G. J., Miller, J. R., & Radue, E. W. (2004). The use of magnetic resonance imaging in the diagnosis and long-term management of multiple sclerosis. *Neurology, 63*(Suppl. 5), S3–11.

Baloh, R. W. (1997). *Dizziness, hearing loss, and tinnitus.* New York, NY: Oxford University Press.

Beasley, N. J., & Jones, N. S. (1996). Menière's disease: Evolution of a definition. *Journal of Laryngology and Otology, 110*, 1107–1113.

Boly, M., Faymonville, M. E., Peigneux, P., Lambermont, B., Damas, P., Del Fiore, G., . . . Laureys, S. (2004). Auditory processing in severely brain injured patients: differences between the minimally conscious state and the persistent vegetative state. *Archives of Neurology, 61*, 233–238.

Bonneville, F., Savatovsky, J., & Chiras, J. (2007). Imaging of cerebellopontine angle lesions: An update. Part 1: Enhancing extra-axial lesions. *European Radiology, 17*, 2472–2482. Part 2: Intra-axial lesions, skull base lesions that may invade the CPA region, and non-enhancing extra-axial lesions. *European Radiology, 17*, 2908–2920.

Brandt, T, & Strupp, M. (2005). General vestibular testing. *Clinical Neurophysiology, 116*, 406–426.

Campbell, K. C., & Abbas, P. J. (1993). Electrocochleography with postural changes in perilymphatic fistula and Menière's disease: Case reports. *Journal of the American Academy of Audiology, 4*, 376–383.

Chiappa, K. H. (1997). *Evoked potentials in clinical medicine*. Philadelphia, PA: Lippincott Williams & Wilkins.

Claes, G. M., Wyndaele, M., De Valck, C. F., Claes, J., Govaerts, P., Wuyts, F. L., & Van de Heyning, P. H. (2008). Travelling wave velocity test and Ménière's disease revisited. *European Archives of Otorhinolaryngology, 265*, 517–523.

Coats, A. C., & Alford, B. R. (1981). Ménière's disease and the summating potential. III. Effect of glycerol administration. *Archives of Otolaryngology, 107*, 469–473.

Colletti, V., Fiorino, F. G., Carner, M., Cumer, G., Giarbini, N., & Sacchetto, L. (2000). Intraoperative monitoring for hearing preservation and restoration in acoustic neuroma surgery. *Skull Base Surgery, 10*, 187–195.

Comi, G., Leocani, L., Medaglini, S., Locatelli, T., Martinelli, V., Santuccio, G., & Rossi, P. (1999). Measuring evoked responses in multiple sclerosis. *Multiple Sclerosis, 5*, 263–267.

Committee on Hearing and Equilibrium (American Academy of Otolaryngology-Head and Neck Surgery). (1995). Guidelines for the diagnosis and evaluation of therapy in Ménière's disease. *Otolaryngology-Head and Neck Surgery, 113*, 181–185.

Conlon, B. J., & Gibson, W. P. (2000). Electrocochleography in the diagnosis of Meniere's disease. *Acta Otolaryngologica, 120*, 480–483.

Cueva, R. A. (2004). Auditory brainstem response versus magnetic resonance imaging for the evaluation of asymmetric sensorineural hearing loss. *Laryngoscope, 114*, 1686–1692.

Cueva, R. A., Morris, G. F., & Prioleau, G. R. (1998). Direct cochlear nerve monitoring: First report on a new atraumatic, self-retaining electrode. *American Journal of Otology, 19*, 202–207.

Daltrozzo, J., Wioland, N., Mutschler, V., & Kotchoubey, B. (2007). Predicting coma and other low responsive patients' outcome using event-related brain potentials: A meta-analysis. *Clinical Neurophysiology, 118*, 606–614.

Daniels, R. L., Swallow, C., Shelton, C., Davidson, H. C., Krejci, C. S., & Harnsberger, H. R. (2000). Causes of unilateral sensorineural hearing loss screened by high resolution fast spin echo magnetic resonance imaging: Review of 1,070 consecutive cases. *American Journal of Otology, 21*, 173–180.

Dauman, R., Aran, J.-M., Charlet de Sauvage, R., & Portmann, M. (1988). Clinical significance of the summating potential in Ménière's disease. *American Journal of Otology, 9*, 31–38.

De Valck, C. F., Claes, G. M., Wuyts, F. L., & Van de Heyning, P. H. (2007). Lack of diagnostic value of high-pass noise masking of auditory brainstem responses in Ménière's disease. *Otology & Neurotology, 28*, 700–707 (with response 2008 *Otology & Neurotology 29*, 1211–1213, and reply 1213–1215).

Don, M., Kwong, B., & Tanaka, C. (2005). A diagnostic test for Ménière's disease and cochlear hydrops: Impaired high-pass noise masking of auditory brainstem responses. *Otology & Neurotology, 26*, 711–722.

Don, M., Kwong, B., & Tanaka, C. (2007). An alternative diagnostic test for active Ménière's disease and cochlear hydrops using high-pass noise masked responses: The complex amplitude ratio. *Audiology and Neurotology, 12*, 359–370.

Don, M., Kwong, B., Tanaka, C., Brackmann, D., & Nelson, R. (2005). The stacked ABR: A sensitive and specific screening tool for detecting small acoustic tumors. *Audiology and Neurotology, 10*, 274–290.

Don, M., Masuda, A., Nelson, R., & Brackmann, D. (1997). Successful detection of small acoustic tumors using the stacked derived-band auditory brain stem response amplitude. *American Journal of Otology, 18*, 608–621.

Donaldson, G. S., & Ruth, R. A. (1996). Derived-band auditory brain-stem response estimates of travelling wave velocity in humans: II. Subjects with noise-induced hearing loss and Ménière's disease. *Journal of Speech and Hearing Research, 39*, 534–545.

Dort, J. C., Cook, E. F., Watson, C., Shaw, G., Brown, D. K., & Eggermont, J. J. (2009).

Power spectrum auditory brainstem response: Novel approach to the evaluation of patients with unilateral auditory symptoms. *Journal of Otolaryngology-Head and Neck Surgery, 38,* 59–66.

Elidan, J., Sohmer, H., Gafni, M., & Kahana, E. (1982). Contribution of changes in click rate and intensity on diagnosis of multiple sclerosis by brainstem auditory evoked potentials. *Acta Neurologica Scandinavica, 65,* 570–585.

Eggermont, J. J. (1976). Electrocochleography. In W. D. Keidel & W. D. Neff (Eds.), *Handbook of sensory physiology. Vol. 3. Auditory system. Clinical and special topics* (pp. 625–705). Berlin, Germany: Springer-Verlag.

Eggermont, J. J, & Don, M. (1986). Mechanisms of central conduction time prolongation in brain-stem auditory evoked potentials. *Archives of Neurology, 43,* 116–120.

Ferraro, J. A., & Durrant, J. D. (2006). Electrocochleography in the evaluation of patients with Ménière's disease/endolymphatic hydrops. *Journal of the American Academy of Audiology, 17,* 45–68.

Fischer, C., Luauté, J., Némoz, C., Morlet, D., Kirkorian, G., & Mauguière, F. (2006). Improved prediction of awakening or non-awakening from severe anoxic coma using tree-based classification analysis. *Critical Care Medicine, 34,* 1520–1524.

Fischer, C., Morlet, D., & Giard, M. (2000). Mismatch negativity and N100 in comatose patients. *Audiology and Neuro-Otology, 5,* 192–197.

Fortnum, H., O'Neill, C., Taylor, R., Lenthall, R., Nikolopoulos, T., Lightfoot, G., . . . Mulvaney, C. (2009). The role of magnetic resonance imaging in the identification of suspected acoustic neuroma: A systematic review of clinical and cost effectiveness and natural history. *Health Technology Assessments, 13,* 1–154.

Ge, X., & Shea, J. J., Jr. (2002). Transtympanic electrocochleography: A 10-year experience. *Otology and Neurotology, 23,* 799–805.

Gibson, W. P. (1992). Electrocochleography in the diagnosis of perilymphatic fistula: Intraoperative observations and assessment of a new diagnostic office procedure. *American Journal of Otology, 13,* 146–151.

Gibson, W. P. (2009). A comparison of two methods of using transtympanic electrocochleography for the diagnosis of Meniere's disease: Click summating potential/action potential ratio measurements and tone burst summating potential measurements. *Acta Otolaryngologica, 129*(Suppl. 560), 38–42.

Gordon, M. A., & Cohen, N. L. (1995). Efficacy of auditory brainstem response as a screening test for small acoustic neuromas. *American Journal of Otology, 16,* 136–139.

Gronseth, G. S., & Ashman, E. J. (2000). Practice parameter: the usefulness of evoked potentials in identifying clinically silent lesions in patients with suspected multiple sclerosis (an evidence-based review). *Neurology, 54,* 1720–1725.

Guérit, J. M. (2005). Evoked potentials in severe brain injury. *Progress in Brain Research, 150,* 415–426.

Halliday, A. M., McDonald, W. I., & Mushin, J. (1972). Delayed visual evoked response in optic neuritis. *Lancet, 1,* 982–985.

Harper, C. M., Harner, S. G., Slavit, D. H., Litchy, W. J., Daube, J. R., Beatty, C. W., & Ebersold, M. J. (1992). Effect of BAEP monitoring on hearing preservation during acoustic neuroma resection. *Neurology, 42,* 1551–1553.

Häusler, R., Kasper, A., & Demierre, B. (1992). Intraoperative electrically evoked vestibular potentials in humans. *Acta Otolaryngologica, 112,* 180–185.

Inglese, M., Makani, S., Johnson, G., Cohen, B. A., Silver, J. A., Gonen, O., &. Grossman, R. I. (2005). Diffuse axonal injury in mild traumatic brain injury: A diffusion tensor imaging study. *Journal of Neurosurgery, 103,* 298–303.

Iragui-Madoz, V. (1990). Electrophysiology of multiple sclerosis. In D. D. Daly & T. A. Pedley (Eds.), *Current practice of clinical electroencephalography* (2nd ed., pp. 707–738). New York, NY: Raven Press.

Iseli, C., & Gibson, W. (2010). A comparison of three methods of using transtympanic electrocochleography for the diagnosis of Meniere's disease: Click summating potential measurements, tone burst summating potential amplitude measurements, and biasing of the summating potential using a low frequency tone. *Acta Otolaryngologica, 130,* 95–101.

Jacobson, J. T., Murray, T. J., & Deppe, U. (1987). The effects of ABR stimulus repetition rate in multiple sclerosis. *Ear and Hearing, 8,* 115–120.

Japaridze, G., Shakarishvili, R., & Kevanishvili, Z. (2002). Auditory brainstem, middle-latency, and slow cortical responses in multiple sclerosis. *Acta Neurologica Scandinavica, 106,* 47–53.

Johnson, K. L., Nicol, T. G., & Kraus, N. (2005). Brain stem response to speech: A biological marker of auditory processing. *Ear and Hearing, 26,* 424–434.

Jones, S. J., Vaz Pato, M., Sprague, L., Stokes, M., Munday, R., & Haque, N. (2000) Auditory evoked potentials to spectrotemporal modulation of complex tones in normal subjects and patients with severe brain injury. *Brain, 123,* 1007–1016.

Jung, P., Beyerle, A., & Ziemann, U. (2008). Multimodal evoked potentials measure and predict disability progression in early relapsing-remitting multiple sclerosis. *Multiple Sclerosis, 14,* 553–556.

Kane, N. M., Butler, S. R., & Simpson, T. (2000). Coma outcome prediction using event-related potentials: P3 and mismatch negativity. *Audiology and Neuro-Otology, 5,* 186–191.

Kato, T., Shiraishi, K., Eura, Y., Shibata, K., Sakata, T., Morizono, T., & Soda, T. (1998). A 'neural' response with 3-ms latency evoked by loud sound in profoundly deaf patients. *Audiology and Neuro-Otology, 3,* 253–264.

Kevanishvili, Z. (2000). The detection of small acoustic tumors: The stacked derived-band ABR procedure. *American Journal of Otology, 21,* 148–149.

Kim-Lee, Y., Ahn, J. H., Kim, Y. K., & Yoon, T. H. (2009). Tone burst vestibular evoked myogenic potentials: Diagnostic criteria in patients with Meniere's disease. *Acta Otolaryngologica, 129,* 924–928.

Kjaer, M. (1987). Evoked potentials in the diagnosis of multiple sclerosis. *Electroencephalography and Clinical Neurophysiology, 98* (Suppl. 39), 291–296.

Kotchoubey, B. (2005). Event-related potential measures of consciousness: Two equations with three unknowns. *Progress in Brain Research, 150,* 427–444.

Kotchoubey, B., Lang, S., Mezger, G., Schmalohr, D., Schneck, M., Semmler, A., . . . Birbaumer, N. (2005). Information processing in severe disorders of consciousness: Vegetative state and minimally conscious state. *Clinical Neurophysiology, 116,* 2441–2453.

Kuroki, A., & Møller, A. R. (1995). Microsurgical anatomy around the foramen of Luschka in relation to intraoperative recording of auditory evoked potentials from the cochlear nuclei. *Journal of Neurosurgery, 82,* 933–939.

Lang, J. (1985). Anatomy of the brainstem and the lower cranial nerves, vessels, and surrounding structures. *American Journal of Otology, 6*(Suppl.), 1–19.

Legatt, A. D. (2002). Mechanisms of intraoperative brainstem auditory evoked potential changes. *Journal of Clinical Neurophysiology, 19,* 396–408.

Levine, R. A., Gardner, J. C., Fullerton, B. C., Stufflebeam, S. M., Furst, M., & Rosen, B. R. (1994). Multiple sclerosis lesions of the auditory pons are not silent. *Brain, 117,* 1127–1141.

Levine, S. C., Antonelli, P. J., Le, C. T., & Haines, S. J. (1991). Relative value of diagnostic tests for small acoustic neuromas. *American Journal of Otology, 12,* 341–346.

Lightfoot, G. R. (1992). ABR screening for acoustic neuromata: The role of rate-induced latency shift measurements. *British Journal of Audiology, 26,* 217–227.

Linden, R. D., Tator, C. H., Benedict, C., Charles, D., Mraz, V., & Bell, I. (1988). Electrophysiological monitoring during acoustic neuroma and other posterior fossa surgery. *Canadian Journal of Neurological Sciences, 15,* 73–81.

Lustig, L. R., Niparko, J., Minor, L. B., & Zee, D. S. (Eds.). (2003). *Clinical neurotology: Diagnosing and managing disorders of hearing, balance and the facial nerve.* London, UK: Martin Dunitz (Taylor-Francis Group).

Machado, C., Valdés, P., García-Tigera, J., Virues, T., Biscay, R., Miranda, J., . . . García, O. (1991). Brain-stem auditory evoked potentials and brain death. *Electroencephalography and Clinical Neurophysiology, 80,* 392–398.

Maitland, C. G. (2001). Perilymphatic fistula. *Current Neurology and Neuroscience Reports, 1,* 486–491.

Margolis, R. H., Rieks, D., Fournier, E. M., & Levine, S. E. (1995). Tympanic electrocochleography for diagnosis of Menière's disease. *Archives of Otolaryngology-Head and Neck Surgery, 121,* 44–45.

Markand, O. N., Garg, B. P., DeMeyer, W. E., Warren, C., & Worth, R. M. (1982) Brain stem auditory, visual and somatosensory evoked potentials in leukodystrophies. *Electroencephalography and Clinical Neurophysiology, 54,* 39–48.

Martin, W. H., Pratt, H., & Schwegler, J. W. (1995). The origin of the human auditory brain-stem response wave II. *Electroencephalography and Clinical Neurophysiology, 96,* 357–370.

Martin, W., & Shi, B. Y. (2007). Intraoperative monitoring. In R. F. Burkard, M. Don, & J. J. Eggermont (Eds.), *Auditory evoked potentials: Basic principles and clinical applications* (pp. 355–384). Baltimore, MD: Lippincott Williams &Wilkins.

Mason, S., Garnham, C., & Hudson, B. (1996). Electric response audiometry in young children before cochlear implantation: A short latency component. *Ear and Hearing, 17,* 537–543.

Maurer, K., & Lowitzsch, K. (1982). Brainstem auditory evoked potentials in reclassification of 143 MS patients. *Advances in Neurology, 32,* 481–486.

McDonald, W. I., Compston, A., Edan, G., Goodkin, D., Hartung, H. P., Lublin, F. D., . . . Wolinsky, J. S. (2001). Recommended diagnostic criteria for multiple sclerosis: Guidelines from the international panel on the diagnosis of multiple sclerosis. *Annals of Neurology, 50,* 121–127.

Meyerhoff, W. L., & Yellin, M. W. (1990). Summating potential/action potential ratio in perilymph fistula. *Otolaryngology-Head and Neck Surgery, 102,* 678–682.

Møller, A. R. (2006). *Intraoperative neurophysiological monitoring* (2nd ed.). Totowa, NJ: Humana Press.

Møller, A. R., Jannetta. P. J., & Jho, H. D. (1994). Click-evoked responses from the cochlear nucleus: A study in human. *Electroencephalography and Clinical Neurophysiology, 92,* 215–224.

Morawski, K. F., Niemczyk, K., Bohorquez, J., Marchel, A., Delgado, R. E., Ozdamar, O., & Telischi, F. F. (2007). Intraoperative monitoring of hearing during cerebellopontine angle tumor surgery using transtympanic electrocochleography. *Otology and Neurotology, 28,* 541–545.

Murofushi, T., Iwasaki, S., Takai, Y., & Takegoshi, H. (2005). Sound evoked neurogenic responses with short latency of vestibular origin. *Clinical Neurophysiology, 116,* 401–405.

Murofushi, T., Shimizu, K., Takegoshi, H., & Cheng, P. W. (2001). Diagnostic value of prolonged latencies in the vestibular evoked myogenic potential. *Archives of Otolaryngology-Head and Neck Surgery, 127,* 1069–1072.

Murofushi, T., Takegoshi, H., Ohki, M., & Ozeki, H. (2002). Galvanic-evoked myogenic responses in patients with an absence of click-evoked vestibulocollic reflexes. *Clinical Neurophysiology, 113,* 305–309.

Murray, J. G., Cohn, E. S., Harker, L. A., & Gorga, M. P. (1998). Tone burst auditory brain stem response latency estimates of cochlear travel time in Meniere's disease, cochlear hearing loss, and normal ears. *American Journal of Otology, 19,* 854–859.

Musiek, F. E., Gollegly, K. M., Kibbe, K. S., & Reeves, A. G. (1989). Electrophysiologic and behavioral auditory findings in multiple sclerosis. *American Journal of Otology, 10,* 343–350.

Naganawa, S., Sugiura, M., Kawamura, M., Fukatsu, H., Sone, M., & Nakashima, T. (2008). Imaging of endolymphatic and perilymphatic fluid at 3T after intratympanic administration of gadolinium-diethylenetriamine pentaacetic acid. *American Journal of Neuroradiology, 29*, 724–726.

Nakashima, T., Naganawa, S., Pyykko, I., Gibson, W. P., Sone, M., Nakata, S., & Teranishi, M. (2009). Grading of endolymphatic hydrops using magnetic resonance imaging. *Acta Otolaryngologica, 129*(Suppl. 560), 5–8.

Narayan, R. K., Greenberg, R. P., Miller, J. D., Enas, G. G., Choi, S. C., Kishore, P. R., . . . Becker, D. P. (1981). Improved confidence of outcome prediction in severe head injury. A comparative analysis of the clinical examination, multimodality evoked potentials, CT scanning, and intracranial pressure. *Journal of Neurosurgery, 54*, 751–762.

Nong, D. X., Ura, M., Kyuna, A., Owa, T., & Noda, Y. (2002). Saccular origin of acoustically evoked short latency negative response. *Otology and Neurotology, 23*, 953–957.

Noseworthy, J. H., Miller, J., Murray, T. J., & Regan, D. (1981). Auditory brainstem responses in postconcussion syndrome. *Archives of Neurology, 38*, 275–278.

Nowé, V., Michiels, J. L., Salgado, R., De Ridder, D., Van de Heyning, P. H., De Schepper, A. M., & Parizel, P. M. (2004). High-resolution virtual MR endoscopy of the cerebellopontine angle. *American Journal of Roentgenology, 182*, 379–384.

Ochi, K., & Ohashi, T. (2001). Sound-evoked myogenic potentials and responses with 3-ms latency in auditory brainstem response. *Laryngoscope, 111*, 1818–1821.

Ohashi, T., Nishino, H., Arai, Y., Hyodo, M., & Takatsu, M. (2009). Clinical significance of the summating potential-action potential ratio and the action potential latency difference for condensation and rarefaction clicks in Meniere's disease. *Annals of Otology, Rhinology and Laryngology, 118*, 307–312.

Ojemann, R. G., Levine, R. A., Montgomery, W. M., & McGaffigan, P. (1984). Use of intraoperative auditory evoked potentials to preserve hearing in unilateral acoustic neuroma removal. *Journal of Neurosurgery, 61*, 938–948.

Orchik, D. J., Ge, N. N., & Shea, J. J. Jr. (1998). Action potential latency shift by rarefaction and condensation clicks in Ménière's disease. *Journal of the American Academy of Audiology, 9*, 121–126.

Ordóñez-Ordóñez, L. E., Rojas-Roncancio, E., Hernández-Alarcón, V., Jaramillo-Safón, R., Prieto-Rivera, J., Guzmán-Durán, J., . . . Angulo-Martínez, E. S. (2009). Diagnostic test validation: Cochlear hydrops analysis masking procedure in Ménière's disease. *Otology and Neurotology, 30*, 820–825.

Osei-Lah, V., Ceranic, B., & Luxon, L. M. (2008). Clinical value of tone burst vestibular evoked myogenic potentials at threshold in acute and stable Ménière's disease. *Journal of Laryngology and Otology, 122*, 452–457.

Owen, A. M., Coleman, M. R., Menon, D. K., Berry, E. L., Johnsrude, I. S., Rodd, . . . Pickard, J. D. (2005). Using a hierarchical approach to investigate residual auditory cognition in persistent vegetative state. *Progress in Brain Research, 150*, 457–471.

Papathanasiou, E. S., Piperidou, C., Pantzaris, M., Iliopoulos, I., Petsa, M., Kyriakides, . . . Papacostas, S. S. (2005). Vestibular symptoms and signs are correlated with abnormal neurogenic vestibular evoked potentials in patients with multiple sclerosis. *Electromyography and Clinical Neurophysiology, 45*, 195–201.

Papathanasiou, E. S., Zamba-Papanicolaou, E., Pantziaris, M., Kleopas, K., Kyriakides, T., Papacostas, S., . . . Piperidou, C. (2004). Neurogenic vestibular evoked potentials using a tone pip auditory stimulus. *Electromyography and Clinical Neurophysiology, 44*, 167–173.

Papathanasiou, E., Zamba-Papanicolaou, E., Pantziaris, M., Kyriakides, T., Papacostas, S., Myrianthopoulou, P., . . . Piperidou, C. (2003). Click evoked neurogenic vestibular potentials (NVESTEPs): A method of assessing the function of the vestibular system. *Electromyography and Clinical Neurophysiology, 43*, 399–408.

Patkó, T., Simó, M., & Arányi, Z. (2007). Vestibular click-evoked myogenic potentials: Sensitivity and factors determining abnormality in patients with multiple sclerosis. *Multiple Sclerosis, 13,* 193–198.

Paty, D. W., Oger, J. J., Kastrukoff, L. F., Hashimoto, S. A., Hooge, J. P., Eisen, A. A., . . . Li, D. K. B. (1988). MRI in the diagnosis of MS: A prospective study with comparison of clinical evaluation, evoked potentials, oligoclonal banding, and CT. *Neurology, 38,* 180–185.

Phelan, J. A., Lowe, L. H., & Glasier, C. M. (2008). Pediatric neurodegenerative white matter processes: leukodystrophies and beyond. *Pediatric Radiology, 38,* 729–749.

Picton, T. W. (1986). Abnormal brainstem auditory evoked potentials: A tentative classification. In R. Q. Cracco & I. Bodis-Wollner (Eds.), *Evoked potentials* (pp. 373–378). New York, NY: Alan R. Liss.

Picton, T. W. (1990). Auditory evoked potentials. In D. D. Daly & T. A. Pedley (Eds.), *Current practice of clinical electroencephalography* (2nd ed., pp. 625–678). New York, NY: Raven Press.

Picton, T. W. (1991). Clinical usefulness of auditory evoked potentials: A critical review. *Journal of Speech-Language Pathology and Audiology, 15,* 3–18 (with commentaries by J. J. Eggermont, B. S. Herrmann, A. R. Thornton, & M. L. Hyde, pp 19–29).

Picton, T. W., & Durieux-Smith, A. (1988). Auditory evoked potentials in the assessment of hearing. *Neurologic Clinics, 6,* 791–808.

Picton, T. W, Durieux-Smith, A., Champagne, S. C., Whittingham, J., Moran, L. M., Giguère, C., & Beauregard Y. (1998). Objective evaluation of aided thresholds using auditory steady-state responses. *Journal of the American Academy of Audiology, 9,* 315–331,

Picton, T. W., Suranyi, L., Guberman, A., & Broughton, R. J. (1982). The neurophysiological investigation of stuporous and comatose patients. In L. P. Ivan. & D. Bruce (Eds.), *Coma: Physiopathology, diagnosis and management* (pp. 31–70). Springfield, IL: Charles Thomas.

Picton, T. W., Taylor, M. .J., & Durieux-Smith, A. (2005). Brainstem auditory evoked potentials in pediatrics. In M. J. Aminoff (Ed.), *Electrodiagnosis in clinical neurology* (5th ed., pp. 525–552). Philadelphia, PA: Elsevier Churchill Livingstone.

Pillion, J. P., Kharkar, S., Mahmood, A., Moser, H., & Shimizu, H. (2006). Auditory brainstem response findings and peripheral auditory sensitivity in adrenoleukodystrophy. *Journal of the Neurological Sciences, 247,* 130–137.

Pillion, J. P., Moser, H. W., & Raymond, G. V. (2008). Auditory function in adrenomyeloneuropathy. *Journal of the Neurological Sciences, 269,* 24–29.

Podoshin, L., Ben-David, Y., Fradis, M., Pratt, H., Sharf, B., & Schwartz, M. (1990). Brainstem auditory evoked potential with increased stimulus rate in minor head trauma. *Journal of Laryngology and Otology, 104,* 191–194.

Qin, P., Di, H., Yan, X., Yu, S., Yu, D., Laureys, S., & Weng, X. (2008). Mismatch negativity to the patient's own name in chronic disorders of consciousness. *Neuroscience Letters, 448,* 24–28.

Raudzens, P. A., & Shetter, A. G. (1982). Intraoperative monitoring of brain-stem auditory evoked potentials. *Journal of Neurosurgery, 57,* 341–348.

Robinette, M. S., Bauch, C. D., Olsen, W. O., & Cevette, M. J. (2000). Auditory brainstem response and magnetic resonance imaging for acoustic neuromas: Costs by prevalence. *Archives of Otolaryngology-Head and Neck Surgery, 126,* 963–966.

Robinson, K., & Rudge, P. (1977). Abnormalities of the auditory evoked potentials in patients with multiple sclerosis. *Brain, 100,* 19–40.

Rupa, V., Job, A., George, M., & Rajshekhar, V.. (2003). Cost-effective initial screening for vestibular schwannoma: Auditory brainstem response or magnetic resonance imaging? *Otolaryngology-Head and Neck Surgery, 128,* 823–828.

Sajjadi, H., & Paparella, M. M. (2008). Meniere's disease. *Lancet, 372,* 406–414.

Sass, K., Densert, B., & Arlinger, S. (1998). Recording techniques for transtympanic electrocochleography in clinical practice. *Acta Otolaryngologica (Stockholm), 118*, 17–25.

Sass, K., Densert, B., & Magnusson, M. (1997). Transtympanic electrocochleography in the assessment of perilymphatic fistulas. *Audiology and Neuro-Otology 2*, 391–402.

Sass, K., Densert, B., Magnusson, M., & Whitaker, S. (1998). Electrocochleographic signal analysis: Condensation and rarefaction click stimulation contributes to diagnosis in Ménière's disorder. *Audiology, 37*, 198–206.

Scherg, M., & von Cramon, D. (1990). Dipole source potentials of the auditory cortex in normal subjects and in patients with temporal lobe lesions. In F. Grandori, M. Hoke, & G. L. Romani (Eds.), *Advances in audiology, Vol. 6. Auditory evoked magnetic fields and electric potentials* (pp. 165–193). Basel, Switzerland: Karger.

Schmidt, R. J., Sataloff ,R. T., Newman, J , Spiegel, J. R., & Myers, D. L. (2001). The sensitivity of auditory brainstem response testing for the diagnosis of acoustic neuromas. *Archives of Otolaryngology-Head and Neck Surgery, 127*, 19–22.

Schoenhuber, R., Gentilini, M., & Orlando, A. (1988). Prognostic value of auditory brainstem responses for late postconcussion symptoms following minor head injury. *Journal of Neurosurgery, 68*, 742–744.

Schoonhoven, R. (2007). Responses from the cochlea: Cochlear microphonic, summating potential and compound action potential. In R. F. Burkard, M. Don, & J. J. Eggermont (Eds.), *Auditory evoked potentials: Basic principles and clinical application* (pp. 180–198). Philadelphia, PA: Lippincott Williams & Wilkins.

Selters, W. A., & Brackmann, D. E. (1977). Acoustic tumor detection with brain stem electric response audiometry. *Archives of Otolaryngology, 103*, 181–187.

Shimizu, H., Moser, H. W., & Naidu, S. (1988). Auditory brainstem response and audiologic findings in adrenoleukodystrophy: Its variant and carrier. *Otolaryngology-Head and Neck Surgery, 98*, 215–220.

Smith, K. J., & McDonald, W. I. (1999). The pathophysiology of multiple sclerosis: The mechanisms underlying the production of symptoms and the natural history of the disease. *Philosophical Transactions of the Royal Society. B Biological Sciences, 354*, 1649–1673.

Soustiel, J. F., Hafner, H., Chistyakov, A. V., Yarnitzky, D., Sharf, B., Guilburd, J. N., & Feinsod, M. (1996) Brain-stem trigeminal and auditory evoked potentials in multiple sclerosis: Physiological insights. *Electroencephalography and Clinical Neurophysiology, 100*, 152–157.

Starr, A. (1976). Auditory brainstem responses in brain death. *Brain, 99*, 543–554.

Symon, L., Sabin, H. I., Bentivoglio, P., Cheesman, A. D., Prasher, D., & Barratt, H. (1988). Intraoperative monitoring of the electrocochleogram and the preservation of hearing during acoustic neuroma excision. *Acta Neurochirurgica Supplement (Wien), 42*, 27–30.

Thornton, A. R., & Farrell, G. (1991). Apparent travelling wave velocity changes in cases of endolymphatic hydrops. *Scandinavian Audiology, 20*, 13–18.

Timmer, F. C., Zhou, G., Guinan, J. J., Kujawa, S. G., Herrmann, B. S., & Rauch, S. D. (2006). Vestibular evoked myogenic potential (VEMP) in patients with Ménière's disease with drop attacks. *Laryngoscope, 116*, 776–779.

Ushio, M., Iwasaki, S., Murofushi, T., Sugasawa, K., Chihara, Y., Fujimoto, C., . . . Yamasoba, T. (2009). The diagnostic value of vestibular-evoked myogenic potential in patients with vestibular schwannoma. *Clinical Neurophysiology, 120*, 1149–1153.

Versino, M., Ranza, L., Colnaghi, S., Alloni, R., Callieco, R., Romani, A., . . . Cosi, V. (2007). The N3 potential compared to sound and galvanic vestibular evoked myogenic potential in healthy subjects and in multiple sclerosis patients. *Journal of Vestibular Research, 17*, 39–46.

Welgampola, M. S., & Colebatch, J. G. (2005). Characteristics and clinical applications of vestibular-evoked myogenic potentials. *Neurology, 64,* 1682–1688.

Wijnen, V. J., van Boxtel, G. J., Eilander, H. J., & de Gelder, B. (2007). Mismatch negativity predicts recovery from the vegetative state. *Clinical Neurophysiology, 118,* 597–605.

Wilkins, R. H., Radtke, R. A., & Erwin, C. W. (1991). Value of intraoperative brainstem auditory evoked potential monitoring in reducing the auditory morbidity associated with microvascular decompression of cranial nerves. *Skull Base Surgery, 1,* 106–109.

Yamamoto, T., Katayama, Y., & Tsubokawa, T. (1994). Persistent absence of auditory brainstem responses with preserved hearing and recovery from a prolonged comatose state. *Brain Injury, 8,* 623–629.

Young, G. B., Wang, J. T., & Connolly, J. F. (2004). Prognostic determination in anoxic-ischemic and traumatic encephalopathies. *Journal of Clinical Neurophysiology, 21,* 379–390.

Young, Y. H., Huang, T. W., & Cheng, P. W. (2003). Assessing the stage of Meniere's disease using vestibular evoked myogenic potentials. *Archives of Otolaryngology-Head and Neck Surgery, 129,* 815–818.

15

Auditory Neuropathy: When Time Is Broke

> How sour sweet music is
> When time is broke and no proportion kept.
> So is it in the music of men's lives.
> And here have I the daintiness of ear
> To check time broke in a disordered string;
> But for the concord of my state and time
> Had not an ear to hear my true time broke.
>
> Shakespeare, *Richard II*, Act V, 5:42–48

This chapter considers one particular type of hearing disorder, auditory neuropathy, in greater depth than has been our custom. One reason is that this disorder was detected on the basis of physiologic testing. Another is that it allows us to see the different ways that pathology might interfere with auditory processing.

Auditory neuropathy initially was identified when otoacoustic emissions (OAEs) and cochlear microphonics (CMs) were measured in patients with absent or abnormal auditory brainstem responses (ABRs). The key features of this disorder are an abnormal auditory nerve response to sound as demonstrated by absence or abnormality of the ABR despite the presence of functioning hair cells as demonstrated by OAEs or CMs. Although several patients with absent ABR but preserved hearing for pure tones had been reported previously (e.g., Kraus, Ozdamar, Stein, & Reed, 1984; Worthington & Peters, 1980), the nature of the disorder remained unknown. The first patient in whom the disorder was fully demonstrated by recording preserved CMs in the absence of ABRs was described by Starr et al. (1991). Normal OAEs were demonstrated in the patient after the paper was submitted, and these were reported in a brief addendum to the final publication. Two similar patients were reported by Berlin, Hood, Cecola, Jackson, and Szabo (1993) as "type I afferent neuron dysfunction." (Type I afferent neurons are the myelinated neurons that receive input from the inner hair cells and carry the main afferent information, as opposed to type II afferent neurons that come from the external hair cells and have uncertain function). Starr, Picton, Sininger, Hood, and Berlin (1996) then reported 10 cases, 8 of whom had an accompanying peripheral neuropathy, and coined the term "auditory neuropathy." At about the same time, Kaga et al. (1996) reported two adult patients with absent ABRs and preserved OAEs, calling the disorder "auditory nerve disease," Konradsson (1996) described four children with a disorder involving "the inner hair cell and/or the first neuron," and Stein et al. (1996) found similar findings in four newborn infants with hyperbilirubinemia.

Auditory neuropathy is a disorder that affects the afferent transmission of auditory information from the cochlea. Concern has been expressed about the name "auditory neuropathy" because the disorder may affect the inner hair cell or its synapse rather than the auditory nerve fibers. Some have objected that the syndrome may include disorders of the central nervous system (Rapin & Gravel, 2003), although this was never the intent of the original proposal, which insisted that the ABR be abnormal beginning at wave I (Starr et al., 1996). Other names have been proposed. Although having the advantage that it sounds almost as distorted as what the patient hears, the name "auditory dyssynchrony" (Berlin, Morlet, & Hood, 2003) proposes a pathophysiology that may or may not be present in the disorder. "Neural hearing loss" (Rapin & Gravel, 2003) is far too nonspecific, as it includes disorders all the way from the auditory nerve to the cortex, and excludes disorders of the inner hair cell or its synapse. A committee putting together guidelines for the identification and management of infants and young children with auditory neuropathy proposed that the disorder be called "auditory neuropathy spectrum disorder" (Hayes, Sininger, & Northern, 2008). This adds to the widely accepted term "auditory neuropathy" the concept of different presentations and different etiologies.

We will continue to use "auditory neuropathy" to describe the disorder, creatures of habit that we are. We note that usage often overcomes exactitude; the term "acoustic neuroma" is still used to describe a tumor that usually is neither acoustic nor a neuroma. Ultimately, the different disorders that comprise auditory neuropathy will be distinguished, and we can call each by the name of the gene or toxin that causes the hearing problem.

DIAGNOSIS

Essential Diagnostic Features

The diagnosis requires two findings, one negative and one positive. First, there must be evidence of abnormal processing in the auditory nerve fibers. This is demonstrated by showing that the neural components of the click-ABR are either absent or severely abnormal beginning at wave I. Typically, the neural components of the ABR waveform are not recognizable. However, in milder cases of auditory neuropathy, the ABR is present but smaller in amplitude, later in latency, and much less defined in terms of recognizable waves than what would be expected from the patient's pure-tone audiogram. When recording the ABRs, we must record separate responses to condensation and rarefaction clicks (Berlin et al., 1998). If we record ABRs using only one polarity of click, sometimes we may record a CM waveform that can mimic the ABR. This can be a problem in children as some children with auditory neuropathy show a CM that is larger and more persistent than in normal subjects (Starr, Sininger, & Pratt, 2000; Starr, Sininger, et al., 2001). If we record ABRs using alternating click-polarity in a patient with auditory neuropathy, both the ABR and the CM will be absent from the recording. The ABR is absent because of the disorder, but the CM is absent because of cancellation rather than pathology. This might obscure the diagnosis if the OAEs are absent, because the CM would then be the only clear evidence for preserved function in the outer hair cells.

Second, there must be evidence for preserved function in the outer hair cells. This is most clearly demonstrated by recording the OAEs, either to transient click stimuli or using pairs of tones and measuring distortion products. OAEs are absent in about a quarter of the patients with auditory neuropathy. In these cases, preservation of function in the outer hair cells can be demonstrated by recording the CM. We must be careful to differentiate the CM from electrical stimulus artifact. This can be done by distancing the transducer from the ear, typically by connecting the transducer to a tube leading to an ear-insert. The sound then has to travel an extra distance before reaching the ear, and this takes time. The stimulus artifact, caused by the transducer setting up an electromagnetic field that induces currents in the recording circuits, would then occur significantly earlier than the CM. The CM also can be distinguished from the artifact by closing off the tube between the transducer and ear without moving the transducer:

the artifact remains but the CM vanishes (because the ear receives no sound).

Figure 15–1 shows the findings in a typical case of auditory neuropathy (Starr et al., 1996). The pure-tone audiogram shows a mainly low-frequency hearing loss. Click-evoked and distortion-product OAEs are clearly present. A striking feature in this particular patient is that the OAEs are present at frequencies (such as 2 kHz) where the audiogram shows a significant hearing loss. The ABR is not recognizable. A definite CM that changes polarity as the stimulus changes from a rarefaction to condensation click can be recognized early in the ABR recording.

The CM also must be distinguished from normal or abnormal neural responses. One way to demonstrate this involves recording separate responses to condensation and rarefaction clicks and then adding or subtracting the two responses (Deltenre, Mansbach, Bozet, Clercx, & Hecox, 1997). If the response is bigger with subtraction, then it is likely the CM (provided stimulus artifact has been ruled out). If the response is bigger with addition, then its origin is likely the summating potential, auditory nerve, or brainstem. In calculating the addition and subtraction waveforms to use with this logic, we should be careful that the computer does not automatically divide by 2 (as would normally be done when averaging two responses together). Typically, however, we do divide by 2 to keep the voltage calibration correct. Figure 15–2 compares the ABR recordings in a patient with auditory neuropathy to those in a normal subject (Starr, 2001), and demonstrates how the CM and the summating potential (SP) can be distinguished from the ABR by the addition and subtraction of responses to condensation and rarefaction clicks.

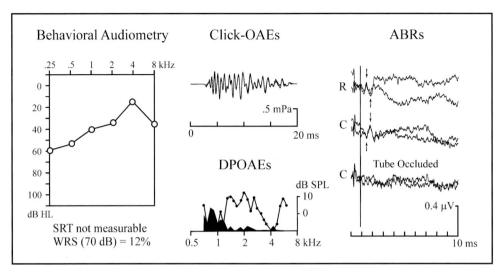

Figure 15–1. *Findings in a patient with auditory neuropathy. The pure-tone audiogram on the left shows a hearing loss mainly at the lower frequencies. The word recognition score (WRS) was very low and no speech reception threshold (SRT) could be measured because the patient could not discriminate the words. The OAEs are shown in the center column. The click OAEs are normal; the distortion product (DP) OAEs show an isolated loss of emissions near 4 kHz (paradoxically where behavioral hearing is best). The ABRs shown on the right were evoked separately by condensation (C) and rarefaction (R) clicks. They show a CM (*arrows*) that reverses polarity with the change in stimulus. The stimuli were presented with an insert and tube; the electrical stimulus artifact occurs before the stimulus reaches the eardrum (*line*). Occlusion of the tube leaves the stimulus artifact but removes the CM. Data are for right ear of patient 2 from Starr et al. (1996).*

Other Findings

Many other findings help to confirm that a patient has auditory neuropathy, but are not crucial to the diagnosis. The degree of pure-tone loss as measured by the pure-tone-average threshold varies from normal to severe, although most patients have a moderate loss. The pure-tone audiogram can have a variety of patterns (Sininger & Oba, 2001). Figure 15–3 shows audiograms from several patients with auditory neuropathy. There is a tendency for the audiogram to show elevated thresholds at high or low frequencies or both. Often there is some preservation of hearing near 2 kHz (Zeng, Kong, Michalewski, & Starr, 2005). This type of audiogram ("peaked"

or "tent") was found in almost half of the patients reported by Kumar and Jayaram (2006) but only in 5% of patients in Starr et al. (2000). Generally, speech discrimination is reduced, with word recognition scores (WRS) significantly worse than what might be expected in patients with a sensory hearing loss and equivalent pure-tone audiograms (Yellin, Jerger, & Fifer, 1989). Speech reception thresholds (SRT) are difficult to evaluate as the patients may hear the words but be unable to recognize them. This fits with the clinical presentation of the disorder in older children or adults with auditory neuropathy. These patients typically complain of difficulties in understanding speech despite being able to hear the sounds.

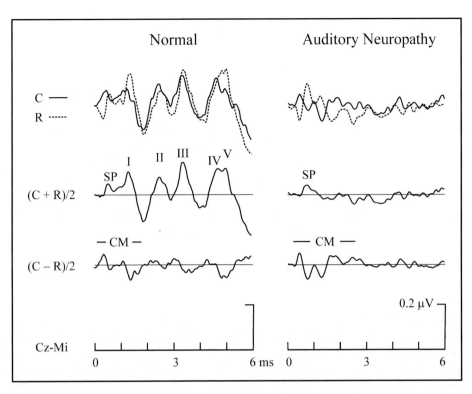

Figure 15–2. *ABRs in a patient with auditory neuropathy compared to recordings in a normal subject. Responses were evoked separately by condensation (C) and rarefaction (R) clicks. Those on the left are from a normal subject and those on the right from a patient with auditory neuropathy. The C + R waveform shows both the summating potential (SP) and the different waves of the ABR. The CM shows up best in the C – R difference waveform. The patient with auditory neuropathy shows both an SP and a CM, but no ABR components. Data from Starr (2001).*

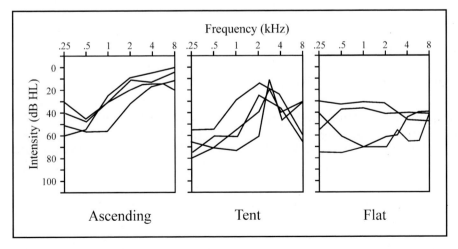

Figure 15–3. *Audiograms in patients with auditory neuropathy. Audiograms have been selected to illustrate the most common patterns from Zeng et al. (2001), Wang, Gu, Han, and Yang (2003), and Berlin et al. (1993).*

Acoustic reflexes are abnormal in auditory neuropathy. This can help to distinguish the hearing loss from a cochlear loss of mild or moderate degree, where reflexes are usually preserved. The middle-ear muscle reflexes in auditory neuropathy are absent in about 90% of the cases and have elevated thresholds in the other 10% (Berlin et al., 2005). Very occasionally the reflexes can be normal (1/44 patients in Starr et al., 2000). Most likely, the lack of reflexes is due to dysfunction in the afferent part of the reflex arc, as the reflexes can be evoked by tactile stimulation (e.g., Starr et al., 1998). Furthermore, in unilateral auditory neuropathy, the reflexes are absent in both ears when the affected ear is stimulated but present in both ears when the normal ear is stimulated (Berlin et al., 2005). Therefore, auditory neuropathy can be quickly indicated if the OAEs are present, tympanometry is normal, and the acoustic reflexes absent (Berlin et al., 2002). The presence of the OAEs indicates auditory thresholds (at least in the cochlea) of less than 35 dB relative to hearing level (HL), and with such thresholds, middle ear muscle reflexes should occur if the disorder is a sensorineural hearing loss. The normal tympanograms would eliminate the possibility of a mild conductive loss, which could elevate the reflex thresholds yet still allow recordable OAEs.

In addition to its effect on the middle-ear muscle reflexes, auditory neuropathy disables the efferent suppression of OAEs (Berlin et al., 1993; Hood, Berlin, Bordelon, & Rose, 2003). Normally, the amplitude of the OAEs is decreased when the olivocochlear bundle is activated by contralateral sounds (Collet et al., 1990). Studies of a patient with unilateral auditory neuropathy show that the disorder is in the afferent part of the reflex arc, as contralateral suppression occurred normally in the ear with auditory neuropathy and was absent in the normal contralateral ear (Hood et al., 2003). Figure 15–4 shows the normal suppression response and its absence in patients with auditory neuropathy.

Although the ABRs are absent or severely abnormal in auditory neuropathy, the later auditory evoked potentials may be within normal limits. In the original report of Starr et al. (1996), the middle-latency responses (MLRs) were absent or abnormal in five of six patients and the late auditory evoked potentials (LAEPs) abnormal in two of three patients. The LAEPs (N1, P2, and SP) may be helpful in evaluating the ability of the subject to recognize speech and in determining the prognosis for treatment (Cone, 2008; Golding et al., 2007; Michalewski, Starr, Zeng, & Dimitrijevic, 2009; Narne & Vanaja, 2008a; Rance et al., 1999; Rance, Cone-Wesson, Wunderlich, & Dowell, 2002). The N1-P2 complex can be evoked by gaps in an ongoing noise in patients with auditory neuropathy, but only for long duration gaps (Michalewski, Starr, Nguyen, Kong, & Zeng, 2005). Auditory steady-state responses (ASSRs) at stimulus rates of 80 to 100 Hz are either absent or show thresholds that are significantly elevated above the behavioral thresholds (Emara & Gabr, 2010; Rance et al., 1999; Raveh, Buller, Badrana, & Attias, 2007). ASSRs at slower stimulus rates may be recorded more easily, but these have not yet been reported.

Vestibular function may be normal or abnormal in patients with auditory neuropathy. The tests are caloric testing and, more recently, vestibular evoked muscle reflexes (see Chapter 9). Caloric testing was found to be abnormal in two of four patients tested in the original series of Starr et al. (1996). Fujikawa and Starr (2000) found abnormal caloric responses in 9 of

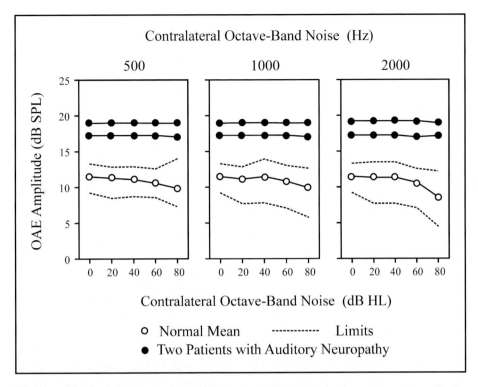

Figure 15–4. Suppression of OAEs by contralateral noise. *Presentation of noise in the contralateral ear begins to reduce the click-evoked OAE when the intensity of the noise exceeds 40 dB HL (and before any clear effects of the middle-ear muscle reflexes). The amount of the suppression is between 2 and 4 dB. This figure shows some of the results in normal subjects and in two patients with auditory neuropathy (Berlin et al., 1993). The normal subjects show suppression as the intensity of the contralateral noise increases; their graphs curve downward as they progress to the right. The amount of suppression is small but the graphs differ from those of the patients with neuropathy which show no evidence of suppression; their graphs stay flat. Both patients show particularly large OAEs.*

14 patients with auditory neuropathy even though none of the patients had experienced vestibular symptoms. Later papers report isolated cases of auditory neuropathy with either abnormal or normal vestibular function (Akdogan, Selcuk, Ozcan, & Dere, 2008; Sheykholeslami, Kaga, Murofushi, & Hughes, 2000; Sheykholeslami, Schmerber, Kermany, & Kaga, 2005). The vestibular evoked myogenic potential (VEMP) is absent in many patients with auditory neuropathy, indicating involvement of the vestibular afferent fibers from the saccule (Sazgar, Yazdani, Rezazadeh & Yazdi, 2010; Sheykholeslami et al., 2005).

Many patients with auditory neuropathy show evidence of a generalized neuropathy on clinical and electrophysiologic tests of peripheral nerve function (80% of adult patients tested by Starr et al., 2000). This finding led to the original proposal by Starr et al. (1996) that the predominant disorder might be a neuropathy, with the auditory nerve affected either as an isolated mononeuropathy or as part of a generalized neuropathy. Sometimes the patient has a well-defined neuropathic syndrome such as Charcot-Marie-Tooth disease (hereditary sensorimotor neuropathy). This disorder is quite common (affecting about 1 in 5000 individuals) and has a variety of subtypes, each of which is associated with one or more genetic abnormalities, a particular clinical history, and a characteristic set of physiologic findings. Involvement of the auditory nerve is common, and hearing impairment may occur before other signs or symptoms (Seeman et al., 2004).

Another ancillary test that can distinguish different types of auditory neuropathy is magnetic resonance imaging (MRI) of the auditory nerve. Buchman et al. (2006) found that the cochlear nerves were deficient or absent in 9 of 51 children with physiologic evidence for auditory neuropathy. Walton, Gibson, Sanli, and Prelog (2008), who found a slightly higher incidence (15 out of 54 children) of cochlear nerve deficiency, reported that children with such cochlear nerve deficiency did not do well with a cochlear implant. Therefore, MRI studies are a necessary part of the workup of a patient with auditory neuropathy who is being considered for implantation.

The course of the disorder is variable. Sininger and Oba (2001) report that, in most patients, the findings are either stable or fluctuate over time. Patients with an underlying genetic disorder tend to show progression. Some newborn infants show distinct improvements with time, particularly if hyperbilirubinemia has been implicated in the etiology (Attias & Raveh, 2007; Madden, Rutter, Hilbert, Greinwald, & Choo, 2002). This means that the diagnosis of auditory neuropathy should be considered with caution in the newborn period. Attias and Raveh (2007) suggest that treatment should not be initiated until some behavioral measure of hearing disorder is available to confirm the abnormal ABR findings.

Differential Diagnosis

The diagnostic criteria for auditory neuropathy are clear and are based on objective physiologic tests. Disorders to be considered in a differential diagnosis therefore usually depend on the interpretation of the physiologic recordings.

As already discussed, the CM must be clearly distinguished from stimulus artifact. In addition, the CM must be distinguished from an ABR. If we record the ABR to clicks of only one polarity, the CM, which can be both large and long-lasting in auditory neuropathy, can mimic the waves of the ABR. Usually, the waveform is abnormal for an ABR, and one can mistakenly interpret the results as indicating a brainstem lesion. The CM is differentiated from the ABR by separately recording responses to condensation and rarefaction clicks as demonstrated in Figures 15–1 and 15–2. Figure 15–5 shows recordings from an adolescent with a prolonged CM response.

A steep high-frequency hearing loss theoretically can cause the latencies of the click-ABR to change significantly between condensation and rarefaction clicks (Coats & Martin, 1977). As in Chapter 8, the ABR latency difference between condensation and rarefaction clicks is determined by the resonant characteristics of the basilar membrane where the response is generated. If there is no hearing at 2000 Hz and higher, the click-ABR will derive mainly from the regions of the basilar membrane responding to about 1000 Hz. The rarefaction response from this region will be ini-

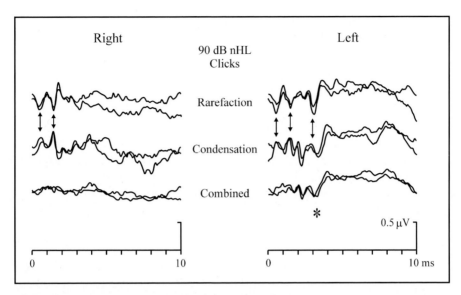

Figure 15–5. *Prolonged cochlear microphonic. These recordings were obtained from a 17-year-old girl with a history of neonatal jaundice and a mild to moderate hearing loss (recordings from Picton et al., 1998). The ABR recordings show no consistent wave V but reliable waveforms out to about 4 ms when using high-intensity clicks. These waves reverse in polarity* (two-headed arrows) *when the stimulus is changed from a rarefaction to a condensation click. This suggests that the findings largely represent a prolonged CM. The remaining waves when the condensation and rarefaction responses are combined for the left ear* (asterisk) *may represent some distorted SP and CAP response, some nonlinearity in the cochlear microphonic, or perhaps a vestibular response (such as reported by Mason et al., 1996).*

tiated one-half cycle (0.5 ms) before the condensation response. Because the successive negative and positive waves of the ABR are separated by about one half a millisecond, this could lead to the positive waves of the condensation response occurring at the same time as the negative waves of the rarefaction response. The recordings could then mimic a CM. The main way to determine if this is happening would be to observe the steep high-frequency loss in the audiogram or the absent high-frequency OAEs.

An acoustic neuroma may present with electrophysiologic findings very similar to those seen in auditory neuropathy. The symptoms of the two disorders often are similar, particularly the decreased speech discrimination out of keeping with the pure-tone audiogram. Wave I of the ABR often is preserved in cases of acoustic neuroma, whereas the diagnostic criteria for auditory neuropathy require wave I to be abnormal. However, as the acoustic neuroma develops, abnormalities of wave I may occur and the electrophysiologic findings can then become very similar in the two disorders. Acoustic neuromas most frequently present in adults, and often are associated with tinnitus, something that is not commonly reported in auditory neuropathy, although it may occur occasionally (e.g., Starr et al., 2004). Radiologic examination provides the definitive demonstration of the tumor or other lesions of the cerebellopontine angle. Boudewyns et al. (2008) present an interesting case of an arachnoid cyst of the cerebellopontine angle presenting as auditory neuropathy in a newborn infant.

In many of the patients diagnosed with auditory neuropathy, there are no OAEs and the CM is taken as evidence of preserved function in the outer hair cells. OAES are preserved in about 75% of patients diagnosed with auditory neuropathy (Berlin et al., 2010; Sininger & Oba, 2001). The incidence of preserved OAEs may be lower in young children with auditory neuropathy, Mo, Yan, Liu, Han, and Zhang (2010) reporting only 40%. Withnell (2001) has shown that the CM may not be the best way to demonstrate normal functioning in the outer hair cells. Most of the CM recorded using electrodes outside of the cochlea derives from the basal turn of the cochlea. Therefore, the presence or absence of a CM says little about the function of the outer hair cells in other regions of the cochlea. A recordable CM can occur in association with a widespread abnormality of outer hair cells, provided there is some sparing of the basal region. Indeed, the absence of any recordable OAEs clearly indicates this. Ahmmed, Brockbank, and Adshead (2008) present an intriguing case of an infant who presented as an auditory neuropathy but was finally diagnosed as having a hereditary sensorineural hearing loss, probably of the Waardenburg type. OAEs were absent and the CM recorded may not have occurred at levels lower than hearing thresholds. In this case, the hair cells were widely affected and the CM simply indicated some residual hair-cell function.

Gibson and Graham (2008) have noted that many patients with sensorineural hearing loss have a disorder that affects both inner and outer hair cells. In some of these patients, there may be a sufficient number of remaining outer hair cells to generate a recordable CM. The absent ABR may be caused both by a direct pathologic effect on the inner hair cells or by pathologic outer hair cells somehow disrupting the normal activation of the inner hair cell system. This type of abnormality might be present in those few patients with the syndrome of auditory neuropathy that do well with hearing aids. It would be highly unlikely to find normal or near-normal OAEs in these patients, as this would indicate a large number of normally functioning outer hair cells.

A particular diagnostic problem in the evaluation of infants for possible auditory neuropathy is the fact that the ABR may be transiently abnormal in premature infants or in infants who have suffered hypoxia (Stockard, Stockard, Kleinberg, & Westmoreland, 1983). If the OAEs are normal, the picture may look like auditory neuropathy, but the ABR can return to normal in a month or so. In these children, repeat ABR testing when they have attained a normal conceptional age or one month after the resolution of the neonatal respiratory problems is essential. As already discussed, ABR improvement also can occur in infants with hyperbilirubinemia.

The main hearing problem that occurs in auditory neuropathy—an impairment of speech recognition disproportionate to any abnormality of the pure-tone audiogram—is very similar to the symptoms of patients with central auditory processing disorders. These disorders may be caused by lesions of the central nervous system but, more often than not, the exact pathology is unknown. Physiologic testing can differentiate auditory neuropathy from cortical auditory processing disorders.

Patients with cortical auditory processing disorders will have normal ABRs and normal middle-ear muscle reflexes. Patients with central auditory processing disorders related to brainstem abnormalities can be distinguished from auditory neuropathy by their normal wave I and electrocochleography (CAP, SP, CM).

ELECTROCOCHLEOGRAPHY (ECOCHG)

The main diagnostic tests that lead to the diagnosis of auditory neuropathy—ABR and OAEs—do not distinguish between different subtypes of the disorder. A major question is whether the disorder is presynaptic, involving the inner hair cell or its synapse, or postsynaptic, involving the afferent neurons (Starr et al., 2004). In recent years, we have turned to the ECochG for more information (McMahon, Patuzzi, Gibson, & Sanli, 2008; Santarelli & Arslan, 2002: Santarelli, Starr, Michalewski & Arslan, 2008). As reviewed in Chapter 7, ECochG recordings can be taken from the mastoid, external auditory meatus, promontory, or round window using both clicks and tones as stimuli. The response becomes larger the closer one gets to the generators, and the recorded waveforms will vary in their morphology with both the location of the electrode and the type of stimulus. The most important information comes from the compound action potential (CAP) and the summating potential (SP). These usually are obtained by calculating the difference between responses to stimuli of opposite polarity.

Recordings from the external auditory meatus in patients with auditory neuropathy show a broad negative click-evoked response that appears to represent a negative SP with either an absent or delayed CAP (Lu et al., 2008). Interestingly, the waveforms in the ABR evoked by a 4-kHz tone in an infant with auditory neuropathy also showed a large broad SP (Dunkley, Farnsworth, Mason, Dodd, & Gibbin, 2003).

More information has been obtained from transtympanic ECochG recordings. Click-evoked responses recorded from the promontory showed a broad (and sometimes delayed) negative SP (Santarelli et al., 2008; see right side of Figure 15–6). The large CAP (N1 and N2 waves) that was normally superimposed on the SP was not found. The click-evoked broad negative wave in patients with auditory neuropathy (middle tracing on the right of Figure 15–6) could contain both neural and receptor components. The neural component (a delayed and distorted N1 wave of the CAP) could be demonstrated by its attenuation with increased stimulus rate (the SP normally not being affected by rate). In some patients, there was just a broad negative SP and no evidence for any neural components (see tracing at bottom right of Figure 15–6). Later recordings in a group of patients with mutations of the otoferlin gene showed similar findings (Santarelli et al., 2009). These results point to a disorder in the activation of the nerve endings. In the otoferlin patients, this may be caused specifically by a disorder in the release of synaptic vesicles at the synapse between the hair cell and afferent nerve fibers (Glowatski, Grant, & Fuchs, 2008).

McMahon et al. (2008) recorded responses from an electrode on the round window using brief tones as well as to clicks. The positive SP response to an 8-kHz tone (different from the negative SP to a click) showed evidence for activation of the inner hair cells. A negative potential following this response was recorded

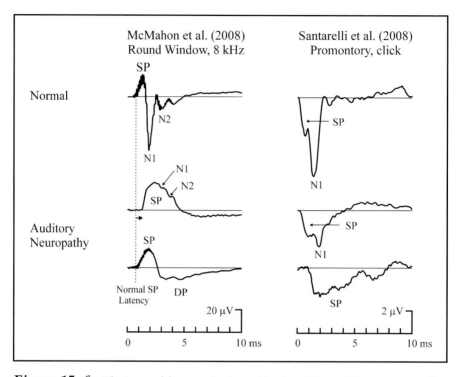

Figure 15–6. *Electrocochleography in patients with auditory neuropathy. Data from two different studies are shown. All responses combine responses to rarefaction and condensation stimuli and thus cancel most of the CM (although a small residual remains in some responses due to asymmetry of the CM waveforms). The waveforms on the left are recorded from the round window in response to 8-kHz tones (MacMahon et al. 2008) and those on the right from the promontory in response to clicks (Santarelli et al., 2008). McMahon et al. reported two patterns, a presynaptic one with a delayed and very broad positive SP (middle tracing) and a postsynaptic one with a dendritic potential (DP) but no action potentials (lower tracing). Santarelli et al. (2008) reported a broad negative SP with or without a small and delayed CAP.*

in some subjects and might represent a dendritic potential (DP, see bottom left tracing in Figure 15–6). Finally, delayed and distorted action potentials could be recognized in some subjects. McMahon and her colleagues proposed that a presynaptic auditory neuropathy would show a delayed SP with no DP but sometimes with delayed and distorted CAPs. On the other hand, a postsynaptic disorder would show a normal latency SP with or without a dendritic potential, but no action potentials. A key distinguishing feature is the delayed onset of the positive sustained potential in patients with a presynaptic abnormality.

Further ECochG studies need to be performed in patients with auditory neuropathy. McMahon et al. (2008) found two main patterns of abnormality (the middle and lower right patterns on the left of Figure 15–6) and attributed them to pre- and postsynaptic disorders. There may be several other patterns of abnormality, each associated with a different underlying etiology. It also would be important to explain more fully the differences between the promontory and round window recordings.

During transtympanic ECochG, one can apply electrical stimulation and see whether an electrically elicited ABR can be recorded. Although this might seem a logical way to distinguish patients for whom an implant will beneficial, extensive studies have found that the ABR electrically evoked during transtympanic ECochG does not really correlate well with outcome measures after cochlear implantation (Nikolopoulos, Mason, Gibbin, & O'Donoghue, 2000). A good response to transtympanic stimulation usually means that the implant will work well, but an absent or abnormal response carries little meaning.

Runge-Samuelson, Drake, and Wackym (2008) found the ABR electrically evoked through the implant was quite variable in patients with auditory neuropathy, although Walton et al. (2008) found that it did correlate with outcome measurements after implantation. This type of recording is available only after the implant is in situ and clearly cannot be used to decide on whether or not to insert the implant.

EPIDEMIOLOGY OF AUDITORY NEUROPATHY

The prevalence of auditory neuropathy in the newborn period has been studied in infants who have been tested with ABRs during neonatal screening. Unfortunately, the data are reported for different populations (babies in a neonatal intensive care unit, all babies, babies at different gestational ages, babies at risk for hearing loss, babies with hearing loss, etc.) and are very difficult to compare. Furthermore, it is not clear that babies who have been diagnosed on the basis of present OAEs (and absent ABRs) and babies who have been diagnosed on the basis of present CMs (and absent ABRs) represent the same diagnostic entity. Rance et al. (1999) found 12 of 5199 at-risk babies (0.23%) presented with signs of auditory neuropathy (compared to 2% found to have a permanent sensorineural hearing loss). Ngo, Ran, Balakrishnan, Lim, and Lazaroo (2006) found 9 cases of auditory neuropathy of 14,807 babies (0.6 per 1000) screened in the neonatal period as part of a universal screening program. These cases were 17% of the total number of babies found to have abnormal hearing. Dowley et al. (2009) reviewed the screening of 45,050 infants in a neonatal intensive care unit who were tested with both OAEs and ABRs. They found 30 infants with a severe or profound hearing impairment, and 12 of these had an auditory neuropathy. Significant risk factors for auditory neuropathy were hyperbilirubinemia, sepsis, and exposure to the antibiotic gentamicin.

Another way to determine how frequently auditory neuropathy occurs is to see how many children diagnosed as hearing-impaired by absent ABRs or elevated ABR-thresholds show signs of outer hair cell function. Rance (2005) reviewed multiple studies and found that approximately 7% (range 1.7–15%) of such children have auditory neuropathy. More recently, Foerst et al. (2006) found an overall prevalence of the disorder in 0.9% of children at risk for hearing loss and in 8.4% of children with a severe hearing loss. Uus and Bamford (2006) reported that auditory neuropathy occurred in 10% (17/169) of infants with a permanent hearing loss that were detected by neonatal screening. Declau, Boudewyns, van den Ende, Peeters, and van den Heyning (2008), however, found that auditory neuropathy occurred in only 2 out of 68 infants with bilateral hearing loss found by screening.

As rough rules of thumb, we might estimate that about 2 in 1000 children are born with a significant sensorineural hearing loss, and that about 1 in 10 of these has auditory neuropathy. However, as we have seen, both incidences can vary widely across different populations.

The prevalence of auditory neuropathy in a total population (adults and children) with sensorineural hearing loss may be much lower. Kumar and Jayaram (2006) found that 0.5% of such patients have both absent ABRs and present OAEs. This low incidence may be related, in part, to using just OAEs rather than either OAEs or CMs as diagnostic criteria for hair cell function. It also is possible that many of the cases showing signs of auditory neuropathy in infancy may have progressed to a more general sensorineural hearing loss by the time they were evaluated.

These low incidences stand in stark contrast to those reported by Berg, Spitzer, Towers, Bartosiewicz, and Diamond (2005), who found that about a quarter of infants from a neonatal intensive care unit (115/477) who were examined with ABRs (and subsequently followed up with OAEs) showed the characteristic findings of auditory neuropathy. Apparently, none of the screened infants had a sensorineural hearing loss. This extremely high incidence of auditory neuropathy might be related to the large number of premature babies tested (cf. Xoinis, Weirather, Mavoori, Shaha, & Iwamoto, 2007), the high incidence of hyperbilirubinemia and hypoxia in their population, or possible effects of antibiotics and other medications.

One problem in assessing the prevalence of auditory neuropathy in infancy is the possibility that the recorded abnor-

malities may resolve over the first few months of life. As already discussed, transient ABR abnormalities can occur in premature newborns (Stockard et al., 1983). Psarommatis et al. (2006) reported that 13 of 20 babies in an intensive care unit found with absent or distorted ABRs and present OAEs showed normal ABRs on retesting several months later. Many of these were born at gestational ages below 38 weeks. Other studies have also found transient ABR problems in infancy (Attias & Raveh, 2007; Madden et al., 2002).

Although auditory neuropathy typically involves both ears, about 1 in 20 cases have involvement of only one ear (4% in Starr et al., 2000; 6% in Berlin et al., 2005). The reported prevalence of unilateral auditory neuropathy may be lower than the actual prevalence, as subjects with normal hearing in one ear may not notice the disorder in the other ear.

PATHOLOGY AND PATHOGENESIS

Types of Hearing Loss

The mammalian peripheral auditory system contains both afferent and efferent systems. The afferent system involves the inner hair cells and the afferent nerve fibers that receive synaptic input from these hair cells (Felix, 2002; Moore & Linthicum, 2001). Approximately 90% of the afferent nerve fibers in the human auditory nerve come from the inner hair cells. Each fiber connects with only one hair cell and each hair cell connects to between 6 and 12 afferent fibers. Dendritic fibers from the inner hair cells become myelinated as they pass through the spiral lamina, and lead over a variable distance to cell bodies in the spiral ganglion. These auditory neurons are truly bipolar with activation traveling through the cell body. Unlike other species, the cell bodies of the human spiral ganglion are unmyelinated. Some afferent fibers come from the outer hair cells but the function of these fibers is not understood.

The peripheral auditory system also contains an efferent system. Most of these neurons synapse on the outer hair cells, although some synapse on the afferent nerve terminals near the inner hair cells. Neurons from the superior olive in the pons travel to the cochlea to synapse on the outer hair cells. These efferent neurons adjust the contractility of the outer hair cells, which act as a special amplifier to modulate the sensitivity of the afferent system. Figure 15–7 shows the organ of Corti of the normal human cochlea.

Hearing can be affected by disorders of either the afferent or efferent auditory system. If the afferent system is affected, information flow from cochlea to the brain is disrupted or distorted. Auditory neuropathy is primarily a disorder of the afferent auditory system. If the efferent system is affected, sounds of low or moderate

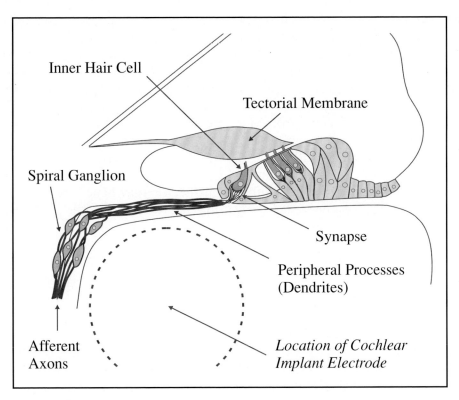

Figure 15–7. Possible locations of pathology in auditory neuropathy. This diagram shows the organ of Corti (light shading) resting on the basilar membrane. The sensory and neural elements are shown with darker shading. The syndrome of auditory neuropathy can result from disorders in any of the elements indicated using normal script. The approximate location of the electrode of a cochlear implant as it coils around the central modiolus is indicated with dashed line (and italic script). More details about the structure of the organ of Corti are provided in Figure 7–2.

intensities are not perceived because the cochlear amplifier in the outer hair cells cannot increase the sensitivity of the afferent system to process them. However, loud sounds still may be able to activate the inner hair cells. The hearing loss caused by disorders of the efferent auditory system combines a loss of low-level hearing with recruitment at higher levels. The physiologic findings are absent OAEs with normal ABRs and normal middle-ear reflexes for stimuli of high intensity.

Many hearing losses have pathology in both afferent and efferent systems. The disorder coud begin in either the afferent or efferent system and then gradually spread to the other system. A disorder that begins as an auditory neuropathy may wind up involving the efferent system and becoming indistinguishable from a severe cochlear hearing loss. Deltenre et al. (1999) first reported that some patients with auditory neuropathy lose their otoacoustic emissions on follow-up testing. Sininger and Oba (2001) found that this happened in 20% of their patients. In an extensive investigation of a family with a dominantly inherited deafness, Starr et al. (2004) showed that the disorder progresses through different stages. It presents with difficulties hearing and the typical physiologic findings of auditory neuropathy: abnormal ABRs and present OAEs. The disorder then progresses to a stage in which the OAEs are abnormal, becoming either absent or present only at low frequencies. Finally, it reaches a stage in which the hearing loss is profound and neither ABRs nor OAEs are recordable.

Within the group of purely afferent hearing disorders, a variety of different pathologies may occur. These can occur at each level of the afferent system, as indicated in Figure 15–7. The inner hair cell may be abnormal or its interaction with the tectorial membrane might be disrupted. The synapse between the inner hair cell and the dendrite of the afferent nerve fiber might not function properly (a synaptopathy). Abnormalities may affect the activation of the peripheral processes (dendrites) of the afferent nerve fiber or the axon leading from the spiral ganglion to the brainstem (axonopathy). Transmission along the afferent fiber may be affected by loss of the myelin that normally surrounds the axon (myelinopathy). Starr et al. (2004) have suggested that auditory neuropathy might be categorized as either postsynaptic or presynaptic. This differentiation may have implications for treatment, as electrical stimulation of the afferent fibers by means of a cochlear implant should be more effective in the presynaptic type of the disorder. In this type of disorder, the electrical stimulation would bypass the abnormality in the inner hair cell or its synapse. However, even cases that primarily involve the nerve fibers, such as the hearing loss that accompanies Friedreich's ataxia, may benefit from a cochlear implant (Miyamoto, Kirk, Renshaw, & Hussain, 1999). In these cases, it is possible that many of the dendritic processes of the neurons have died back and are no longer functionally connected to the inner hair cells. The implant might still be able to stimulate the neurons at the level of the spiral ganglion.

Etiologies

Auditory neuropathy can be caused in many different ways. The disorder presents at two different ages: in infancy the patients are referred when abnormal ABRs are found during newborn hearing screening, and in later years patients present to audiologists or physicians because they are experiencing difficulty understanding speech. At both times, genetic abnormalities can be the root cause. In infancy, hyperbilirubinemia and hypoxia are the most common other etiologic factors. Older patients presenting with auditory neuropathy often have hereditary sensorimotor neuropathy. Other causes are acquired neuropathies, infections, or toxicity (e.g., xylene, Draper & Bamiou, 2008). Often the etiology is unknown.

Many animal models of auditory dysfunction show findings similar to those recorded in human auditory neuropathy (Cacace & Burkard, 2009; Matsumoto, Sekiya, Kojima, & Ito, 2008; Sawada, Mori, Mount, & Harrison, 2001). The main models are based on pharmacologic effects (e.g., glutamate, ouabain or carboplatin toxicity), chronic anoxia, auditory nerve compression, and various genetic defects.

Starr, Zeng, Michalewski, and Moser (2008) reviewed many of the different genetic abnormalities associated with auditory neuropathy in human subjects and animal models. As more and more familial cases of auditory neuropathy are studied and characterized, more genes likely will be implicated. Table 15–1 shows some of the genetic deficits that have been shown in human subjects and their possible pathologic mechanisms. Two of the gene loci identified on the basis of auditory neuropathy are named after the disorder: AUNA1 with autosomal dominant inheritance (Kim et al., 2004) and AUNX1 with X-linked recessive inheritance (Wang et al., 2006). The auditory neuropathy occurring in association with autosomal dominant optic atrophy responds well to cochlear implantation (Huang, Santarelli, & Starr, 2009).

Multiple cases of familial auditory neuropathy have been associated with defects in the OTOF gene at the DFNB9 locus controlling otoferlin (Smith, Gurrola, & Kelley, 2008; Varga et al., 2006). This protein is localized in inner hair cells and probably contributes to efficient synaptic function. Interestingly, one particular mutation of this gene causes an auditory neuropathy that is temperature-sensitive. Patients with this disorder have a transient hearing loss when they become febrile. During the hearing loss, the ABR becomes abnormal or absent while the OAEs remain (Gorga, Stelmachowicz, Barlow, & Brookhouser, 1995; Starr et al., 1998). Figure 15–8 shows data from a patient with this disorder. These patients also show an increased sensitivity of the ABR to stimulus rate, with wave V decreasing significantly at click rates of around 20/s (Starr et al., 2000).

The deafness associated with Mohr-Tranebjaerg syndrome is caused by a rare mutation or deletion in the TIMM8A gene (Roesch, Curran, Tranebjaerg, & Koehler, 2002; Tranebjaerg, 2009). The hearing impairment in this X-linked disorder is rapidly progressive over the first few years of life, at which time the infants show characteristic findings of absent ABRs and preserved OAEs (Richter et al., 2001). As the child grows older, the deafness becomes profound and other manifestations of the syndrome such as vision loss, dystonia, and dementia develop. Cochlear implantation provides only fair assistance (Brookes et al., 2008). Some patients with this syndrome show an associated reduction in the gamma-globulins in the blood, caused by an associated abnormality of a contiguous gene (Richter et al., 2001). Several patients with this disorder have had their temporal bones evaluated after death (Bahmad, Merchant, Nadol, &

Table 15–1. Genetic Causes of Auditory Neuropathy

Disorder	Gene or Locus	Pathogenesis	References
Charcot-Marie-Tooth disease (Hereditary sensorimotor neuropathy)	Peripheral myelin protein (PMP22), Myelin protein zero (MPZ)	Demyelination of axons (causing slow nerve conduction), and secondary depletion of neurons	Starr et al., 2003 Seeman et al., 2004
	Neurofilament light (NF-L)	Mainly axonal degeneration	Butinar et al., 1999, 2008
Friedreich's ataxia	Frataxin (FXN)	Mitochondrial dysfunction leading to spinocerebellar degeneration and peripheral neuropathy	Rance et al., 2008
Autosomal dominant auditory neuropathy	locus AUNA1	Unknown, perhaps involving both inner and outer hair cells	Kim et al., 2004
X-linked recessive auditory neuropathy	locus AUNX1	Unknown, possibly synaptic problems	Wang et al., 2006
Familial auditory neuropathy with temperature sensitivity	Otoferlin (OTOF) DFNB9	Unknown, possibly synaptic problems with temperature-sensitivity	Varga et al. 2006
Autosomal recessive auditory neuropathy	Pejvakin, DFNB59	Unknown, may affect both afferent nerve fibers and hair cells	Delmaghani et al., 2006 Ebermann et al., 2007
Autosomal dominant optic atrophy	OPA1	Mitochondrial dysfunction affecting unmyelinated nerve terminals in optic and auditory nerves	Huang et al., 2009
Mohr-Tranebjaerg syndrome (X-linked deafness-dystonia syndrome)	DDP (deafness dystonia protein) TIMM8A	Mitochondrial dysfunction affecting cerebral neurons, auditory and optic nerves	Tranebjaerg, 2009 Bahmad et al., 2007

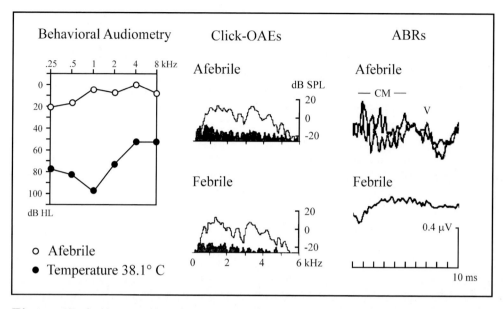

Figure 15–8. Temperature-sensitive auditory neuropathy. Data taken from Starr et al. (1998) for the left ear of the patient identified as "sister." The audiogram shows the results for the left ear. The click-OAEs (middle column) were normal in the afebrile state and remained essentially the same when the patient experienced a severe hearing loss during a fever. The ABRs separately recorded using condensation and rarefaction clicks at 80 dB (normal hearing level) when the patient was afebrile (upper right) showed a cochlear microphonic and a delayed wave V. During the febrile state there was no recordable ABR response even at 90 dB nHL. This recording was obtained using a different transducer and the large stimulus artifact might have obscured the CM.

Tranebjaerg, 2007). The sections showed a near-total loss of auditory nerve fibers, a severe loss of vestibular nerve fibers, and at least partial preservation of the hair cells (even thought the organs of Corti underwent some degree of autolysis prior to fixation).

The recently described DFNB59 deafness is interesting because it shows that genetic disorders might affect both nerve fibers and hair cells. The initial description of the disorder showed the classic findings of auditory neuropathy with abnormal ABRs and preserved OAEs (Delmaghani et al., 2006). However, a later study showed that a different mutation of the DFNB59 gene can also affect hair cell function and

cause a primarily cochlear hearing loss (Ebermann et al., 2007). Genetic mutations have complex manifestations.

TEMPORAL BONE STUDIES

The papers that have reported on the temporal bones of patients with auditory neuropathy provide support for two distinct pathologies. Amatuzzi et al. (2001) studied the temporal bones of infants with abnormal ABRs and found an isolated loss of inner hair cells with preservation of spiral ganglion cells and outer hair cells. This fits with the experimental work of Sawada et al. (2001), showing that the inner hair cells may be particularly sensitive to chronic hypoxia during development.

Other studies have shown loss of neurons. Starr et al. (2003) studied the temporal bones of an adult whose auditory neuropathy was associated with a peripheral neuropathy (caused by an abnormality in the myelin protein zero gene). There was a marked depletion of spiral ganglion cells and nerve fibers with preservation of both inner and outer hair cells. Similar pathologic findings were reported in previous studies of afferent auditory dysfunction before the clinical diagnosis of auditory neuropathy became feasible (Hallpike, Harriman, & Wells, 1980; Nadol, 2000; Spoendlin, 1974). Bahmad et al. (2007) showed a total loss of auditory nerve fibers along with preservation of the hair cells in Mohr-Tranebjaerg syndrome.

Pathophysiology

The pathophysiology of auditory neuropathy must explain why thresholds for hearing are less affected than the ability to discriminate complex sounds such as speech, and why the ABR is absent or distorted (Starr, Picton, & Kim, 2001). Two different explanations are possible, one involving the number of afferent nerve fibers and the other involving the synchrony of their firing. If there are only a small number of functioning afferent fibers, the thresholds for their activation may be normal but their ability to carry information about complex sounds will be limited. This is particularly true about timing information; portraying the envelope patterns of a sound requires multiple neurons as single neurons cannot fire rapidly enough. A small number of fibers would reduce the amplitude of the recorded ABR.

If there is a normal number of functioning afferent fibers, their ability to carry complex information, especially about timing, can be disrupted if the fibers are unable to synchronize their firing with the stimulus. Any jitter in firing could then cancel out both the recorded ABR and the envelope information carried by multiple afferent neurons. Either neuronal depletion or neuronal desynchrony can explain the difficulty experienced by the auditory nervous system in following rapidly changing sounds (Figure 15–9). In many pathologies, both depletion and desynchrony occur simultaneously.

In terms of auditory neuropathy occurring as part of a familial neuropathy such as Charcot-Marie-Tooth, both the axonal and the demyelinating variants thus could cause problems. Axonal neuropathies lead to a decreased number of afferent fibers; demyelinating neuropathies, in addition to the slowing of nerve conduction velocity, also disrupt the synchrony of firing among a group of fibers.

Dual pathophysiologies also could occur with a presynaptic disorder that disrupts the transmission of information from inner hair cell to afferent dendrite. Inner hair cell disorders could lead to a decreased release of synaptic transmitter so that only a few afferent fibers become activated. The synaptic abnormality also could lead to variability in the timing of the postsynaptic potentials and then to desynchronization of the afferent fiber discharges.

PERCEPTUAL CONSEQUENCES

The most significant perceptual consequence of auditory neuropathy is decreased speech recognition (Rance et al.,

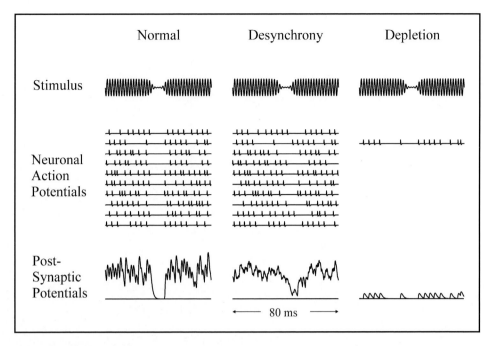

Figure 15–9. Desynchrony and depletion. *This figure diagrams what might happen if the brainstem neurons activated during the processing of a brief gap in a 500-Hz tone are either desynchronized (center column) or depleted (right column). The action potentials follow a stochastic firing pattern in response to the tone with rates of around 150 Hz when the sound is on. The excitatory postsynaptic potentials in the brainstem neurons are modeled with rise and fall time-constants of 1 and 9 ms (individual postsynaptic potentials are seen at the bottom right where only one neuron is firing). In the normal situation, these postsynaptic potentials (summed over all 10 neurons) follow the frequency of the ongoing tone (and therefore would generate a frequency-following response) and clearly demarcate the gap. The model for desynchrony includes a variable delay of between 0 and 10 ms for each of the action potentials. This could occur either at the synapse between inner hair cell and afferent fiber or in the conduction of the afferent fibers to the brainstem. In the desynchronized situation, there is no frequency-following response and the representation of the gap has become delayed and less clear-cut. When only one neuron (rather than 10) responds, the postsynaptic potentials cannot reliably portray either the tonal frequency or the gap.*

2007; Zeng & Liu, 2006). This is much worse when speech occurs in noise. Electric stimulation via a cochlear implant improves speech recognition in most subjects with auditory neuropathy. Figure 15–10 shows results of speech discrimination testing in patients with auditory neuropathy.

Much of the difficulty in recognizing speech signals may result from problems in temporal processing (Starr et al., 1991; Zeng et al., 2005). Perhaps the clearest demonstration of this occurs during the localization of sounds. Patients with auditory neuropathy can localize on the basis of interaural level differences but not on the basis of interaural timing differences (Zeng et al., 2005). Another simple test for disordered temporal processing is the

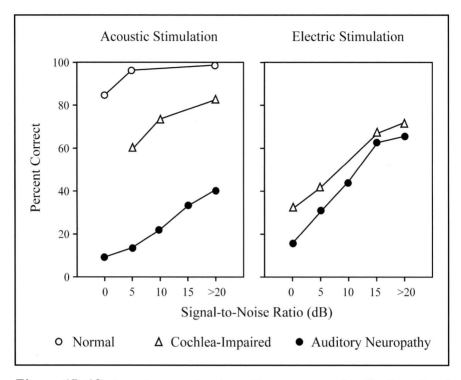

Figure 15–10. *Speech perception in auditory neuropathy. The data plotted are the approximate average data estimated from graphs 9 and 10 in the paper by Zeng and Liu (2006). The dependent variable was the percent correct keywords recognized in sentences spoken in a conversational voice at a comfortable hearing level. The left graph compares the performance of four patients with auditory neuropathy to the performance of five normal subjects and two patients with cochlear impairment. The speech perception of the patients with auditory neuropathy is very low. The right graph compares the performance of two groups of patients who had received a cochlear implant: eight subjects with cochlear impairment and four subjects with auditory neuropathy. The patients with auditory neuropathy show improved speech perception (compared to left graph). The results in patients with auditory neuropathy who were implanted are close to those found in patients implanted for severe to profound cochlear hearing loss (right graph).*

detection of a gap in an ongoing broadband noise (Zeng et al., 2005) or pure tone (Yalçinkaya, Muluk, Ataş, & Keith, 2009). The temporal modulation transfer function also is very abnormal: the threshold for detecting an amplitude modulation is much higher than normal and the function begins to fall off at a lower frequency (Zeng et al., 2005). Figure 15–11 shows the results

of gap detection and temporal modulation detection in auditory neuropathy.

Michalewski, Starr, Zeng, and Dimitrijevic (2009) found that the N1 wave of the late auditory evoked potential (LAEP) was decreased in amplitude and significantly delayed in patients with auditory neuropathy. The extent of the latency delay was related to the deterioration in

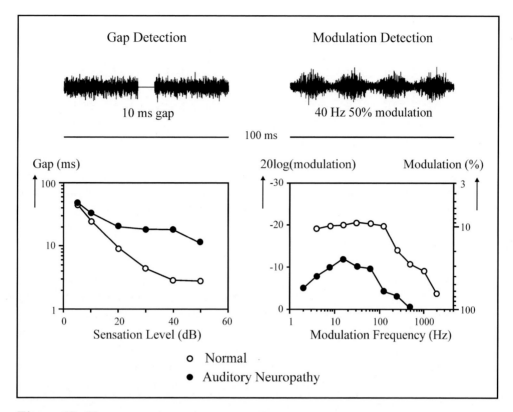

Figure 15–11. *Temporal perception in auditory neuropathy. The upper part of the figure represents the stimuli that must be discriminated from continuous unmodulated noise when determining gap detection thresholds and amplitude modulation. The graphs at the bottom compare the performance of patients with auditory neuropathy to that of normal subjects (data from Zeng et al. 2005). The patients with neuropathy can only perceive gaps when they have a much larger duration than normal. Their threshold for detecting modulation occurs at greater depths of modulation (lower on the right graph) and begins to fall off at a lower cutoff frequency (below rather than above 100 Hz).*

the patient's ability to detect gaps in white noise. Therefore, the N1 latency might provide an objective measure of the temporal processing disorder in auditory neuropathy.

Frequency discrimination is particularly affected at the lower frequencies in patients with auditory neuropathy. Therefore, a possible treatment idea might be to transpose frequencies from low to high, the opposite of what is usually done in a frequency-transposing hearing aid, or to filter out low-frequency sounds that may mask the information at higher frequencies (Zeng et al., 2005).

Speech sounds perceived by patients with auditory neuropathy can be more distracting than helpful. Zeng, Oba, Garde, Sininger, and Starr (2001) have simulated what may be happening in auditory neuropathy by changing the stimulus envelopes to fit with the temporal modulation functions observed in patients with auditory neuropathy. Speech sounds tinny and distorted, and with greater degrees of simulated neuropathy, the speech becomes unintelligible. Samples are available at http://www.healthaffairs.uci.edu/hesp/Simulations/simulationsmain.htm. In the second simulation you can hear Arnold Starr quoting from T. S. Eliot's *Four Quartets*: "Time present and time past . . . "

Many members of the kindred described by Starr et al (2004) have taken to "silent talking" as a way of communication. In this way, they get the benefit of lip-reading cues without the distraction of the distorted sound.

MANAGEMENT

Once the diagnosis of auditory neuropathy is confirmed, hearing aids are usually tried (Hayes et al., 2008; Roush, 2008). In adults and older children, fitting can be based on the pure-tone thresholds obtained in the audiogram with the proviso that such thresholds may not be that meaningful for discrimination and that the aid should be further adjusted on the basis of speech perception. In infants, we have to adjust the hearing aids on the basis of behavioral observations of speech awareness. Some fear has been expressed that amplification in infants with auditory neuropathy may lead to hair cell dysfunction, thereby compounding their neural problem with a noise-induced hearing loss. Nevertheless, the consensus has been to provide amplification within reasonable limits. We should not deprive the infant of audibility unless hearing and general behavior become demonstrably worse with amplification.

Unfortunately, most patients with auditory neuropathy do not do well with hearing aids, and some patients consider them more hindrance than help. Berlin et al. (2010) found that 85% of patients found hearing aids to be of little of no benefit. Young children with auditory neuropathy may perhaps do better with hearing aids (Rance & Barker, 2008). The outcome may be determined largely by the particular etiology of the disorder. Systems that use frequency-modulated (FM) radio transmission to provide speech sounds with a high signal-to-noise ratio (SNR) are helpful in situations where the communication is from one person (e.g., teacher or caregiver). We must not forget that language can develop in the absence of auditory input, and that patients with auditory neuropathy can be provided with visual means of communication such as sign language and cued speech (Berlin et al., 2010).

The compression that typically occurs in hearing aids may make the speech envelope less easy to follow. Narne and Vanaja (2008b, 2009) have found that speech discrimination in some patients with auditory neuropathy can be improved by electronically enhancing the speech envelope. These results certainly deserve follow-up.

Cochlear implantation has been used with good success in some patients with auditory neuropathy. The first implant in a patient with auditory neuropathy (child E in Trautwein, Shallop, Fabry, & Friedman, 2001) was performed before OAEs were routinely used to evaluate infants with hearing loss. A year after implantation, OAEs were detected in the nonimplanted ear. The measurements were obtained since the child's younger brother had been diagnosed with auditory neuropathy. The implanted child, who likely had a bilateral auditory neuropathy, has progressed well with the implant. Since then, many patients with auditory neuropathy have been implanted and the results are promising (e.g., Buchman, Roush, Teagle, & Zdanski, 2009; Buss et al., 2002; Peterson et al., 2003; Teagle et al., 2010; Walton et al., 2008).

Rance and Barker (2008, 2009) compared the effects of hearing aids and cochlear implants in children with auditory neuropathy. They found that both means of management improved the child's ability to perceive speech with no significant difference between amplification and implantation. Furthermore, implanted children with auditory neuropathy did not perform as well as children who received an implant because of severe cochlear hearing loss. However, using the same tests of speech perception as Rance and Barker, Shallop (2008) found that implanted patients with auditory neuropathy did as well or better than patients implanted for cochlear hearing loss. Auditory neuropathy has many etiologies and it is likely that some etiologies will show better outcomes with implants than others.

The infant with auditory neuropathy poses special problems in management (Uus, 2008). As reviewed, some infants born with an absent ABR may develop a normal ABR as they grow older. Clearly, we need to wait before initiating therapy to see if there is any return of auditory function. Many questions remain unanswered. How long should we wait to see if the ABRs return? Once we have decided that the auditory neuropathy is not going to spontaneously remit, what management protocol do we initiate? Although they work well for cochlear hearing loss, hearing aids may not be beneficial for some types of auditory neuropathy. Which infants should be provided with cochlear implants and when should this be done? If the ABRs remain absent on repeated testing over at least a year and if hearing aids provide no clear benefit in terms of beginning speech, then an implant might be considered. However, such possible criteria need to be evaluated in controlled studies. We have to get some handle on the heterogeneity of the disorder. As we become more familiar with the various etiologies, we may be better able to fit each disorder to an appropriate management protocol. At the present time, we must realize that our lack of knowledge about what to do can lead to anxiety and confusion in the child and the parents. Kindness and caution are absolutely necessary at all times.

CONCLUSIONS

Auditory neuropathy is a disorder of the afferent hearing system composed of the inner hair cells and the afferent fibers of the auditory nerve. However, many different disorders may present in this way, and some of these disorders will overlap with cochlear hearing losses that affect both inner and outer hair cells. Probably, this overlap is more likely when the OAEs are absent and preserved function of the outer hair cells is demonstrated only by the presence of the CM. Much work needs to be done to distinguish the different underlying disorders and to determine the best treatments for each. Until now, we have been more concerned with diagnosis than with treatment. Clinical trials are needed to assess different treatment protocols: How long should hearing aids be tried? When are cochlear implants warranted? What are the best means for language development? We must broaden our focus to find some better concord between our diagnostic achievements and our therapeutic abilities. Shakespeare's Richard II realized too late he should have considered the state of his whole kingdom and not just the affairs of his court.

ABBREVIATIONS

ABR	Auditory brainstem response
ASSR	Auditory steady-state response
CAP	Compound action potential
CM	Cochlear microphonic
DP	Dendritic potential
DPOAE	Distortion product otoacoustic emission
ECochG	Electrocochleography
LAEP	Late auditory evoked potential
MLR	Middle-latency response
MRI	Magnetic resonance imaging
OAE	Otoacoustic emission
SNR	Signal-to-noise ratio
SP	Summating potential
SRT	Speech reception threshold
WRS	Word recognition score

REFERENCES

Ahmmed, A., Brockbank, C., & Adshead, J. (2008). Cochlear microphonics in sensorineural hearing loss: Lesson from newborn hearing screening. *International Journal of Pediatric Otorhinolaryngology, 72*, 1281–1285.

Akdogan, O., Selcuk, A., Ozcan, I., & Dere, H. (2008). Vestibular nerve functions in children with auditory neuropathy. *International Journal of Pediatric Otorhinolaryngology, 72*, 415–419.

Amatuzzi, M. G., Northrop, C., Liberman, M. C., Thornton, A., Halpin, C., Herrmann, B., . . . Eavey, R. D. (2001). Selective inner hair cell loss in premature infants and cochlea pathological patterns from neonatal intensive care unit autopsies. *Archives of Otolaryngology-Head and Neck Surgery, 127*, 629–636.

Attias, J., & Raveh, E. (2007) Transient deafness in young candidates for cochlear implants. *Audiology & Neurootology, 12*, 325–333.

Bahmad, F., Jr., Merchant, S. N., Nadol, J. B., Jr., & Tranebjaerg, L. (2007). Otopathology in Mohr-Tranebjaerg syndrome. *Laryngoscope, 117*, 1202–1208.

Berg, A. L., Spitzer, J. B., Towers, H. M., Bartosiewicz, C., & Diamond, B. E. (2005). Newborn hearing screening in the NICU: Profile of failed auditory brainstem response/passed otoacoustic emission. *Pediatrics, 116*, 933–938. Erratum in (2006) *Pediatrics, 117*, 997.

Berlin, C. I., Bordelon, J., St. John, P., Wilensky, D., Hurley, A., Kluka, E., & Hood, L. J. (1998). Reversing click polarity may uncover auditory neuropathy in infants. *Ear and Hearing, 19*, 37–47.

Berlin, C. I., Hood, L. J., Cecola, R. P., Jackson, D. F., & Szabo, P. (1993). Does type I afferent neuron dysfunction reveal itself through lack of efferent suppression? *Hearing Research, 65*, 40–50.

Berlin, C. I., Hood, L. J., Jeanfreau, J., Morlet, T., Brashears, S., & Keats, B. (2002). The physiological bases of audiological management. In C. I. Berlin, L. J. Hood, & A. Ricci (Eds.), *Hair cell micromechanics and otoacoustic emissions* (pp. 139–154). San Diego, CA: Singular Publishing.

Berlin, C. I., Hood, L. J., Morlet, T., Wilensky, D., Li, L., Mattingly, K. R., Taylor-Jeanfreau, J., . . . Frisch, S. (2010). A. Multi-site diagnosis and management of 260 patients with auditory neuropathy/dys-synchrony (auditory neuropathy spectrum disorder). *International Journal of Audiology, 49*, 30–43.

Berlin, C. I., Hood, L. J., Morlet, T., Wilensky, D., St. John, P., Montgomery, E., & Thibodaux, M. (2005). Absent or elevated middle ear muscle reflexes in the presence of normal otoacoustic emissions: A universal finding in 136 cases of auditory neuropathy/dys-synchrony. *Journal of the American Academy of Audiology, 16,* 546–553.

Berlin, C. I., Morlet, T., & Hood, L. J. (2003). Auditory neuropathy/dyssynchrony: Its diagnosis and management. *Pediatric Clinics of North America, 50,* 331–340.

Boudewyns, A. N., Declau, F., De Ridder, D., Parizel, P. M., van den Ende, J., & Van de Heyning, P. H. (2008). Case report: "Auditory neuropathy" in a newborn caused by a cerebellopontine angle arachnoid cyst. *International Journal of Pediatric Otorhinolaryngology, 72,* 905–909.

Brookes, J. T., Kanis, A. B., Tan, L. Y., Tranebjaerg, L., Vore, A., & Smith, R. J. (2008). Cochlear implantation in deafness-dystonia-optic neuronopathy (DDON) syndrome. *International Journal of Pediatric Otorhinolaryngology, 72,* 121–126.

Buchman, C. A., Roush, P. A., Teagle, H. F., Brown, C. J., Zdanski, C. J., & Grose, J. H. (2006). Auditory neuropathy characteristics in children with cochlear nerve deficiency. *Ear and Hearing, 27,* 399–408.

Buchman, C. A., Roush, P. A., Teagle, H. F. B., & Zdanski, C. J. (2009). Clinical management of children with "auditory neuropathy." In L. S. Eisenberg (Ed.), *Clinical management of children with cochlear implants* (pp. 633–654). San Diego, CA: Plural Publishing.

Buss, E., Labadie, R. F., Brown, C. J., Gross, A. J., Grose, J. H., & Pillsbury, H. C. (2002). Outcome of cochlear implantation in pediatric auditory neuropathy. *Otolaryngology and Neurotology, 23,* 328–332.

Butinar, D., Starr, A., Zidar, J., Koutsou, P., & Christodoulou, K. (2008). Auditory nerve is affected in one of two different point mutations of the neurofilament light gene. *Clinical Neurophysiology, 119,* 367–375.

Butinar, D., Zidar, J., Leonardis, L., Popovic, M., Kalaydjieva, L., Angelicheva, D., . . . Starr, A. (1999). Hereditary auditory, vestibular, motor, and sensory neuropathy in a Slovenian Roma (Gypsy) kindred. *Annals of Neurology, 46,* 36–44.

Cacace, A. T., & Burkard, R. F. (2009). Auditory neuropathy: Bridging the gap between basic science and current clinical problems. In A. T. Cacace & D. J. McFarland (Eds.), *Controversies in central auditory processing disorder* (pp. 305–343). San Diego, CA: Plural Publishing.

Coats, A. C., & Martin, J. L. (1977). Human auditory nerve action potentials and brain stem evoked responses. Effects of audiogram shape and lesion locations. *Archives of Otolaryngology, 103,* 605– 622.

Collet, L., Kemp, D. T., Veuillet, E., Duclaux, R., Moulin, A., & Morgon, A. (1990). Effect of contralateral auditory stimuli on active cochlear micro-mechanical properties in human subjects. *Hearing Research, 43,* 251–261.

Cone, B. (2008). The electrophysiology of auditory neuropathy spectrum disorder. In D. Hayes, Y. Sininger, & J. Northern, N. (Eds.), *Guidelines for identification and management of infants and young children with auditory neuropathy spectrum disorder. (Report of a Conference at NHS2008, Como, Italy)* (pp. 20–27). Aurora, CO: The Children's Hospital-Colorado.

Declau, F., Boudewyns, A., Van den Ende, J., Peeters, A., & van den Heyning, P. (2008). Etiologic and audiologic evaluations after universal neonatal hearing screening: Analysis of 170 referred neonates. *Pediatrics, 121,* 1119–1126.

Delmaghani, S., del Castillo, F. J., Michel, V., Leibovici, M., Aghaie, A., Ron, U., . . . Petit, C. (2006) Mutations in the gene encoding pejvakin, a newly identified protein of the afferent auditory pathway, cause DFNB59 auditory neuropathy. *Nature Genetics, 38,* 770–778.

Deltenre, P., Mansbach, A. L., Bozet, C., Christiaens, F., Barthelemy, P., Paulissen, D., & Renglet, T. (1999). Auditory neuropathy with preserved cochlear microphonics and secondary loss of otoacoustic emissions. *Audiology, 38,* 187–195.

Deltenre, P., Mansbach, A. L., Bozet, C., Clercx, A., & Hecox, K. E. (1997). Auditory neuropathy: A report on three cases with early onsets and major neonatal illnesses. *Electro-encephalography and Clinical Neurophysiology, 104,* 17–22.

Dowley, A. C., Whitehouse, W. P., Mason, S. M., Cope, Y., Grant, J., & Gibbin, K. P. (2009). Auditory neuropathy: Unexpectedly common in a screened newborn population. *Developmental Medicine and Child Neurology, 51,* 642–646.

Draper, T. H., & Bamiou, D. E. (2008). Auditory neuropathy in a patient exposed to xylene: Case report. *Journal of Laryngology and Otology, 28,* 1–4.

Dunkley, C., Farnsworth, A., Mason, S., Dodd, M., & Gibbin, K. (2003). Screening and follow up assessment in three cases of auditory neuropathy. *Archives of Diseases in Children, 88,* 25–26.

Ebermann, I., Walger, M., Schol, H. P., Charbel Issa, P., Lüke, C., Nürnberg, G., . . . Bolz, H. J. (2007). Truncating mutation of the DFNB59 gene causes cochlear hearing impairment and central vestibular dysfunction. *Human Mutation, 28,* 571–577.

Emara, A. A., & Gabr, T. A. (2010). Auditory steady state response in auditory neuropathy. *Journal of Laryngology and Otology, 14,* 1–7.

Felix, H. (2002). Anatomical differences in the peripheral auditory system of mammals and man. A mini review. *Advances in Otorhinolaryngology, 59,* 1–10.

Foerst, A., Beutner, D., Lang-Roth, R., Huttenbrink, K. B., von Wedel, H., & Walger, M. (2006). Prevalence of auditory neuropathy/synaptopathy in a population of children with profound hearing loss. *International Journal of Pediatric Otorhinolaryngology, 70,* 1415–1422.

Fujikawa, S., & Starr, A. (2000). Vestibular neuropathy accompanying auditory and peripheral neuropathies. *Archives of Otolaryngology-Head and Neck Surgery, 126,* 1453–1456.

Gibson, W. P., & Graham, J. M. (2008). 'Auditory neuropathy' and cochlear implantation—myths and facts. *Cochlear Implants International, 9,* 1–7.

Glowatzki, E., Grant, L., & Fuchs, P. (2008). Hair cell afferent synapses. *Current Opinion in Neurobiology, 18,* 389–395.

Golding, M., Pearce, W., Seymour, J., Cooper, A., Ching, T., & Dillon, H. (2007). The relationship between obligatory cortical auditory evoked potentials (CAEPs) and functional measures in young infants. *Journal of the American Academy of Audiology, 18,* 117–125.

Gorga, M. P., Stelmachowicz, P. G., Barlow, S. M., & Brookhouser, P. E. (1995). Case of recurrent, reversible, sudden sensorineural hearing loss in a child. *Journal of the American Academy of Audiology, 6,* 163–172.

Hallpike, C. S., Harriman, D. G., & Wells, C. E. (1980). A case of afferent neuropathy and deafness. *Journal of Laryngology and Otology, 94,* 945–964.

Hayes, D., Sininger, Y., & Northern, J. (2008). *Guidelines for identification and management of infants and young children with auditory neuropathy spectrum disorder. (Report of a Conference at NHS2008, Como, Italy).* Aurora, CO: The Children's Hospital-Colorado.

Hood, L. J., Berlin, C. I., Bordelon, J., & Rose, K. (2003). Patients with auditory neuropathy/dys-synchrony lack efferent suppression of transient evoked otoacoustic emissions. *Journal of the American Academy of Audiology, 14,* 302–313.

Huang, T., Santarelli, R., & Starr, A. (2009). Mutation of OPA1 gene causes deafness by affecting function of auditory nerve terminals. *Brain Research, 1300,* 97–104.

Kaga, K., Nakamura, M., Shinogami, M., Tsuzuku, T., Yamada, K., & Shindo, M. (1996). Auditory nerve disease of both ears revealed by auditory brainstem responses, electrocochleo-graphy and otoacoustic emissions. *Scandinavian Audiology, 25,* 233–238.

Kim, T. B., Isaacson, B., Sivakumaran, T. A., Starr, A., Keats, B. J., & Lesperance, M. M. (2004). A gene responsible for autosomal dominant auditory neuropathy (AUNA1) maps to 13q14-21. *Journal of Medical Genetics, 41,* 872–876.

Konradsson, K. S. (1996). Bilaterally preserved otoacoustic emissions in four children with profound idiopathic unilateral sensorineural hearing loss. *Audiology, 35,* 217–227.

Kraus, N., Ozdamar, O., Stein, L., & Reed, N. (1984). Absent auditory brain stem response:

peripheral hearing loss or brain stem dysfunction? *Laryngoscope, 94,* 400–406.

Kumar, U. A., & Jayaram, M. M. (2006). Prevalence and audiological characteristics in individuals with auditory neuropathy/auditory dys-synchrony. *International Journal of Audiology, 45,* 360–366.

Lu, Y., Zhang, Q., Wen, Y., Ji, F., Chen, A., Xi, X., & Li, X. (2008). The SP-AP compound wave in patients with auditory neuropathy. *Acta Otolaryngologica, 128,* 896–900.

Madden, C., Rutter, M., Hilbert, L., Greinwald, J. H. Jr., & Choo, D. I. (2002). Clinical and audiological features in auditory neuropathy. *Archives of Otolaryngology-Head and Neck Surgery, 128,* 1026–1030.

Mason, S., Garnham, C., & Hudson, B. (1996). Electric response audiometry in young children before cochlear implantation: A short latency component. *Ear and Hearing, 17,* 537–543.

Matsumoto, M., Sekiya, T., Kojima, K., & Ito, J. (2008). An animal experimental model of auditory neuropathy induced in rats by auditory nerve compression. *Experimental Neurology, 210,* 248–256.

McMahon, C. M., Patuzzi, R. B., Gibson, W. P., & Sanli, H. (2008). Frequency-specific electrocochleography indicates that presynaptic and postsynaptic mechanisms of auditory neuropathy exist. *Ear and Hearing, 29,* 314–325.

Michalewski, H. J., Starr, A., Nguyen, T. T., Kong, Y. Y., & Zeng, F. G. (2005). Auditory temporal processes in normal-hearing individuals and in patients with auditory neuropathy. *Clinical Neurophysiology, 116,* 669–680.

Michalewski, H. J., Starr, A., Zeng, F. G., & Dimitrijevic, A. (2009). N100 cortical potentials accompanying disrupted auditory nerve activity in auditory neuropathy (AN): Effects of signal intensity and continuous noise. *Clinical Neurophysiology, 120,* 1352–1363.

Miyamoto, R. T., Kirk, K. I., Renshaw, J., & Hussain, D. (1999). Cochlear implantation in auditory neuropathy. *Laryngoscope, 109,* 181–185.

Mo, L., Yan, F., Liu, H., Han, D., & Zhang, L. (2010). Audiological results in a group of children with auditory neuropathy spectrum disorder. *ORL Journal of Otorhinolaryngology and Related Specialties, 72,* 75–79.

Moore, J. K., & Linthicum, F. H. (2001). Anatomy of the human cochlea and auditory nerve. In Y. Sininger & A. Starr (Eds.), *Auditory neuropathy: A new perspective on hearing disorders* (pp. 83–97). San Diego, CA: Singular Publishing Group.

Nadol, J. B. (2001). Primary cochlear neuronal degeneration. In Y. Sininger & A. Starr (Eds.), *Auditory neuropathy: A new perspective on hearing disorders* (pp. 99–140). San Diego, CA: Singular Publishing Group.

Narne, V. K., & Vanaja, C. (2008a). Speech identification and cortical potentials in individuals with auditory neuropathy. *Behavior and Brain Function, 4,* 15.

Narne, V. K., & Vanaja C. (2008b). Effect of envelope enhancement on speech perception in individuals with auditory neuropathy. *Ear and Hearing, 29,* 45–53.

Narne, V. K., & Vanaja, C. S. (2009). Perception of speech with envelope enhancement in individuals with auditory neuropathy and simulated loss of temporal modulation processing. *International Journal of Audiology, 48,* 700–707.

Ngo, R. Y., Tan, H. K., Balakrishnan, A., Lim, S. B., & Lazaroo, D. T. (2006). Auditory neuropathy/auditory dys-synchrony detected by universal newborn hearing screening. *International Journal of Pediatric Otorhinolaryngology, 70,* 1299–1306.

Nikolopoulos, T. P., Mason, S. M., Gibbin, K. P., & O'Donoghue, G. M. (2000). The prognostic value of promontory electric auditory brain stem response in pediatric cochlear implantation. *Ear and Hearing, 21,* 236–241.

Peterson, A., Shallop, J., Driscoll, C., Breneman, A., Babb, J., Stoeckel, R., & Fabry, L. (2003). Outcomes of cochlear implantation in children with auditory neuropathy. *Journal of the American Academy of Audiology, 14,* 188–201.

Picton, T. W, Durieux-Smith, A., Champagne, S. C., Whittingham, J., Moran, L. M., Giguère, C., & Beauregard, Y. (1998). Objective evaluation of aided thresholds using auditory steady-state responses. *Journal of the American Academy of Audiology, 9,* 315–331.

Psarommatis, I., Riga, M., Douros, K., Koltsidopoulos, P., Douniadakis, D., Kapetanakis, I., & Apostolopoulos, N. (2006). Transient infantile auditory neuropathy and its clinical implications. *International Journal of Pediatric Otorhinolaryngology, 70,* 1629–1637.

Rance, G. (2005). Auditory neuropathy/dyssynchrony and its perceptual consequences. *Trends in Amplification, 9,* 1–43.

Rance, G., & Barker, E. J. (2008). Speech perception in children with auditory neuropathy/dyssynchrony managed with either hearing AIDS or cochlear implants. *Otology and Neurotology, 29,* 179–182.

Rance, G., & Barker, E. J. (2009). Speech and language outcomes in children with auditory neuropathy/dys-synchrony managed with either cochlear implants or hearing aids. *International Journal of Audiology, 48,* 313–320.

Rance, G., Barker, E., Mok, M., Dowell, R., Rincon, A., & Garratt, R. (2007). Speech perception in noise for children with auditory neuropathy/dys-synchrony type hearing loss. *Ear and Hearing, 28,* 351–360.

Rance, G., Beer, D. E., Cone-Wesson, B., Shepherd, R. K., Dowell, R. C., King, A. M., . . . Clark, G. M. (1999) Clinical findings for a group of infants and young children with auditory neuropathy. *Ear and Hearing, 20,* 238–252.

Rance, G., Cone-Wesson, B., Wunderlich, J., & Dowell, R. (2002). Speech perception and cortical event related potentials in children with auditory neuropathy. *Ear and Hearing, 23,* 239–253.

Rance, G., Fava, R., Baldock, H., Chong, A., Barker, E., Corben, L., & Delatycki, M. B. (2008). Speech perception ability in individuals with Friedreich ataxia. *Brain, 131,* 2002–2012.

Rapin, I., & Gravel, J. (2003). "Auditory neuropathy": Physiologic and pathologic evidence calls for more diagnostic specificity. *International Journal of Pediatric Otorhinolaryngology, 67,* 707–728.

Raveh, E., Buller, N., Badrana, O., & Attias, J. (2007). Auditory neuropathy: clinical characteristics and therapeutic approach. *American Journal of Otolaryngology, 28,* 302–308.

Richter, D., Conley, M. E., Rohrer, J., Myers, L. A., Zahradka, K., Keleciç, J., . . . Stavljeniç-Rukavina, A. (2001). A contiguous deletion syndrome of X-linked agammaglobulinemia and sensorineural deafness. *Pediatric Allergy and Immunology, 12,* 107–111.

Roesch, K., Curran, S. P., Tranebjaerg, L., & Koehler, C. M. (2002). Human deafness dystonia syndrome is caused by a defect in assembly of the DDP1/TIMM8A-TIMM13 complex. *Human Molecular Genetics, 11,* 477–486.

Roush, P. (2008). Management of children with auditory neuropathy spectrum disorder: Hearing aids. In D. Hayes, Y. Sininger, & J. Northern (Eds.), *Guidelines for identification and management of infants and young children with auditory neuropathy spectrum disorder. (Report of a Conference at NHS2008, Como, Italy)* (pp. 28–29). Aurora, CO: The Children's Hospital-Colorado.

Runge-Samuelson, C. L., Drake, S., & Wackym, P. A. (2008). Quantitative analysis of electrically evoked auditory brainstem responses in implanted children with auditory neuropathy/dyssynchrony. *Otology and Neurotology, 29,* 174–178.

Tranebjaerg, L. (updated 2009). Deafness-dystonia-optic neuronopathy syndrome (DFN-1, Deafness-dystonia syndrome, Mohr-Tranebjaerg syndrome). In *GeneReviews* at GeneTests: Medical Genetics Information Resource. Available from: http://www.gene tests.org

Santarelli, R., & Arslan, E. (2002). Electrocochleography in auditory neuropathy. *Hearing Research, 170,* 32–47.

Santarelli, R., Del Castillo, I., Rodríguez-Ballesteros, M., Scimemi, P., Cama, E., Arslan, E., & Starr, A. (2009). Abnormal cochlear potentials from deaf patients with mutations in the otoferlin gene. *Journal of the Association for Research in Otolaryngology, 10,* 545–556.

Santarelli, R., Starr, A., Michalewski, H. J., & Arslan, E. (2008). Neural and receptor cochlear potentials obtained by transtympanic electrocochleography in auditory neuropathy. *Clinical Neurophysiology, 119,* 1028–1041.

Sawada, S., Mori, N., Mount, R. J., & Harrison, R. V. (2001). Differential vulnerability of inner and outer hair cell systems to chronic mild hypoxia and glutamate ototoxicity: Insights into the cause of auditory neuropathy. *Journal of Otolaryngology, 30,* 106–114.

Sazgar, A. A., Yazdani, N., Rezazadeh, N., & Yazdi, A. K. (2010). Vestibular evoked myogenic potential (VEMP) in patients with auditory neuropathy: Auditory neuropathy or audiovestibular neuropathy? *Acta Otolaryngologica,* in press.

Seeman, P., Mazanec, R., Huehne, K., Suslíková, P., Keller, O., & Rautenstrauss, B. (2004). Hearing loss as the first feature of late-onset axonal CMT disease due to a novel P0 mutation. *Neurology, 63,* 733–735.

Shallop, J. K. (2008). Management of children with auditory neuropathy spectrum disorder: Cochlear implants. In D. Hayes, Y. Sininger, & J. Northern, N. (Eds.), *Guidelines for identification and management of infants and young children with auditory neuropathy spectrum disorder. (Report of a Conference at NHS2008, Como, Italy)* (pp. 33–34). Aurora, CO: The Children's Hospital—Colorado.

Sheykholeslami, K., Kaga, K., Murofushi, T., & Hughes, W. D. (2000). Vestibular function in auditory neuropathy. *Acta Otolaryngologica, 120,* 849–854.

Sheykholeslami, K., Schmerber, S., Kermany, M. H., & Kaga, K. (2005). Sacculo-collic pathway dysfunction accompanying auditory neuropathy. *Acta Otolaryngologica, 125,* 786–791.

Sininger, Y., & Oba, S. (2001). Patients with auditory neuropathy: Who are they and what can they hear? In Y. Sininger & A. Starr (Eds.), *Auditory neuropathy: A new perspective on hearing disorders* (pp. 15–35). San Diego, CA: Singular Publishing Group.

Smith, R. J. H., Gurrola, J. G., & Kelley, P. M. (2008). OTOF-related deafness. In *Gene-*

Reviews at GeneTests: Medical Genetics Information Resource. Available from: http://www.genetests.org

Spoendlin, H. (1974). Optic cochleovestibular degenerations in hereditary ataxias. II. Temporal bone pathology in two cases of Friedreich's ataxia with vestibulo-cochlear disorders. *Brain, 97,* 41–48.

Starr, A. (2001). The neurology of auditory neuropathy. In Y. Sininger & A. Starr (Eds.), *Auditory neuropathy: A new perspective on hearing disorders* (pp. 37–49). San Diego, CA: Singular Publishing Group.

Starr, A., Isaacson, B., Michalewski, H. J., Zeng, F. G., Kong, Y. Y., Beale, P., . . . Lesperance, M. M. (2004). A dominantly inherited progressive deafness affecting distal auditory nerve and hair cells. *Journal of the Association of Research in Otolaryngology, 5,* 411–426.

Starr, A., McPherson, D., Patterson, J., Don, M., Luxford, W., Shannon, R., . . . Waring, M. (1991). Absence of both auditory evoked potentials and auditory percepts dependent on timing cues. *Brain, 114,* 1157–1180.

Starr, A., Michalewski, H, J., Zeng, F. G., Fujikawa-Brooks, S., Linthicum, F., Kim, C. S., Winnier, D., & Keats, B. (2003). Pathology and physiology of auditory neuropathy with a novel mutation in the MPZ gene (Tyr145->Ser). *Brain, 126,* 1604–1619.

Starr, A., Picton, T. W., & Kim, R. (2001). Pathophysiology of auditory neuropathy. In Y. Sininger & A. Starr (Eds.), *Auditory neuropathy: A new perspective on hearing disorders* (pp. 67–82). San Diego, CA: Singular Publishing.

Starr, A., Picton, T. W., Sininger, Y. S., Hood, L. J., & Berlin, C. I. (1996). Auditory neuropathy. *Brain, 119,* 741–753.

Starr, A., Sininger, Y., Nguyen, T., Michalewski, H. J., Oba, S., & Abdala, C. (2001). Cochlear receptor (microphonic and summating potentials, otoacoustic emissions) and auditory pathway (auditory brain stem potentials) activity in auditory neuropathy. *Ear and Hearing, 22,* 91–99.

Starr, A, Sininger, Y, & Pratt, H. (2000). The varieties of auditory neuropathy. *Journal of*

Basic and Clinical Physiology and Pharmacology, 11, 215–230.

Starr, A., Sininger, Y., Winter, M., Derebery, M. J., Oba, S., & Michalewski, H. J. (1998). Transient deafness due to temperature-sensitive auditory neuropathy. *Ear and Hearing, 19,* 169–179.

Starr, A., Zeng, F. G., Michalewski, H. J., & Moser, T. (2008). Perspectives on auditory neuropathy: Disorders of inner hair cell, auditory nerve, and their synapse. In A. I. Basbaum, A. Kaneko, G. M. Shepherd, & G. Westheimer (Series Eds.), P. Dallos & D. Oertel (Volume Ed.), *The senses: A comprehensive reference. Vol. 3. Audition* (pp. 397–412). San Diego, CA: Academic Press.

Stein, L. K., Tremblay, K., Pasternak, J., Banerjee, S., Lindemann, K., & Kraus, N. (1996). Brainstem abnormalities in neonates with normal otoacoustic emissions. *Seminars in Hearing, 17,* 197–213.

Stockard, J. E., Stockard, J J., Kleinberg, F., & Westmoreland, B. F. (1983). Prognostic value of brainstem auditory evoked potentials in neonates. *Archives of Neurology, 40,* 360–365.

Teagle, H. F., Roush, P. A., Woodard, J. S., Hatch, D. R., Zdanski, C. J., Buss, E., & Buchman, C. A. (2010). Cochlear implantation in children with auditory neuropathy spectrum disorder. *Ear and Hearing, 31,* 325–335.

Tranebjaerg, L. (updated 2009). Deafness-dystonia-optic neuronopathy syndrome (DFN-1, Deafness-dystonia syndrome, Mohr-Tranebjaerg syndrome). In *GeneReviews* at GeneTests: Medical Genetics Information Resource. Available from: http://www .genetests.org

Trautwein, P., Shallop, J., Fabry, L., & Friedman, R. (2001). Cochlear implantation of patients with auditory neuropathy. In Y. Sininger, & A. Starr (Eds.), *Auditory neuropathy: A new perspective on hearing disorders* (pp. 203–231). San Diego, CA: Singular Publishing Group.

Uus, K. (2008). Identification of neonates with auditory neuropathy spectrum disorder. In D. Hayes, Y. Sininger, & J. Northern, N. (Eds.), *Guidelines for identification and management of infants and young children with auditory neuropathy spectrum disorder. (Report of a Conference at NHS2008, Como, Italy)* (pp. 30–32). Aurora, CO: The Children's Hospital-Colorado.

Uus, K., & Bamford, J. (2006). Effectiveness of population-based newborn hearing screening in England: Ages of interventions and profile of cases. *Pediatrics, 117,* e887–e893.

Varga, R., Avenarius, M. R., Kelley, P. M., Keats, B. J., Berlin, C. I., Hood, L. J., . . . Kimberling, W. J. (2006). OTOF mutations revealed by genetic analysis of hearing loss families including a potential temperature sensitive auditory neuropathy allele. *Journal of Medical Genetics, 43,* 576–581.

Walton, J., Gibson, W. P., Sanli, H., & Prelog, K. (2008). Predicting cochlear implant outcomes in children with auditory neuropathy. *Otology and Neurotology, 29,* 302–309.

Wang, Q., Gu, R., Han, D., & Yang, W. (2003). Familial auditory neuropathy. *Laryngoscope, 113,* 1623–1629.

Wang, Q. J., Li, Q. Z., Rao, S. Q., Lee, K., Huang, X. S., Yang, W. Y., . . . Shen, Y. (2006). AUNX1, a novel locus responsible for X linked recessive auditory and peripheral neuropathy, maps to Xq23-27.3. *Journal of Medical Genetics, 43,* e33.

Withnell, R. H. (2001). Brief report: The cochlear microphonic as an indication of outer hair cell function. *Ear and Hearing, 22,* 75–77.

Worthington, D. W., & Peters, J. F. (1980). Quantifiable hearing and no ABR: Paradox or error? *Ear and Hearing, 1,* 281–285.

Xoinis, K., Weirather, Y., Mavoori, H., Shaha, S. H., & Iwamoto, L. M. (2007). Extremely low birth weight infants are at high risk for auditory neuropathy. *Journal of Perinatology, 27,* 718–723.

Yalçinkaya, F., Muluk, N. B., Ataş, A., & Keith, R. W. (2009). Random gap detection test and random gap detection test-expanded results in children with auditory neuropathy. *International Journal of Pediatric Otorhinolaryngology, 73,* 1558–1563.

Yellin, M. W., Jerger, J., & Fifer, R. C. (1989). Norms for disproportionate loss in speech intelligibility. *Ear and Hearing, 10,* 231–234.

Zeng, F. G., Kong, Y. Y., Michalewski, H. J., & Starr, A. (2005). Perceptual consequences of disrupted auditory nerve activity. *Journal of Neurophysiology, 93,* 3050–3063.

Zeng, F. G., & Liu, S. (2006). Speech perception in individuals with auditory neuropathy. *Journal of Speech Language and Hearing Research, 49,* 367–380.

Zeng, F. G., Oba, S., Garde, S., Sininger, Y., & Starr, A. (2001). Psychoacoustics and speech perception in auditory neuropathy. In Y. Sininger & A. Starr (Eds.), *Auditory neuropathy: A new perspective on hearing disorders* (pp. 141–164). San Diego, CA: Singular Publishing Group.

16

Cochlear Implants:
Body Electric

I sing the body electric,
The armies of those I love engirth me and I engirth them,
They will not let me off till I go with them, respond to them,
And discorrupt them, and charge them full with the charge of the soul.

Walt Whitman, *Leaves of Grass*, 1881

The development of the cochlear implant for patients with severe or profound hearing impairment has been one of the greatest biomedical advances of all time. Many initial studies had shown that electrical stimulation could provide auditory sensation. However, with the development of multiple-contact electrodes (Clark et al., 1977; Simmons, 1966), it became possible to perceive speech through the implant without benefit of either lip-reading or semantic context (Clark, Tong, & Martin, 1981).

In general, the implant is a cost-effective treatment for severe to profound hearing loss (Bond et al., 2009). The improvement in communication, the lower expenses for mainstreamed children, and the higher quality of life outweigh the expenses of the implant, surgery, and training. The most marked benefits occur in adults whose deafness began after the development of language and in young children implanted at an age when the brain is developing its ability to process speech and language (Eisenberg, 2009; Papsin & Gordon, 2007).

Cochlear implants can help the infant with severe to profound hearing loss develop hearing and language at levels that would be impossible with amplification alone. Multichannel implants were first used in preschool children in 1990 (Staller, 1991), and have since been shown to be both effective in terms of facilitating communication (Geers, Tobey, Moog, & Brenner, 2008; Stacey, Fortnum, Barton, & Summerfield, 2006) and cost-effective in terms of the savings to the educational system (Barton, Stacey, Fortnum, & Summerfield, 2006; Cheng et al., 2000).

Auditory evoked potentials (EPs) provide helpful information in evaluating hearing, setting the limits for stimulation, and monitoring how well the implant is working. In assessment of a candidate for an implant, auditory EPs can provide objective thresholds to improve or confirm behavioral results. Such objective audiometry is particularly important for infants who may not be able to cooperate with behavioral testing. In Chapter 13, we considered how infants can be evaluated, with auditory EPs providing physiologic thresholds for use in fitting hearing aids. The absence of EPs other than at very high intensities of stimulation can contribute to the final decision to proceed with an implant. The absence of an auditory brainstem response (ABR) combined with evidence of hair-cell function as shown in recordings of the cochlear microphonic (CM) or otoacoustic emissions (OAEs) are essential parts of the diagnosis of auditory neuropathy. We considered this syndrome and how, in certain situations, it might be treated with cochlear implants in Chapter 15.

Programming an implant to provide auditory information optimally to the patient requires measuring threshold levels (T-levels) and either maximum comfort levels (C-levels) or most comfortable listening levels (M-levels) for electrical stimulation at each of the different electrode contacts. These levels then are used to set the minimum and maximum current levels for representing the intensity of incoming acoustic signals. Different implant systems base their stimulus programming on different behavioral measurements, particularly whether we measure the maximum tolerated stimulus levels or the most comfortable listening level. In infants, difficulty in obtaining consistent behavioral responses to electrical stimuli leads to uncertainty implant programming. Some

of this uncertainty can be reduced by recording the electrical EPs, which may be used to derive estimates for T- and C-levels. These physiologic measurements are helpful estimates that must be adjusted to the child's behavior. Most importantly, EPs can be used to predict levels at which the stimuli will be audible, levels at which we can start to obtain more precise behavioral measurements.

Finally, auditory EPs may provide a means to monitor how well the implant is working. They can indicate that auditory information is being processed in the brain and that stimuli are being discriminated.

In this chapter, we briefly introduce the principles whereby a cochlear implant converts sound patterns to electrical stimuli. Then we consider the responses that can be evoked by these electrical stimuli, or by acoustic stimuli processed through the implant.

COCHLEAR IMPLANTS

The components of the cochlear implant can be demonstrated by tracing the path of sound through the implant to the auditory nerve. The external processor receives the sound and codes it into electrical signals that are transmitted to the internal unit through radio frequency (RF) pulses. The internal unit converts these signals into stimuli that are then sent to particular contacts on the electrode array in the cochlea. These stimuli activate the auditory nerve fibers near the particular electrode contact to which the stimuli are directed. Figure 16–1 provides an anatomic view of the different components of the implant, and Figure 16–2 links them together diagrammatically. The technical aspects of converting acoustic energy to electrical stimuli have been covered in

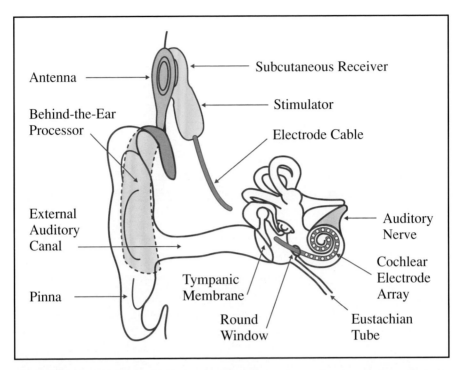

Figure 16–1. *Diagrammatic representation of a typical cochlear implant. The behind-the-ear external processor is attached to the pinna with an ear hook. This processor contains a microphone to pick up sound, electronic circuits to convert the incoming sound to digital electrical signals, and a battery to provide power. The stimulus information is then transmitted as radio-frequency signals through an antenna. An internal receiver is located beneath the skin behind the ear and the antenna is held in place above it by a magnet in the receiver. The stimulator decodes the signals from the receiver, converts the signals into electric currents, and sends them along the wires in the cable to a multicontact electrode that has been threaded through the temporal bone into the middle ear and then through the round window into the cochlea.*

more detail in several reviews (Clark, 2003; Wilson & Dorman, 2008; Zeng, Reb-scher, Harrison, Sun, & Feng, 2008).

External Components

The external components of the implant are a processor that usually hooks onto the pinna and rests behind the ear and an antenna positioned over the internal receiver a little behind and above the ear.

The processor unit contains batteries that provide the power for all of the implant's processes. Sound is picked by a microphone in the processor. Generally, this is set up to give preference to the sounds coming from in front of the subject over those coming from the side or rear. With bilateral implants, more sophisticated directional microphones can be used. Incoming sounds are then amplified using parameters optimized for human speech: typically, a band-pass of 100 to 8000 Hz and a dynamic

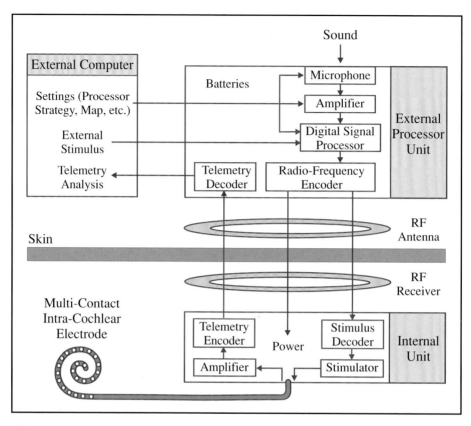

Figure 16–2. Block diagram of cochlear implant system. *The upper part of the figure shows the two external components of the system. The External Computer can be connected to the External Processor Unit to evaluate the thresholds for perceiving the electrical stimuli and thus constructing a map of the different stimulus levels appropriate to each electrode contract. After all the settings have been loaded into the processor the computer is disconnected and the external processor functions independently. The External Computer also may be connected to the External Processor Unit to record electrical compound action potentials (ECAPs) from the implanted electrode contacts. This requires having the digital signal processor initiate stimuli under the control of the computer rather than the sounds coming through the microphone. In normal use, sounds are picked up by the microphone, amplified, and then converted into instructions for electrical stimuli by the digital signal processor. These instructions for the stimulator are encoded and sent to the Internal Unit by radio-frequency (RF) transmission between an Antenna on the scalp and a subcutaneous Receiver. The various components of the External Processor Unit are powered by its batteries. The Internal Unit contains a stimulator to activate the auditory nerve fibers through the intracochlear electrode under the instructions received from the External Processor. The Internal Unit also contains amplifiers to record their ECAP responses. It derives the power to operate these processes from the radio-frequency field.*

range of 60 dB or more. The amplifier can be set up with automatic gain control, to keep the incoming signal within the range of the processor, and can have an adjustable dynamic range that can be optimized for different sound environments. Digital noise reduction algorithms can be used to attenuate continuous background noise and thus facilitate the perception of speech.

The amplified sounds then are analyzed by a digital signal processor. The processor filters the signal using a set of bandpass filters that act something like the tuning curves of auditory neurons (although with nowhere near their precision). This filter bank essentially provides a continuous representation of the spectrum of the auditory signal, a spectrum that has sufficient resolution in the frequency domain to distinguish formants and that varies in time with sufficient resolution to represent important phonemic transitions. However, the spectrum is limited in terms of providing fine frequency selectivity or precise temporal resolution.

The transduction process requires converting the frequency of the sounds to electrical stimuli presented through the array of electrode contacts. Frequency is coded by location. Each electrode contact is linked to a particular frequency of input sound on the basis of its location in the cochlea. High frequencies go to the contacts near the round window and low frequencies to the apical contacts. However, for several reasons, the effective resolution of electrical stimulation along the basilar membrane is less than the number of electrode contacts, which may be more than 20. First, the currents have to return through other electrodes—through a ground electrode with monopolar stimulation and through an adjacent electrode or electrodes with bipolar stimulation. Second, the currents at one electrode-contact diffuse through the fluids in the scala tympani and activate neurons over a range of several electrode contacts. Thus, the typical array of contacts can support somewhere between four and eight independent "channels" of information. The incoming acoustic information therefore is divided into between four and eight channels, which are then distributed over the 20+ available electrodes by grouping them together in sets of two to four adjacent electrodes. Some new electrode designs—spiral spring-electrodes that hold themselves more tightly to the modiolus—may improve the spatial resolution and provide a more precise representation of frequencies along the basilar membrane (Gordin, Papsin, James, & Gordon, 2009).

Stimulus intensity within each filter band is converted to an absolute value by means of rectification and low-pass filtering. As this value changes from moment to moment, an envelope is constructed for each particular frequency band. The temporal resolution of this envelope will depend on how rapidly the processor can clock through the different channels of the sound; this can be anywhere between several hundred to several thousand times a second. The intensity values are scaled exponentially to fit into the range available for each electrode. The envelope then modulates the amplitude of the pulses generated in the stimulator. The intensity of the auditory stimulus at a particular frequency thus is coded by the amplitude of the current pulses passed through an electrode contact.

After connecting the processor to an external computer to control the stimulator, the audiologist can measure a threshold level and a maximum comfort level for the current pulses at each electrode. These measurements form a "map" that is then loaded into the processor so that all the electrical stimuli fit within its limits. Any electrode that is not working can be switched off. Furthermore, if stimulation at an electrode causes twitching in the facial muscles or spurious sensations such as dizziness, that electrode can be inactivated. The connection from the external computer to the processor also allows the audiologist to change between different stored stimulus maps and to set various parameters of the amplifier and the microphone.

Exactly how the spectrum of the incoming sound is sent out over the array of electrode contacts in the cochlea is determined by the processor's programming "strategy" (Loizou, 1998; Wilson & Dorman, 2008; Zeng et al., 2008). The main processes used to convert the incoming sound waveform to a set of pulses in an array of electrodes are diagrammed in Figure 16–3. Basically, peaks in the spectrum with the highest amplitudes are

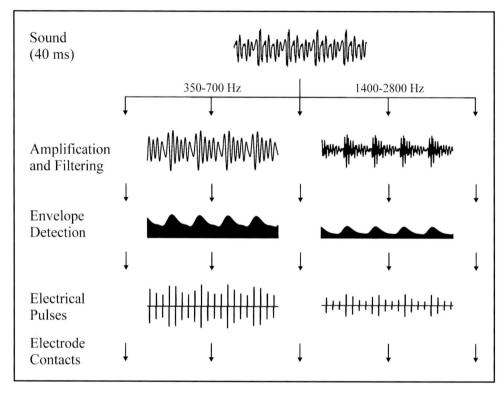

Figure 16–3. Signal processing. *This figure illustrates the conversion of sound into current pulses which are then sent to the different electrode contacts of the implant. The sound is taken from the vowel "a" spoken by a male speaker. The sound is amplified and then filtered using a set of band-pass filters. Only two of the filtered signals are shown—we can imagine multiple such signals each representing the incoming sound in a particular frequency band. The envelope of the filtered activity is then determined, for example, by full-wave rectification and low-pass filtering. The envelope then controls the amplitude of the biphasic current pulses that are presented to the appropriate electrode contacts. The higher frequency channels are directed to the more basal electrodes. The current pulses are scaled by using a power relationship and fit within the limits of each electrode contact (as determined by the T-levels and C-levels of the implant "map"). The pulses going to each contact are interleaved so that only one contact is activated at one time; in this particular illustration, the high-frequency channel follows the low-frequency channel. The filtering and timing characteristics in this illustration are arbitrary and do not represent those of any particular implant.*

selected and sent out as electrical stimuli to the appropriate electrode-contacts. One approach is to filter the acoustic signal into a number of bands equal to the number of channels; another approach ("n of m") is to filter the acoustic signal into a larger number (m) of bands, and then select only some of these (n) on the basis of spectral amplitude peaks. To convert the bandpassed signal to electric stimuli, the ongoing envelope of each bandpassed signal is used to modulate a biphasic pulse generator that has a set frequency of several hundred to several thousand pulses per second per electrode. The sound envelope within a particular bandpass thus determines the amplitude of the pulses going to a particular location on the basilar membrane. In general, pulses are presented only to one electrode-contact at a time to prevent distortion of the currents; simultaneous pulses on two electrode contacts would cause current to flow in the region between them. The system then cycles through the different electrodes one at a time using a procedure known as "continuous interleaved sampling." The electrodes may be activated in sequential (1,2,3 . . .) or staggered (1,4,2,5) order. Some implant systems can use simultaneous stimulation at different electrodes to steer the current to locations between the electrodes and thus give more precise stimulus localization.

The most important information sent to the internal receiver at each moment in time is which electrode to be stimulated and the amplitude and duration of the current pulse to be presented by that electrode. This information can be coded using a small number of bits, which are transmitted through an antenna using RF pulses. The RF unit also must allow transmission of power to the internal stimulator, and receive back-transmission if the system is set up to record from the electrode contacts ("telemetry") in addition to presenting stimuli through them.

Internal Components

The receiver is located under the scalp behind the ear. As well as the receiving coil, this unit contains a small magnet that holds the external antenna in place. RF signals are decoded by the stimulator and converted to electrical pulses, which are then sent to the appropriate contacts on the electrode array, which has been threaded into the scala tympani of the cochlea. Typically, the pulses are biphasic (negative-positive). This prevents polarization (and slow deterioration) of the electrode contact. The amount of current passing through the electrode contact varies with the device but is of the order of 0-1 mA. The current level typically is resolved with a precision of 8 bits and reported in terms of arbitrary current units (1–255), although different manufactures use different scales. These current units usually are related to current level using a power function (Gordin et al., 2009; Shallop, Carter, Feinman, & Tabor, 2003). The stimulus pulses are presented through the electrode contacts using either a monopolar or bipolar configuration. In a monopolar configuration, the current return is through a reference electrode near the internal unit, whereas in a bipolar configuration, the current returns through a selected nearby electrode.

The location of the electrode relative to the organ of Corti is shown diagrammatically in Figure 15–7. When optimally positioned, the electrode contacts are close to the spiral ganglion. Therefore, the electric currents directly stimulate the nerve at the level of the cell body or even the proximal portion of the bipolar nerve cell (the axon going from the cell body to the cochlear brainstem). This means that the stimulus bypasses the hair cell, the synapse between the hair cell and the afferent fiber, and the peripheral process of the afferent fiber. Bypassing the hair cell is important when we are treating common cochlear hearing losses. However, bypassing the synapse or the peripheral process of the afferent fiber is important when we are treating auditory neuropathy. New electrode designs have been developed to make the electrode array coil more tightly around the modiolus, thereby bringing the electrode closer to the spiral ganglion cells and reducing the level of stimulation needed to activate the nerve cells (Gordin et al., 2009).

ELECTRICAL ABR

We begin our discussion of the responses that can be evoked by electrical stimulation of the cochlea with the "electrical auditory brain response" or EABR. This was the first electrical response to be recorded in human subjects (Starr & Brackmann, 1979) and it is still widely studied. Furthermore, it illustrates both the basic principles of these responses and the technical difficulties involved in recording them. Figure 16–4 presents and compares EABRs that have been reported by various investigators.

Recording EABRs

The response is recorded following stimulation of one or several contacts on the implanted electrode array using software in the computer that connects to the external processor. We do not present an acoustic click to the processor, as that would cause all sorts of transduction problems. The software allows us to choose the electrode contact (or contacts), stimulus intensity (measured in current units), polarity, and duration. We usually select a duration between 50 and 200 μs (measured as the width of the initial phase) and a biphasic stimulus. The initial stimulus polarity of this biphasic pulse can be alternated to cancel the artifact but this might cause problems because of the different latencies of the response to the different polarities. Because the artifact is brief, using a consistent (negative going to positive) pulse usually provides acceptable recordings. The stimulus is presented to one electrode using a monopolar electrode configuration. The recording generally is taken between the vertex and the mastoid contralateral to the implanted ear. This montage attenuates any response coming from the auditory nerve, but this is of little consequence since the first millisecond of the recording is overwhelmed by stimulus artifact. The other recording parameters are the same as for the acoustic ABR. We probably should choose a low setting for the high-pass filter—10 or 20 Hz rather than 100 Hz. This will allow us to see small delayed responses and will decrease the temporal spread of the artifact. Mason (2003) provides a clear summary of EABR procedures.

The first thing that we note about the response in the upper left of Figure 16–4 is the huge size of the stimulus artifact. Because the stimulus directly injects electrical current into the cochlea, the recorded artifact is much larger than that caused by electromagnetic induction in the recording circuits from an earphone. Generally, the artifact overwhelms the first 1 to 2 ms of the recording and often tails off through the rest of the ABR. Several procedures are needed to allow the recording to proceed

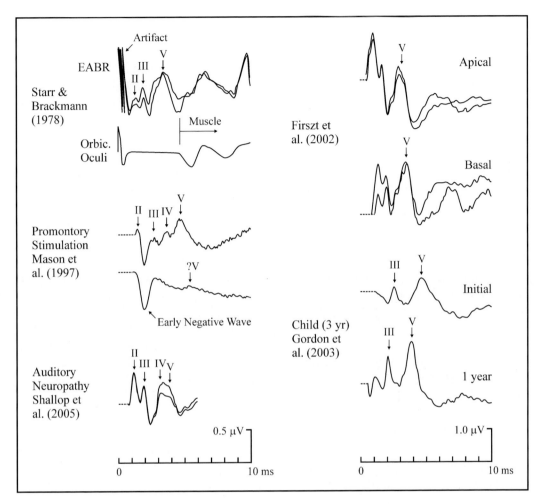

Figure 16–4. *Auditory brainstem responses to electrical stimulation. This figure compares the EABR waveforms from different studies. The tracings in the upper left show the large stimulus artifact at the beginning. In the other EABR waveforms, this artifact has been attenuated. The late potentials in the EABR derive from the facial muscles activated by spread of the stimulus to the facial nerve. The recordings from the oribicularis oculi in the upper left (Starr & Brackmann, 1978) were performed at a much lower sensitivity than the EABR. The Mason et al. (1997) responses to promontory stimulation are from two different subjects. The first shows a normal waveform. The second shows an early negative wave and only a questionable wave V. The recordings in the lower left represent the EABR from a patient with auditory neuropathy (Shallop et al, 2005). Before the implant, there were no recognizable ABR to an acoustic click. The recordings in the upper right compare EABRs to apical and basal stimulation (Firszt et al., 2002). The apical response has earlier latencies. The EABR to apical stimulation typically has larger amplitudes though this is not as evident (for wave V) in this particular subject. The tracings in the lower right (Gordon et al., 2003) show the EABRs of a young child (3 years old at time of implant). The waves are much larger and earlier 1 year after the implant than at the time of initial implant activation.*

with such a large artifact and to decrease its effect. First, any artifact rejection protocol must skip first 2 ms of the recording or every trial would be considered artifact-contaminated leaving no trials to be averaged. Second, we need to prevent the amplifier from blocking and therefore not working properly for some period after the artifact. Some systems have used a blanking procedure that disconnects the amplifier from the input signal for the first millisecond. Without this capability, it may be necessary to decrease the amplification factor in order to prevent blocking. Third, we can consider using stimuli of alternating polarity. This will not completely remove the artifact and it may distort the response but the advantages of alternating stimuli often outweigh the problems. Fourth, using a low high-pass filter setting on the amplifier can limit the temporal extent of the artifact so that it does not spread too far into the recorded response.

Although it can interfere with the recording of the EABR, the stimulus artifact can provide important information about the integrity of the implant (Shallop et al., 2003). Recording the voltage generated at the scalp by stimulating each electrode, we can see whether the stimuli are being delivered properly to the cochlea. This "device integrity check" can be performed quickly by presenting low-intensity electrical pulses at a rapid rate (several hundred stimuli per second). Recordings from the vertex to ipsilateral mastoid are averaged over several hundred trials. The average stimulus voltage recorded at the scalp for stimuli at an intensity just above T-level is lower for the more apical electrodes, varying from 200 µV at the base to 5 µV at the apex. This is between 10 and several hundred times larger than the amplitude of the EABR.

Another large part of the recorded waveform may be generated by various muscles activated by the stimulus current spreading to the facial nerve (Cushing, Papsin, & Gordon, 2006; Kelsall, Shallop, Brammeier, & Prenger, 1997). The facial nerve travels alongside the vestibular and cochlear nerves in the internal auditory meatus, passes close to the cochlea, enters the facial canal behind the middle ear, and then exits from the skull behind and below the earlobe. Activation of the facially innervated muscles is associated with muscle twitches in the face that are perceptible to the patient and sometimes visible to the examiner. The electrical activity from these muscles typically begins around 3 to 5 ms after the stimulus and therefore can obscure the later part of the EABR recording. With high-intensity stimulation, the responses can begin around 2 ms (Cushing, Papsin Strantzas, & Gordon, 2009). If the recording is performed under anesthesia (during the implantation, for example), the muscle responses can be prevented with muscle relaxants. Muscle responses generally are not present at lower stimulus intensities and occur only with stimulation of some electrode-contacts. As the electrode coils around the cochlea, the distances between the contacts and the facial nerve will vary. In adults, otosclerosis is a risk factor for facial nerve stimulation (Kelsall et al., 1997), probably because of changes to the flow of current in the ear. The threshold for facial nerve stimulation will set an upper limit to the useful stimulation levels at each electrode. Some electrodes may need to be turned off or the electrode pairs altered to allow optimal stimulation of the cochlea without facial-nerve side effects. Monitoring the electromyogram (EMG) from the muscles of the face may help ensure that cochlear stimulus levels are not activating the facial nerve at levels below observable twitching. This would be very helpful in children who may not be able to report the facial sensations (Cushing et al., 2006).

Normal EABR

In between the stimulus artifact (always present) and the muscle response (sometimes present), an EABR generally can be recognized. The EABR consists of three main waves named after homologous waves II, III, and V in the ABR to an acoustic stimulus. We often use a lowercase "e" to indicate the electrical stimulus—eII, eIII, and eV. Different EABR waveforms are illustrated in Figure 16–4. The acoustic and electrical responses are compared in the left section of Figure 16–5. The EABR waves occur about 1.5 ms earlier than those evoked acoustically by moderate to high intensity stimuli. Some reported latencies are given in Table 16–1. Just as in the acoustic response, a wave eIV sometimes can be distinguished from

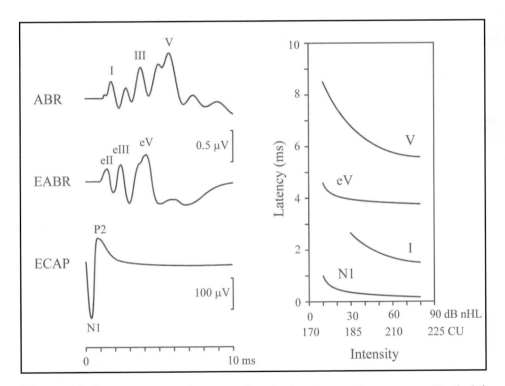

Figure 16–5. ***Comparisons between electrical and acoustic responses.*** *On the left are typical waveforms for the acoustic ABR to a click presented at 70 dB nHL (normal hearing level) and the EABR and ECAP (to a stimulus near C-level). The EABR is similar to the acoustic ABR shifted about 1.5 ms earlier. On the right are typical latency-intensity functions. Wave V and wave I of the acoustic ABR show a large increase in latency with decreasing intensity. The homologous waves eV of the EABR and N1 of the ECAP change very little with intensity until very close to threshold. The intensities of the electrical stimulus in current units (CU) are representative levels for a typical subject using an 8-bit scale.*

Table 16–1. Electrical Auditory Brainstem Response: Peak Measurements

Study	eII		eIII		eV	
	Lat	*Amp*	*Lat*	*Amp*	*Lat*	*Amp*
Abbas & Brown (1988)	1.4±0.2		2.0±0.2		4.0±0.2	
Shallop et al. (1990)					3.9±0.2	
Firszt et al. (2002)[a]						
apical	1.3±0.1	0.6±0.5	2.1±0.1	0.9±0.5	3.7±0.2	1.2±0.6
basal	1.3±0.1	0.5±0.1	2.1±0.3	0.4±0.3	3.9±0.2	0.8±0.4
Gordon et al. (2006)						
children[b]	1.4±0.2		2.3±0.2		4.0±0.2	
Gordon et al. (2007)[c]						
apical	1.5±0.3		2.3±0.2	0.7±0.3	4.2±0.3	1.2±0.6
basal	1.5±0.3		2.4±0.2	0.4±0.2	4.4±0.3	0.8±0.4
Normal ABR[d]	2.8±0.2	0.2±0.1	3.8±0.2	0.3±0.2	5.6±0.2	0.6±0.3

Means and standard deviations. Latencies in millisecond and amplitudes in microvolts.
[a]Measurements for stimulation at 75% of behavioral dynamic range.
[b]The asymptote after developmental changes.
[c]Children, measurements taken at initial device activation.
[d]See Table 8–1 (70 dB nHL alternating click).

wave eV at high stimulus levels. Waves eII to eIV are no longer recognizable and the waveform only shows wave eV at lower levels. Electrical stimulation through the cochlear implant activates the nerve fibers at the level of the spiral ganglion cells. Thus, the latency of the response does not include the delay required to convey sound acoustically from the transducer to the oval window, the delay involved in the traveling wave and hair-cell filtering (cochlear delay), the delay necessary for synaptic transmission across the synapse between hair cell and afferent fiber, and whatever delay is needed to depolarize the afferent fiber sufficiently to initiate an action potential.

Other than the absolute latency, the main difference between the acoustic and the electric response is the relative stability of the EABR latencies with changes in stimulus intensity or rate. The change of eV latency from near threshold to maximum intensity is about 0.5 ms compared to the changes of 3 to 5 ms for the ABR to an acoustic stimulus (Shallop, Beiter, Goin, & Mischke, 1990). Most of the EABR latency change occurs near threshold; once the stimulus is several current units above threshold, the latencies change little. These differences are illustrated in the right section of Figure 16–5. This means that these parameters affect the acoustic response by means of physiologic processes that occur before neuronal activation at the level of the spiral ganglion. We discussed these processes in Chapter 8. The increase in latency with decreasing intensity of an acoustic click likely is related in part to a shift of the dominant activation pattern on the basilar membrane from the 4-kHz region to the 1-kHz region and in part to some change in the AP discharge patterns as the intensity is decreased. The increase in latency with increasing rate of an acoustic click probably is related to greater adaptation of the regions of the basilar membrane processing the higher frequencies.

The waves of the EABR following stimulation of an apical electrode generally are larger and earlier than those evoked by stimulation of a basal electrode (Firszt, Chambers, Kraus, & Reeder , 2002; Gordon, Papsin, & Harrison, 2007; Shallop et al., 1990). This is illustrated in the upper right of Figure 16–4. As shown in Table 16–1, the latency changes are less than 0.1 ms for eII and eIII and are about 0.2 ms for eV (Firszt et al., 2002). In addition, the threshold for the apical response generally is lower in terms of stimulus current than that for the basal response. Exactly why the apical responses tend to be earlier and larger is not known. Patients with GJB2-related deafness (involving connexin abnormalities) show no significant differences between apical and basal stimulation (Propst, Papsin, Stockley, Harrison, & Gordon, 2006). This connexin disorder affects gap junctions equally along the length of the cochlea and leaves the spiral ganglion cells well preserved. Other causes of hearing loss that lead to implantation may affect the basal regions of the cochlea more than the apical and lead to fewer basal spiral ganglion cells. Stimulation would generate smaller and later EABRs from basal region and larger and earlier EABRs through the better preserved apical ganglion cells.

Patients with auditory neuropathy who are implanted may show a normal EABR after there has been no preoperative response to acoustic stimulation (Shallop, Jin, Driscoll, & Tribesar, 2004). These waveforms are shown in the lower left of Figure 16–4. Further study is needed to see whether the EABR after implantation reflects the various diagnostic categories that may cause auditory neuropathy.

Although the latency of the EABR changes little, the amplitude of the response increases rapidly with increasing stimulus intensity (Abbas & Brown, 1988). The threshold for evoking a recognizable response — typically between 0.1 and 0.2 mA although this will vary with the implant (Abbas & Brown, 1991; Gordin et al., 2009) — is higher than the behavioral threshold for perceiving the stimulus. The slope of the amplitude-intensity function is greater for apical electrodes than for basal electrodes. The eV response reaches maximum amplitudes near 1 µV (ranging from 0.5 to 3 µV) at stimulus intensities near the C-level. There often is a leveling off at these amplitudes, although this does not occur in all subjects and cannot easily be used as a means to set the C-level because of patient discomfort (Abbas & Brown, 1988; Allum, Shallop, Hotz, & Pfalz, 1990). It is difficult to compare the intensity of the electrical stimulus to that of an acoustic stimulus. However, the electric response is mediated through only one electrode and the acoustic click response mediated through the whole basilar membrane. A better comparison might be the tone-ABR, and then the EABR is much larger than the acoustic response. This difference is related mainly to the synchronization of the discharges in the afferent neurons when electrical stimulation is used.

The EABR is reasonably stable in its latency and amplitude when stimuli are presented rapidly. When stimuli are presented in brief trains at rates of 500 Hz, the

EABR is distorted by the superimposed stimulus artifacts (occurring every 2 ms) during the train but can be recognized following the last stimulus. The EABR is unaffected by the duration of the train—from 1 to 50 stimuli (Davids, Valero, Papsin, Harrison, & Gordon, 2008a).

When originally recorded, the EABRs were evaluated as a means for estimating the T- and C-levels for programming the processor. EABR thresholds typically are somewhere between these two levels. Behavioral thresholds usually are assessed using a brief burst of stimuli whereas the EABRs are evoked by single stimuli. However, the ability of the patient to benefit from temporal integration varies and recording behavioral thresholds using single stimuli does not improve the relationship between physiologic and behavioral thresholds (Davids, Valero, Papsin, Harrison, & Gordon, 2008b). Therefore, the EABR thresholds can only give a rough approximation of where the stimulus limits might be set (Brown et al., 2000). In this context, EABRs have been superseded by the recordings of the electrical compound action potential (ECAP), which can be obtained more rapidly.

Amplitude, latency, and threshold measurements of the EABR do not correlate highly with measurements of speech perception in implanted subjects (Abbas & Brown, 1991; Firszt, Chambers, & Kraus, 2002). Threshold measurements correlate with measurements of the behavioral threshold but, as we have discussed, the variability is such that they cannot be used to set stimulus limits without other information. Speech perception involves cortical processes and perhaps we will find higher correlations when we examine the later components of the electrical EP.

Changes in the EABR with Implant Use

The EABR in young children changes significantly as the implant is used. The latencies of the waves decrease and the amplitude increases (Gordon, Papsin, & Harrison, 2003, 2006; Gordon, Valero, Jewell, Ahn, & Papsin, 2010). Most of the changes occur within the first 2 months after implantation. The use-dependant changes are greater for wave eV than for the earlier waves, the eIII-eV latency difference decreasing significantly by about 0.25 ms. These results are similar to the changes in the acoustic ABR with normal development but occur after the implant rather than after birth, and therefore reflect the effects of "time in sound." The changes in the EABR with device use may be used to indicate that the auditory brainstem pathways are affected by the stimuli presented through the implant. The changes may be due to both increased myelination and synaptic changes.

Pre- and Intraoperative EABR Recordings

In the early days of cochlear implants, preoperative recordings to electrical stimulation through a transtympanic electrode —promontory or round window EABRs —were evaluated as a possible means to determine whether a cochlear implant would be beneficial (Mason, O'Donoghue, Gibbin, Garnham, & Jowett, 1997). The EABR evoked by this means is similar to that evoked by stimulation of the electrode contacts in an implant except that the latencies tend to be few tenths of a millisecond later (see middle tracings in the left section of Figure 16–4).

An EABR recorded in this manner clearly can indicate that the auditory nerve and brainstem are responsive to electrical stimulation. However, the absence of a response is difficult to interpret. Patients can gain useful auditory information from the implant even when stimulation of the cochlear implant in situ elicits no clear EABR. Nikolopoulos, Mason, Gibbin, and O'Donoghue (2000) reviewed their experience with preoperative promontory stimulation and found no significant difference in hearing performance in children with or without a recognizable EABR on preoperative testing. Nevertheless, the fact that a recognizable EABR does indicate responsive auditory nerve fibers can be helpful as part of the assessment battery for children with congenital malformations of the ear, suspected cochlear nerve aplasia, or narrow internal auditory canal (Kim et al., 2008). The effectiveness of EABR recording with transtympanic stimulation will vary with the location of the electrode. A round window electrode placed after myringotomy may be better than the usual promontory electrode (Pau, Gibson, & Sabli, 2006), though the EABR recorded with this electrode requires further evaluation in terms of its prognostic implications.

During the surgical placement of the implant, EABRs and the electrically evoked compound action potential (ECAPs) are recorded to test the system. Once the electrode is positioned and connected, simple tests of the integrity of the electrode contacts are performed. Then, EABR and ECAP thresholds are estimated. These recordings can be performed rapidly, because background EEG/EMG noise is much reduced under anesthesia. The absence of any recognizable ECAP or EABR, which can occur in about 10% of cases, does not indicate that the implant will not provide any benefit. Subjects can perceive the stimuli even when there is no clear physiologic response. Furthermore, response thresholds typically decrease between the operation and the activation of the implant several weeks later.

Early Vestibular Response

In some patients, a negative wave with a peak-latency near 2 ms can be recorded in the EABR. This can occur with stimulation of the implanted electrode, but tends to be more frequent and prominent with transtympanic stimulation, particularly when the stimulus intensity is high (Mason, 2003; Mason et al, 1997). The middle left waveforms in Figure 16–4 illustrate this wave. This is probably homologous to the negative wave with a peak latency near 3 to 4 ms that is recorded following intense acoustic stimulation. As we discussed in Chapter 14, this wave probably is generated in the vestibular system, although exactly where—vestibular nerve or nucleus—is unknown.

ELECTRICAL COMPOUND ACTION POTENTIAL (ECAP)

In the EABR, the response of the auditory nerve fibers in the cochlea—wave I of the acoustic ABR—is impossible to recognize because of the stimulus artifact. Two developments made it possible to record the ECAP from human cochlear implant users (Brown, Abbas, & Gantz, 1990). The first was recording from the electrode contacts on the implanted array in the cochlea rather than from electrodes on the scalp. The stimulus was applied to one electrode contact (or between two contacts) and the response was recorded from another. Recording from the cochlea rather than the scalp made the response much larger; the response typically reaches 100 to 500 μV at higher levels of stimulation. This is about a thousand times larger than the response recorded from the scalp. Furthermore, the background noise in the cochlear recording was much lower than on the scalp. The second development was a masking technique to remove the artifact. First, the response (and the artifact) was recorded normally. Then, in a second recording, a pair of stimuli was presented. The response to the second stimulus is reduced (optimally to zero) by the masking stimulus occurring about 0.7 ms earlier. This recording (which contains the artifact and no response) is then subtracted from the response to the stimulus alone (which contains the artifact and the response) to give the response without any artifact. Various techniques to remove the stimulus artifact are illustrated in Figure 7–9, and the most commonly used present technique (Brown, 2003; Brown et al., 2009) is illustrated in the left section of Figure 16–6. Other refinements are possible (e.g., Alvarez et al., 2008).

The procedures reported by Brown et al. (1990) were quickly incorporated into the commercial implants. The recordings, which originally were performed using a direct percutaneous connection between the implant and an external amplifier, are now obtained using telemetry, the electrical activity at a selected electrode is transmitted back through the radio-frequency link between the internal and external components of the implant (Abbas et al., 1999). The stimulation and masking protocols are now automatically programmed into the software that externally controls the processor. The responses usually are recorded following monopolar stimulation at a single electrode contact and are recorded from a nearby electrode contact, typically two or three contacts away as immediately adjacent electrodes can show distorted responses (Brown, 2003). In general, the size of the response is larger for contacts closer to the stimulating electrode (Brown, 2003). Like the EABR, the response generally is larger for stimulation at apical electrode contacts compared to stimulation at basal contacts (Gordon et al., 2007), although this will vary with the patient. Programs are available that automatically assess ECAP thresholds without the need for any subjective interpretation of the responses (Gärtner, Lenarz, Joseph, & Buchner, 2010; van Dijk et al., 2007).

Normal ECAP Findings

The ECAP consists of a large N1 wave followed by a smaller and more prolonged P2 wave. At moderate to high intensities, the N1 wave peaks between 0.2 and 0.4 ms after the stimulus and the P2 peak occurs about 0.3 ms later. The latencies of these peaks increase by a small amount (between 0.1 and 0.2 ms) as the stimulus intensity is decreased and by an extra few tenths of a millisecond very close to threshold. The amplitude of the response increases rapidly and regularly with increasing intensity. The slope of the amplitude-intensity function is steeper in children than in adults (Brown, Abbas, Etler, O'Brien, & Oleson, 2010). The cause of this difference is unknown. It may relate to the different types of hearing loss treated with implants in adults and children or to differences in the placement of the electrode contacts relative to the modiolus. The higher thresholds and steeper growth functions in children lead

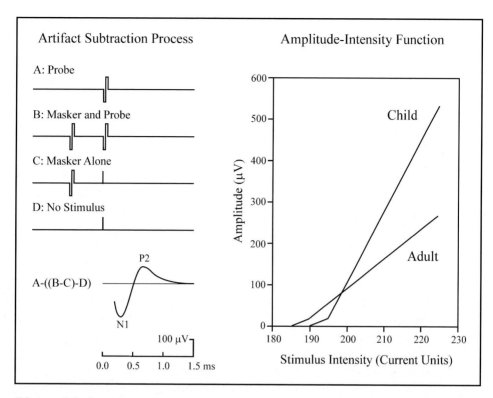

Figure 16–6. *Electrical compound action potential (ECAP). The left section of the figure shows the procedures to remove the artifact when recording from the electrode contacts of the cochlear implant. In condition B, the response to the probe is masked by an immediately preceding stimulus. Thus, subtracting B from A should remove the artifact related to the probe stimulus. Condition C is to control for any residual effect (artifact and response) from the masker and condition D controls for any switching artifacts that can occur when changing between the stimuli* (thin line). *This diagram derives from Brown (2003). The graph on the right shows the growth in the N1-P2 amplitude as the stimulus intensity is increased. The thresholds and slopes are representative growth functions based on the average data from Brown et al. (2010). On average, children show a higher threshold and a steeper growth function compared to adults.*

to more restricted limits for the stimulus intensity in children than adults; using the 8-bit scale, the limits are typically around 160 to 200 in children and 140 to 220 in adults. Typical growth functions are shown in the right section of Figure 16–6.

The threshold for detecting the ECAP varies with different subjects. ECAP thresholds usually are higher in children than in adults (Brown, Abbas, Etler, O'Brien, & Oleson, 2010). Generally, the ECAP threshold is slightly lower than the EABR threshold. ECAP thresholds typically occur somewhere between the T-levels and the C-levels determined behaviorally, although in some subjects the thresholds will be close to the T-levels and in others close to the C-levels. These results are similar for implants from different manufacturers (Alvarez et al., 2010; Jeon et al., 2010). Because of the intersubject variability in their relationship to behavioral thresholds, ECAP thresholds cannot be directly used to set C- and T-levels. ECAP thresholds do indicate a level at which the stimulus will be audible, and therefore can suggest a reasonable level to start behavioral testing. Furthermore, they run roughly parallel to the C- and T-levels as we move from electrode to electrode. Therefore, if we are able to get behavioral C- and T-levels at one electrode, we can use the differences between C- and T-levels and the ECAP threshold at that electrode contact to estimate C- and T-levels at other electrode contacts (Botros & Psarros, 2010; Brown et al., 2009).

Long-term studies of the ECAP have found that the threshold and the slope of the amplitude-intensity function do not change significantly over periods of up to 6 years (Brown et al., 2010). This fits with the general stability of the implant map once it has been adjusted and evaluated over the first few months of use.

STAPEDIUS REFLEXES

As well as the ECAP and EABR, we can record stapedius reflexes in response to brief bursts of electrical stimuli (Hodges, Butts, & King, 2003). These recordings can be obtained using normal impedance measurements. Because the reflex is bilateral, the measurement can be in the ear contralateral or ipsilateral to the implanted ear. When performed at the time of implantation, the recording would be contralateral. Stapedius reflexes must be distinguished from direct activation of the facial nerve, which usually is associated with observable muscle twitches in the facial muscles. Latency measurements are available if we record directly from the stapedius during the operation to insert the implant (Pau et

al., 2009). Reflexes occur with a latency of 10 ms or more (often several tens of ms) whereas direct activation of the facial nerve shows a latency of less than 2 ms. The electrical stapedius reflex threshold generally is close to the behavioral C-level but the relationship is variable and the reflex is not measurable in about a third of the patients.

PROGRAMMING IMPLANT STIMULUS LEVELS IN AN INFANT

In an adult or older child, the implant is programmed behaviorally. For each electrode contact, we determine the threshold level for sensation and the maximum comfort level and then adjust the processor settings so that stimuli only occur within these limits. This is not easily possible when the patient is a young infant. Several physiologic tests can give us some direction about what levels to start testing. Intraoperative EABR and ECAP and stapedius reflex recordings can be obtained when the implant is inserted into the cochlea and these may guide the audiologist when the implant is "turned on" (typically about 3 weeks after the operation). The relationships between physiologic and behavioral measurements are shown in Figure 16–7, which presents some of the data from Gordon, Papsin, and Harrison (2004).

Physiologic measurements are helpful only when used together with some behavioral measurements of the infant's response. The initial activation of the implant is crucial. In the best of all possible worlds, the infant stops playing and looks around when the stimulus goes above threshold and pulls a wry face

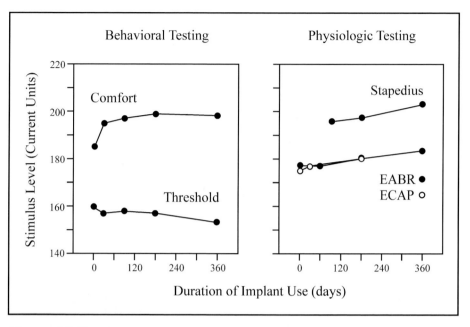

Figure 16–7. **Fitting stimulus levels for cochlear implant.** *The left graph plots the behavioral thresholds and comfort levels over the first year of implant use for a group of implanted children (mean age of implantation 5 years). The right graph represents the thresholds for detecting the stapedius reflex, EABR, and ECAP. All results are from evaluation of an apical electrode. These data are replotted from a more extensive set of data (including the results of different electrodes) from Gordon et al. (2004).*

when the stimulus becomes uncomfortable. In the real world, the infant may cry as soon as stimulation begins and multiple sessions may be required to get some estimate of stimulus limits for just a few electrode contacts. Ultimately, the infant will learn to provide behavioral responses indicating both the perception of the sound or the feeling of discomfort and the examiner will learn to recognize these responses. The ability to store multiple maps is helpful as this allows the parents to change maps based on how well the infant is doing. In general, the infant's ability to tolerate higher levels of stimulation increases as he or she becomes more used to the implant.

ELECTRIC MIDDLE LATENCY RESPONSES

Electrical middle latency responses (EMLRs) can be easily recorded from implanted subjects using either a single pulse or a brief train of pulses. If a brief train is used, the Nb-Pb components of the EMLR increase in amplitude with increasing duration of the train up to 2 ms (Davids et al, 2008a). The latencies of the EMLR waves are determined by the onset of the train. Thus, if we record both an EABR and EMLR to a brief train of pulses, the EABR that we recognize is evoked by the last stimulus in the train and the EMLR by the first. The latency between wave V and the EMLR thus decreases with increasing train duration.

The waveform of the EMLR is variable from subject to subject. Figure 16–8 shows some of this variability. This variability may relate to different degrees of cortical development. The EMLR in children increases in amplitude and decreases in latency over time since implantation (Gordon, Papsin, & Harrison, 2005). Part of this change may relate to the normal development of the cortical connections during childhood and part may relate to the activation of the auditory pathways by the electrical stimulation. The fact that the amplitudes increased in both young and old children supports the idea of use-dependent maturation.

The EMLR components recorded in implanted adults have earlier latencies and tend to be larger than the middle-latency responses (MLRs) evoked by clicks in nor-

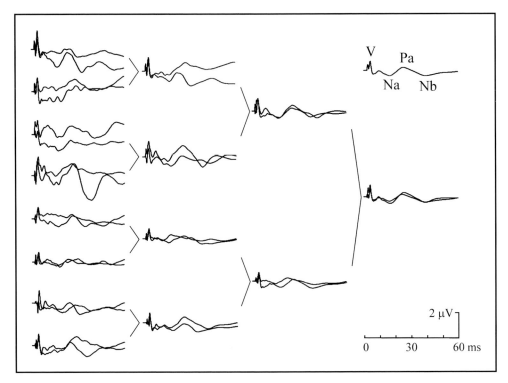

Figure 16–8. *Middle-latency responses to electrical stimulation (EMLRs). On the left are the EMLRs from 16 different implanted children (arbitrarily superimposed in 8 pairs). The artifact contaminated initial portion (1.8 ms) of the recording has been zeroed and the residual effect of the artifact on the later recording has been subtracted out. The responses are paired and then warp-averaged together to give the eight waveforms in the second column. The principles of warping and warp-averaging are described in Chapter 6. Warping prevents the distortion caused by averaging responses that occur with different latencies in different subjects. The warp-averaging procedure is repeated until only two responses are present at the middle right of the figure. These are then warp-averaged to give the final EMLR template plotted at the upper right. This figure derives from some unpublished research using waveforms supplied by Karen Gordon.*

mal adults (Firszt & Kileny, 2003). The latency differences likely are related in part to the absence of any cochlear delay when electrical stimulation is used and also to increased synchronization as the response travels through the brainstem and thalamus to the cortex. The amplitude differences likely are related to the increased synchronization of the response to electrical stimulation.

The Na-Pa amplitude of the EMLR shows significant correlations with tests of speech perception in implanted patients (Firszt, Chambers, &, Kraus, 2002). This makes sense because speech perception is cortical and the EMLR represents the amount of information reaching the cortex.

Steady-State Responses to Electrical Stimulation

Auditory steady-state responses (ASSRs) can be recorded when amplitude-modulated tones are presented in free field and processed through the implant speech processor, or when the electric stimulus signal is connected to the audio input of the speech processor (Yang, Chen, & Hwang, 2008). These responses have thresholds similar to the patient's behavioral thresholds. However, the electric artifact resulting from the stimulator is an almost insurmountable problem. The processor determines the envelope of incoming sounds and then uses that envelope to control the amplitude of the stimulus. We should expect an electrical artifact at the frequency of modulation and we should expect that the threshold for recording this artifact should be at the lower limits that are programmed into the stimulator. True physiologic response may perhaps be differentiated from stimulus artifact on the basis of their different responses to manip-

ulating different processor parameters. Ménard et al. (2004), for example, used different durations of the stimulus pulse to dissociate the artifact. The recorded response then can be shown to contain components of physiologic origin (and not to be simply artifactual). However, disentangling exactly what is physiologic from what is artifactual is almost impossible.

If we directly activate the stimulator to present stimulus pulses at a constant rate (rather than using auditory signals), we can use some of the techniques we have already considered to reduce the artifact. For example, we can present single brief biphasic pulses lasting about 100 µs (like an acoustic click) at 40 Hz and alternate the polarity of the pulses. This will not completely remove the artifact as the RF transmission of the stimulus information to the internal unit also generates artifacts. Hofmann and Wouters (2010) found that the artifact could be reduced from 100 µV to around 20 µV by using stimuli of alternating polarity, this still being much larger than the 40-Hz response, which attains amplitudes of around 0.5 µV. Because the stimulus is a brief pulse, however, it does not last through the stimulus and can thus be cut from the recording with little effect on the entrained ASSR. Hofmann and Wouters (2010) then showed that the 40-Hz following response was differently affected by stimulus intensity than the artifact, supporting a physiologic rather than artifactual origin.

Jeng et al. (2007, 2008) have proposed an interesting technique to distinguish stimulus from response. They bypass both the processor and stimulator and use an amplitude-modulated sinusoid as the stimulus. Large artifacts occur at the carrier frequency and at the sidebands, but no artifact should occur at the modulation frequency itself. This can result only from some nonlinearity in the processing of the stimulus, and nonlinearities are typical of the physiologic response. Recently, Gräbel, Hirschfelder, Scheiber, and Olze (2009) used this stimulus for preoperative promontory stimulation. This type of stimulus needs to be evaluated further in human subjects both as a preoperative assessment and as a means for assessing the responsiveness of the brain to stimulation through the implant.

ELECTRICAL LATE AUDITORY EVOKED POTENTIALS

Electrical late auditory evoked potentials (ELAEPs) can be evoked easily using single pulses, trains of pulses lasting a few tens of milliseconds, or acoustic stimuli presented though the speech processor. If the stimulus is brief, we can zero the period of the artifact in the recording and leave the later ELAEP waves.

Longer stimuli cause more significant problems with artifact. If the stimulus lasts longer than the latencies of the LAEP peaks, the artifact can obscure the response and make it difficult to determine what comes from the brain and what comes from the implant. Several approaches to removing the artifact have been investigated. One technique is to use independent component analysis (Gilley et al., 2006; Ponton & Don, 2003), which dissociates the artifact and the response on the basis of their scalp topographies. Another approach uses beamformer algorithms to suppress the artifact (Wong & Gordon, 2009).

A simple technique to distinguish the artifact is to record the response under two conditions where the response changes but the artifact remains the same. Martin (2007) recorded responses to a change a synthetic vowel when the subject was ignoring the stimuli or attending to them. The response to the change was much larger in the attend condition. Friesen and Picton (2010) recorded ELAEPs to speech stimuli and tones using two different stimulus onset asynchronies (SOAs). The LAEP was much larger at longer SOA whereas the electrical artifact is the same. The difference waveform calculated by subtracting the response at the short SOA (1.1 s) from the response at the long SOA (3.6 s) then showed a clear LAEP with little if any residual artifact.

The ELAEP in adults with postlingual deafness who have been implanted is similar to that recorded in normal adults in response to acoustic stimuli. The main ELAEP components to a brief stimulus— P1, N1, and P2—occur with similar morphology and amplitude but with latencies that are 10 to 20 ms earlier than the homologous acoustic responses (Firszt & Kileny, 2003). Like the normal LAEP, responses can be recorded not just to the onset but also to changes in an ongoing sound (Friesen & Tremblay, 2006) or changes from stimulation of one electrode to another (Brown et al., 2008). Electrical source analysis (Debener, Hine, Bleeck, & Eyles, 2008) and magnetoencephalography (MEG: Hari et al., 1988), which is possible only if the implant does not contain a magnet to hold the RF antenna in place, have clearly shown that the ELAEP is generated in auditory cortex. Furthermore, MEG studies found that the amplitude of the response increases with implant use—the response was not really recognizable for several months after the implant was activated, but then grew dramatically in amplitude (Pantev, Dinnesen, Ross, Wollbrink, & Knief, 2006).

In normal young children, the main component of the late auditory evoked potential (LAEP) is a large vertex-positive

P1 wave. The normal N1 wave only begins to develop around age 10 years, and this wave attenuates and shortens the latency of the P1. The ELAEP in implanted children show the same P1 wave as in normal children but this is delayed in latency. Ponton, Don, Eggermont, Waring, and Masuda (1996a, 1996b) showed that the P1 latency was best predicted by how long the child had been using the implant —"time in sound." The developmental curve for the P1 wave in the implanted child was delayed by the time that the child had not experienced any activation of the central auditory system. The amount of change in the P1 after the implant is much greater when the implant occurs at a younger age (Sharma, Dorman, & Kral, 2005). This suggests that there is a sensitive period for the LAEP during the first few years of life age, and this is consistent with the better performance of children implanted at a younger age. The rapid decrease in the P1 latency in infants also is associated with the development of babbling, an early communicative behavior (Sharma et al., 2004). Plots of the course of the P1 latency with increasing age vary with the age of implantation in prelingually deaf children (Sharma, Gilley, Dorman, & Baldwin, 2007). Most of change in P1 occurs within the first 6 months after implantation and the earlier the implant the faster the P1 latency decreases. Furthermore, children implanted at ages older than 6 years do not reach normal P1 latencies. The effects of time in sound and age of implantation are illustrated in Figure 16–9.

In addition to the increased latency of the P1, an implanted child may not develop the N1 wave in the same way as the normal child. Ponton and Don (2003) found that the N1 failed to develop in implanted children, with the ELAEP showing only the large P1 wave. Perhaps the proper development of the N1 requires some synchronization between activation and myelination in central auditory neurons. More recent data have found that an N1 can develop in children who are implanted before age 3.5 years (Sharma, Gilley, Dorman, & Baldwin, 2007). Most of the children in the earlier studies of Ponton and Don were older.

Sometimes the N1 that develops in implanted children is abnormal. Gordon, Tanaka, Wang, and Papsin (2008) found a wave similar to the N1 in scalp topography in some implanted children. However, this wave was earlier than the usual N1 and did not show any change with stimulus frequency whereas the acoustic response is larger for lower frequency sounds. Interestingly, children who showed this unusual negative wave did not do as well on speech perception tests as children with ELAEPs showing just the simple P1. Gordon et al. (2008) therefore suggested that this negative wave may indicate abnormal cortical development. The nature of this abnormality is unknown. It might represent information in the auditory cortex being read out before it has been fully processed. It also could represent activation of different regions of the auditory cortex than those activated in normal subjects (Gilley Sharma, & Dorman, 2008). Some of the waveforms from Ponton et al. (1996b) and Gordon et al. (2008) are presented in Figure 16–10.

Mismatch Negativity (MMN)

The MMN is a small negative wave that occurs in the LAEP to an improbable deviant stimulus occurring in a train of standard stimuli (reviewed in Chapter 11). It is an appealing response to study in patients with cochlear implants as it

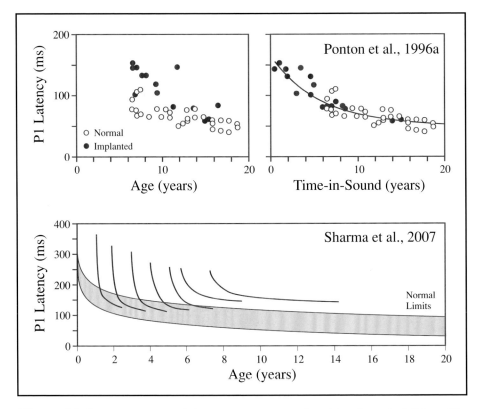

Figure 16–9. *Maturation of the LAEPs in normal and implanted children. The data for the two upper graphs are taken from Ponton et al. (1996a). The upper left graph plots the P1 latency against the age of the child. The latency is longer in the children with implants. The upper right graph plots the latencies against "time-in-sound." For the normal child, this is the same as the age of the child, but for the children who are implanted, this is the age at the time of recording minus the age at the time of implantation. The data then fit a simple exponential maturation curve. The data in the lower graph show representative maturation curves for children implanted at different ages. These data are from Sharma et al. (2007), who present the longitudinal development of the P1 wave for 231 implanted children. This paper includes children implanted at much earlier ages than those evaluated by Ponton et al. The P1 latency decreases to within normal limits for the younger children, with the rate of decrease decreasing with increasing age. The P1 waves of children implanted after age 6 years tend not to reach normal limits.*

indicates that the brain can discriminate between the standard and deviant stimuli. Therefore, it might be useful as an objective measurement of discrimination in implanted patients.

Kraus et al. (1993) demonstrated that adult patients with implants showed a MMN to a deviant "ta" syllable occurring in a train of "da" syllables. The MMN showed a peak latency near 220 ms and an amplitude between 0.5 and 4 µV. Ponton and Don (1995) demonstrated an MMN when using longer stimuli (pulse trains directly through the implant to two different electrode contacts). Because discrimination of these stimuli was much simpler

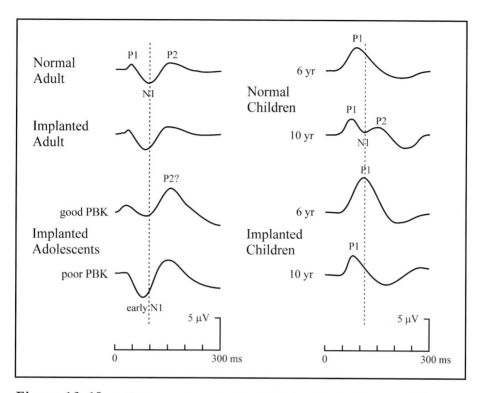

Figure 16–10. **LAEP waveforms in implanted patients.** *The upper left waveforms are diagrammatic. The lower left waveforms were traced from Gordon et al. (2008) and the waveforms on the right come from Ponton and Don (2003). The responses in normal subjects were obtained with acoustic stimulation. The upper left responses show the typical responses in normal adults and in implanted postlingually deafened adults. The responses are similar in waveform but the response in the implanted subject is slightly earlier. The vertical dotted line gives the normal N1 latency in adults. The lower tracings on the left show responses in implanted adolescents who had been using implants for 2 to 15 years. The subjects were divided into those with good perceptual performance on the Phonetically Balanced Kindergarten (PBK) word list and those with poor performance. The poor performers had a large early N1 wave (Gordon et al., 2008). The waveforms on the right show the maturation of responses from normal and implanted children (Ponton & Don, 2003). Implanted children show a later P1 wave which then decreases in latency with increasing age. The normal children show a small N1 wave beginning at about age 10 years. This is not apparent in many of the implanted children at the same age. Here the vertical dotted line shows the N1 latency in normal older children.*

than the discrimination of the phonemic contrast of Kraus et al., the MMN latency was much earlier—between 100 and 120 ms. In order to remove the artifact, they recorded the responses with the same stimulus acting as the deviant in one condition and as the standard in another. They then subtracted the standard response from the response to the same stimulus when it was a deviant. This controlled for difference in the artifact caused by stimulating different electrodes.

Ponton et al. (2000) studied the development of the MMN in children with cochlear implants. The discrimination was between brief trains of pulses of durations 18 ms and less. The MMN was remarkably similar in children of different ages and in children with implants compared to normal children. This differs from the other waves of the LAEP like the P1 which show large changes with maturation. However, the signal-to-noise ratio of the response was small and special statistics were necessary to be sure that a significant MMN was occurring (Ponton, Don, Eggermont, & Kwong, 1997). One interesting finding was that the threshold for detecting a significant MMN was sometimes lower than the behavioral discrimination threshold. The auditory cortex was perhaps detecting differences that were not available to conscious perception.

The MMN remains a way to check discrimination in children with implants who cannot cooperate with behavioral testing. However, it does require some degree of collaboration. The child must at least sit still and stay awake during the test. Because the response is small, the test is time-consuming. Checking several levels of discrimination may take an hour or more. Furthermore, the fact that a MMN can be measured when the subject does not behaviorally discriminate the sounds is difficult to understand. It may represent a discrimination that the subject has not yet learned to categorize perceptually, resulting in a dissociation between sensory information and perceptual usefulness.

P300

Several early studies of patients with cochlear implants demonstrated a P300 wave in response to an actively detected oddball target in a train of standard stimuli (Kaga, Kodera, Hirota, & Tsuzuka, 1991; Micco et al., 1995; Oviatt & Kileny, 1991). The amplitude and latency of the P300 varies with the ability of the subjects to discriminate the sounds used as targets and standards. Thus, the P300 may be helpful in assessing the benefit of the implant (Beynon, Snik, & van den Broek, 2002) or in deciding among different processor strategies (Beynon, Snik, Stegeman, & van den Broek, 2005). However, because it takes much longer to record a P300 than to perform simple discrimination tests, this approach has not been widely used. Implanted children who get greater benefit from their implant show P300 waves and those who have poor perception do not (Beynon et al., 2002; Kileny, Boerst, & Zwolan, 1997). Further studies might show whether the development of the P300 in implanted children follows a normal or abnormal course.

OVERVIEW

The auditory EPs are very helpful in patients with implants. They are an essential part of the evaluation of candidates for implantation. Once the implant is in place, the EPs can be used to check the integrity of the stimulator, and to help set the lower and upper limits for the stimulus intensity at each electrode contact. Following the development of the EPs once the implant is working can give us insight to how the human brain changes with sensory input.

The cochlear implant has been very successful in providing hearing to severe and profoundly deaf patients. The information provided by the implant is much less than that which is available to the normally functioning cochlea (Shannon,

Zeng, Kamath, Wygonski, & Ekelid, 1995). The ability of patients to do so well with so little indicates both that speech is a highly redundant signal and that the human auditory system is an amazingly powerful learning system. Provided the implant is in a subject who has developed reasonable language before their deafness or in a child under the age of about 6 years, the auditory system can quickly learn to use the highly impoverished input provided by implants to interpret speech. Recently, Moore and Shannon (2009) pointed out the importance of this learning process. Now that we have become more comfortable fitting the implant, we need to design better ways to help the implanted subjects learn to use them. The EPs might be helpful in monitoring these learning processes, showing how the brain changes as it learns and suggesting which learning strategies are best suited to the different signal processing strategies available in the implant.

The cochlear implant is one of our greatest biomedical achievements. It can provide patients without any useful hearing with the ability to hear and to communicate. Walt Whitman sang the body electric. Now we can electrify the song.

ABBREVIATIONS

ABR	Auditory brainstem response
ASSR	Auditory steady-state response
ECAP	Electrical compound action potential
C-level	Maximum comfort level
CM	Cochlear microphonic
CU	Current unit
EABR	Electrical auditory brainstem response
ELAEP	Electrical late auditory evoked potential
EMLR	Electrical middle-latency response
EP	Evoked potential
LAEP	Late auditory evoked potential
MEG	Magnetoencephalography
M-level	Most comfortable listening level
MLR	Middle-latency response
MMN	Mismatch negativity
nHL	Normal hearing level
OAE	Otoacoustic emission
PBK	Phonetically balanced kindergarten word list
RF	Radio frequency
SOA	Stimulus onset asynchrony
T-level	Threshold level

REFERENCES

Abbas, P. J., & Brown, C. J. (1988). Electrically evoked brainstem potentials in cochlear implant patients with multi-electrode stimulation. *Hearing Research, 36,* 153–162.

Abbas, P. J., & Brown, C. J. (1991). Electrically evoked auditory brainstem response: Growth of response with current level. *Hearing Research, 51,* 123–128.

Abbas, P. J., Brown, C. J., Shallop, J. K., Firszt, J. B., Hughes, M. L., Hong, S. H., & Staller, S. J. (1999). Summary of results using the nucleus CI24M implant to record the electrically evoked compound action potential. *Ear and Hearing, 20,* 45–59.

Allum, J. H., Shallop, J. K., Hotz, M., & Pfaltz, C. R. (1990). Characteristics of electrically evoked "auditory" brainstem responses elicited with the nucleus 22-electrode intracochlear implant. *Scandinavian Audiology, 19*, 263–267.

Alvarez, I., de la Torre, A., Sainz, M., Roldán, C., Schoesser, H., & Spitzer P. (2008). An improved masker-probe method for stimulus artifact reduction in electrically evoked compound action potentials. *Journal of Neuroscience Methods, 175*, 143–147.

Alvarez, I., de la Torre, A., Sainz, M., Roldán, C., Schoesser, H., & Spitzer P. (2010). Using evoked compound action potentials to assess activation of electrodes and predict C-levels in the Tempo+ cochlear implant speech processor. *Ear and Hearing, 31*, 134–145.

Barton, G. R., Stacey, P. C., Fortnum, H. M., & Summerfield, A. Q. (2006). Hearing-impaired children in the UK, IV: Cost-effectiveness of paediatric cochlear implantation. *Ear and Hearing, 27*, 575–588.

Beynon, A. J., Snik, A. F., Stegeman, D. F., & van den Broek, P. (2005). Discrimination of speech sound contrasts determined with behavioral tests and event-related potentials in cochlear implant recipients. *Journal of the American Academy of Audiology, 16*, 42–53.

Beynon, A. J., Snik, A. F., & van den Broek, P. (2002). Evaluation of cochlear implant benefit with auditory cortical evoked potentials. *International Journal of Audiology, 41*, 429–435.

Bond, M., Mealing, S., Anderson, R., Elston, J., Weiner, G., Taylor, R. S., . . . Stein, K. (2009). The effectiveness and cost-effectiveness of cochlear implants for severe to profound deafness in children and adults: A systematic review and economic model. *Health Technology Assessment, 13*(44), 1–330.

Botros, A., & Psarros, C. (2010). Neural response telemetry reconsidered: I. The relevance of ECAP threshold profiles and scaled profiles to cochlear implant fitting. *Ear and Hearing, 31*, 367–379.

Brown, C. J. (2003). The electrically-evoked whole nerve action potential. In H. E. Cullington (Ed.), *Cochlear implants: Objective measures* (pp. 96–129). London, UK: Whurr Publishers.

Brown, C. J., Abbas, P. J., Etler, C. P., Larson, A. K., Musser, K. E., & O'Brien, S. N. (2009). Electrically evoked auditory potentials: Clinical applications. In L. S. Eisenberg (Ed.), *Clinical management of children with cochlear implants* (pp. 133–156). San Diego, CA: Plural Publishing.

Brown, C. J., Abbas, P. J. Etler, C. P., O'Brien, S., & Oleson, J. J. (2010). Effects of long-term use of a cochlear implant on the electrically evoked compound action potential. *Journal of the American Academy of Audiology, 21*, 5–15.

Brown, C. J., Abbas, P. J., & Gantz, B. J. (1990). Electrically evoked whole-nerve action potentials: Data from human cochlear implant users. *Journal of the Acoustical Society of America, 88*, 1385–1391.

Brown, C. J., Etler, C., He, S., O'Brien, S., Erenberg, S., Kim, J.R., Dhuldhoya, A. N., & Abbas, P. J. (2008). The electrically evoked auditory change complex: Preliminary results from nucleus cochlear implant users. *Ear and Hearing, 29*, 704–717.

Brown, C. J., Hughes, M. L., Luk, B., Abbas, P. J., Wolaver, A., & Gervais, J., 2000. The relationship between EAP and EABR thresholds and levels used to program the Nucleus 24 speech processor: Data from adults. *Ear and Hearing, 21*, 151–163.

Cheng, A. K., Rubin, H. R., Powe, N. R., Mellon, N. K., Francis, H. W., & Niparko J. K. (2000). Cost-utility analysis of the cochlear implant in children. *Journal of the American Medical Association, 284*, 850–856.

Clark, G. M. (2003). *Cochlear implants: Fundamentals and applications*. New York, NY: Springer Science.

Clark, G. M., Tong, Y. C., Black, R. C., Forster, I. C., Patrick, J. F., & Dewhurst, D. J. (1977). A multiple electrode cochlear implant. *Journal of Laryngology and Otology, 91*, 935–945.

Clark, G. M., Tong, Y. C., & Martin, L. F. (1981). A multiple-channel cochlear implant. An evaluation using open-set CID sentences. *Laryngoscope, 91*, 628–634.

Cushing, S. L., Papsin, B. C., & Gordon, K. A. (2006). Incidence and characteristics of facial nerve stimulation in children with cochlear implants. *Laryngoscope, 116*, 1787–1791.

Cushing, S. L., Papsin, B. C., Strantzas, S., & Gordon, K. A. (2009). Facial nerve electromyography: A useful tool in detecting nonauditory side effects of cochlear implantation. *Journal of Otolaryngology-Head and Neck Surgery, 38*, 157–165.

Davids, T., Valero, J., Papsin, B. C., Harrison, R. V., & Gordon, K. A. (2008a). Effects of stimulus manipulation on electrophysiological responses in pediatric cochlear implant users. Part I: Duration effects. *Hearing Research, 244*, 7–14.

Davids, T., Valero, J., Papsin, B. C., Harrison, R. V., & Gordon, K. A. (2008b). Effects of stimulus manipulation on electrophysiological responses of pediatric cochlear implant users. Part II: Rate effects. *Hearing Research, 244*, 15–24.

Debener, S., Hine, J., Bleeck, S., & Eyles, J. (2008). Source localization of auditory evoked potentials after cochlear implantation. *Psychophysiology, 45*, 20–24.

Eisenberg, L. S. (Ed.). (2009). *Clinical evaluation of children with cochlear implants*. San Diego, CA: Plural Publishing.

Firszt, J. B., Chambers, R. D., & Kraus, N. (2002). Neurophysiology of cochlear implant users II: Comparison among speech perception, dynamic range and physiological measures. *Ear and Hearing, 23*, 516–531.

Firszt, J. B., Chambers, R. D., Kraus, N., & Reeder, R. M. (2002). Neurophysiology of cochlear implant users I: Effects of stimulus current level and electrode site on the electrical ABR, MLR, and N1-P2 response. *Ear and Hearing, 23*, 502–515.

Firszt, J. B., & Kileny, P. R. (2003). Electrically-evoked middle latency and cortical auditory-evoked potentials. In H. E. Cullington (Ed.), *Cochlear implants: Objective measures* (pp. 160–186). London, UK: Whurr Publishers.

Friesen, L. M., & Picton, T. W. (2010). A method for removing cochlear implant artifact. *Hearing Research, 259*, 95–106.

Friesen, L. M., & Tremblay, K. L. (2006). Acoustic change complexes recorded in adult cochlear implant listeners. *Ear and Hearing, 27*, 678–685.

Gärtner, L., Lenarz, T., Joseph, G., & Büchner, A. (2010) Clinical use of a system for the automated recording and analysis of electrically evoked compound action potentials (ECAPs) in cochlear implant patients. *Acta Otolaryngologica, 130*, 724–732.

Geers, A., Tobey, E., Moog, J., & Brenner, C. (2008). Long-term outcomes of cochlear implantation in the preschool years: From elementary grades to high school. *International Journal of Audiology, 47*(Suppl. 2), S21–S30.

Gilley, P. M., Sharma, A., & Dorman, M. (2008). Cortical reorganization in children with cochlear implants. *Brain Research, 1239*, 56–65.

Gilley, P. M., Sharma, A., Dorman, M., Finley, C. C., Panch, A. S., & Martin, K. (2006). Minimization of cochlear implant stimulus artifact in cortical auditory evoked potentials. *Clinical Neurophysiology, 117*, 1772–1782.

Gordin, A., Papsin, B., James, A., & Gordon, K. (2009). Evolution of cochlear implant arrays result in changes in behavioral and physiological responses in children. *Otology and Neurotology, 30*, 908–915.

Gordon, K. A., Papsin, B. C., & Harrison, R. V. (2003). Activity-dependent developmental plasticity of the auditory brainstem in children who use cochlear implants. *Ear and Hearing, 24*, 485–500.

Gordon, K. A., Papsin, B. C., & Harrison, R. V. (2004). Toward a battery of behavioral and objective measures to achieve optimal cochlear implant stimulation levels in children. *Ear and Hearing, 25*, 447–463.

Gordon, K. A., Papsin, B. C., & Harrison, R. V. (2005).Effects of cochlear implant use on the electrically evoked middle latency response in children. *Hearing Research, 204*, 78–89.

Gordon, K. A., Papsin, B. C., & Harrison, R. V. (2006). An evoked potential study of the developmental time course of the auditory nerve and brainstem in children using cochlear implants. *Audiology and Neurootology, 11*, 7–23.

Gordon, K. A., Papsin, B. C., & Harrison, R. V. (2007). Auditory brainstem activity and development evoked by apical versus basal cochlear implant electrode stimulation in children. *Clinical Neurophysiology, 118*, 1671–1684.

Gordon, K. A., Tanaka, S., Wong, D. D. E., & Papsin, B. C., (2008). Characterizing responses from auditory cortex in young people with several years of cochlear implant experience. *Clinical Neurophysiology, 119*, 2347–2362.

Gordon, K. A., Valero, J., Jewell, S. F., Ahn, J., & Papsin, B. C. (2010). Auditory development in the absence of hearing in infancy. *NeuroReport, 21*, 163–167.

Gräbel, S., Hirschfelder, A., Scheiber, C., & Olze, H. (2009). Evaluation of a novel, non-invasive, objective test of auditory nerve function in cochlear implant candidates. *Otology and Neurotology, 30*, 716–724.

Hari, R., Pelizzone, M., Mäkelä, J. P., Hällström, J., Huttunen, J., & Knuutila, J. (1988). Neuromagnetic responses from a deaf subject to stimuli presented through a multichannel cochlear prosthesis. *Ear and Hearing, 9*, 148–152.

Hodges, A. V., Butts, S. L., & King, J. E. (2003). Electrically-evoked stapedial reflexes, utility in cochlear implant patients. In Cullington, H. E. (Ed.), *Cochlear implants: Objective measures* (pp. 81–95). London, UK: Whurr Publishers.

Hofmann, M., & Wouters, J. (2010).Electrically evoked auditory steady state responses in cochlear implant users. *Journal of the Association for Research in Otolaryngology, 11*, 267–282.

Jeng, F. C., Abbas, P. J., Brown, C. J., Miller, C. A., Nourski, K. V., & Robinson, B. K. (2007). Electrically evoked auditory steady-state responses in Guinea pigs. *Audiology and Neurotology, 12*, 101–112

Jeng, F. C., Abbas, P. J., Brown, C. J., Miller, C. A., Nourski, K. V., & Robinson, B. K. (2008). Electrically evoked auditory steady-state responses in a guinea pig model: Latency estimates and effects of stimulus parameters. *Audiology and Neurotology, 13*, 161–171.

Jeon, E. K., Brown, C. J., Etler, C. P., O'Brien, S., Chiou, L. K., & Abbas, P. J. (2010). Comparison of electrically evoked compound action potential thresholds and loudness estimates for the stimuli used to program the Advanced Bionics cochlear implant. *Journal of the American Academy of Audiology, 21*, 16–27.

Kaga, K., Kodera, K., Hirota, E., & Tsuzuku, T. (1991). P300 response to tones and speech sounds after cochlear implant: A case report. *Laryngoscope, 101*, 905–907.

Kelsall, D. C., Shallop, J. K., Brammeier, T. G., & Prenger, E. C. (1997). Facial nerve stimulation after Nucleus 22-channel cochlear implantation. *American Journal of Otology, 18*, 336–341.

Kileny, P. R., Boerst, A., & Zwolan, T. (1997). Cognitive evoked potentials to speech and tonal stimuli in children with implants. *Otolaryngology-Head and Neck Surgery, 117*, 161–169.

Kim, A. H., Kileny, P. R., Arts, H. A., El Kashlan, H. K., Telian, S. A., & Zwolan, T. A. (2008). Role of electrically evoked auditory brainstem response in cochlear implantation of children with inner ear malformations. *Otology and Neurotology, 29*, 626–634.

Kraus, N., Micco, A. G., Koch, D. B., McGee, T., Carrell, T., Sharma, A., . . . Weingarten, C. Z. (1993). The mismatch negativity cortical evoked potential elicited by speech in cochlear-implant users. *Hearing Research, 65*, 118–124.

Loizou, P. C. Mimicking the human ear: An overview of signal-processing strategies for converting sound into electrical signals in cochlear implants. *IEEE Signal Processing Magazine, 15*(5), 101–130.

Martin, B. A. (2007). Can the acoustic change complex be recorded in an individual with a cochlear implant? Separating neural responses from cochlear implant artifact. *Journal of the American Academy of Audiology, 18*, 126–140.

Mason, S. (2003). The electrically-evoked auditory brainstem response. In H. E. Cullington (Ed.), *Cochlear implants: Objective measures* (pp. 130–159). London, UK: Whurr Publishers.

Mason, S. M., O'Donoghue, G. M., Gibbin, K. P., Garnham, C. W., & Jowett, C. A. (1997). Perioperative electrical auditory brain stem response in candidates for pediatric cochlear implantation. *American Journal of Otology, 18,* 466–471.

Ménard, M., Gallego, S., Truy, E., Berger-Vachon, C., Durrant, J. D., & Collet, L. (2004). Auditory steady-state response evaluation of auditory thresholds in cochlear implant patients. *International Journal of Audiology, 43*(Suppl. 1), S39–S43.

Micco, A. G., Kraus, N., Koch, D. B., McGee, T. J., Carrell, T. D., Sharma, A, . . . Wiet, R, J. (1995). Speech-evoked cognitive P300 potentials in cochlear implant recipients. *American Journal of Otology, 16,* 514–520.

Moore, D. R., & Shannon, R. V. (2009). Beyond cochlear implants: awakening the deafened brain. *Nature Neuroscience, 12,* 686–691.

Nikolopoulos, T. P., Mason, S. M., Gibbin, K. P., & O'Donoghue, G. M. (2000). The prognostic value of promontory electric auditory brain stem response in pediatric cochlear implantation. *Ear and Hearing, 21,* 236–241.

Oviatt, D. L., & Kileny, P. R. (1991). Auditory event-related potentials elicited from cochlear implant recipients and hearing subjects. *American Journal of Audiology, 1,* 48–55.

Pantev, C., Dinnesen, A., Ross, B., Wollbrink, A., & Knief, A. (2006). Dynamics of auditory plasticity after cochlear implantation: A longitudinal study. *Cerebral Cortex, 16,* 31–36.

Papsin, B. C., & Gordon, K. A. (2007). Cochlear implants for children with severe-to-profound hearing loss. *New England Journal of Medicine, 357,* 2380–2387.

Pau, H., Gibson, W. P., & Sanli, H. (2006). Trans-tympanic electric auditory brainstem response (TT-EABR): The importance of the positioning of the stimulating electrode. *Cochlear Implants International, 7,* 183–187.

Pau, H. W., Zehlicke, T., Sievert, U., Schaudel, D., Behrend, D., & Dahl, R. (2009). Electromyographical recording of the electrically elicited stapedius reflex via a bipolar hook electrode. *Otology and Neurotology, 30,* 1–6.

Ponton, C. W., & Don, M. (1995). The mismatch negativity in cochlear implant users. *Ear and Hearing, 16,* 131–146.

Ponton, C. W., & Don, M. (2003). Cortical auditory-evoked potentials recorded from cochlear implant users, methods and applications In H. E. Cullington (Ed.), *Cochlear implants: Objective measures* (pp. 187–230). London, UK: Whurr Publishers.

Ponton, C. W, Don, M., Eggermont, J. J., & Kwong, B. (1997). Integrated mismatch negativity (MMNi): A noise-free representation of evoked responses allowing single-point distribution-free statistical tests. *Electroencephalography and Clinical Neurophysiology, 104,* 143–150. Erratum (1997) *Electroencephalography and Clinical Neurophysiology, 104,* 381–382.

Ponton, C. W., Don, M., Eggermont, J. J., Waring, M. D., & Masuda, A. (1996a). Auditory system plasticity in children after long periods of complete deafness. *NeuroReport, 8,* 61–65.

Ponton, C. W., Don, M., Eggermont, J. J., Waring, M. D., & Masuda, A. (1996b). Maturation of human cortical auditory function: Differences between normal-hearing children and children with cochlear implants. *Ear and Hearing, 17,* 430–437.

Ponton, C. W., Eggermont, J. J., Don M., Waring, M. D., Kwong, B., Cunningham, J., & Trautwein, P. (2000). Maturation of the mismatch negativity: effects of profound deafness and cochlear implant use. *Audiology & Neuro-Otology, 5,* 167–185.

Propst, E. J., Papsin, B. C., Stockley, T. L., Harrison, R. V., & Gordon, K. A. (2006). Auditory responses in cochlear implant users with and without GJB2 deafness. *Laryngoscope, 116,* 317–327.

Shallop, J. K., Beiter, A. L., Goin, D. W., & Mischke, R. E. (1990). Electrically evoked auditory brainstem responses (EABR) and middle latency responses (EMLR) obtained from patients with the Nucleus Multichannel cochlear implant. *Ear and Hearing, 11,* 5–15.

Shallop, J. K., Carter, P., Feinman, G., & Tabor B. (2003). Averaged electrode voltage measurements in patients with cochlear implants. In

H. E. Cullington (Ed.), *Cochlear implants: Objective measures* (pp. 40–80). London, UK: Whurr Publishers.

Shallop, J. K., Jin, S. H., Driscoll, C. L. W., & Tibesar, R. J. (2004). Characteristics of electrically evoked potentials in patients with auditory neuropathy/auditory dys-synchrony. *International Journal of Audiology, 43*(Suppl. 1), S22–S27.

Shannon, R. V., Zeng, F. G., Kamath, V., Wygonski, J., & Ekelid, M. (1995). Speech recognition with primarily temporal cues. *Science, 270,* 303–304.

Sharma, A., Dorman, M. F., & Kral, A. (2005). The influence of a sensitive period on central auditory development in children with unilateral and bilateral cochlear implants. *Hearing Research, 203,* 134–143.

Sharma, A., Gilley, P.M., Dorman, M. F. & Baldwin, R. (2007). Deprivation-induced cortical reorganization in children with cochlear implants. *International Journal of Audiology, 46,* 494–499.

Sharma, A., Tobey, E., Dorman, M., Bharadwaj, S., Martin, K., Gilley, P., & Kunkel, F., 2004. Central auditory maturation and babbling development in infants with cochlear implants. *Archives of Otolaryngology-Head and Neck Surgery, 130,* 511–516.

Simmons, F. B. (1966). Electrical stimulation of the auditory nerve in man. *Archives of Otolaryngology, 84,* 2–54.

Stacey, P. C., Fortnum, H. M., Barton, G. R., & Summerfield A. Q. (2006). Hearing-impaired children in the UK, I: Auditory receptive capabilities, communication skills, educational achievements, and quality of life. *Ear and Hearing, 27,* 161–186.

Staller, S. J. (1991) Special issue—multichannel cochlear implants in children. *Ear and Hearing, 12*(4), 1S–89S.

Starr, A., & Brackmann, D. E. (1979). Brain stem potentials evoked by electrical stimulation of the cochlea in human subjects. *Annals of Otology, Rhinology and Laryngology, 88,* 550–556.

van Dijk, B., Botros, A. M., Battmer, R. D., Begall, K., Dillier, N., Hey, M., . . . Offeciers, E. (2007). Clinical results of AutoNRT, a completely automatic ECAP recording system for cochlear implants. *Ear and Hearing, 28,* 558–570.

Wilson, B. S., & Dorman, M. F. (2008). Cochlear implants: Current designs and future possibilities. *Journal of Rehabilitation Research and Development, 45,* 695–730.

Wong, D. D., & Gordon, K. A. (2009). Beamformer suppression of cochlear implant artifacts in an electroencephalography dataset. *IEEE Transactions in Biomedical Engineering, 56,* 2851–2857.

Yang, C. H., Chen, H. C., & Hwang, C. F. (2008). The prediction of hearing thresholds with auditory steady-state responses for cochlear implanted children. *International Journal of Pediatric Otorhinolaryngology, 72,* 609–617.

Zeng, F. G., Rebscher, S., Harrison, W. V., Sun, X., & Feng, H. (2008). Cochlear implants: System design, integration and evaluation. *IEEE Reviews in Biomedical Engineering, 1,* 115–142.

17

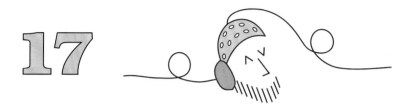

Concluding Comments: Beginning to Live

> A word is dead, when it is said
> Some say—
> I say it just begins to live
> That day.
>
> Emily Dickinson, 1862

This book has not reviewed all that is known about how the human brain perceives sounds. If you are coming to this chapter after dutifully reading through the book, you may not wish to know how much is missing—given how long it took to get this far. If you are quickly checking whether the conclusions might justify reading the preceding chapters more closely, you may not wish to hear about their shortcomings. The book provides the general principles about the auditory evoked potentials and reviews much of the current literature. However, there are unwritten chapters.

Our understanding is always compromised by what is not known. Science is always changing and never complete. However, what we know now will transform itself into future understanding, and this book can provide a base to build on.

New findings will be both experimental and clinical. We need to know more about the nature of the auditory evoked potentials (EPs) and we need to understand more fully how best to use them for our patients. There are prizes to be won and much enjoyment to be had in their winning. This final chapter mentions some of the areas where we need to know more and point to some directions that might be helpful.

SPEECH

How sounds make words, how words make sense, and how sense is understood by someone else remain mysterious. Nevertheless, because the human auditory system has evolved to perceive speech, how it does so may be the key to all its processes. At present, we do not really know the basic organization of human hearing. We can conceive of the visual system in terms of a 2½-dimensional sketch, arrayed in the visual cortex, colored, moved, and topographically altered to provide us with visual objects. However, we have no clear organizing principle for the auditory system. Is the incoming sound wave arrayed in time or in frequency? How does it determine our perceptions of auditory objects? How is it parsed into syllables and words?

We have spent much time trying to piece together how complex auditory perception works from studying how simple stimuli—clicks and tones—are processed. In recent years, we have been moving toward studying complex perceptions more directly using words and sentences as stimuli. Some of this new research with speech sounds was mentioned briefly in the preceding chapters of this book. However, we have only scratched the surface. Most of our work with speech stimuli has looked at the late auditory evoked potentials (LAEPs). Speech stimuli also can be used to elicit early brainstem responses (Skoe & Kraus, 2010). Furthermore, these brainstem responses can adapt themselves to perceive the particular aspects of speech in the language we grow up with (Krishnan, Xu, Gandour, & Cariani, 2005).

Several studies have investigated whether the responses of the human auditory cortex are especially sensitive to the human voice in the same way that the visual cortex is sensitive to the human face. Early studies reported a positive wave with a latency around 320 ms for voice but not other sounds, but this varied with both the task and the direction of attention (Levy, Granot, & Bentin, 2001,

2003). MEG studies found an increased sustained field for voice stimuli (Gunji et al., 2003). Recent studies have shown a voice-specific frontotemporal positivity peaking much earlier than in the original studies (Charest et al., 2009). In children, EPs to voice differentiate from the responses to other stimuli as early as 60 ms, with this difference being greatest over the right temporal scalp (Rogier, Roux, Belin, Bonnet-Brilhaut, & Bruneau, 2010). The many different aspects of the human voice need further investigation. How does vocal periodicity affect the processing of other information in the sound, such as formant frequencies? How do particular voices get categorized and remembered?

LANGUAGE

Human language initially develops in association with what we hear and speak. How this development occurs in the child's brain is not known. Both the extent that our genes unroll the structure of our language and the way that our experience alters that structure remain to be determined.

Many fascinating experiments have looked at language processing in the human brain with the event-related potentials (ERPs). Probably the most famous of these is the discovery of a negative wave with a peak latency of around 400 ms— the N400—that is evoked by semantic incongruities such as the last word in the sentence, "He spread the warm bread with socks" (Kutas & Hillyard, 1980). The brain expects the word "butter" and is discombobulated by the incongruous "socks." The N400 has allowed us to study many aspects of human language processing, and has led to the discovery of other ERP components related to other processes such as lexical access during word perception and the detection of syntactic violations. Kutas and her colleagues have presented excellent reviews of these ERP findings under the title "Psycholinguistics Electrified" (Kutas & Van Petten, 1994; Kutas, Van Petten, & Kluender, 2006).

Most language ERP work has used visual stimuli. The words in a sentence are presented using rapid serial visual presentation; each word is displayed for a brief time and then replaced by the next. This type of presentation facilitates the recording and measurement of ERPS, averaging being time-locked to the onset of the display. Language-related ERPs also can be evoked using spoken words and sentences (e.g., Connolly & Phillips, 1994; Newman & Connolly, 2009), but the responses are distorted by the variable latencies at which spoken words are perceived. Nevertheless, an N400-like wave can be elicited by semantic incongruity, and an earlier "phonological mapping negativity" (PMN) can occur if the first phoneme differs from that expected in the context of the sentence. For example, if the sentence beginning "They left the dirty dishes in the . . . " is completed by the word "kitchen" a PMN occurs but no N400. Although initial phoneme of "kitchen" is not the same as that of the expected word "sink," the word is semantically correct. If the final word is "sister," there would be no PMN because the initial phoneme is as expected, but an N400 would occur because of the semantic incongruity.

We are learning more and more about how spoken words are processed. We need to find out how sounds are processed as phonemes, how our lexicon of word patterns is consulted to provide the meaning of the word, and how we keep adjusting our expectancies for what will be heard next. The technical difficulties related to the variability in timing are immense. Since each spoken word has its own particular time pattern, it is hard to set up averaging protocols that work when words are changing. Listening to the same word repeated over and over does not really involve linguistic processing. Nevertheless, we need to understand how language is processed in the auditory domain. Our language normally is learned through sound. Reading comes later.

CENTRAL AUDITORY PROCESSING DISORDER

Many patients with hearing problems show no obvious abnormalities on basic audiometric testing. Deficits occur only when they are asked to perform more complicated tasks than simply detecting whether a stimulus is present. Their problems often are attributed to "central auditory processing disorder" (CAPD) although this is not a clear diagnostic entity (Cacace & McFarland, 2009; Dawes & Bishop, 2009).

Difficulty in understanding speech is the most common symptom of CAPD, and abnormalities in processing speech in noise the most prominent finding on examination. However, exactly how to diagnose the disorder or disorders is complicated by the lack of any gold standard that tells us when a particular person has CAPD. Probably, there are many different kinds of processing disorders. Some may affect simple brainstem mechanisms such as those used to localize a particular speaker and thus differentiate that person's speech from others. Others may affect higher levels of perception such as the ability to follow rapid stimulus changes.

Some may be specific to the auditory system whereas others may involve supramodal language impairments that affect reading as well as hearing. The syndrome of attention deficit disorder often overlaps with CAPD and it then is difficult to determine whether one leads to the other or both coexist. The diagnosis of patients with disorders of attention, language, or hearing often depends on who is doing the evaluation and what tests are performed (Dawes & Bishop, 2009).

Many different pathophysiologies may lead to CAPD. The auditory EPs should be able to distinguish these, for example, by demonstrating abnormalities in some EP components but not in others. However, EPs may be abnormal only in certain situations. We certainly should evaluate the effects of stimulus rate and of masking noise. Furthermore, abnormalities may only show up clearly when we actually use speech stimuli.

Patients with auditory neuropathy have a type of auditory processing disorder that we now understand more fully. Before we began to recognize this disorder, many patients with auditory neuropathy probably were diagnosed as having some central hearing disorder. No one thought to look at their ABRs because their basic hearing thresholds were normal. Auditory neuropathy, itself, is a diagnosis with many different etiologies, but it restricts the location of the abnormality to the inner hair cell and its afferent auditory nerve fibers. Furthermore, there are clear diagnostic criteria for the disorder and, as reviewed in Chapter 15, we are slowly feeling our way toward management protocols. Some patients can be helped with cochlear implants but others cannot. Other distinct syndromes within the category of CAPD probably exist. We need to find objective ways to diagnose them.

TINNITUS

In this book, we have been concerned mainly with the negative symptoms of the auditory system: elevated thresholds and decreased discrimination. Auditory EPs have become very helpful in objectively assessing the degree of hearing loss and in localizing the causes of this loss. We have not paid attention to the positive symptoms of auditory system. One of the great unclaimed prizes is an objective measurement of tinnitus.

The nature of tinnitus is not known. The basic pathophysiology likely is related to increased firing and synchrony in auditory neurons following the removal of afferent input—"neuronal hyperactivity due to loss of afferent inhibition" (Eggermont, 2007). Although the trigger point may be anywhere the in the auditory system, the final effects will cause changes in the topographical organization of the cortex and in the firing patterns of its neurons. Tinnitus is subjective and its treatment can never be divorced from psychological factors (Noble & Tyler, 2007). Nevertheless, new treatments may be possible with transcranial magnetic stimulation (Kleinjung, Vielsmeier, Landgrebe, Hajak, & Langguth, 2008) or acoustic manipulations of the auditory input (Okamoto, Stracke, Stoll, &, Pantev, 2010).

The auditory EPs in patients with tinnitus show complex results. The electrical N1 of the LAEP is smaller than in control patients (Attias, Urbach, Gold, & Shemesh, 1993; Jacobson & McCaslin, 2003). However, magnetic studies indicate that the N1 may be larger in the right hemisphere in patients with tinnitus (Weisz, Wienbruch, Dohrmann, & Ebert, 2005). The 40-Hz auditory steady state response (ASSR) in patients with tinnitus has a higher threshold, a larger amplitude, and an abnormal source distribution compared to normal subjects (Wienbruch, Paul, Weisz, Elbert, & Roberts, 2006). Another recent study evaluated subjects with tinnitus using ASSRs to multiple simultaneous tones amplitude-modulated at rates near 40 Hz (Diesch, Andermann, Flor, & Rupp, 2010). Normal subjects showed a decrease the response amplitude when three stimuli with different carrier frequencies were presented simultaneously compared to when the stimuli were presented separately. Subjects with tinnitus showed an increase in amplitude during simultaneous stimulation. These results suggest decreased lateral inhibition in the auditory cortex in tinnitus.

CORTICAL PLASTICITY

One of the characteristics of the auditory cortex is its plasticity. This can occur over both short (Weinberger, 2007) and long time periods (Irvine, Rajan, & McDermott, 2000). In the short term, we can adapt our perceptions to the context of what we are listening to, and in the long term, we can learn to hear sounds we have not previously understood. Plasticity also may underlie some of our abnormal perceptions. Certain types of tinnitus may relate to de-afferented regions of the cortex becoming activated by other input.

Plasticity is the basis for the infant developing into an adult with speech and language. A wealth of information can be gained from studying the ERPs of children (Stevens & Neville, 2009). Studying how the brain changes during development should help us understand how the adult brain does what it does—watching how a machine is put together can help us to understand how it works. Recording the auditory EPs of children as they are learning to produce and perceive speech should help us see how speech and language work in the adult brain.

As well as showing how the brain learns about the world, ERP studies of children also may demonstrate how the world can affect the brain's ability to learn. Children of lower socioeconomic status do not attend to the world in the same way as more privileged children (D'Anguilli, Herdman, Stapells, & Hertzman, 2008; Stevens, Lauinger, & Neville, 2009).

Music is another intriguing area of study. Almost everybody learns to perceive a spoken language but only some individuals go on to learn as much about the sounds of music as normal people know about their mother tongue. The brain of the musician becomes different from that of the nonmusician (Dalla Bella et al., 2009; Tervaniemi, 2003). Auditory EPs can describe some of these differences and show how they develop.

Plasticity occurs in adult brains as well as developing brains (Eggermont, 2008). Our aging auditory cortex must learn to cope with input that is much less precise than when all our hair cells were exactly tuned and all our neurons rapidly responsive. Auditory EPs can show both the decreased amount of sensory information reaching the cortex (Tremblay & Burkard, 2007), and the compensatory mechanisms brought to bear to ensure that perception still occurs (Alain, McDonald Ostroff, & Schneider, 2004). Much can be learned from how elderly brains adapt to their own deterioration and still develop wisdom.

THE INTERACTIVE BRAIN

Over the past few decades, the way in which we look at the brain has changed. We no longer consider the brain in terms of discrete centers, each responsible for specific processes. The neurons of the brain—cortical neurons, in particular—function as an interacting network. The meaning is not in the centers but in the connections between them. Thus, we may be mistaken in trying to localize discrete sources for the electrical events that we record from the scalp. We need a much greater understanding of how networks of interacting neurons might create electric fields.

Over recent years, we have become more aware of cross-modal processing, auditory cortex processing visual information and visual cortex processing auditory information (Schroeder, Lakatos, Smiley, & Hackett, 2007). Sensory systems do not work in isolation. An obvious demonstration occurs when we see the mouth moving differently from what we might expect from the sounds we hear (Sams et al., 1991; Sams, Möttönen, & Sihvonen, 2005). What we hear is affected by what we see.

An interactive brain functions through its connections. One way to transfer information in a network involves the rhythmic synchronization between neurons. These activities generate the rhythms that make up the electroencephalogram (EEG). In this book, we considered the EEG mainly as noise to be removed so that we can measure the specific responses to stimuli. What we have considered as noise may be more meaningful than we thought. However, exactly how to examine these rhythms remains to be determined.

FAREWELL

I have had my say—the book is done. This final chapter has asked many questions and provided no answers. Nevertheless, if you have read through the rest of the book, you should have a good understanding of the principles for recording and interpreting auditory EPs. It is now time to learn more about what we do not know by studying these waveforms in the laboratory or in the clinic. Once you finish reading, you must begin to live. Life is learning.

ABBREVIATIONS

ASSR Auditory steady-state response

CAPD Central auditory processing disorder

EEG Electroencephalogram

EP Evoked potential

LAEP Late auditory evoked potential

PMN Phonological mapping negativity

REFERENCES

Alain, C., McDonald, K. L., Ostroff, J. M., & Schneider, B. (2004). Aging: A switch from automatic to controlled processing of sounds? *Psychology and Aging, 19*, 125–133.

Attias, J., Urbach, D., Gold, S., & Shemesh, Z. (1993) Auditory event related potentials in chronic tinnitus patients with noise induced hearing loss. *Hearing Research, 71,* 106–113.

Cacace, A. T., & McFarland, D. J. (Eds.). (2009). *Controversies in central auditory processing disorder.* San Diego, CA: Plural Publishing.

Charest, I., Pernet,.C. R., Rousselet, G. A., Quinones, I., Latinus, M., Fillion-Bilodeau, S., Chartrand J-P., & Belin, P. (2009). Electrophysiological evidence for an early processing of human voices. *BMC Neuroscience, 10,* 127.

Connolly, J. F., & Phillips, N. A., 1994. Event-related potential components reflect phonological and semantic processing of the terminal word of spoken sentences. *Journal of Cognitive Neuroscience, 6,* 256–266.

Dalla Bella, S., Kraus, N., Overy K., Pantev, C., Snyder , J. S., Tervaniemi, M., . . . Schlaug, G. (2009). *The neurosciences and music III: Disorders and plasticity, Annals of the New York Academy of Sciences, Vol. 1169.* New York, NY: Wiley.

D'Angiulli, A., Herdman, A., Stapells, D., & Hertzman, C. (2008). Children's event-related potentials of auditory selective attention vary with their socioeconomic status. *Neuropsychology, 22,* 293–300.

Dawes, P., & Bishop, D. (2009). Auditory processing disorder in relation to developmental disorders of language, communication and attention: A review and critique. *International Journal of Language and Communication Disorders, 44,* 440–465.

Diesch, E., Andermann, M., Flor, H., & Rupp, A. (2010). Interaction among the components of multiple auditory steady-state responses: Enhancement in tinnitus patients, inhibition in controls. *Neuroscience, 167,* 540–553.

Eggermont, J. J. (2007). Pathophysiology of tinnitus. *Progress in Brain Research, 166,* 19–35.

Eggermont, J. J. (2008). The role of sound in adult and developmental auditory cortical plasticity. *Ear and Hearing, 29,* 819–829.

Gunji, A., Koyama, S., Ishii, R., Levy, D., Okamoto, H., Kakigi, R., & Pantev, C. (2003). Magnetoencephalographic study of the cortical activity elicited by human voice. *Neuroscience Letters, 348,* 13–16.

Irvine, D. R., Rajan, R., & McDermott, H. J. (2000). Injury-induced reorganization in adult auditory cortex and its perceptual consequences. *Hearing Research, 147,* 188–199.

Jacobson, G. P., & McCaslin, D. L. (2003). A re-examination of the long latency N1 response in patients with tinnitus. *Journal of the American Academy of Audiology, 14,* 393–400.

Kleinjung, T., Vielsmeier, V., Landgrebe, M., Hajak, G., & Langguth, B. (2008). Transcranial magnetic stimulation: A new diagnostic and therapeutic tool for tinnitus patients. *International Tinnitus Journal, 14,* 112–118.

Krishnan, A., Xu, Y., Gandour, J., & Cariani, P. (2005). Encoding of pitch in the human brainstem is sensitive to language experience. *Cognitive Brain Research, 25,* 161–168.

Kutas, M., & Hillyard, S. A. (1980). Reading senseless sentences: brain potentials reflect semantic incongruity. *Science, 207,* 203–205.

Kutas, M., & Van Petten, C. (1994). Psycholinguistics electrified: Event-related potential investigations. In: M. A. Gernsbacher (Ed.), *Handbook of psycholinguistics* (pp. 83–143). New York, NY: Academic Press.

Kutas, M., Van Petten, C., & Kluender, R. (2006). Psycholinguistics electrified II: 1994–2005. In M. Traxler & M. A. Gernsbacher (Eds.), *Handbook of psycholinguistics* (2nd ed., pp. 659–724). New York, NY: Elsevier.

Levy, D. A., Granot, R., & Bentin, S. (2001). Processing specificity for human voice stimuli: Electrophysiological evidence. *NeuroReport, 12,* 2653–2657.

Levy, D. A., Granot, R., & Bentin, S. (2003). Neural sensitivity to human voices: ERP evidence of task and attentional influences. *Psychophysiology, 40,* 291–305.

Newman, R. L., & Connolly, J. F. (2009). Electrophysiological markers of pre-lexical speech processing: Evidence for bottom-up and top-down effects on spoken word processing. *Biological Psychology, 80,* 114–121.

Noble, W., & Tyler, R. S. (2007). Physiology and phenomenology of tinnitus: Implications for treatment. *International Journal of Audiology, 46,* 569–574.

Okamoto, H., Stracke, H., Stoll, W., & Pantev, C. (2010). Listening to tailor-made notched music reduces tinnitus loudness and tinnitus-related auditory cortex activity. *Proceedings of the National Academy of Science (USA). 107,* 1207–1210.

Rogier, O., Roux, S., Belin, P., Bonnet-Brilhault, F., & Bruneau, N. (2010). An electrophysiological correlate of voice processing in 4- to 5-year-old children. *International Journal of Psychophysiology, 75,* 44–47.

Sams, M., Aulanko, R., Hämäläinen, M., Hari, R., Lounasmaa, O. V., Lu, S. T., & Simola, J.

(1991). Seeing speech: visual information from lip movements modifies activity in the human auditory cortex. *Neuroscience Letters, 127*, 141–145.

Sams, M., Möttönen, R., & Sihvonen, T. (2005). Seeing and hearing others and oneself talk. *Cognitive Brain Research, 23*, 429–435.

Schroeder, C. E. Lakatos, P., Smiley, J., & Hackett, T. A. (2007). How and why is auditory processing shaped by multisensory convergence. In R. F. Burkard, M. Don, & J. J. Eggermont (Eds.), *Auditory evoked potentials: Basic principles and clinical applications* (pp. 441–462). Baltimore, MD: Lippincott Williams & Wilkins.

Skoe, E., & Kraus, N. (2010) Auditory brain stem response to complex sounds: A tutorial. *Ear and Hearing, 31*, 302–324.

Stevens, C., Lauinger, B., & Neville, H. (2009). Differences in the neural mechanisms of selective attention in children from different socioeconomic backgrounds: An event-related brain potential study. *Developmental Science, 12*, 634–646.

Stevens, C., & Neville, H. (2009). Profiles of development and plasticity in human neurocognition. In M. Gazzaniga (Ed.), *The cognitive neurosciences IV* (pp. 165–181). Cambridge, MA: MIT Press.

Tervaniemi, M. (2003). Cortical representations for music sounds–EEG and MEG evidence. In I. Peretz & R. J. Zatorre (Eds.), *Cognitive neuroscience of music* (pp. 294–309). Oxford, UK: Oxford University Press.

Tremblay, K. L., & Burkard, R. F. (2007). The aging auditory system. In R. F. Burkard, M. Don, & J. J. Eggermont (Eds.), *Auditory evoked potentials: Basic principles and clinical application* (pp. 403–425). Philadelphia, PA: Lippincott Williams & Wilkins.

Weinberger, N. M. (2007). Auditory associative memory and representational plasticity in the primary auditory cortex. *Hearing Research, 229*, 54–68.

Weisz, N., Wienbruch, C., Dohrmann, K., & Elbert, T. (2005) Neuromagnetic indicators of auditory cortical reorganization of tinnitus. *Brain, 28*: 2722–2731.

Wienbruch, C., Paul, I., Weisz, N., Elbert, T. & Roberts, L.E. (2006) Frequency organization of the 40-Hz auditory steady-state response in normal hearing and in tinnitus. *NeuroImage, 33*, 180–194.

Index

Notes: Two- and three-word expressions are generally indexed by the initial word ("facial nerve" rather than "nerve, facial"), unless the last term is clearly more important ("attention, selective" rather than "selective attention"). The most prominent components of the different auditory evoked potentials a (such as Pa and N1) are indexed separately. Names beginning with numeric expressions (e.g., "40-Hz response") are listed at the beginning. Roman numerals (the peaks of the auditory brainstem response) follow Arabic numerals.

(±) reference, also known as (±) average, 38, 157–159

40-Hz response
  absence in infants, 18–19, 297
  aging, 297–299
  amplitude, 297–298
  anesthesia, 301–302
  apparent latency, 293–294, 297–298, 300
  attention, 302–303
  choice of stimuli, 320
  carrier frequency, 303–304
  development, 297, 299
  electrical stimuli (cochlear implant), 589–590
  frequency of maximum amplitude, 297–298
  hemispheric asymmetry, 295, 303
  intensity, 310
  mechanisms, 18–19, 293–295
  MEG studies, 299, 304
  minute rhythms, 302
  multiple simultaneous stimuli, 308, 314
  relation to MLR, 18–19, 293–295, 299
  sleep, 300–301
  sources, 295
  temporal integration, 310–311
  thresholds, 312–314
  tinnitus, 604–605
  tuning curve, 304–308
80-Hz response
  aging, 299
  anesthesia, 302
  apparent latency, 291, 293,
  attention, 303
  carrier frequency, 303–304
  choice of stimuli, 320
  infants, 19, 297, 299
  intensity, 310, 312–313
  multiple simultaneous stimuli, 175–177, 308–310
  sedatives, 302
  sleep, 300–301
  SNR, 300, 316–320
  temporal integration, 310–311
  thresholds, 308, 314–320
  tuning curve, 304–308

I (ABR), *See also* Compound action potential
  abnormal in auditory neuropathy, 536
  acoustic neuroma, 501–503
  intensity, 222, 228–234
  intracranial recordings, 109
  latency, 219, 228–230
  optimum stimulus rate, 172–173
  recorded from external auditory meatus, 214, 222
  relation to eI of EABR, 579–580
  relation to N1 of ECochG, 214
  stimulus polarity, 222
  stimulus rate, 222
I' (ABR), 216

II (ABR), 88, 99–100
III (ABR)
  acoustic neuroma, 501–503
  components, 216
  contralateral vs. ipsilateral recordings,
    216–217, 468–469
  intracranial recordings, 109
  Lissajous trajectory, 218–219
  scalp distribution, 215–216
  stimulus rate, 234–235
IV (ABR)
  intracranial recordings, 109
  lemniscal pathways, 111
  morphology of IV–V complex, 221–222
V (ABR)
  acoustic neuroma, 501–503
  amplitude measurement, 219–220
  anesthetics, 237
  contralateral vs. ipsilateral recordings,
    216–217, 468–469
  filter effects, 220
  gender, 220, 235–237
  head size, 236
  infancy, 14, 238–240
  intensity, 14, 222, 228–234
  intracranial recordings, 109
  latency-intensity functions, 229–233
  lemniscal pathways, 111
  maximum length sequences, 235, 252
  morphology of IV–V complex, 221–222
  neck reference electrode, 222
  normative data, 219–222
  notched noise, 228–229
  optimum stimulus rate, 172–173
  relation to eV of EABR, 579–581
  sleep, 237
  sedatives, 237
  spectrum, 27–28
  stimulus rate, 14, 222, 234–235
  temperature, 237
  threshold, 128–130, 231
  tone, 228–229
  undermasking, 487–498

A

ABR, *See* Auditory brainstem response
Accessory nerve (also known as spinal
    accessory nerve), 264, 268, 271

Acetylcholine, 257, 259
Acoustic calibration
  brief stimuli, 126–128
  infant-adult differences, 462
  intensity measurements, 126–128
  issues in infants, 460–463
  spectral measurements, *See* Acoustic
    spectrum
Acoustic change complex, 336, 340
Acoustic coupler, 124–126, 482
Acoustic delay (ear inserts), 125, 286, 288,
    537–538
Acoustic neuroma, 88, 500–510
  ABR patterns, 501–503
  intraoperative monitoring, 506–509
  mechanisms of hearing loss during
    surgery, 506
  MRI, 502–503
  neurofibromatosis, 501
  stacked ABR, 138–140, 503–505
  VEMP, 275, 523
Acoustic spectrum
  2–1–2 tone, 131–132, 471
  amplitude modulation, 142
  beats, 142
  chirps, 141
  derived response technique, 137–138
  envelope effects, 131–132
  exponential modulation, 142
  frequency modulation, 142
  skirts (spread of energy), 131–132, 136, 228
  tone in notched noise, 136
Acoustic tumors, 138–140, 500–510, *See also*
    Acoustic neuroma
Action potential (AP), *See also* Compound
    action potential (CAP)
  auditory neuropathy, 555
  conduction block, 511–512
  generation, 95–96
  muscle fiber, 259
  saltatory conduction, 96, 510–512
  voltage sensitive channels, 95, 512
AD, *See* Analog-to-digital
Adaptation, *See* Selective adaptation
Adrenoleukodystrophy, 516–517
Aging,
  ABR, 240
  ASSR, 297–300
  LAEP, 378, 431–433

MLR, 254
VEMP, 275
Aliasing, 34, 36, 287–288
Alps (Bernese), 214
Alzheimer's disease, 259, 433–435
AM, *See* Amplitude modulation
Amp, 94
Amplifiers, 31
  Common-mode rejection, 31
  differential, 31
  at electrodes, 29
  input impedance, 197
  inverting and noninverting input, 31
Amplitude
  measurement, 45–46
  replications, 182–183
  spectrum, 61–63
  unbiased estimate, 162
Amplitude-intensity function
  ASSR, 82, 313
  CAP, 13, 203
  ECAP, 584–586
  LAEP, 344, 374
  MLR, 254
  SP, 374
Amplitude-modulation (AM), 140–143
  acoustic spectra, 142
  broadband noise, 143
  exponential, 141–142, 320, 474
Analog-to-digital (AD) conversion, 34–37
  amplitude resolution, 36–37
  frequency resolution, 36
  recommended settings, 35
Anatomy
  auditory cortex, 92–94
  brain, 88–94
  brainstem, 88–92
  cerebellopontine angle, 507
  ear, 189–194
Anesthesia, 254–257
  40-Hz response, 301–302
  ABR, 237, 256
  ASSR, 301–302
  end–tidal concentration, 255–256
  goals, 254–255
  intra-operative awareness, 254, 301–302
  MLR, 255–257
Animal EP studies, 7, 9, 20, 109–112
Anterior cingulate cortex, 425–426

Anticipation, 415–416
AP, *See* Action potential
Apex (cochlea), 134, 190, 580–581, 584
Apparent latency, 64, 73–75
  40-Hz response, 293–294, 297–298
  80-Hz response 293–294
  envelope following responses, 291,
    293–294
  graphic analysis, 74
  problems of interpretation, 75
Area measurements, 46
Artifact, 9, 49–54
  blink, 50, 52–53, 347
  classification, 49–50
  electrical stimulus (ECAP recording),
    206–207, 584–585
  electrocardiogram, 51
  imaging, 51
  independent component analysis, 54, 590
  muscle, 54
  ocular, 52–54
  pulse 51
  rejection, 40–41, 577–578
  rider, 54
  source components, 52–54
  stimulus, 52, 125–126, 158, 288
  tongue, 50
ASSR, *See* Auditory steady state response
Atmospheric tide, 37
Attention, 14–18, 399–438
  ABR, 237–238, 400–402
  active and passive, 406
  architecture, 429
  control, 399
  dichotic listening, 403–415
  differentiation from phasic arousal,
    400–403
  direction, 399
  divided, 406
  expectant, 415–418
  FFR, 237–238
  fMRI, 409–410
  frontal negativity, 415
  LAEPs, 399–438
  MLR, 254, 400–402
  MMN, 410–414
  Nd, 405–410
  P3, 424–426
  parasol, 408

Attention *(continued)*
  Pd, 408–409
  selective, 403–415
  socioeconomic status, 605
  spotlight, 399
  stimulus set vs. response set, 14–15, 405, 407
  strategy, 399
  supervisory, 427–429
  switching, 400
  target discrimination, 400–402
Attention deficit disorder, 604
Audera instrument, 315, 318–319
Audiogram, *See also* Thresholds
  acoustic neuroma, 500
  ascending, 539
  auditory neuropathy, 538–539
  estimating from EP thresholds, 179–182
  Ménière's disease, 494
  multiple sclerosis, 515–516
  tent-shaped audiogram, 538–539
Audiological evaluation of infant, 465–485
  acoustic transducers, 466
  ASSR, 472–477
  auditory neuropathy, 480–481
  bone-conduction, 477, 479–481
  click-ABRs, 467–470
  genetic evaluation, 482
  hearing aids, 482–485
  LAEPs, 377, 450, 452, 484
  OAEs, 478–480
  PAM reflexes, 269, 481
  pneumatic otoscopy, 465, 480, 482
  protocols, 479–482
  referral from screening, 457–458, 465–467
  threshold evaluation, 466–467
  time available, 466
  tone-ABRs, 470–473, 477
  tympanometry, 466, 477–478
Auditory brainstem pathways, 88–91
Auditory brainstem response (ABR), 2, 213–241,
    See also specific waves (I, II, III, IV, V)
  acoustic neuroma, 501–503
  aging, 240
  anesthetics, 237, 508–509
  animal studies, 109–110
  anoxia, 464
  attention, 237, 400–402

auditory neuropathy, 535–539
basilar membrane length, 236
binaural interaction component, 143–144
bone-conducted stimuli, 477
chirps, 140–141
chloral hydrate, 466
coma, 520
contralateral vs. ipsilateral recordings,
    216–217, 468–469
delayed maturation, 464, 544, 559
derived responses, 222–225
ear asymmetry, 219
early recordings, 11–15
early vestibular response, 543
electrical ABR, 547, 576–583, *See also* main
    entry
filter settings, 35, 215, 248, 250
gap, 240
gender, 220, 235–237
head size, 236
hydrocephalus, 469–470
identification of peaks, 213–214, 220–222
infants, 14, 238–240, 467–473
intensity, 14, 228–234
interpeak latencies, 219–220, 240
intracranial recordings, 109–110
intraoperative monitoring, 506–509
lesion studies, 111
Lissajous trajectory, 217–219
maximum length sequences, 173–175, 235,
    239, 251–252, 471
multiple sclerosis, 512–516
normative data, 219–222, 239–240
power spectrum ABR, 504–505
premature infants, 239, 464
rate, 14, 234–235, 239, 471, 513–514
recognition, 165
recording parameters, 35, 471
scalp topography, 215–219, 239
sedatives, 237, 468
sleep, 237
SOA, 14, 234–235, 239, 471, 513–514
spectrum, 27–28
speech, 148–149, 290, 602
stacked ABR, 138–140, 503–505
stimulus polarity, 226–227
temperature, 237, 508–509
threshold, 128–130, 231–234, 472–473

tone, 227–229, 470–473
warp–averaging, 184, 214, 221
Auditory cortex, 92–94
core, belt and parabelt, 92–93
development of N1 (LAEP), 377, 384
dipole tracking, 349, 382
dipoles, 103–106
electrophysiology, 103–106, 380–381
fMRI, 92, 380
hemispheric asymmetry, 92
LAEPs, 380–381
latency, 361
lateral inhibition, 384
progressive excitation, 349,
patchwork activation, 381–382
pulsatile activation, 381–382
tonotopicity, 92–94, 248–249
what and where processing streams, 92,
94, 380–382, 386
Auditory nerve (also known as cochlear
nerve)
action potentials, 194, 555
anatomy, 88–91,190, 507
afferent fibers, 191, 193
cochlear nerve action potential
(intracranial), 506–508
compound action potential, *See* main entry
efferent fibers , *See also* Olivocochlear
bundle, 193–194
MRI evaluation, 502–503, 505, 542
myelin, 549
post-stimulus-time histograms for afferent
fibers, 223, 225
potentials, *See* Compound action potential,
I, II
stimulus polarity, 225–226
Auditory neuropathy, 535–559
ABRs, 535–539
animal models, 551
arachnoid cyst, 544
ASSRs, 540
audiogram, 538–239
axonopathy, 550
caloric testing, 540–541
central auditory processing disorder,
544–545, 604
CM, 535–539, 547–548, 559
cochlear implants, 547, 550, 558–559

condensation and rarefaction clicks,
537–539,542–543
contralateral suppression of OAEs,
540–541
course of the disorder, 542
delayed maturation of ABR, 464, 544, 559
diagnosis, 536–542
differential diagnosis, 542–545
dys-synchrony, 536
ECochG, 545–547
electrical ABR, 547, 577
etiologies, 550–553
FM system, 558
genetic abnormalities, 551–553
hearing aids, 544, 558–559
history, 536–537
infants, 457–458, 464, 547–548
LAEPs, 540
management, 558–559
middle ear muscle reflexes, 540
MLRs, 540
MRI of auditory nerve, 542
myelinopathy, 550
neonatal intensive care unit, 457–458, 548
neuronal depletion, 554–555
neuronal desynchrony, 554–555
newborn hearing screening, 457–458, 464,
547
nomenclature, 536
OAEs, 535–539, 547–548, 550, 559
otoferlin, 545, 551–552
pathogenesis, 548–544
perceptual consequences, 554–558
peripheral neuropathy, 541–542, 552
prematurity, 548
presynaptic vs. postsynaptic, 545–547
prevalence, 547–548
progression, 550
silent talking, 558
SP, 537–539
spectrum disorder, 536
speech perception, 538, 554–556
temperature–sensitivity, 551–553
temporal bone studies, 554–555
unilateral, 548
Auditory object, 124, 349–350, 368–370, 407
Object-related negativity, 349–350
relation to Nd, 407

Auditory pathways, 88–91
Auditory steady state response (ASSR), 285–325. *See also* 40-Hz response and 80-Hz response
  aging, 297–299
  Amplitude-modulated white noise, 459
  anesthesia, 301–302
  auditory neuropathy, 540
  binaural masking level difference, 296
  binaural stimuli, 296
  bone conducted stimuli, 477
  compared to transient, 72, 289
  chloral hydrate, 466
  development in children, 297–298
  early recordings, 18–19
  electrical stimuli (cochlear implant), 589–590
  exponential amplitude modulation, 474
  harmonics, 296
  infants, 472–477
  intensity, 310, 312–313
  interaural correlation, 143–145
  interaural timing, 143–145
  mechanisms, 18–19, 293–295
  model for rate-effects, 293–295
  modulation frequency, 290–297
  multiple simultaneous stimuli (MASTER), 175–177, 308–310
  newborn infants, 452, 456, 458–459
  phase-weighting, 165–167
  relation to transient EPs, 18–19, 296
  rate, 290–297
  sleep, 19–20, 300–301
  slow rates, 295
  sources, 115, 295
  SNR, 161–167, 316–320
  spectrogram, 70–71
  speech–weighted noise, 295
  superimposition of transient responses, 18–19
  temporal integration, 310–311
  thresholds, 130, 312–320, 472–477
  tinnitus, 604–605
  tonotopicity, 92–94
  tuning curve, 304–308
Augmenting-reducing, 344
Autocorrelation techniques, 165, 321
Automatic processing, *See* Bottom–up processing

Averaging, 25, 37–41
  assumptions, 37
  coherent, 75–76
  induced activity, 65–66
  initial application to EPs, 9
  latency jitter, 37–39
  recommended number of trials, 35
  selective or sorted, 40–41
  spectral averaging, 75–76
  square–root rule, 37
  weighted, 40, 231
Axon, 88–91, 95–97
  hillock, 95–97
  terminals, 101
  multiple sclerosis, 510–512

B

Basilar membrane, 133–134, 139, 191
  activation pattern, 134, 136, 138–140, 303–304, 306–307, 306, 308–309
  frequency, 131, 134, 308–309
  gender differences, 236–237
  length, 134
  Ménière's disease, 494–495, 497
  perilymphatic fistula, 500
Bayesian probability, 425
Beats, 142–143, 292
BERAphone, 459–460
Bereitschaftspotential (also known as readiness potential), 415–416
BESA, *See* Brain Electric Source Analysis
Binaural interaction component, 143–145
Binaural masking level difference, 296, 517
Binaural stimulation, 143–147, 296, 301
Bipolar affective disorder, 258
Blackman envelope, 132, 273
Blink, 50, 52–54, 277, 347
Blink reflex, 268, 277
Bone conduction, 125–126
  ABR, 233, 456, 464, 477–481
  ASSR, 315, 477–481
  infants, 460–461
  VEMP, 273, 275
Bonferroni correction, 160, 177–178
Bottom-up processing, 337, 387, 414
Brain Electric Source Analysis (BESA), 113–116
  ASSR, 295

LAEP, 116
MLR, 113
Brainstem tumors, 510
Broca's area, 93
Butler paradigm, 354–359
Butterfly plot, 44

C

Caloric testing, 275, 494, 540–541
CAP, *See* Compound action potential
CAPD, *See* Central auditory processing disorder
Caregiver concern (about infant hearing loss), 463–464
Central auditory processing disorder (CAPD), 603–604
  differentiation from auditory neuropathy, 543–544, 604
  relation to attention deficit disorder, 604
Central pontine myelinolysis, 519
Cerebellopontine angle, 99
  intraoperative monitoring, 506–509
  tumors, *See also* Acoustic neuroma, 500–510
  view through operating microscope, 507
Cerebrospinal fluid, 88, 98–100, 109, 112, 192, 510, 519
CHAMP, *See* Cochlear Hydrops Analysis Masking Procedure
Change, *See also* onset response, 2, 335–342
  change-1 vs. change-2, 340, 385
  level, 340
  rate of change, 338
  rest-motion, 337–338
Characteristic frequency, 133, 135, 223, 225, 304–308
Charcot-Marie-Tooth disease, 464, 542, 552, 554
Chirps, 140–141, 266, 320
Circular T^2, 161–163
C–level, *See* Maximum comfort level
Click, 124, 126–127
  alternating, 199, 203
  condensation and rarefaction, 197–198, 215, 225–227, 272, 536–539, 542–543, 546, 553
  normal behavioral thresholds, 128
  spectrum, 126

CM, *See* Cochlear microphonic
CNAP, *See* Cochlear nerve action potential
CNV, *See* Contingent negative variation
Cochlear amplifier, 134, 192, 549–550
Cochlear delay, 134, 138, 139, 204, 223, 348
Cochlear Hydrops Analysis Masking Procedure (CHAMP), 497–499
Cochlear implant, 206–208, 569–595
  amplitude resolution, 573
  antenna, 571–572, 575
  auditory neuropathy, 547, 550, 558–559, 570
  channels, 573–575
  components, 570–576
  continuous interleaved sampling, 574–575
  cost–effectiveness, 569
  current pulses, 574–575
  device integrity check, 578
  EABR, 578–583, *See also* main entry
  ECAP, 206–208, 583–587, *See also* main entry
  ELAEP, 590–594, *See also* main entry
  EMLR, 587–590, *See also* main entry
  external processor, 570–575
  facial nerve stimulation, 578
  frequency resolution, 573–574
  learning, 595
  location of electrode in cochlea, 549, 573, 576
  map, 572, 586–587
  MMN, 591–594
  multiple-contact electrode array, 569, 571–576
  "n of m" strategy, 575
  otosclerosis, 578
  P300, 594
  radio-frequency transmission, 206, 571–572, 575
  speech perception, 554–556, 591, 595
  stimulus programming, 573–575, 581–582, 585–587
  telemetry, 572, 575, 583–586
  time in sound, 591–592
  turning on, 586
Cochlear microphonic (CM), 197–199
  auditory neuropathy, 198, 535–539, 547–548
  differentiation from CAP, 197–199
  differentiation from FFR, 228, 286

Cochlear microphonic (CM) *(continued)*
   generation in hair cells, 193, 287
   initial human recordings, 7
   masking, 197
Cochlear nerve, *See* Auditory nerve
Cochlear nerve action potential (CNAP),
   intraoperative recordings, 506–508
Cochlear nucleus, 88–91, 117, 501, 506–507
Cochlear promontory, 195–196, 545–547
Cocktail party problem, 403–415
Coherence, 80, 161–163, 164
Coma, 518–520
Common mode rejection, 31
Components, 6–7, 45–49, 336–337, 403–405
   endogenous and exogenous, 10–11, 336
   independent component analysis, 49
   mesogenous, 336
   principal component analysis, 47–49
   source components, 45–49, 112–116, 405
Compound action potential (CAP), 2, 98–100,
      194, 202–203
   auditory neuropathy, 545–547
   differentiation from summating potential, 6
   ear asymmetry, 202
   electrical (ECAP), 206–208, *See also* main
      entry
   frequency, 204
   gender, 202
   intensity, 202–204
   intracranial (cochlear nerve action
      potential), 506–508
   stimulus polarity, 204, 495, 497
   stimulus rate, 197–198, 204
   threshold estimation, 203–204
   tuning curve, 204–206
Computers (for averaging), 9
Concatenation, 75–76
Conditioned orientation response
      audiometry, 452
Conductance, 94
Conduction block, 511–512
Confidence limits, *See* Normal limits
Connexin, 465, 581
Consciousness, 428, 438, 518–520
Consonant, 148–149, 321, 371–372
Contingent negative variation (CNV), 415–416
   component structure, 415
   initial recordings, 10
   orientation and expectancy waves, 415

Controlled processing, *See* Top–down
      processing,
Contour plot, 44–45, 48, 53, 79
Convolution, 223
Corollary discharge, 417–418
Correlation, 40–41, 84, 158, 177–178, 266, 286,
      323–324
Corti, *See* Organ of Corti
Cortical plasticity, 605
C-level (also known as maximum comfort
      level), 570, 581–582
C-process, 339–340
Criterion (statistical), 155–156, 168–171
   problems with multiple tests, 177–178
Cross-modal processing, 606
CU, *See* Current unit
Curare, 247
Current, 94
   cochlear implant stimuli, 575
   sources and sinks, 95, 98, 101–106
Current source density, 45
Current unit (CU) (cochlear implant), 575,
      579, 585, 587

D

Debriefing, 403
Decision, 167–171
   criterion, 155–156, 168–171
   problems with multiple tests, 177–178
Deconvolution, 175, 251
Definitions for EP terms, 1–2
Degrees of freedom, 158–159, 161, 165
Dementia, 433–435
Demyelinating lesions, 510–517, *See also*
      Multiple sclerosis
Dendrite, 88, 95–96
   apical, 101–106
Dendritic potential (DP) in ECochG, 546
Derived responses,
   ABR, 137–140, 222–225, 503–505
   ASSR, 307–308
   center frequency, 138
   latency-intensity functions (ABR), 223–224
   stacked ABR, 138–140, 503–505
Dieter's cells, 191
Difference waveforms, 46–47
   attend-ignore, 15, 405–410
   condensation and rarefaction, 197–198, 289

initial use, 15–17
integrated difference waveform, 160
negative difference waveform (Nd), 15, 405–410
positive difference waveform (Pd), 408–409
SNR issues, 159–161
target-standard, 17, 411
Diffusion tensor imaging, 518
Dipole, 97–98
  equivalent, 103–104
  layer, 103–104
  MEG current dipole , 108
  radial and tangential, 108
  stationary, 99–100
Dishabituation, 352–353
Disinhibition, 254, 378
Distortion products,
  OAEs, 194–195, 456–457, 469, 478–479, 481, 537–538
  FFR, 288
DP, *See* Dendritic potential
DPOAE, *See* Otoacoustic emissions, Distortion product
Dynamic causal modeling, 385
Dynamic time warping, 183–184, 221, 588

E

eII, eIII, eV, 6, 576–577, 579–580
EABR, *See* Electrical auditory brainstem response,
EAM, *See* External auditory meatus
Ear,
  anatomy, 189–193, 549, 571
  physiology, 189–208
Ear canal, *See* External auditory meatus
Ear inserts, 125–126, 195–196
  size in infants, 460–462
Early right anterior negativity, 373, 386
Early vestibular response, 543, 521–522, 543, 577, 583
Earphone, 124–126, 460–463
ECAP, *See* Electrical compound action potential
ECG, *See* Electrocardiogram
Echo (reverberation), 124, 253
ECochG, *See* Electrocochleogram
Echoic memory, 367, 383
EEG, *See* Electroencephalogram

Efference copy, 417
Efficiency, 171–179, 234–235, 319–320, 362–363
ELAEP, *See* Electrical late auditory evoked potential
Electrical auditory brainstem response (EABR)
  apical and basal electrodes, 580–581
  artifact, 576–579
  auditory neuropathy, 547
  changes with implant use, 582
  comparison to acoustic ABR, 579–581
  eII, eIII, eV, 576–577, 579–580
  electrodes, 576
  first recording from cochlear implant, 576
  latency-intensity function, 579–580
  pre- and intraoperative recordings, 582–583
  threshold, 581–582
  transtympanic, 576, 582–583
  stimuli, 576–578
  stimulus rate, 581
  vestibular response, 577, 583
Electrical compound action potential (ECAP)
  artifact, 206–207, 584–585
  amplitude-intensity function, 584–586
  changes with time, 586
  estimating T- and C-levels, 585–587
  latency-intensity function, 579, 584
  N1 wave (also known as eI), 579, 584–587
  stimulus artifacts, 206–208
  threshold, 584–585
Electrical late auditory evoked potentials (ELAEP), 590–594
  artifacts, 590
  development, 590–594
  latency, 590
  MEG, 590
  MMN, 591–594
  normal and abnormal N1, 591–593
  P1, 590–592
  P300, 594
  SOA, 590
  source analysis, 590
  time in sound, 591–592
Electrical middle-latency responses (EMLR), 587–589
  speech perception, 589
  use-dependent maturation, 588

Electrical stimuli,
  amplitude modulated sinusoid, 589–590
  cochlear implants, 570–576
  EABR, 576–583
  ECAP, 583–587
  ELAEP, 590–594
  EMLR, 587–590
  somatosensory, 6
  transtympanic, 547, 577, 582–583
  VEMP, 273, 523
Electric charge, 94
Electric fields, 87
  extracellular, 98–109
  open and closed, 102–103
Electrocardiogram (ECG)
  artifact, 51
Electrocochleogram (ECochG), 2, 189–208,
    See also components (cochlear
    microphonic; summating potential;
    compound action potential)
  auditory neuropathy, 545–547
  dendritic potential, 546
  initial human recordings 7, 11–13
  intra-operative monitoring, 208, 506–508
  Ménière's disease, 494–497
  promontory recordings, 545–546
  recording electrodes, 195–197
  round window recordings, 545–546
Electrode, 27–31
  active and reference, 31
  amplifier, 29
  butterfly (ECochG), 195
  fixation, 28–29
  golf club (round window), 195, 583
  impedance, 29, 197
  montage, 42
  needle (EMG), 260–261, 270
  nomenclature, 29–31
  pop, 29
  recommended, 35
  round window, 195, 583
  scalp location, 29–30
  transtympanic, 12, 195–197
  tympanic (tymptrode), 195–196
  reference, 42–43
  vertex, 10, 30
  virtual, 49
Electroencephalogram (EEG), 59
  anesthesia, 255

background noise for EP recording, 37,
    295–296, 606
  brain death, 518
  degenerative diseases in childhood, 517
  frequency components, 26
  initial recordings, 7–8
  isoelectric, 518
  rhythms, 26, 77, 606
  sleep, 251, 373, 375–376
Electromyogram (EMG)
  acoustic monitoring, 260, 274–275
  background levels for VEMP, 274–275
  background noise for EP recording, 37
  general principles, 259–262
EMG, *See* Electromyogram
EMLR, *See* Electrical middle–latency response
Endogenous components, 10–11, 336
Endolymph, 190–193
Endolymphatic hydrops, 199, 202, 494, *See
    also* Ménière's disease
Endplate, 259–261
End–tidal concentration (anesthetics), 255–256
Envelope-following response, 6, 83, 285–287,
    See also ASSR
  models, 294–295
  modulation frequency, 290–297
EP, *See* Evoked potential (auditory,
    somatosensory, or visual)
Epoch (also known as recording sweep)
  recommended settings, 35
EPSP, *See* Postsynaptic potential, excitatory
Equivocation, 422–424
ERD, *See* Event-related desynchronization
ERP, *See* Event-related potential
Error-related negativity (Ne), 425–426
Error-related positivity (Pe), 425–426
Errors (statistical), 167–171
  Type I and II, 167, 169–171
ERS, See Event-related synchronization
Eustachian tube, 190, 237
Event-related desynchronization (ERD), 2,
    69, 77–78
  alpha ERD, 78–79
  beta ERD, 78–79
Event-related potential (ERP), 2
Event-related synchronization (ERS), 2,
    69–72, 77–78
  alpha ERS, 78–79
  theta ERS, 78–79

Evoked potential audiometry, 453, *See also*
    Objective audiometry or thresholds
    ABR, 228–234, 465–472, 477
    ASSR, 312–320, 472–477
    ECochG, 203
    MLR, 251–254
    LAEP, 345–348
Evoked potential (EP), auditory (*See also* the
    different components such as auditory
    brainstem response, middle–latency
    response, late auditory evoked potential)
    classification, 2–4
    components, 6–7, 9–10
    early, 2–3
    historical recordings, 7–21
    nomenclature, 4–6, 9–10
    slow, 2–3, 5
Evoked potential (EP), somatosensory, 9
Evoked potential (EP), vestibular, 521–522,
    543, 577, 583
Evoked potential (EP), visual, 18, 175
Expectancy wave, 415, *See also* CNV
External auditory meatus (EAM, also called
    ear canal), 12, 190, 195–196, 215–216
    electrodes, 35, 195–197
    size in infants, 460–462
Exogenous components, 336
Eyeblink, *See* Blink
Eye movements, 53–54, *See also* Saccade
    roving, 269

F

Facial nerve, 88–89, 262, 264, 268–269,
    507–508
    monitoring in acoustic neuroma surgery,
    508
    stimulation in cochlear implant, 578–579
False alarm, *See* False positive
False discovery rate, 177
False negative (FN), 167–169
False positive (FP), 167–171
    ASSRs, 316
Far fields, 101
Fast Fourier Transform (FFT), 26, *See also*
    Fourier Transform
Feedback, 415–416, 425–426
FFR, *See* Frequency–following response
FFT, *See* Fast Fourier Transform

Fibrillation (muscle), 259–260
Fields, *See* Electric fields, Magnetic fields, or
    Far fields
Filters, 9, 31–34
    adaptive, 38–39, 432
    analog vs. digital, 33
    bandpass, 311
    notch, 32, 251
    optimum, 32, 215
    phase distortion, 33
    recommended settings, 34–35
    time-varying, 34
    Woody, 38–39
Flutter (sensation), 292–293
FM, *See* Frequency modulation
FM system, 558
Fmp, *See* F-ratio at multiple points
fMRI, *See* Functional magnetic resonance
    imaging
FN, *See* False negative
Following response, 285, *See also* Frequency-
    following response and Envelope-
    following response terminology
    speech-following responses, 321–324
Foramen of Luschka, 506–507
Formant, 124, 147–149, 321, 573
Forward solution, 87, 112,
Fourier analyzer, 81–83, 286, 290–293,
    321–322
Fourier Transform, 25–27, 60–64
    frequency resolution, 27, 60–61, 66–72
    Hanning window, 64, 67
    leakage, 64
    real and imaginary values, 27, 60–61
    short-term, 67–69
    spectrogram, 66–72
FP, *See* False positive
F-ratio at a single point (Fsp), 158–159
F-ratio at multiple points (Fmp), 159
F-test, 161–162, 171
Free-field speaker, 124
Frequency, 124
    ASSRs, 304
    LAEPs, 374
    place coding (labeled line), 191, 573
    SPs, 373–374
    temporal coding, 192
Frequency change, 337–338
Frequency domain, 25–27, 59–66, 161–167

Frequency modulation (FM), 141–142
ASSR, 296
Frequency-following response (FFR), 228,
286–290
attention, 237, 289–290
components, 288
differentiation from CM, 286
differentiation from transient response,
228, 289
distortion products, 288
early recordings, 14–15
frequency, 288–289
intensity, 288
speech, 148–149, 290
threshold, 288–289
vowels, 290
Frequency specificity, 131–132
relation to place specificity, 131–132
Frequency selectivity, 206, *See also* Tuning
curve.
Fresh afferents, 340, 356, 383, *See also*
Selective adaptation
Friedreich's ataxia, 550
Frontal lobe, 93
MMN, 410
N1, 115, 117, 337, 383
Nd wave (processing negativity), 337, 407
P3a, 411–412
P50, 258
what and where processing, 410
Fsp, *See* F-ratio at a single point
Functional magnetic resonance imaging
(fMRI), 92, 380
attention, 409–410
locked-in syndrome, 520
oddball paradigm, 410–411, 427
seeding source analysis, 114
what and where processing, 92, 94, 379–382

G

GA, *See* Gestational age
Galvanic stimulation, 273
Gamma-amino butyric acid, 254
Gamma-band response (GBR), 64–66, 69–72,
77–78, 310–311
Gap detection,
ABR, 240
auditory neuropathy, 540, 556–557

MMN, 362–363, 378–379
N1 (LAEP), 339, 540
GBR, *See* Gamma–band response
Gender
ABR, 220, 235–237
ASSR, 300
CAP, 202
menstrual cycle, 237
P3, 432
Gestational age (GA), 239
GJB2 (gap junction protein beta 2), 465, 581,
Global field power, 44
Glycerol, 495–496
Group delay, 74, *See also* Apparent latency

H

Habituation, 352–353
Hair cell, 192–195
auditory neuropathy, 535–536, 548–550,
553–554, 559
cochlear amplifier, 134, 192
cochlear microphonic, 198–199
compression and rectification, 287
filter, 134, 138
inner, 191–194, 550
Ménière's disease, 499
outer, 191–193
summating potential, 194, 203
suppression, 133, 135
synaptic bar (ribbon synapse), 193–194
tuning curve, 135
Hanning window, 64, 67
Harmonics, 124
ASSR, 287, 296, 312
mistuned, 349–350
voice, 147–149, 321–322
Head injury,
ABR patterns, 518–519
perilymphatic fistula, 500
postnatal hearing loss in childhood, 464
Hearing aids, 124
ASSRs, 312, 320–321, 484–485
compression, 484–485
fitting, 452, 482–485
LAEPs, 345, 424, 484
long term average speech spectrum, 482
physiologic threshold estimates, 482–484
SNR issues, 345

Hearing impairment, *See* Hearing loss
Hearing Level (HL), 128
Hearing loss,
  acoustic neuroma, 500
  afferent vs. efferent auditory systems, 548–550
  childhood, 453–456,463–464
  conductive, 232–233, 240, 464–465, 518
  congenital, 453–456
  family history, 455
  functional, 347
  head trauma, 463–464
  high-frequency, 232–233, 240
  Ménière's disease, 494
  meningitis, 463–464
  middle ear effusions, 464–465
  ototoxic medication, 463–464
  permanent bilateral sensorineural, 454–455, 463–464
  presbycusis, 240
  retrocochlear, 232–233
  sensorineural, 232, 317
  unilateral, 88, 465, 500–501
  Waardenburg syndrome, 544
Hearing screening, *See also* Newborn hearing screening
  after newborn period, 458, 463–464
Hedgehog and fox, 386
Helium, liquid (MEG), 108
Hensen's cells, 191
Heschl's gyrus, 92–93, 248, 258
History (of EP studies), 7–21
  lessons of history, 19–21
HL, *See* Hearing Level
Hotelling's T^2, 161, 163
Huntington's disease, 435
Hydrocephalus, 469–470
Hyperbilirubinemia, 454–455, 542, 547, 551
Hypotheses, 21, 169, 223

I

Impedance matching, 190
Incus (anvil), 190
Independent component analysis, 49
  artifacts, 54
Induced activity, 2, 64–65, 78–80
Infant hearing tests, *See* Audiological evaluation of infant or Newborn hearing screening

Inferior colliculus, 89–92, 293
Inion, 29–30, 248, 255–256, 264, 270
  reflex, *See* Vestibular evoked myogenic potential
Intensity measurements, *See also* Acoustic calibration, 126–128
Interaural attenuation, 125
Interaural correlation, 143–145
Interaural phase difference, 145–147
Interaural timing, 143–145
Internal auditory meatus, 88, 99, 506–507
Interstimulus interval, 123–124. *See also* Stimulus onset asynchrony (SOA)
Interweaving, 175
Intraoperative monitoring, 506–509
  mechanisms of hearing loss during acoustic neuroma surgery, 506
Intraoperative awareness, 254, 301–302
Inserts, *See* Ear inserts
Inverse solution, 87, 112
Ions, 94–95
IPSP, *See* Postsynaptic potential, inhibitory
Isolated forearm, 254–255

J

Jaw reflex, 270, 276
Jitter, *See also* Synchrony
  change response, 338
  during averaging, 37–39, 183–184
  motor unit, 260
  muscle potential, 260
  N1 (LAEP), 342
  rest–motion response, 337–338

K

K-complex, 4–5, 8–9, 373, 375–376
Ketamine (anesthetic), 302
Krabbe's disease, 517

L

Labeled lines (place coding), 131, 223, 325, 573
LAEP, *See* Late auditory evoked potential
Language,
  difficulty studying spoken language, 603

Language *(continued)*
    N400, 602–603
    phonemic prototypes, 370
    phonological mapping negativity (PMN),
        603
    tonal, 321–322
Late auditory evoked potential (LAEP), 2, *See
        also* different components (such as N1,
        N2, N145, P2, P50)
    adaptation, 352–359
    aging, 431–433
    arousal, 400–403
    attention, 399–438
    auditory neuropathy, 540
    binaural interaction component, 143–144
    clinical uses, 428–437
    components, 403–405
    corollary discharge, 417–418
    development, 377–379
    early recordings, 9–10
    electrical, 590–594, *See also* main entry
    filters, 35, 347–348
    frequency, 374
    hearing aids, 345, 424
    infancy, 347–348, 450
    intensity, 343–345, 374
    interaural correlation, 143–145
    interaural phase difference, 145–147
    interaural timing, 143–145
    intracranial recordings, 110–111
    lesions, 115–117
    limitations of clinical use, 429–430
    maximum length sequences, 173
    MEG, 417
    multiple component view, 379–383
    multiple stimulus paradigms, 347–348,
        359
    noise, 345
    optimum stimulus rate, 172
    predictability, 417
    recognition using phase coherence,
        162–164, 347
    refractory period, 175
    selective adaptation, 340–342, 354–359
    self–initiated stimuli, 417
    sleep, 347, 373, 375–376
    SNR, 345
    SOA, 350–352, 367, 374

source analysis, 112–113, 115, 117,
        379–383
    speech, 377
    spectrogram, 70–71
    spectrum, 27–28
    streaming, 369
    threshold, 343–348
    tonotopicity, 92–94, 348–349
    topography, 348
    underlying processes, 429, 437
    voice, 602
Latency
    classification of EPs, 2, 5
    intensity function, *See* main entry
    interpeak, 219–220
    jitter during averaging, 37–39, 183–184
    measurement, 45–46
    nomenclature, 4
    replications, 182–183
Latency-intensity functions, 13, 82, 203
    ABR, 229–233
    EABR, 579–580
    ECAP, 579–580, 584
    CAP, 13, 203
    LAEP (N1 and P2), 344
    MLR, 253–254
Latency jitter, *See* Jitter
Late positive wave, *See* P3
Lateral inhibition, 133, 384, 604–605
Lateral lemniscus 89–91, 111, 117, 268, 513
Lateralization, 143–145, 338–339
Learning, 370–373
    cochlear implants, 595
    training and experience, 371
Leukodystrophies, 516–517
Line noise, 31, 251
    notch filtering, 32, 251
    removing, 51–52
Lissajous trajectory, 217–219
Locked-in syndrome, 520
Logarithmic axes, 2–3
LORETA, *See* Low-resolution electromagnetic
        tomography
Loudness, 124
    ASSR, 312
    LAEP, 343
Low-resolution electromagnetic tomography
        (LORETA), 114

M

Magnetic fields, 106–109
Magnetic resonance imaging (MRI), *See also*
    Functional magnetic resonance imaging
    acoustic neuroma, 502–503, 504–505
    auditory neuropathy, 542
    brainstem tumors, 510
    gadolinium, 494, 503
    head injury, 518
    leukodystrophies, 517
    Ménière's disease, 494, 499
    multiple sclerosis, 510, 516
    neurology, 523–524
Magnetoencephalography (MEG), 5, 106–109
    ASSRs, 299, 304
    binaural processing, 146–147
    cochlear implants, 590
    LAEPs (N1m and MMN), 108, 342, 348,
        352, 354, 368, 371, 373, 379, 382
    MLR, 248–249
    tonotopicity of auditory cortex, 92–94,
        248–249
Magnitude squared coherence, 161–163
Malleus (hammer), 190, 196
Masking. *See also* Derived responses
    asymmetry, 133
    central, 133
    forward, 205, 286
    function (ASSRs), 305–308
    high-pass noise, 137, 497–499
    simultaneous, 205
    spread of masking, 135–136
    tone on tone, 133
Masseter muscle, 264, 286
MASTER, *See* Auditory steady-state
    responses, multiple
    instrument, 308
Maximum comfort level (C-level, cochlear
    implants), 206, 570, 574, 578, 581–582,
    585–587
Maximum length sequence (MLS), 173–175
    anesthesia, 255
    ABR, 235, 239, 251–253
    MLR, 251–253
    SNR effects, 174, 235
Medial geniculate, 89–91
Median, 467

MEG, *See* Magnetoencephalography
Membrane potential, 94–96
    channels, 95
    depolarization, 95–96
    hyperpolarization, 95–96
    polarization, 95
Ménière's disease, 199–204, 494–500
    ABR, 497–499
    clinical presentation, 494
    cochlear hydrops analysis masking
        procedure (CHAMP), 497–499
    differentiation from perilymphatic fistula,
        494, 500
    ECochG, 494–497
    endolymphatic hydrops, 494
    MRI, 494, 499
    N1, (CAP) latency condensation-
        rarefaction difference, 495, 497
    SP, 495–496
    SP/CAP ratio, 199–204, 495–496, 499
    traveling wave velocity, 497
    undermasking, 498–499
    VEMP, 275, 499, 523
Mesogenous components, 336
Mho, 94
Microreflexes, *See* Muscle reflexes
Middle ear muscle reflexes, *See* Stapedius
    reflex
Middle ear effusions, 465
Middle latency response (MLR), 2, 248–259
    aging, 254
    ASSR, 251
    attention, 254, 400–402, 413–414
    auditory neuropathy, 540
    binaural interaction component, 143–144,
        251–252
    chirps, 140–141
    clicks and tones, 252–253
    differentiation from PAM, 248–249
    early recordings, 9–10
    echoes, 253
    electrodes, 35, 250
    electrical, 587–589, *See also* main entry
    filters, 35, 250–251
    hemispheric asymmetries, 250
    infants, 253–254, 450
    intensity, 249, 251
    intracranial recordings, 110–111

Middle latency response (MLR) *(continued)*
  muscle relaxants, 247
  maximum length sequences, 173, 175,
    251–252, 255
  sleep, 251, 254
  SNR issues, 250–251
  SOA, 251–252
  source analysis, 112–113, 115, 117, 248–250
  spectrum, 27–28
  stimulus rate, 251
  temporal lobe lesions, 250
  threshold, 251–252
  tonotopicity, 92–94, 248–249
Minimum norm solution, 114
Minute rhythms (40-Hz response), 302
Mismatch negativity (MMN), 336, 359–371
  abstract features,364–365, 384
  aging, 378–379, 384
  attention, 410–414
  automatic processing, 411–413
  "change-2," 340, 386
  children, 362–364, 384
  cochlear implants, 591–594
  coma, 520
  conjunction, 361
  controls for selective adaptation of N1,
    342, 359–360
  development, 377
  differentiation from N1, 340–342
  differentiation from N2b, 411, 413
  discrimination, 362–364, 592–594
  double deviant, 361
  duration change, 362
  dynamic causal modeling, 385
  fMRI, 410–411
  frequency difference, 340–342
  frontal activation, 410
  gap, 363, 378
  hemispheric asymmetry, 371
  infants, 362
  initial recordings, 15–17
  integrated difference waveform, 160
  intensity decrement, 361
  interaural correlation, 143–145
  interaural timing, 143–145
  latency, 361
  lateral inhibition, 384
  learning, 370–371

MEG, 342, 361
memory comparison, 383–386
multimodal interactions, 414
optimum paradigm, 179, 362–363
pattern, 364–365
phonemic prototype, 370–371
polarity, 378
probability, 366–367
refractory period, 367
relation to N1, 383–386
relation to P3a, 411–412
roving standard, 366, 384
selective adaptation, 383–386
sleep, 370, 376
SNR issues, 362–364, 594
SOA, 384
sources, 361
temporal integration, 343, 368
topography, 362, 384
trace duration, 365–368, 376–378
varying standard, 360, 370
ventriloquism effect, 414
Mismatch response (MMR), 377
Miss, *See* False negative
Missing fundamental, 349
Mistuned harmonic, 349–350
Mixed modulation (MM), 141–142
M-level, *See* Most comfortable listening level
MLR, *See* Middle latency response
MLS, *See* Maximum length sequence
MM, *See* Mixed modulation
MMN, *See* Mismatch negativity
MMR, *See* Mismatch response
Mode, 9, 423, 432
Modiolus, 88, 191, 549, 584
Mohr-Tranebjaerg syndrome, 551–554
Monte Carlo simulations, 177–178
Most comfortable listening level (M-level), 570
Motor preparation, 415–416
Motor potential (MP), 427
Motor unit, 259–262
Morlet wavelet, 69, 71,
MP, *See* Motor potential
MRI, *See* Magnetic resonance imaging
Multiple looks, 128, 343
Multiple sclerosis, 510–516
  ABR patterns, 512–516
  cerebrospinal fluid, 510

conduction block, 511–512
LAEPs, 524
MLR, 524
MRI, 516
oligoclonal bands, 510
retrobulbar neuritis, 510, 512, 514–515
visual EPs, 512–513
VEMP, 523
Musical experience, 323, 349, 605
early right anterior negativity, 373
P2 (LAEP), 349
right hemisphere, 349
Muscle fibers, 259–260
action potential, 259
fibrillation, 259–260
Muscle reflexes, 9, 54, 262–277
excitatory, 262
inhibitory, 260, 262–263
Muscle relaxants, 247, 254, 257
Muscles (head and neck), 264
Myelin, 95–96
auditory nerve, 549
development, 240
multiple sclerosis, 510–512
saltatory conduction, 96, 510–512

N

N1 (CAP), 202–206
condensation and rarefaction clicks,
197–198, 204, 495–497
ear asymmetry, 202
frequency, 204
gender, 202
intensity, 13
Ménière's disease, 495–497
relation to wave I of ABR, 216
stimulus polarity, 197–198, 204
stimulus rates, 197–198, 204
N1 (ECAP), 579
N1 (LAEP, also referred to as N1b, N100 and
N1m), 3, 5, 8, 335–387, 405–415
adaptation, 352–359
adolescence, 377
anterior and posterior sources, 352, 354,
379–383
attention, 15–17, 405–415
audibility, 424

auditory neuropathy, 556–557
change-1 response, 340, 386
cochlear implants, 591–593
component analysis, 47–49
corollary discharge, 417–418
current source density, 45
dendritic activation, 380
development, 377
differentiation from MMN, 340–341, 405
dipole tracking, 349
duration, 343–344
enhancement at short SOA, 354
frequency, 373–374
frontal lobe, 352, 382
gating, 379
intensity, 343–344, 374
interaural correlation, 143–145
interaural timing, 143–145
intracranial recordings, 110–111
latency, 336, 342
MEG, 108, 342, 349, 352, 354, 368, 371, 373,
379, 382
monkey recordings, 111
musical experience, 373
planum temporale, 382
predictability, 417
refractory period, 339–341, 350–359
relation to Nd, 405–410
rise-time, 343
selective adaptation, 340–341, 354–359
self-initiated stimuli, 417
sensitization, 354, 379
sleep, 11, 373, 375–376
SOA, 350–352, 374
source analysis, 115–116, 379–383
spectrogram, 70–71
speech stimuli, 417–418
time constant, 351
tonotopicity, 92–94, 348
topography, 42–43, 45, 405
tuning, 379
N1a, 379
N1c, *See* N145
N2, 336, 405, *See also* N300, N550
component structure, 405
N2a and N2b, 405
sleep, 375–376. 405
N2a, 405

N2b, 405, 406
  aging, 431–433
  relation to MMN, 405, 413
  sources, 413
  topography, 413
N145 (also referred to as N1c, N140, N150
    and Tb), 379
  component analysis, 47–49
  development, 377
  intracranial recordings, 110
  source analysis, 115–116, 382
  streaming, 369
N300, 375–376
N400, 520, 602–603
N550, 375–376
Na, 249–250
Narrowband derived responses, *See* Derived
    responses
Narrowband noise, 142
Nasion, 29–30, 264
NBN, *See* Narrowband noise
Nd, 405–410, *See also* Difference waveform,
    negative
  blindness, 414
  early and late, 407–410
  hierarchy of processing, 407
  lesions, 407
  sources, 407,
  timing, 407
  voice, 406, 414
Ne, *See* Error-related negativity/positivity
Nerve conduction. 95–96
  auditory neuropathy, 541–542, 552
  Charcot-Marie-Tooth disease, 552
  saltatory, 96
Networks, *See* Neuronal networks
Neurofibromatosis, 501
Neurology and neurotology, 493–524
Neuromuscular junction (NMJ), 259–261
Neuron
  basic structure, 96
  bipolar, 88, 102
  physiology, 94–97
  pyramidal, 101–103
  stellate, 102–103
Neuronal networks, 6, 357, 368, 383, 385–386,
    428, 606
Newborn hearing screening, 450–465
  ABR, 451–452, 456–457, 460

ASSR, 452
audiological evaluation of infant, 465–485,
    See also main entry
auditory neuropathy, 457–458
automated ABR, 165, 451–452, 460
conductive hearing loss, 464–465
contralateral suppression of OAE, 460
cost-benefit evaluations, 454
genetic screening, 465
history, 450–451
justification, 453–456
missing mild hearing losses, 460
OAE, 451–452, 456
postnatal hearing loss, 463–464
protocols, 454–458
referral from screening, 457–458, 465–467
risk factors, 454–455
sensitivity and specificity, 457–458
stimulus calibration issues, 460–463
unilateral hearing loss, 465
universal screening, 450–451
nHL, *See* Normal hearing level
NMDA (N-methyl–D-aspartic acid), 385
NMJ, *See* Neuromuscular junction
NN, *See* Notched noise
Node of Ranvier, 95–96, 510–512
Normal hearing level (nHL)
  clicks, 128
  physiological threshold level (PTL), 128–131
  relation to HL, 129
  tones, 128
Normal limits (also known as upper and
    lower limits of normal), 160, 166, 182,
    524
  ABR, 220, 231, 240, 501–502, 505
  ASSR, 291, 317, 322
  ECochG, 495–496
  SP/CAP ratio, 495–496
Normative data, *See* Normal limits
Notched noise (NN), 133–136, 228–229, 471
Novelty, 411–412, 435
Null hypothesis, 169
Nyquist frequency, 27, 36, 60

O

OAE, *See* Otoacoustic emission
Objective audiometry, 179, 208, 262, 269,
    345–348, 452–453

Object-related negativity, 349–350, 386
Occiput, 264
Offset response, 2, 4, 337–339
Ohm's law, 94, 98
Olivocochlear bundle, 91, 192
Onset response, 2, 4, 99, 337–339
  butterfly plot, 44
Orbicularis oculi, 264
Organ of Corti, 189–195, 549, 571
Oscillopsia, 276
Otitis media, 464–465
Otoacoustic emission (OAE), 194–195
  auditory neuropathy, 535–540, 553
  contralateral suppression, 195, 452,
    540–541
  distortion product (DPOAE), 194–195,
    456–457, 478–479, 537–538
  infants, 478–479
  maximum length sequence, 173–174
  newborn hearing screening, 450–452,
    456–457
  transient, 194, 456
Otolith, 270–271, 275, *See also* Saccule
Ototoxic medication, 195, 454–455, 463–464,
    547–548
Oval window, 196
Overlapping, 175

P

Po, 247–248
P1 (adults), *See* P50
P1 (childhood)
  cochlear implants, 591–593
  developmental changes, 376–377, 591, 593
P2
  cortical output, 380
  current source density, 45
  latency, 336
  learning, 371–373
  musical experience, 349, 372–373
  predictability, 417
  principal components analysis, 48
  spectrogram, 70–71
  streaming, 368–370
  topography, 45
P3 (LAEP, also known as late positive wave,
    P3b, P300, P400), 418–437
  aging, 431–433

Alzheimer's disease, 433–435
amplitude, 433–435
attention, 408, 424–426
attentional blink, 428
Bayesian probability, 425
blindness, 414
category probability, 419–420
closure, 427–428
cochlear implants, 594
coma, 520
components, 427–428
consciousness, 428, 438, 518–520
contingent probability, 425
context–updating, 427–428
controlled processing, 427
dementia, 433–435
differentiation into P3a and P3b, 411–412
discriminability, 424
discrimination of targets, 402–405, 422–424
dopamine, 427
early recordings 10–12
equivocation, 422–424
feedback, 425
first stimulus in train, 353
fMRI, 427
frequency difference, 422–424
hearing aids, 424
intensity, 422
meaning, 424–426
mistuned harmonic, 350
neighborhood, 427
norepinephrine, 427
oddball paradigm, 418–422
probability, 419–422
reaction time, 422–424, 432–433
recording parameters, 418–419
response selection, 424
salience, 422, 425
schizophrenia, 435–437
short intervals, 421
SOA, 420–422
stimulus evaluation, 424, 427
target-standard differences, 17, 404
target-target interval, 420–422
task-relevance, 422, 424–426
temporal probability, 419–422
topography, 405, 433
uncertainty, 418
waltzing oddball, 422

P3a (also known as novelty P3), 160, 411–412
  Alzheimer's disease, 434–435
  dopamine, 427
  hippocampus, 412
  novelty 411–412, 435
  relation to MMN, 411–412
  salience, 425
  vascular dementia, 435
P3b, *See* P3
P4 (in feedback response), 425
P300, *See* P3
P400, *See* P3
P900, 376
P50 (also known as Pb or P1), 257–259, 311, 336
  aging, 254, 259, 378
  Alzheimer's disease, 258–259
  bipolar affective disorder, 258
  nomenclature, 247–248, 257
  post-traumatic stress disorder, 258
  schizophrenia, 257–258
  sensory gating, 257–259
  suppression, 257
Pa (MLR), 10, 19, 248–250
  attention, 254
  echo, 253
  frequency, 248–249
  maximum length sequences, 175
  sources, 248–250
PAM, *See* Post–auricular muscle
Paradigm, 123
  Butler, 354–359
  dichotic listening (cocktail party), 403–415
  oddball, 359
  omitted stimulus, 365–366
  roving standard, 366, 384
  varying standard, 360, 370
  waltzing oddball, 422
Parkinson's disease, 435
Partial least squares, 49
Pattern analysis, 183
Pb, *See* P1
PBK (phonetically balanced kindergarten
    word list), 591, 593
PCA, *See* Principal component analysis
Pd, 408–409, *See also* Difference wave, positive
Pe, *See* Error-related positivity
Peaks, 6
  measurements, 45–46
Pejvakin, 552

Pelizaeus-Merzbacher disease, 517
Perception, 368–370
  bottom-up and top-down processing, 337,
    387, 414
  EEG rhythms, 77–80, 605–606
  object perception, 349–350, 386
Perceptual binding, 77–80, 310, 325
Perilymph, 190–193
Perilymphatic fistula, 494, 500
Periodicity pitch, 349
Persistent vegetative state, 519–520
peSPL, *See* Sound pressure level, peak-to-peak
Phase, 27, 60–64
  ambiguity, 72
  coherence, 80, 161–164, 347
  delay, 72
  intensity function, 82
  locking, 64, 77, 288
  relation to latency, 63–64, 72–75
  resetting, 78–80
  spectrum, 61–62
  synchronization, 80
  weighting, 165–167, 171
Phonological mapping negativity (PMN), 603
Physiology, 20
  EMG, 259–262
  nerves, 94–97
Physiologic threshold level (PTL), 130–131
Pinna, 189–190, 262, 264–267, 571
Pitch, 83, 124
Plasma concentration, 255–256
PMN , *See* Phonological mapping negativity
Place specificity, 131, 325, 573
Planum temporale, 93–94
  role in LAEP generation, 112, 372, 382
Play audiometry, 452
Pneumatic otoscopy, 465, 480, 482, 500
Point-optimized variance ratio, 165
Polar plot, 60–61, 63, 161–163, 176, 322
Polarity
  plotting convention (EEG), 5
  plotting convention (EMG), 262
  principal component, 47
  stimulus, 52, 197–198, 204, 225–227,
    536–539, 542–543,
Post-auricular muscle (PAM), 262–269
  ABR, 235–236
  absence, 264–265
  amplitude, 266–267

anesthesia, 255, 302
attention, 269
bilateral, 267–268
cochlear origin of reflex, 262
coma, 519
correlation, 266
differentiation from cortical MLR, 262
electrodes, 249, 264
filters, 266
gaze, 264, 267–269
infants, 269, 481
location, 248, 264
MLR, 248–249
muscle relaxants, 262
rate, 266
reflex mechanism, 263, 269
reflex pathway, 268
single trials, 265
sleep, 269
source, 115
threshold, 265, 269
Postconcussion syndrome, 518
Postnatal hearing loss, 463–464
Post-stimulus-time histograms, 223, 225
Postsynaptic potential,
excitatory (EPSP), 101, 104–106
inhibitory (IPSP), 101, 104–106
Post-traumatic stress disorder, 258
Potential, 1–2, 94
Power spectrum, 66
Power spectrum ABR, 504–505
Prematurity, 239, 454–455, 464
Prestin, 192
Presbycusis, 240
Principal component analysis, 47–49
artifacts, 54
LAEPs, 47–49
SNR measurements, 161
spatial and temporal, 47–49
Probability
Bayesian, 425
category, 419–420
contingent, 425
density, 170
global and local, 419
statistical criterion, 155–156
temporal, 419–421
Processing negativity, 15–17, 337, 375, 406,
See also Nd

pSPL, *See* Sound pressure level, peak
Psychoacoustics, 20
binaural processing, 143–147, 296, 517
flutter and roughness, 292–293
loudness, 124, 312, 343
multiple looks, 128, 343
temporal integration, 128–129, 181–182
PTL, *See* Physiologic threshold level
Pure tone average threshold, 346, 455
Pyramidal cell, 101–106

Q

Q_{10dB}, 205
Quadripole, 98–99

R

Radio frequency (RF) (cochlear implant), 206,
571–572, 575
Rate codes, 293
Reaction time,
MMN, 360–361
N2, 424
P3, 422–424
Readiness potential (RP), 415–416
Receiver operating characteristic (ROC),
169–171
Recruitment, 181, 232, 312, 317–318, 484–485,
497
Rectification, 65–66
hair cell synapse, 287
induced activity, 65–66
Reference electrode, 35, 42–44
average, 43
linked mastoid, 43
mastoid, 35, 216–217, 248–249, 286, 288,
290, 468–469
neck, 35, 290
noncephalic, 42
Refractory period
auditory nerve fibers, 206–207
evoked potentials, 175, 340, 352–359
frequency specificity, 175
MMN, 365–368
N1 (LAEP), 352–359
neuron, 95–96
specificity, 175, 340

Regression
   aging P3 latency, 431–432
   apparent latency calculations, 293–294
   threshold estimation, 318
   VEMP vs. EMG, 274
Reissner's membrane, 190–191, 494
Rejection positivity, *See* Pd
Replications, 38, 157–159, 182–183
Resistance, 94
Resolution
   amplitude, 36
   frequency, 27, 60–61, 68
Response selection, *See* Attention
Rest-motion change, 337–338
Reticular formation, 91, 277, 335
Retrobulbar neuritis, 510, 512, 514–515
Reverberation, 124, 253
RF, *See* Radio frequency
Rhythms, 26, 285–325, 606
   alpha, 7–8, 26, 301
   idling, 77
   minute, 302
   mu, 77
   tau, 7, 77
Right-hand rule, 106–107
Rise time (of tone), 227, 342–343
rms, *See* Root-mean-square
Rock and roll, 272
Rolandic fissure, 93
ROC, *See* Receiver operating characteristic
Root-mean-square (rms)
   amplitude of EP, 44
   muscle activity, 260, 274
   sound pressure level, 127
Roughness, 292–293
Round window, 190, 192, 196, 545–546, 571
RP, *See* Readiness potential
RT, *See* Reaction time

S

Saccade, 53–54
Saccule, 190, 268, 499
   early vestibular response, 521–522, 577, 583
   VEMP, 268, 270–271, 274, 523
Salience
   P3 wave, 425
   partial least squares analysis, 49
Saltatory conduction, 96, 510–512

SAM, *See* Amplitude modulation, sinusoidal
SC, *See* Semicircular canal
Scala media, 190–192
Scala tympani, 190–191
Scala vestibuli, 190–191
Scalp
   head model, 112
   potentials, 29
   preparation, 29
   topography, 41–45, 215–216, 286–288, 295, 405–407, 416, 433–434
Schemata, 427–429
Schizophrenia
   attentional control, 437
   hallucinations, 437
   N1, 435–437
   P3, 435–437
   P50, 257–258
Schwann cell, 95–96, *See also* Myelin
SD, *See* Standard deviation
SDR, *See* Standard deviation ratio
Selective adaptation theory (also known as specificity of refractory period), 340, 354–359
Semicircular canal (SC), 190, 275
Sensation level (SL), 219–220
Sensitivity and specificity, 168–171
   acoustic neuroma, 503–504
   Ménière's disease, 496–497, 499
   multiple sclerosis, 516
   newborn hearing screening, 450, 457
   VEMP testing of vestibular dysfunction, 275
Sensory gating, 257–259
Serendipity, 21
Shielding, 51
Sidebands, 140, 142, 287
Signal-to-noise ratio (SNR), 9, 156–166
   acoustic, 345
   amplitude and variance measurements, 156
   ASSRs, 300, 318–320
   averaging, 37
   difference waveform, 159–161
   envelope-following responses, 291
   frequency domain, 63, 160–166
   maximum length sequences, 174, 235
   time domain, 157–160
Silent talking, 558

Simultaneous stimuli, 175–177, *See also* ASSR, multiple simultaneous
Sinks, *See* Current sources and sinks
Skin
  potentials, 29, 50
  preparation, 29, 50
SL, *See* Sensation level
Sleep, 8–11, 20
  ABR, 237, 457, 466, 478–479
  ASSR, 300–302, 466, 478–479
  LAEPs, 11, 273, 375–376
  MLR, 248, 251, 254
  MMN, 376
  muscle relaxation, 300–301
  physiologic thresholds, 181
  REM and NREM, 373, 375–376
  stages, 11, 373, 375–376
  spindles, 11, 301, 373
Slow auditory evoked potentials, 2, 336. *See also* Late auditory evoked potentials
Slow wave (SW), 425
SN10 (slow negative wave at 10 ms), 34
SNHL, *See* Hearing loss, sensorineural
SNR, *See* Signal–to–noise ratio
SOA, *See* Stimulus onset asynchrony
Socioeconomic status, 605
Sound pressure level (SPL), 126–128
  impulse, 127
  peak-to-peak sound pressure level (peSPL), 127
  peak sound pressure level (pSPL), 127
Sources, intracerebral, 6, *See also* Current sources or Source analysis
Sources, auditory, 124
Source analysis (electric), 112–117
  ABR, 215–219
  ASSR, 295
  constraints, 114
  discrete and distributed , 112–113
  LAEP, 116, 379–383
  MLR, 113
  iterative fitting, 114
  relation to fMRI activations, 114–115
  seeded, 114
SP, *See* Summating potential (cochlea) or Sustained potential (cortex)
SP/CAP ratio, 199–201
  electrode effects, 200
  Ménière's disease, 495–496

relation to CAP amplitude, 199–200
Specificity, *See* Sensitivity
Spectrogram, 66–72
  color scaling, 69
  time-frequency trade-offs, 68–69
  wavelet, 69–72
  windowing, 67, 69
Speech, 147–149, 321–324, 601–602
  ABR, 148–149, 290, 602
  compression, 323
  envelope, 84, 323–324, 558
  fundamental, 321
  FFR, 321–322, 602
  LAEPs, 377, 602
  phonemic prototypes, 370
  phonological mapping negativity (PMN), 603
  pitch–tracking, 322
  tonal languages, 321–322
  voice, 602, *See also* main entry
Speech perception
  acoustic neuroma, 500
  auditory neuropathy, 538, 554–556
  cochlear implants, 554–556, 582, 595
  redundancy, 595
Speech reception threshold (SRT), 538
Spherical spline, 45
Spinal accessory nerve, *See* Accessory nerve
Spiral ganglion, 88, 117, 191, 194, 549
SPL, *See* Sound pressure level
SPN, *See* Stimulus preceding negativity
SRT, *See* Speech reception threshold
Stacked ABR, 138–140, 503–505
Standard deviation (SD), 180, 182
  relation to standard error, 233
Standard deviation ratio (SDR), 158–159
Stapedectomy, 500
Stapedius muscle, 190
Stapedius reflex, 269, 456
  acoustic neuroma, 500–501
  auditory neuropathy, 540
  electrical (cochlear implant) 586
Stapes, 134, 190
Startle reflex, 268, 276–277, 450, 452
Sternocleidomastoid muscle, *See* Sternomastoid
Sternomastoid muscle, 248, 264, 268
  reflex, *See* Vestibular evoked myogenic potential

Sternum, 264, 271
Stereocilia, 192–193
Stimulus artifact, 52, 125–126, 158, 288
Stimulus onset asynchrony (SOA), 123–124
  ABR, 14, 234–235, 239, 471, 513–514
  CAP, 197–198
  EABR, 581
  LAEPs, 350–352, 367, 374
  MLR, 251–253
  MMN, 340
  optimum, 172–173
  recommended settings, 35
  SP, 374
  VEMP, 272–273
Stimulus polarity
  alternating, 126, 215, 272, 576
  condensation vs. rarefaction, 197–198, 215,
    225–227, 272, 536–539, 542–543, 546, 553
Stimulus preceding negativity (SPN),
  415–416
Stimulus rate, *See also* Stimulus onset
  asynchrony (SOA)
  recommended settings, 35
Stimulus set, *See* Attention
Streaming, 368–370
Stria vascularis, 191–192, 494
Stopping rules, 167, 177–178
Subject option, 400–403
Succinylcholine, 247
Summating potential (SP), 2, 194, 199–202,
    See also SP/CAP ratio,
  absolute amplitude, 201–202, 496
  auditory neuropathy, 545–547
  biasing, 202, 495–496
  broad waveform in auditory neuropathy,
    544–546
  differentiation from CAP, 6, 197–199
  delayed in presynaptic auditory
    neuropathy, 546
  generation, 194
  glycerol, 495–496
  hair cell damage, 203
  masking, 197
  Ménière's disease, 495–497
  perilymphatic fistula, 500
  polarity, 197, 200
Superior olive, 89–91
  synaptic delay, 111

Superior canal dehiscence, 276
Suppression
  cochlear, 133, 135, 206
  cortical, 257
Sustained potential (SP), 2, 4, 5, 311, 373–374
  butterfly plot, 44
  early recordings, 18
  frequency, 374
  intensity, 374
  source analysis, 115–116
  SOA, 374
  spectrogram, 70–71
  topography, 42–43
SW, *See* Slow wave
Sweep technique, 80–83
  intensity, 80–82, 312–313
  masking function, 307
  modulation frequency, 83, 290–297
Sylvian fissure, 93
Synapse, 96–97, *See also* Postsynaptic
    potentials
  hair cell, 193
  superior olive, 111
Syllable, 148–149
Synchrony
  muscle, 260–261, 263
  neuron, 99, 101–102, 194, 237, 293, 325, 606

T

T-complex (Ta and Tb), 380
T-level (threshold level, cochlear implants),
    570, 581–582
Tectorial membrane, 191–192, 550–551
Telemetry
  ABR recording, 29
  ECAP, 572, 575, 583–586
Temperature
  circadian rhythms, 237
  effects on ABR, 237
  gender effects, 236–237
  intraoperative monitoring, 508
  menstrual cycle, 237
Temporal acuity, 292
Temporal integration,
  ASSRs, 310–311
  hearing thresholds, 128–129, 181–182, 347
  multiple looks, 343

MMN, 365, 368, 370
  N1(LAEP), 343, 347, 354
Temporal lobe, 93
  lesions, 115–116, 250
Temporalis muscle, 264
Temporal modulation transfer function, 290, 292
Tensor tympani, 190
Threshold, *See also* Evoked potential audiometry
  behavioral, 128–131
  binary search procedure, 466
  estimated behavioral, 180
  exaggerated, 347
  extrapolation, 347
  physiologic, 179–180
  physiologic-behavioral, 130, 179–182, 472–477
  regression estimates, 317–319, 347, 475
Threshold level (T-level, cochlear implants), 207, 570, 574, 578, 585–587
Timbre, 124, 349
Time-codes, 293, 325
Time domain, 25–26, 59–66
Time-frequency uncertainty principle, 68
Tinnitus, 273, 604–605
  acoustic neuroma, 500–501
  ASSRs, 604–605
  auditory neuropathy, 543
  lateral inhibition, 604–605
  Ménière's disease, 494
  pathophysiology, 604
  transcranial magnetic stimulation, 604
  treatment with acoustic manipulations, 604
Tympanic membrane (eardrum), 190, 195–196
Tymptrode (tympanic membrane electrode), 195–196
T-level , *See* Threshold level
TN, *See* True negative
TOA , *See* Train onset asynchrony
Tone
  2–1–2 tone, 128, 131–132, 227, 251, 470–471
  acoustic spectrum, 132, 136, 471
  notched noise, 135, 471
Tonotopicity, 92–94, 248–249, 348–349
Top-down processing, 337, 378, 387, 414

Topography, 41–45
  ABR, 215–216
  ASSR, 286–288, 295
  color scales, 45
  interpolation, 44
  LAEPs (N1, Nd, P2, P3), 405–407, 416, 433–434
  spherical spline, 45
TORCH (toxoplasmosis, rubella, cytomegalovirus, herpes), 455
TP, *See* True positive
TP41 (MLR), 250
Train onset asynchrony (TOA), 352–353
Transfer function, 124
  vocal tract, 147
Transtympanic electrode, 12, 195–197
  golf club electrode, 195
  stimulation, 547, 577, 582–583
Trapezius muscle, 264, 270
Trapezoid body, 90–91
Traveling wave, 131, 192
  delay, 138
Trigeminal nerve, 264
True negative (TN), 168–169
True positive (TP), 168–171
TT, *See* Trans-tympanic (electrode)
t-test, 160
  phase-weighted, 166, 171
Tullio phenomenon, 276
Tuning curve, 133, 135, 223
  ASSR, 304–308
  CAP, 204–206
  detuning, 305
  forward masking, 205, 305
  Q_{10dB}, 205
  suppression, 135, 205, 305
Tympanometry, 452, 456
Tympanostomy tubes, 465
Type I afferent neuron dysfunction, 535–536, *See also* Auditory neuropathy

U

Uncertainty,
  diagnosis, 155–156, 183, 524
  hearing aid fitting, 482–484
  P3, 418–424
Utricule, 190

V

Vascular dementia, 435
Vector, 59–63, *See also* Polar plots
　vector averaging, 291
Vegetative state, 519–520
VEMP, *See* Vestibular evoked myogenic
　potential
Ventriloquism effect, 414
Vertigo, 276
　Ménière's disease, 494
　philosophical, 493–524
Vertex, 30
　response, 335, *See also* Late auditory
　　evoked potentials
　sharp waves during sleep, 373
Vestibular evoked myogenic potential
　(VEMP), 270–277, 523
　accessory nerve, 271
　aging, 272, 275
　amplitude, 276
　asymmetry ratio, 275
　auditory neuropathy, 541
　bilateral stimulation, 275
　bone conduction, 273
　clinical testing, 275–276
　electrical stimulation. 273, 523
　electrodes, 271–272
　EMG level, 274–275
　filters, 272
　frequency, 272–273, 523
　galvanic stimulation, 273, 523
　infants, 275
　inhibition, 263, 270
　inion response, 248, 270
　intensity, 272
　ipsilateral vs. bilateral, 271
　latency, 275
　reference electrode, 271, 272
　reflex pathway, 268, 271
　rock and roll, 272
　saccule, 267, 270, 272
　sensitivity and specificity, 275
　SOA, 272–273
　sternomastoid muscle, 270
　stimulus rate, 272–273
　threshold, 272
　trapezius, 270
Vestibular evoked potential (also known as
　early vestibular response), 521–522, 543,
　577, 583
Vestibular nerve, 88–89, 190, 268, 521
Vestibular neuritis, 275
Vestibular schwannoma, 88, *See also* Acoustic
　neuroma
Vestibulocollic reflex, *See* Vestibular evoked
　myogenic potential
Vestibulo-ocular reflex, 277, 521
Vestibulospinal tract, 268
Vocal folds, 145–146, 321–324
Voice, 147
　cocktail party problem, 406, 414
　envelope-following response, 323–324
　FFR, 321–322
　voice evoked potentials, 602
　voice onset time, 321, 371–372
Volume-conductor, 43–44, 98, 100
Vowel, 83, 124, 147–149, 371–372

W

Waardenburg syndrome, 544
Warping, 183–184, 221, 588
Wavelets, 69–72
Wernicke's area, 93
What and where processing streams, 92, 94,
　379–382, 386, 407, 410
Window (also known as envelope)
　exponential, 142
　Hanning, 64, 67
　rectified sine, 142
Woody filter (also known as adaptive filter),
　38–39, 432
Working memory, 383
Word recognition score (WRS), 538